Emergency laparoscopic surgery in the elderly and frail patient

Ferdinando Agresta • Mauro Podda
Fabio Cesare Campanile
Carlo Bergamini • Gabriele Anania
Editors

Emergency laparoscopic surgery in the elderly and frail patient

Springer

SICE
Società Italiana
di Chirurgia Endoscopica
e Nuove Tecnologie

Editors
Ferdinando Agresta
Department of General Surgery
ULSS2 Trevigiana del veneto
Vittorio Veneto (TV)
Italy

Fabio Cesare Campanile
General Surgery
Ospedale San Giovanni
Decollato - Andosilla
Civita Castellana, Viterbo
Italy

Gabriele Anania
UO di chirurgia Generale e Toracica
AOU Ferrara
Ferrara
Italy

Mauro Podda
Policlinico Universitario Duilio Casula
AOU Cagliari, Department of
Emergency Surgery
Monserrato
Italy

Carlo Bergamini
Department of Emergency Surgery
AOU Careggi
Firenze
Italy

ISBN 978-3-030-79989-2 ISBN 978-3-030-79990-8 (eBook)
https://doi.org/10.1007/978-3-030-79990-8

This Springer imprint is published by the registered company Springer Nature Switzerland AG
The registered company address is: Gewerbestrasse 11, 6330 Cham, Switzerland

Thinking of our elders, from a professional, personal, and human point of view; taking into account our young people—the reason for our being professional, personal, and human; without forgetting us, with our frailties: professional, personal, and human.

Foreword

Randomized clinical trials (RCTs) are the best way to assess the efficacy and/or toxicity of a therapeutic product. They have been developed and refined particularly for clinical pharmacology. RCTs are seldom used for non-pharmacological interventions, and very rarely in surgery.

Even when there is an improvement, it is hard to find scientific evidence to establish whether a surgical procedure is better than some other one, whether surgery that has achieved good results in adults is also effective in old people and is equally favorable in males and females. This kind of information is very important for supplementing a Health Therapeutic Assessment (HTA) and implementing the guidelines in various areas of surgery.

However, the field of surgery is always very complex because the experience and the manual skills of surgeons and their staff are of paramount importance for the success of any intervention. This means that surgical RCTs must be multicentric in order to randomize the surgeons when comparing, for instance, two surgical procedures. It is even harder to achieve double blindness because the surgeons must be aware of the procedure, while the blindness should be mandatory for the patients. It is instead possible that the results of a surgical intervention are evaluated by surgeons who are not involved in that clinical trial.

This book, written by Italian surgeons, sets out to define and discuss these problems in a specific field: laparoscopy in frail old people. The definition of frailty is particularly relevant for the Italian population. In fact, Italians top the lists for lifespan (81 and 85 years for males and females, respectively), but the drop lower when the healthy lifespan is considered because they often suffer one or more pathologies in the last part of their lives. Probably, scarce attention to good life styles is the main reason.

Therefore, "classic" surgery could be contraindicated in such conditions while laparoscopy, being less invasive, may be tolerated better by frail old people.

The authors of this book are convinced that only RCTs can give answers to a number of questions. Is the treatment urgent and necessary or could it be delayed? Some cases of acute appendicitis can avoid surgery because the infection could be cured by antibiotics. A recent study shows that obese diabetics achieve the same results—loss of body weight—with a well-balanced diet or a gastric bypass.

Most surgical knowledge is based on interventions in adults. Are they transferable to frail old people? Then too, if laparoscopy is really well tolerated in old people, are the results acceptable? Results mean not only in the short term, but also with long enough follow-up to evaluate late or long-term side effects and relapses. All these questions in the various pathological areas call for RCTs to avoid "good intentions" translating to damage. We need to know what is better because we cannot accept that the age of patients and their frailty is a reason to avoid surgery or an excuse to limit them to non-surgical treatments.

The possibility of organizing more RCTs in surgery depends essentially on the availability of adequate resources that national and European governments will make available. This book gives them good reasons.

Frail old people deserve attention!

Silvio Garattini
"Mario Negri" Institute for
Pharmacological Research,
Milan, Italy

Preface

"Science is built of facts the way a house is built of bricks: but an accumulation of facts is no more science than a pile of bricks is a house", wrote the mathematician Henri Poincare.

However, as surgeons and doctors, we have to face and consider our own "facts".

We are ageing! This is the first fact. From a global perspective, it is estimated that the number of people over 65 years old will increase from 5234 million in 2010 to more than 1.5 billion in 2050 and, currently, about 33% of hospital stays and 41% of hospital costs are attributed to patients over 65 years old.

As an example, more than 20% of the Italian population is over 65 years old and this percentage is expected to rise to 34% by 2050. Over the last 20 years, life expectancy in the country has increased from 78 to 80 years for men and from 84 to 85 years for women. About 20% of the elderly and 6% of the country's total population are now over 80 years old.

Second fact: when we think of the elderly, our first thought is chronic medical illness, but it is estimated that 21% of the total population over 60 will need surgery, compared to only 12% of people in the 45–60 age group.

Third fact: we are all well aware of the advantages of laparoscopy in planned surgical procedures, which include elderly and frail patients. However, there are many doubts about emergencies: people over 70 who undergo an emergency laparotomy have a hospital mortality of 21.4%, and older patients, especially octogenarians, have worse outcomes with up to 44% mortality reported.

Fourth fact: an ageing population will put greater financial pressure on elderly care systems. And in an era of budgetary restrictions, this has to be taken into careful consideration.

Fifth fact: we continue to use the term "elderly" only in a chronological sense: 65 years old continues to be adopted as a threshold for old age. This can no longer be the case, just as it can no longer be just a number (age) to define a person's situation. That is why it is better to use and talk about, and define, frailty.

Sixth fact: last but not least, it is no longer the time for the one-man show; surgeons cannot and must no longer ignore multidisciplinarity, especially in the medical profession.

These are the facts. However, on their own, these facts are not science.

"... As doctors and surgeons, our mission is to treat patients to the best of our knowledge and expertise. The exponential knowledge eruption and the nearly daily skill-related technology advances in minimally invasive surgery make it more than ever mandatory that we, surgeons and doctors, humbly examine, analyze and objectively audit our own practice...we have to recognize and discard our acquired biases, and base our diagnostic procedures and surgical therapy on 'hard' evidence..." It is still correct, timeless, and contextual what Dr. Fingerhut wrote.

So these were the ideas that led us to be the Editors of a book about the laparoscopic approach in emergencies in elderly and frail patients.

We tried to work on it with a multitasking approach, involving not only surgeons but also anaesthetists, internists, nurses, and radiologists. As this is an indisputable fact, only together, we could try to summarize the facts in science.

Without forgetting ethics!

The idea for this book was born at the beginning of 2020, and in the meantime another worrying fact has emerged, the SARS-CoV-2 (COVID-19) infection.

There is no real evidence, especially regarding surgery, about this "worrying fact". However, we could not overlook it, especially considering that our elderly were significantly affected during the first wave. On the contrary, in the second wave, younger people became frail.

We have tried to answer the questions listed above, which we want to share with everyone. Perhaps "forcing" the meaning of the Aristotelian syllogism a bit: if the safety and efficacy profiles of laparoscopy in the elderly and frail patient have been confirmed, then it is even more true in the non-elderly and non-frail patient.

Vittorio Veneto, Italy — Ferdinando Agresta
Monserrato, Italy — Mauro Podda
Civita Castellana, Italy — Fabio Cesare Campanile
Firenze, Italy — Carlo Bergamini
Ferrara, Italy — Gabriele Anania

Contents

Part I

Generalities

How to Define an Elderly and Frail Patient?

1

Ferdinando Agresta, Carlo Bergamini, Mauro Podda, Fabio Cesare Campanile, Gabriele Anania, Stefano Volpato, Alessandro Nobili, Gianluca Costa, Alessandro Puzziello, Francesco Corcione, and Gianluigi Melotti

1.1 How to Define Elderly?

The definitions of old age are not consistent from the standpoints of biology, employment, retirement, and sociology. For statistical and public administrative purposes, *elderly is conventionally defined as a person 65 years old or older, while those from 65 through 74 years old are often referred to as "young old" and those over 75 years old as "old."*

With recent advances in medical and public health science, the average life expectancy has

F. Agresta (✉)
Department of General Surgery, ULSS2 Trevigiana del veneto, Vittorio Veneto (TV), Italy

C. Bergamini
Department of Emergency Surgery, Azienda Ospedaliero-Universitaria Careggi, Florence, Italy

M. Podda
Policlinico Universitario Duilio Casula, AOU Cagliari, Department of Emergency Surgery, Monserrato, Italy

F. C. Campanile
Department of General Surgery, San Giovanni Decollato—Andosilla Hospital, Civita Castellana, Italy

G. Anania
Department of General and Thoracic Surgery, Arcispedale Sant'Anna, Ferrara, Italy

S. Volpato
Department of Medical Science, Azienda Ospedaliero-Universitaria di Ferrara, Ferrara, Italy

A. Nobili
Laboratory for Quality Assessment of Geriatric Therapies and Services, Istituto di Ricerche Farmacologiche Mario Negri IRCCS, Milan, Italy

G. Costa
Surgery Center, Campus Bio-Medico University Hospital, Rome, Italy

A. Puzziello
Department of Surgery and Transplants, AOU San Giovanni di Dio e Ruggi d'Aragona, Università of Salerno, Salerno, Italy

F. Corcione
Department of General Surgery and Surgical Speciality, University Federico II, Naples, Italy

Emeritus President of the Italian Society of Surgery, Naples, Italy

G. Melotti
Hon. Fellow of International College of Surgeons, Modena, Italy

F. Agresta et al. (eds.), *Emergency laparoscopic surgery in the elderly and frail patient*,
https://doi.org/10.1007/978-3-030-79990-8_1

increased rapidly. Thus, some studies have systematically addressed the issue of biological age-based descriptions of "elderly" in clinical settings. In the most conspicuous review, the authors recommend limiting the definition to the people over 75 years of age, instead of the current 65, and to reform the social system according to the aging society (1). Others suggest using "pre-old age" from 65 to 74 and "old age" over 75. In addition, people aged 90 years and over can be classified as "oldest-old" or "super-old." There are also regional differences in average life expectancy. Therefore, when defining elderly on the basis of chronological age, we need to take into account also historical, regional, and social variations.

Some studies have systematically addressed the issue of chronological age-based descriptions of "elderly" in clinical settings. The first differs from chronological age because it takes into consideration a number of factors other than just the date of birth. Since aging would occur gradually accumulating damage to various cells and tissues in the body, the concept of "biological age" may be used as a *trait d'union* between elderly and frail. The concept of biological age is quite clear from a speculative and philosophical point of view, but it is difficult to translate in a clear operational definition; it maintains a considerable individual variability and interobserver discrepancy when used in clinical practice. Therefore, when dealing with the concept of elderly in this textbook, we will mainly refer to the strict concept of chronological age, whose theoretical definition, despite having not so clear numerical boundaries, still maintains a certain uniformity among various authors.

1.2 How Often Do We Face an Elderly Patient in the General Population and Surgical Practice?

Globally, the population is aging, and the life expectancy is increasing worldwide. According to the National Institute on Aging, National Institute of Health, and the World Health Organization, the number of people 65 and older is projected to grow from an estimated 524 million in 2010 to nearly 1.5 billion in 2050, while those 80 years or more will number 400 million persons, with most of the increase in developing country (2). In Figs. 1.1, 1.2, and 1.3, we report

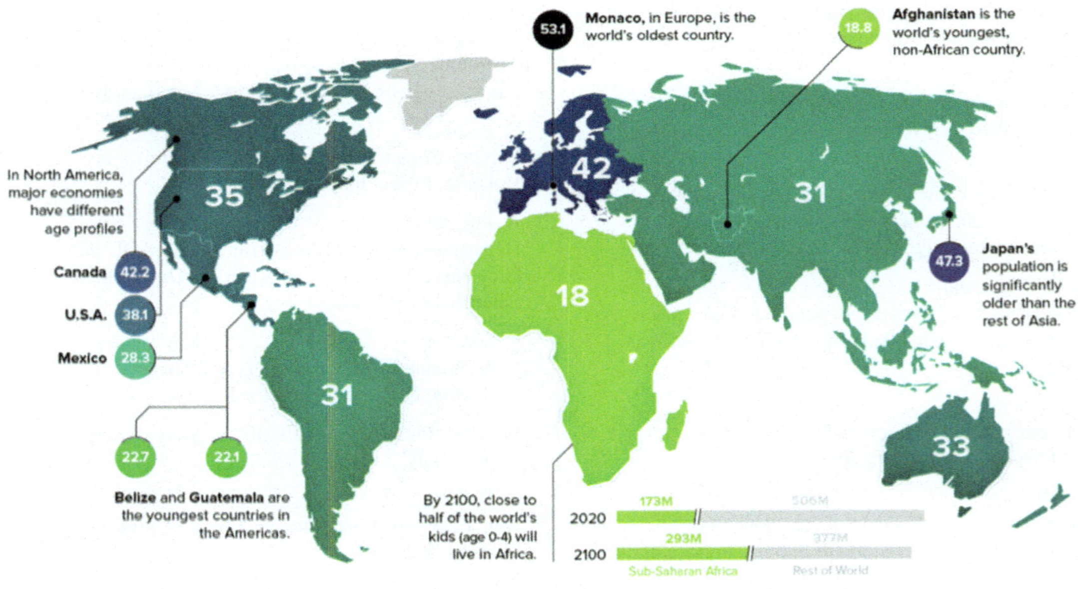

Fig. 1.1 The median age of the population on each continent

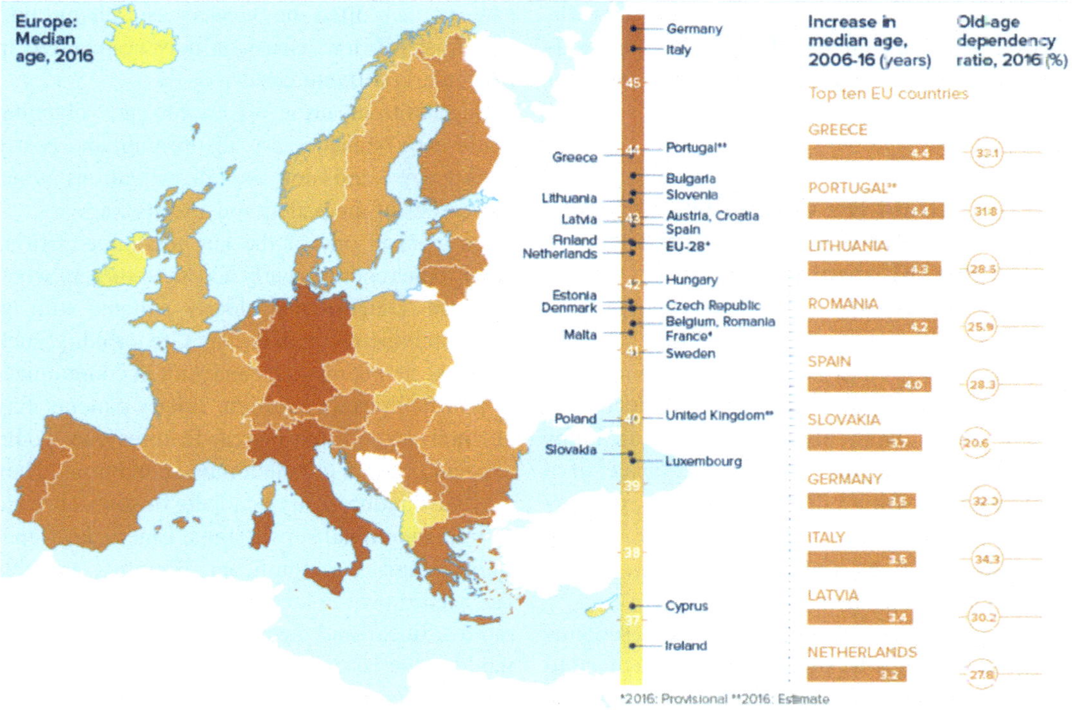

Fig. 1.2 Median age increasing among the European countries in the 2006–2016 decade

Fig. 1.3 Elderly index in Italy during the last 15 years

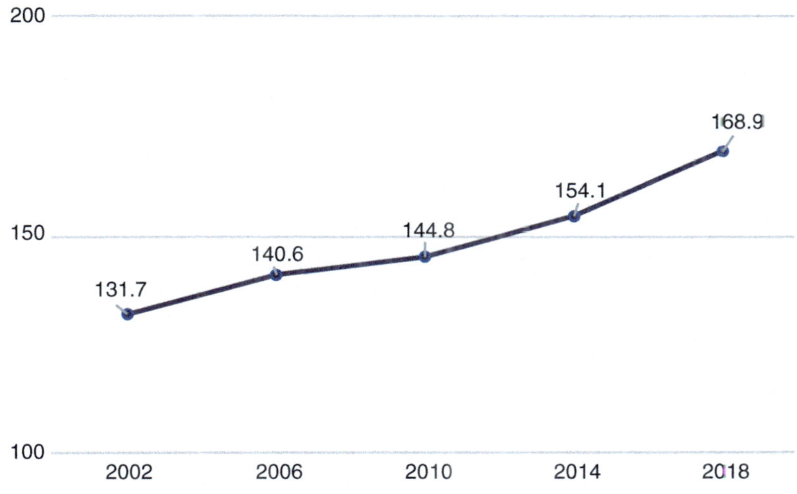

the median age distribution in the world and in Europe, and the increase in elderly index (percentage ratio between the population aged 65 and over and the population aged 0–14) in Italy in the last 15 years. The median age increasing among the European countries in the last decade is evident.

As a result of the increasing number of elderlies worldwide, the conditions that require surgery, such as atherosclerosis, cancer, arthritis, prostatism, and others, are also increasing. This demographic transition has changed the surgeons' definition of older patients, still based on a threshold of 50 in 1907, when surgery was not warranted even in this age group; indeed, nowadays a growing number of complex operations are being successfully performed to patients over 80 years.

1.3 Should the Operative and Perioperative Approach Be Different in Elderly Patients?

Pharmacotherapy has helped people living longer, and patients who need surgery in elective or urgent setting commonly use several medications (polypharmacotherapy) as a consequence of a high level of multimorbidity. Therefore, the surgeon must be able to know and interact with organ dysfunctions and with the adverse side effects of polytherapies.

The clinical presentation of surgical problems in the elderly may be subtle, and this may lead to delay in diagnosis. While the results of elective surgery in the elderly are reproducibly good, it has long been acknowledged that elderly patients having emergency surgery can have worse outcomes. Depending on the specific scenario, these worse outcomes can manifest in different ways: increased risk of peri- or postoperative death, development of postoperative complications, prolonged length of hospital stay, or discharge destination being other than the patient's own home (the need for rehabilitation, care, or nursing home placement). A patient's age should be treated as a scientific fact, not with prejudice, and no particular chronologic age is a contraindication to surgery. However, not all patients with conditions amenable to operative management should be taken to the theater. Futile surgery must be avoided; this requires robust risk assessment and discussion with the patient, family, caregivers, and patient advocates. Some older patients admitted with life-threatening pathology will be aware that they are approaching death and would rather have the focus shifted to palliative measures rather than heroic and unrealistic surgery. Deciding not to operate can be a difficult task and is certainly not the easy option. With patient and family emotions running high, deciding against surgery can often be viewed as "giving up." Multidisciplinary discussion may be required in particularly difficult cases.

In addition, prior advanced care planning could avoid unnecessary, distressing, and costly emergency admission and investigations when the wishes of the patient are already known.

In reverse, one of the key recommendations from some reports is early access to surgery when required. Diagnosis in elderly patients with an acute abdomen is challenging. Comorbidity, such as stroke and dementia, can result in communication difficulties. In addition, elderly patients may not present with the typical features one would expect in certain intraabdominal conditions. They may have reduced, atypical pain or show absence of intraabdominal sepsis signs. Emergency laparotomy carries a significant mortality, and this has been shown to increase with age; therefore, a rapid clinical and instrumental diagnosis must guide to the correct and timely surgical intervention to be performed. If definitive intervention is not timely undertaken, it can result in deterioration, development of adverse events, and poor outcome. In the most severe cases, delays in delivering definitive treatment have contributed to death.

No evidence supports a single standard presurgical assessment for the elderly. Preoperative screening should be guided by the type of surgery and the underlying comorbidities rather than a routine list of tests. Cardiac, pulmonary, liver, and renal function, as well as electrolytes and nutritional status, should be evaluated for any patient, but keeping the physiologic age-related changes into a great consideration.

A report of the Royal College of Surgeons of England on the "Higher Risk General Surgical Patient" includes discussion on the use of risk assessment in emergency surgery (3).

There are many risk predictions models available to the emergency clinician, for example, ASA, P-POSSUM, and APACHE-2. None of these risk scores makes any adjustment for frailty. Some are more complicated and time consuming than others and a balance is required between accuracy of prediction and real-world applicability. Although age-specific risk prediction models do exist, they are often cumbersome, making them of limited practical utility in an emergency. However, it is encouraging to see that attempts to accurately assess the risks in the elderly are being made.

The American College of Surgeons has developed a comprehensive online morbidity and mortality calculator for use in emergency and elective surgery (*http://riskcalculator.facs.org*) using data from 1.4 million operations in American hospitals between 2009 and 2012. It is a very powerful tool to help with informed consent and individual surgical risk. Accurate preoperative risk assessment is crucial in informed consent for operative surgery, and provides valuable information for clinicians (clinical audit and morbidity and mortality meetings), patients, and relatives. It can be used to predict the likelihood of adverse events, and allows steps to be taken to reduce their effects on the patient. Realistic and frank discussion of the risk of dying during or after an intervention may also allow sensible, respectful, and dignified decisions about end-of-life care.

Comorbidity and frailty often coexist with polypharmacy. Polypharmacy itself has been used as a surrogate for frailty: the prescription of more than five medications has been shown to correlate with frailty in elderly patients, and result in poorer outcomes (4). An in-depth discussion of polypharmacy management is beyond the scope of this book. However, the surgeon must be increasingly able to know and interact with organ dysfunctions and with the adverse side effects of polytherapies.

Postoperative care of the elderly patient is extremely important for both decreasing the short- and long-term mortality of the patients and improving the quality of life. There are no standard guidelines for postoperative care of the elderly patient. The care is similar to other patients with special concerns for the respiratory and cardiovascular systems, taking into account the physiologic changes and comorbidities. Also, good oxygenation and hydration of the tissues is necessary for wound healing, so hypoxia, hypovolemia, and hypervolemia should be avoided. The following are worth mentioning when working with elderly patients: hypothermia, pain control, mobilization, rehabilitation, fall prevention, prevention of postoperative delirium and cognitive dysfunction, and intolerance to complications.

In conclusion, the concepts expressed so far can be summarized in the following statements: *surgical patients are increasingly older, and often suffering from multiple diseases. The surgeon must, therefore, be familiar with the physiological, pathological, and clinical changes in this group of people* (5).

Enhanced recovery after surgery (ERAS) programs are evidenced-based protocols designed to standardize and optimize perioperative care to reduce surgical trauma, perioperative physiological stress, and organ dysfunction (metabolic, endocrine, and inflammatory response, as well as to reduce protein catabolism) related to elective procedures. Their application to elderly patients seems to be possible, even in an emergency environment. Several studies have shown shorter hospital stay, more effective discharge to home, and reduced cognitive and physical dysfunction. However, the primary objective remains to improve the morbidity and mortality rates. Further studies that specifically target these problems are needed to establish an evidence-based practice (6).

1.4 How to Define Frailty?

Frailty is defined as a *clinically recognizable state of increased vulnerability, resulting from age-associated decline in functionality across multiple physiologic systems such that the ability to cope with every day or acute stressors is compromised*. Frailty encompasses physical frailty, which is the most widely studied and most easily recognized state (7).

However, there is no clear consensus about the definition of frailty in research and clinical practice. Fried et al. from the Johns Hopkins University produced an operational definition of frailty based on measurable and objective criteria (8). It identifies frailty by five measurable components: (a) unintentional weight loss, greater than 4.5 kg or more than 5% of body weight in the last year; (b) signs of fatigue; (c) reduction in handgrip strength, assessed with a specific instrument and adjusted to the person's sex and body mass; (d) limited physical activity, assessed by calorie consumption and adjusted by sex; and (e) reduction in usual gait speed on a 4.5 m distance adjusted by gender and height. In the absence of a gold standard, frailty has been operationally defined as a condition meeting three of the five criteria (Table 1.1). A prefrail stage, in which one or two criteria are present, identifies a subset at high risk of progressing to frailty. Various adaptations of the clinical phenotype described by Fried have been described (8).

A second definition was formulated by researchers from the Canadian Initiative on Frailty and Aging (CIF-A). Frailty was defined using a more holistic approach, which emphasizes the complex etiology of the phenomenon, meant as not an optimal condition in elderly, multifactorial and dynamic in nature, and relating it to its history or trajectory of life. The indicated trajectory can be shaped by biological, psychological, and social factors; whose interactions result in resources and/or individual deficits in a given context.

A tool was developed to measure frailty in the elderly—the Edmonton Frail Scale (EFS)—contemplating nine domains: (1) cognition, (2) general state of (3) functional independence, (4) support, (5) medication use, (6) nutrition, (7) humor, (8) continence, and (9) functional performance. These authors consider this scale more comprehensive, especially considering aspects of cognition, humor, and social support.

Alternatively, frailty has been defined as a risk index (frailty index: FI) counting the number of deficits accumulated over time, including disability, diseases, physical and cognitive impairments, psychosocial risk factors, and geriatric syndromes (e.g., falls, delirium, and urinary incontinence) (Fig. 1.4).

Compared with the Fried frailty phenotype, the FI is a more sensitive predictor of adverse health outcomes because of its finer graded risk scale, and its robustness in clinical inferences with regard to the number and actual composition of the items (9).

In this book, we will adopt the Fried definition of frailty phenotype for several reasons: (1) the five-component phenotype is more appealing for use in a clinical setting than the FI that typically contains 30–70 items, and it is a better way to define frailty as a precise clinical state; (2) the clinical manifestations of frailty are better evaluated and followed up with simple clinical observations; (3) there are evidences that these manifestations exhibit the typical associations of a syndrome presentation; and (4) this theoretical approach facilitates the investigation of mechanisms underlying the development of frailty (7).

But how is frailty diagnosed? Researchers and clinicians require simple, valid, accurate, and reliable tools to detect frailty.

The Frail Elderly Functional Questionnaire (19 items) was identified as a potential outcome measure for frailty intervention studies as it is suitable for use by telephone or proxy, valid and reliable, and is sensitive to change (Table 1.2). The Groningen Frailty Indicator and the Tilburg Frailty Indicator are other simple and similar questionnaire-based approaches to detecting people with frailty. Aspects of validity have been investigated but, importantly, studies of diagnostic accuracy against well-defined community populations of older people are not yet available (10).

The timed-up-and-go test (TUGT), a simple standardized measure of gait speed that requires a stopwatch, and hand grip strength with a hand-

Table 1.1 Frail scale to evaluate frailty

FRAIL scale		Yes: 1 point No: 0 point
F	atigue: "Do you feel tired?"	
R	esistance: "Are you able to climb one flight of stairs?"	
A	mbulation: "Are you able to walk one block?"	
I	llneses: "Do you have more than five illnesses?"	
L	oss of weight: "Did you lose greater than 5% of your weight in the last 6 months?"	
	Total Score	/5
	Frailty State (0/5: Robust; 1–2/5: Pre-frail; ≥ 3/5: Frail)	

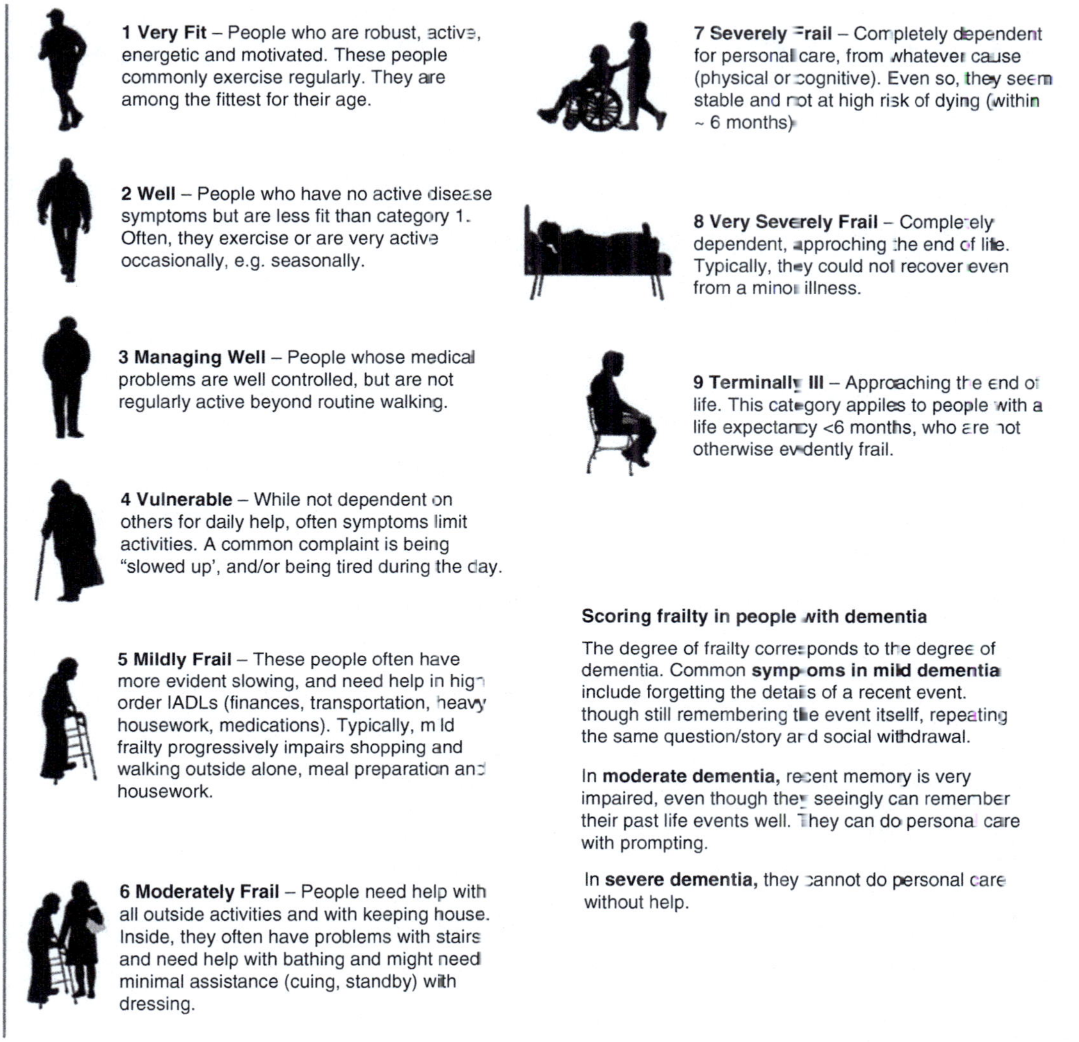

Fig. 1.4 The frailty index scale and system

held dynamometer, has been investigated as potential single assessments to detect frailty. Pulmonary function is associated with frailty and may have utility as a straightforward detection test. However, diagnostic accuracy of these assessments has not been confirmed (Fig. 1.5).

The Edmonton Frail Scale is a multidimensional assessment instrument that includes the TUGT, and a test for cognitive impairment. It is quick to administer (less than 5 min) and is valid, reliable, and feasible for routine use by nongeriatricians but the diagnostic accuracy has not been investigated (Table 1.3).

Nine items are included in the Changes in Health, End-Stage Disease, and Signs and Symptoms (CHESS) Scale. CHESS has been demonstrated to be a strong predictor of mortality and further validation studies are ongoing (Table 1.4) (11).

Comprehensive geriatric assessment (CGA) has become the internationally established method to assess older people in clinical practice.

Table 1.2 Frail elderly functional questionnaire

Individual question reliability
Task
1. Ambulation
2. Transferring
3. Turning in bed
4. Washing dishes
5. Meal preparation
6. Handling finances
7. Using telephone
8. Eating
9. Dressing, day clothes
10. Dressing, night clothes
11. Tub bath
12. Sponge bath
13. Using toilet
14. Using bedside commode
15. Using bedpan
16. Sitting up in bed
17. Grasping
18. Reaching out
19. Taking medication

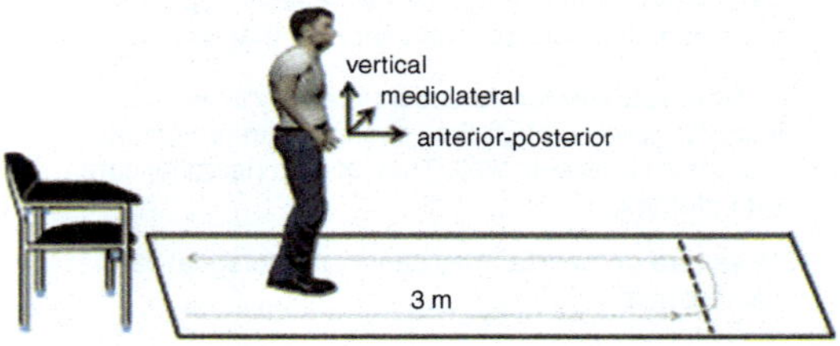

Fig. 1.5 The timed-up-and-go test

It is a multidisciplinary diagnostic process to determine an older person's medical, psychological, and functional capability to develop a plan for treatment and follow up. The process is associated with superior outcomes and has been applied successfully beyond elderly care medicine (Table 1.5) (12).

Table 1.4 Changes in health, end-stage disease, and signs and symptoms (CHESS) scale

Score	Item
0–2, 8	Change in decision making
0–3	Change in ADL status
0–2, 8	Change in ADL status
0–4	Health condition—vomiting
0–4	Health condition—peripheral edema
0–3	Health condition—dyspnea
0, 1	End-stage disease
0, 1	Weight loss
0, 1	Insufficient fluid
0, 1	Dehydrated
0, 1	Decrease in food or fluid
0, 1	Fluid output exceeds input
Range: 0–5	
Scoring:	
0 = No health instability	
1 = Minimal health instability	
2 = Low health instability	
3 = Moderate health instability	
4 = High health instability	
5 = Very high health instability	

Table 1.3 The Edmonton Frail Scale

Cognition	Clock drawing	No errors	Minor spacing	Other errors
Health status	Number of hospital admissions in last year	0	1	>1
	Patient description of overall health	Good	Fair	Poor
Functional dependence activities of daily living?	Help needed with number of	0–1	2–4	5–8
Social support	Reliable support available?	Always	Sometimes	Never
Medication use	>4 regular medications?	No	Yes	–
	Patient forgets to take medicines?	No	Yes	–
Nutrition	Recent weight loss present?	No	Yes	–
Mood	Often sad or depressed?	No	Yes	–
Continence	Urinary incontinence present?	No	Yes	–
Functional performance score out of 17	Timed up-and-go	0–10 s	11–20 s	>20 s or unable

Table 1.5 Comprehensive geriatric assessment (CGA)

Key elements of comprehensive geriatric assessment
Medical assessment
Problem list
Comorbidities
Medications
Nutritional assessment
Functional assessment
Basic activities of daily living
Instrumental activities of daily living
Gait and balance assessment
Exercise/activity assessment
Psychological assessment
Cognitive status
Assessment of mood
Social assessment
Informal social support
Environmental assessment
Care resource eligibility/financial assessment
Home safety
Access to transport facilities

These studies are the first objective confirmation that CGA is sensitive to the reliable detection of degrees of frailty. *CGA is currently the gold standard to detect frailty and it should be more widely deployed.* The practical limitation of CGA is the time and expertise required for the process.

1.5 How Often Can Do Face a Frail Patient in General Population and Surgical Practice?

A recent systematic review investigated the prevalence of frailty. Twenty-one community-based cohort studies involving 61,500 older people were identified. The operational definitions for frailty and the inclusion/exclusion criteria varied between the studies, which largely explained the considerable variation in reported frailty prevalence rates of 4.0–59.1%. However, when the reported rates were restricted to the studies that used the phenotype model, the weighted average frailty prevalence rate was 9.9% and, for pre-frailty prevalence, 44.2%. Frailty was statistically more prevalent in women than men. Most frailty models were developed in Caucasian populations with high prevalence in southern Europe. Similar high prevalence of frailty was observed also in older Hispanic and African Americans.

The prevalence of frailty in patients of all ages presenting for surgical procedures is quoted at between 4.1 and 50.3%. This wide variation relates to the issues of definition, measurement, and varying populations studied. Therefore, it would be useful to define an improved methodology that reduce these variability rates. A recent UK study used the Fried model to define frailty in community-dwelling people aged between 65 and 74 years. Prevalence rates of frailty in this study were 8.5% for women and 4.1% for men. Studies examining older patients undergoing elective cardiac and non-cardiac surgery quote prevalence rates of frailty at between 41.8 and 50.3%. This high prevalence of frailty in older surgical populations, compared with the prevalence rate of less than 10% observed in older community-dwelling individuals, highlights the vulnerability of this patient group (13).

1.6 How Does a Patient Become Frail?

As said above, frailty is a state of increased vulnerability to poor resolution of homeostasis following a stress, which increases the risk of adverse outcomes including falls, delirium, and disability. This is shown in Fig. 1.6, in which an apparently small insult (e.g., a new drug; "minor" infection; or "minor" surgery) results in a dramatic and disproportionate change in health status: from independent to dependent, mobile to immobile, postural stability to falling, and lucid to delirious.

The pathophysiology of frailty is a complex interaction of diseases and age-related decline that leads to a general state of low functional reserve capacities, affecting multiple domains. Frailty is often described as a *transitional phase* between successful aging and disability. Progression of frailty leads to increased risk of falls, disability, immobility, hospitalizations, institutionalization, caregiver burden, decreased

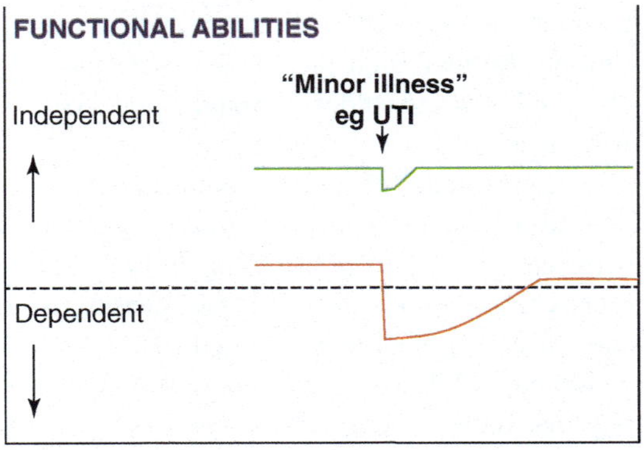

Fig. 1.6 The effect on the human being dependency by an insult that destabilizes normal and frail patient (the red line corrisponds to frail patients, the green one to normal patient)

quality of life, and even death. Therefore, there is a gradual decline in physiological reserve with aging but, in frailty, this decline is accelerated, and homeostatic mechanisms start failing (14).

An important perspective for frailty, therefore, is to consider how the complex mechanisms of aging promote cumulative decline in multiple physiological systems, consequent erosion of homeostatic reserve, and vulnerability to disproportionate changes in health status following relatively minor stressor events. The flipside of frailty is resilience, a newer concept that is highly relevant to successful aging. Resilience has been described in the psychosocial literature as the capacity to maintain or regain well-being during or after adversity. Instead of focusing on the negative aspects of human functioning, there is interest in understanding what fortifies older adults in the face of stressors, as internal and external resources for resilience would be empowering for older adults and serve as important targets for intervention.

These complex aging mechanisms are influenced by underlying genetic and environmental factors in combination with epigenetic mechanisms, which regulate the differential expression of genes in cells and may be especially important in aging (15). Increasing evidence suggests that microbiota plays an important role in stem-cell aging. The tremendous importance of microbiota in microbial homoeostasis, alterations in metabolism, and both innate and adaptive immune systems has been well established. The dysbiosis or compositional changes in gut microbiota are linked to the aging of stem cells in terms of dysregulations of metabolism, aberrant activation of the immune system, as well as promoting epigenetic instability of stem cell.

A schematic representation of frailty is provided in Fig. 1.7.

According to the modern theories, frailty is considered to result from the lifelong accumulation of molecular and cellular damage caused by multiple mechanisms under the regulation of a complex maintenance and repair network. There is uncertainty regarding the precise level of cellular damage required to cause impaired organ physiology but, importantly, many organ systems exhibit considerable redundancy, which provides the physiological reserve required to compensate for age- and disease-related changes.

Therefore, a key question is whether there is a critical threshold of age-related, cumulative decline in multiple physiological systems beyond which frailty becomes evident. The number of abnormal systems seems to be more predictive than abnormalities in any particular system. This provides evidence to suggest that when physiological decline reaches an aggregate critical mass, frailty becomes evident.

The brain, endocrine system, immune system, and skeletal muscle are intrinsically interrelated and are currently the organ systems best studied in the development of frailty; moreover, the physiological reserve in the respiratory, cardiovascular, renal, and hemopoietic/clotting systems and nutritional status are also investigated as potential mediating factors. However, a deeper examination of their involvement in the pathophysiology of the frailty syndrome is beyond our discussion and we refer to the works cited in the references for a more in-depth examination (16).

1.7 Is an Older Patient Always Frail Too and Vice Versa?

The concept of frailty is frequently mentioned in studies related to the older population. In fact, despite elderly does not mean frailty, aging process leads to frailty, which means that there are

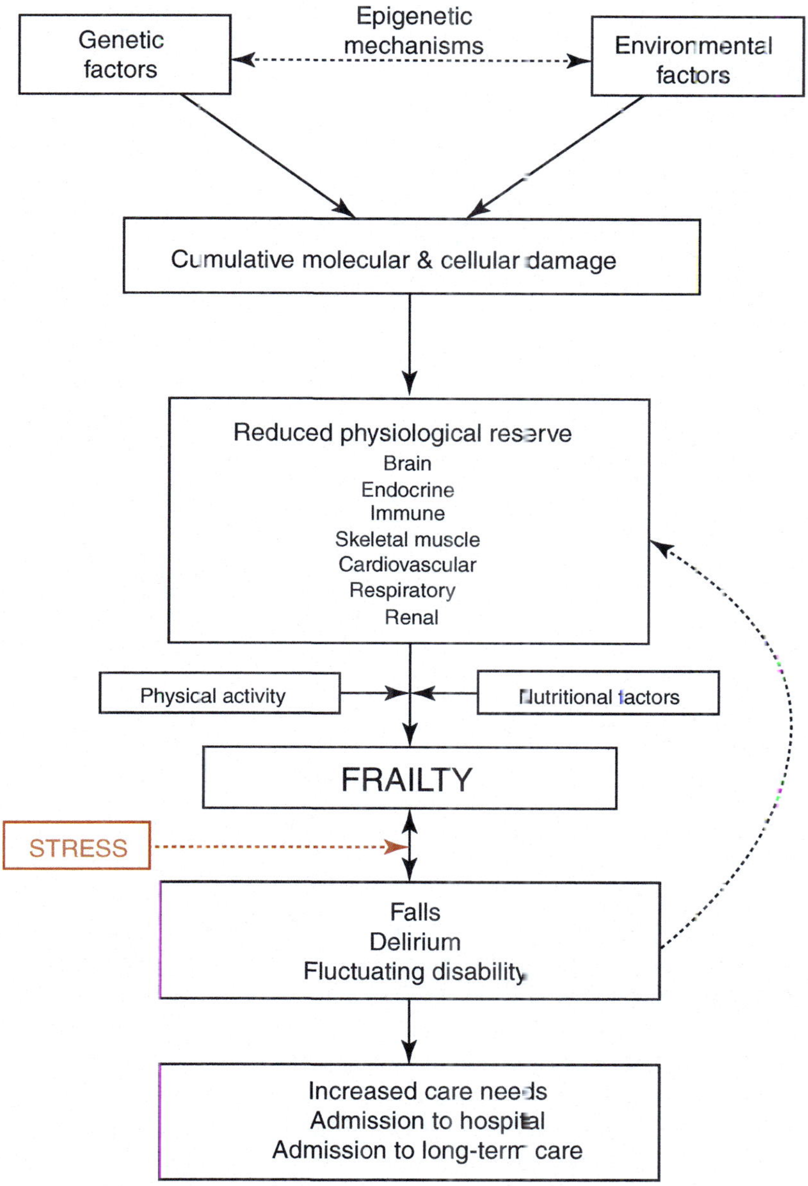

Fig. 1.7 Pathophysiological elements of frailty syndrome

changes that reflect aging-related alterations and involve intrinsic and extrinsic factors which are typical of aging. Frailty increased steadily with age: 65–69 years: 4%; 70–74 years: 7%; 75–79 years: 9%, 80–84 years: 16%; and >85 years: 26% (Canadian data). Rates appear to be higher in studies that employed the graded frailty index (17).

In Fig. 1.8, a possible overlap between frailty and the typical geriatric syndrome is reported.

1.8 What Is the Conceptual Difference Among Frailty, Multimorbidity, and Disability?

Comorbidity is defined by some authors as *two or more of the following nine diseases: myocardial infarction, angina, congestive heart failure, claudication, arthritis, cancer, diabetes, hyper-*

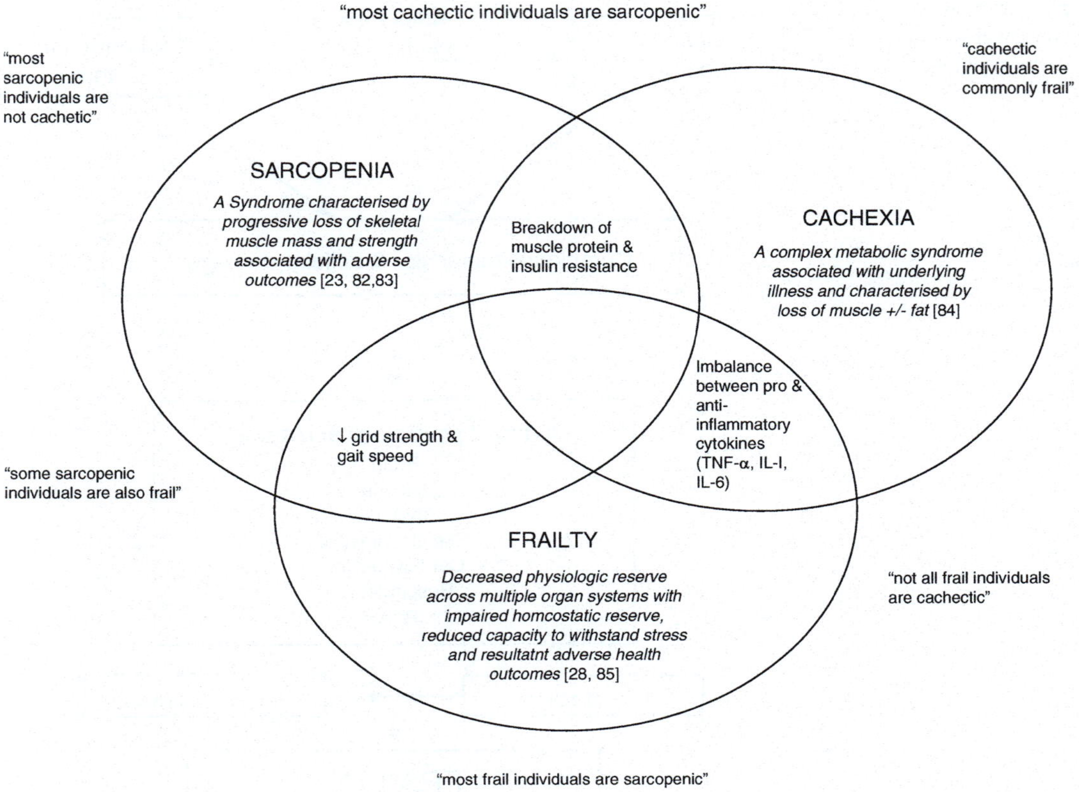

Fig. 1.8 The overlap between different geriatric syndromes

tension, and chronic obstructive pulmonary disease; whereas disability is described as *the presence of restriction in at least one activity of daily living*. In a most important study, the overlap between frailty and comorbidity was present in 46.2% of the population, frailty and disability in 5.7%, and the combination of frailty, disability, and comorbidity in 21.5%. Importantly, frailty was present without comorbidity or disability in 26.6% of the study group. This finding provides support for frailty as an independent concept, distinct from comorbidity and disability. However, more recent work suggests that the overlap is more frequent and increases with greater frailty (18).

1.9 Are There Any Therapeutic Methods to Prevent, Contrast, or Treat the Frailty Process?

Reducing the prevalence or severity of frailty is likely to have large benefits for the individual, their families, and for society. Several approaches have been investigated in clinical trials (19, 20):

- *Interventions based on comprehensive geriatric assessment*

  Frail older people receiving inpatient CGA are more likely to return home, less likely to experience cognitive or functional decline, and have lower in-hospital mortality. Complex interventions based on CGA delivered to older people in the community can increase the likelihood of continuing to live at home, principally through a reduced need for care home admission and reduced falls, but those who are most frail appear to receive least benefit. (12)

- *Exercise interventions*

Exercise has physiological effects on the brain, endocrine system, immune system, and skeletal muscle. Some studies concluded that exercise can improve outcomes of mobility and functional ability. The most effective intensity (duration and frequency) of exercise intervention remains uncertain, but adherence was characteristically high across a range of interventions (21).

A Cochrane review incorporated 49 RCTs of exercise interventions for long-term care (LTC) residents (a group of older people who are likely to be very frail) and concluded that these interventions, particularly those involving strength and balance training, can successfully increase muscle strength and functional abilities. It is, therefore, possible that even small gains in strength of LTC residents translate into important functional gains (22).

- *Nutritional interventions and environmental factors*

Nutritional interventions may have potential to address the impaired nutrition and weight loss of frailty. However, there is a paucity of evidence. One RCT that investigated the effects of exercise and nutritional supplementation in 100 frail older people living in long-term care reported that nutritional supplementation had no effect on muscle strength, gait speed, stair climbing, or physical activity (23). A Cochrane review of nutritional interventions for preventing and treating pressure ulcers in older hospital patients, a group who are likely to be frail, reported that it was not possible to draw any firm conclusions due to the absence of trials of high methodological quality. Moreover, some environmental factors, such as family, home, finances, neighborhood, and health care, interact with individual factors to influence the physical and mental health of older adults (24).

- *Pharmacological agents*

The use of pharmacological agents for the prevention and treatment of frailty is an important area for future research. *Few pharmacological agents have been investigated in frailty. Angiotensin-converting enzyme (ACE) inhibitors* have been demonstrated to improve the structure and biochemical function of skeletal muscle and there is evidence that ACE inhibitors may halt or slow the decline in muscle strength in older age and improve exercise capacity and quality of life (25). *Testosterone* not only improves muscle strength but also increases adverse cardiovascular and respiratory outcomes. *IGFs* have direct effects on skeletal muscle but IGF-1 does not appear to improve muscle strength or bone density in healthy older women (26). *Low vitamin D levels* have been associated with frailty and damages after falls. Although vitamin D prescription for older people who are deficient may reduce falls and fractures, *the general use of vitamin D as treatment for frailty remains controversial.* Indeed a recent meta-analysis suggests that malnutrition and, especially, vitamin deficiencies like vitamin D are associated with immune senescence and could lead to immunodeficiency in the elderly rather than to fractures and cognitive impairment (27).

1.10 How Does Frailty Modify the Surgical Approach and Outcome?

Studies in various surgical populations have identified frailty as an independent risk factor for major morbidity, mortality, protracted length of stay (LOS), and institutional discharge. Within the older and frail surgical population, the process of preoperative assessment provides an opportunity for proactive recognition of the frailty syndrome. The preoperative assessment process can be considered to serve two broad purposes. First, to perform appropriate patient risk stratification to fully inform health professionals, patients, and their relatives or caregivers on the inherent risks in undergoing a procedure. Second, in order that modifiable factors are proactively identified and optimized preoperatively; and thus, improving the patient's likelihood of a successful outcome.

There is a relative paucity of research on the influence of frailty in surgical outcome. Moreover, the disparate approach to the measurement of frailty makes the available researches difficult to be compared. Notably, the two studies by Robinson et al. show a very high incidence of postdischarge institutionalization (26% and 30%, respectively). While the high rate of institutionalization may reflect a difference in the American social care model, the findings of these studies raise two questions. First, was it appropriate to perform surgery in this group with over a quarter subsequently needing institutional care? Second, what is the role for intervention targeted at individual components of the frailty syndrome in improving surgical outcomes? (28).

A recent study examined inflammatory biomarkers, thought to be important in the pathophysiology of frailty, and the association with postoperative complications in older colorectal surgical patients. Patients aged 70 years or over were defined as frail, prefrail, or robust using comprehensive geriatric assessment (CGA) and an approximation to the frailty phenotype.

The inflammatory biomarkers C-reactive protein (CRP), interleukin-6 (Il-6), tumor necrosis factor-α (TNF-α), and D-dimer were examined 2 weeks prior to elective resection for colorectal cancer. Levels of CRP, Il-6, and TNF-α increased significantly with increasing frailty level. Having adjusted for tumor location, which is an established risk factor for postoperative complications, CGA defined frailty and Il-6 were predictive of complications (29, 30).

In summary, frailty is predictive of mortality, postoperative complications, and institutional discharge in older patients undergoing cardiac and noncardiac surgery (31, 32).

To improve morbidity and mortality, several aspects of care need to be addressed. These include accurate and timely preoperative assessment to identify treatable pathology and, where possible, to consider and correct age-specific disease processes. Identification of patients in whom treatment would be futile or associated with high risk is needed to avoid unnecessary interventions and to give patients and cares realistic expectations. The use of multidisciplinary teams to identify common postoperative complications and age-specific syndromes is paramount. Prevention of complications is preferable to rescue treatment due to the high proportion of patients who fail to recover from adverse events. Even with successful surgical treatment, long-term functional decline and increased dependency are common. More research into emergency surgery in the elderly is needed to improve care for this growing group of vulnerable patients.

Five Things You Should Know of on How to Define an Elderly and Frail Patient

- For statistical and public administrative purposes, elderly is conventionally defined as a person 65 years, but in the most conspicuous review, the authors recommend limiting the definition to the people over 75 years of age, instead of the current 65.
- No evidence supports a single standard presurgical assessment for the elderly. Preoperative screening should be guided by the type of surgery and the underlying comorbidities rather than a routine list of tests.
- Postoperative care of the elderly patient is extremely important for both decreasing the short- and long-term mortality of the patients and improving the quality of life. There are no standard guidelines for postoperative care of the elderly patient. The care is similar to other patients with special concerns for the respiratory and cardiovascular systems, taking into account the physiologic changes and comorbidities. Also, good oxygenation and hydra-

tion of the tissues are necessary for wound healing, so hypoxia, hypovolemia, and hypervolemia should be avoided.

- Frailty is defined as a clinically recognizable state of increased vulnerability, resulting from age-associated decline in functionality across multiple physiologic systems, such that the ability to cope with every day or acute stressors is compromised. Reducing the prevalence or severity of frailty is likely to have large benefits for the individual, their families, and for society. Several approaches have been investigated in clinical trials, such as: interventions based on comprehensive geriatric assessment, exercise interventions, nutritional interventions and environmental factors, and pharmacological agents.
- Frailty is predictive of mortality, postoperative complications, and institutional discharge in older patients undergoing cardiac and noncardiac surgery. To improve morbidity and mortality, several aspects of care need to be addressed. These include accurate and timely preoperative assessment to identify treatable pathology and, where possible, to consider and correct age-specific disease processes.

References

1. Ouchi Y, Rakugi H, Arai H, et al. Joint Committee of Japan Gerontological Society (JGLS) and Japan Geriatrics Society (JGS) on the definition and classification of the elderly. Redefining the elderly as aged 75 years and older: proposal from the Joint Committee of Japan Gerontological Society and the Japan Geriatrics Society. Geriatr Gerontol Int. 2017;17(7):1045–7.
2. World Health Organization. 10 facts on ageing and the life course. 2012. http://www.who.int/features/factfiles/ageing/ageing_facts/en/index.html.
3. Anderson I, Eddleston J, Grocott M, et al. The higher risk general surgical patient towards improved care for a Forgotten Group. London: RCS; 2011.
4. British Geriatrics Society. Fit for frailty: consensus best practice guidance for the care of older people living with frailty in community and outpatient settings. 2014.
5. Chen CY, Gan P, How CH. Approach to frailty in the elderly in primary care and the community. Singapore Med J. 2018;59(5):240–5.
6. Paduraru M, Ponchietti L, Casas IM, et al. Enhanced Recovery After Surgery (ERAS)—the evidence in geriatric emergency surgery: a systematic review. Chirurgia. 2017;112:546–57.
7. Xue QL. The frailty syndrome: definition and natural history. Clin Geriatr Med. 2011;27(1):1–15.
8. Fried LP, Tangen CM, Walston J, et al. Frailty in older adults: evidence for a phenotype. J Gerontol A Biol Sci Med Sci. 2001;56(3):M146–56.
9. Rockwood K, Andrew M, Mitnitski A. A comparison of two approaches to measuring frailty in elderly people. J Gerontol A Biol Sci Med Sci. 2007;62:738–43.
10. Michael Gloth F, Scheve AA, Shah S, et al. The frail elderly functional assessment questionnaire: its responsiveness and validity in alternative settings. Arch Phys Med Rehabil. 1999;80:1572–6.
11. Ogarek JA, McCreedy EM, Thomas KS, et al. Minimum data set changes in health, end-stage disease and symptoms and signs scale: a revised measure to predict mortality in nursing home residents. J Am Geriatr Soc. 2018;66(5):976–81.
12. Eamer G, Taheri A, Chen SS, et al. Comprehensive geriatric assessment for older people admitted to a surgical service. Cochrane Database Syst Rev. 2018;1:CD012485.
13. Collard RM, Boter H, Schoevers RA. Prevalence of frailty in community-dwelling older persons: a systematic review. J Am Geriatr Soc. 2012;60:1487–92.
14. Mitnitski AB, Mogilner AJ, Rockwood K. Accumulation of deficits as a proxy measure of aging. Sci World J. 2001;1:323–36.
15. Bishop NA, Lu T, Yankner BA. Neural mechanisms of ageing and cognitive decline. Nature. 2010;464(7288):529–35.
16. Miller RA. The aging immune system: primer and prospectus. Science. 1996;273(5271):70–4.
17. Clegg A, Young J, Iliffe S. Frailty in elderly people. Lancet. 2013;381(9868):752–62.
18. Theou O, Rockwood MR, Mitnitski A, et al. Disability and co-morbidity in relation to frailty: how much do they overlap? Arch Gerontol Geriatr. 2012;55(2):e1–8.
19. Leng S, Chen X, Mao G. Frailty syndrome: an overview. Clin Interv Aging. 2014;9:433–41. https://doi.org/10.2147/cia.s45300.
20. Fried LP, Hadley EC, Walston J, et al. From bedside to bench: research agenda for frailty. Sci Aging Knowl Environ. 2005;2005(31):24.
21. Hassani A, Kubicki A, Brost V, et al. Kinematic analysis of motor strategies in frail aged adults during the timed up and go: how to spot the motor frailty? Clin Interv Aging. 2015;10:505–13.
22. Ellis G, Gardner M, Tsiachristas A, et al. Comprehensive geriatric assessment for older adults admitted to hospital. Cochrane Database Syst Rev. 2017;9(9):CD006211. https://doi.org/10.1002/14651858.cd006211.pub3.
23. Hubbard RE, Fallah N, Searle SD, et al. Impact of exercise in community-dwelling older adults. PLoS One. 2009;4:e6174.
24. Langer G, Fink A. Nutritional interventions for preventing and treating pressure ulcers. Cochrane

Database Syst Rev. 2014;(6):CD003216. https://doi.org/10.1002/14651858.CD003216.
25. Band MM, Sumukadas D, Struthers AD, et al. Leucine and ACE inhibitors as therapies for sarcopenia (LACE trial): study protocol for a randomised controlled trial. Trials. 2018;19:6.
26. Ory MG, Lee Smith M. What if healthy aging is the 'new Normal'? Int J Environ Res Public Health. 2017;14(11):1389.
27. Mailliez A, Guilbaud A, Puisieux F. Circulating biomarkers characterizing physical frailty: CRP, hemoglobin, albumin, 25OHD and free testosterone as best biomarkers. Results of a meta-analysis. Exp Gerontol. 2020;139:111014. https://doi.org/10.1016/j.exger.2020.111014.
28. Dhesi JK, Lees NP, et al. Frailty in the perioperative setting. Clin Med (London). 2019;19(6):485–9.
29. Cable N, Hiyoshi A, Kondo N, et al. Identifying frail-related biomarkers among community-dwelling older adults in Japan: a research example from the Japanese Gerontological evaluation study. Biomed Res Int. 2018;2018:5362948.
30. Tannou T, Koeberle S, Aubri R. Multifactorial immunodeficiences in frail elderly patients: contributing factors and management. Med Mal Infect. 2019;49:167–72.
31. Sundermann S, Dademasch A, Praetorius J, et al. Comprehensive assessment of frailty for elderly high-risk patients undergoing cardiac surgery. Eur J Cardiothorac Surg. 2011;39:33–7.
32. Robinson TN, Wu DS, Pointer L, et al. Simple frailty score predicts postoperative complications across surgical specialties. Am J Surg. 2013;206(4):544–50.

2 Defining the Burden of Emergency General Surgery in the Elderly Today

Elisa Cassinotti, Luigi Boni, and Ludovica Baldari

2.1 Introduction

Emergency general surgery (EGS) represents a considerable workload in most health-care systems and includes very diversified pathologic situations all related by the urgent nature of the condition [1].

In contrast to elective surgery, emergency setting present at inconvenient hours, often without a definite diagnosis, with limited background information, and frequently with little time for planning. This often does not allow a quiet evaluation and an extended assessment: the surgeon who deals with emergency surgery needs proper tools to quickly take the right decisions based on solid data about the chances of success and about the expectations of life after a procedure [2].

Patients undergoing EGS are at highest surgical risk; their outcomes are usually much worse than after elective surgery, with high rate of postoperative morbidity and mortality [1, 3]. This leads to consumption of a substantial amount of health-care resources. In the UK, EGS accounts for 50% of the workload in NHS hospitals and 80% of the surgical-related deaths; in the United States, there are more than three million admissions for EGS and patients are more than 8 times more likely to die compared with their elective surgical counterparts [3, 4].

The increasing age of the population is an unavoidable phenomenon: the number of elderly people has risen by more than 50% over the last 15 years and it will increase dramatically over the next few decades with population projections toward 2040 indicating a 66% increase in the age groups 65–74 years. Currently, there are over 46.3 million (14.5%) geriatric Americans, and this figure is expected to grow to 98 million (24%) by 2060.

More importantly, people aged 85 and older will increase from 2.8% in 2011 to 7.8% in 2050, with an average life expectancy of 85.3 years for males and 90.5 years for females, with obvious implications, both for the health policies and from a clinical standpoint [5, 6].

The aging of population is a major public health issue deeply connected with surgical care: in the UK, it is estimated, for instance, that even though people >65 years of age are currently about 12% of the total population, these individuals undergo over 25% of the annual surgical procedures and that over 33% of the elderly population undergoes surgery within the last year of life [7].

E. Cassinotti (✉) · L. Boni
General Surgery Department, IRCCS Ca' Granda Policlinico Ospedale Maggiore Milano, University of Milan, Milan, Italy
e-mail: elisa.cassinotti@policlinico.mi.it; luigi.boni@unimi.it

L. Baldari
General Surgery Department, Fondazione IRCCS Ca' Granda Policlinico Ospedale Maggiore Milano, Milan, Italy
e-mail: ludovica.baldari@unimi.it

F. Agresta et al. (eds.), *Emergency laparoscopic surgery in the elderly and frail patient*,
https://doi.org/10.1007/978-3-030-79990-8_2

Some studies, focused primarily on elective surgery, indicate that frailty is an important predictor of adverse postsurgical outcomes in elderly patients undergoing vascular, cardiac, and gastrointestinal major interventions. A 2017 meta-analysis including more than one million patients undergoing major abdominal surgery has clearly showed the relation of frailty with increased postoperative mortality and morbidity [8, 9].

As regards emergency surgery, admissions are growing annually in developed countries, with the elderly population making a definite contribution to the overall increase [1]. More unfavorable results are reported for EGS procedures on older patients, with higher rates of postoperative morbidities and mortality; indeed, in emergency setting, age is an independent predictor of adverse postoperative outcomes and high resource use [10, 11].

In elective surgical setting, the issues of comorbidity, polypharmacy, poor nutrition, and poor mobility are well known, with quite established strategies to identify and manage them; on the contrary, it is particularly challenging to manage the elderly in an emergency scenario and, so far in literature, the population-level effect of frailty on EGS is poorly described [9, 12].

2.2 Older Patients and Emergency Surgery

As previously stated, elderly people undergoes emergency surgery at a higher rate than other age groups: despite making up only 15% of the population, more than 30% of EGS cases are performed on aged patients. Certainly, this demographic shift is predicted to have an impact on patient outcomes and increase health system costs.

It is widely accepted that people of different ages have different health-care needs, and the outcomes of surgery and anesthesia can be influenced by age, with the prevalence of frailty increasing exponentially as the age rises [12, 13]. Although clinical outcomes after elective operations are similar in young and older individuals, EGS procedures lead to significant increase in morbidity and mortality rate in elderly and fragile patients [14].

In particular, mortality rate after emergency surgery is considerably higher in the elderly even for surgical conditions usually regarded as "low risk" surgeries: for example, in acute appendicitis, the reported mortality rate in patients aged over 70 years is six to seven times higher than in those aged 20–49 years [15].

As reported in a large retrospective review on JAMA Surgery in 2016, where data on over 420,000 patients on 4-year study period were analyzed, elderly patients represented 28.8% of all major EGS cases with laparotomies, large and small bowel resections, cholecystectomies, operative peptic ulcers repair, lysis of adhesions, and appendectomies collectively accounting for 80% of all procedures. Nevertheless, these procedures also represent 80.3% of deaths, 78.9% of complications, and 80.2% of inpatient nationwide costs [4, 16].

Several other papers, on smaller cohorts, have investigated the prevalence of different abdominal diseases requiring urgent surgical treatment in old patients: in particular, 40–50% of cases are obstructive syndromes, where the most frequent causes of obstruction are incarcerated inguinal hernias and colorectal cancer; especially, colorectal obstructions represent a significant cause of morbidity and mortality in elderly undergoing EGS [16, 17].

The other major causes of elderly EGS are peritonitis (approximately 30% of cases), mainly due to perforated acute diverticulitis, acute cholecystitis, and appendicitis. Even if appendectomies and cholecystectomy could be considered as lower-risk emergency surgeries, overall mortality rates tend to increase exponentially with age. It must also be taken into account that in one of the abovementioned retrospective series, 53% of cholecystitis and 44% of appendicitis were gangrenous [18]; additionally, other studies demonstrated that acute appendicitis in elderly patients might be distinguished by delay in treatment, high perforation rate, and unfavorable outcome [13, 15].

Other than higher 30-day and in-hospital mortality rates (for the most part due to abdominal and pulmonary septic complications), older people also frequently experience higher complications rate after EGS procedures.

Based on health administrative data in United States on 150,000 patients, Kuy and colleagues reported a 27% complication rate after emergency cholecystectomy in people 65–79 years old, rising to a 38% rate in people aged over 80; this resulted in longer length of hospital stay and higher costs; and this study also revealed that longer time from admission to surgery is a significant predictor of poor outcome [19].

2.2.1 Diagnostic and Therapeutic Challenges

In elderly patients presenting with acute condition, the eventual indication for emergency surgery may not be clear to the primary care physician, and specialist consultation should be the next step to improve diagnosis, discuss pros and cons, treatment, and alternatives. The diagnostic process is often more difficult and sometimes totally inconclusive because of communication difficulties and peculiar biochemical and radiographic changes. A retrospective analysis on elderly patients with abdominal pain showed that temperature, physical examination, and basic blood tests have limited sensitivity in discriminating the surgical cases [20]. Another recent article reports that 75% of elderly patients evaluated in the emergency room for abdominal pain were discharged with a final diagnosis of NSAP (nonspecific abdominal pain) [8]. In this group of patients, the diagnostic path is often aggressive and is often completed with a CT scan. CT scan is generally characterized by a good ability to identify the source of the problem, taking into consideration that long-term side effect of radiation is less of a concern in the elderly [21].

In particular, as the population grows older, the number of added organs with disease conditions that may need treatment or support become more prevalent, yet also with an increasing associated additional risk burden by surgery. This burden may be related to comorbidity that may require particular attention. Will the patient need dialysis? Will the heart tolerate the surgical stress? Will the pulmonary condition require ventilator support, and, if yes, when will the patient be able to be weaned off the ventilator, if at all? Clearly, the number and severity of other underlying conditions, as well as the impact of the acute surgical disease on further function and quality of life, is a complex picture to handle.

In the decision, clinical issues (chance of recovery, procedure-related risks, and available therapeutic alternatives), ethical aspects, and health policy considerations (what resources are right to employ against a limited life expectancy?) need to be considered.

It has been well described that older patients undergoing emergency surgery have poorer outcomes [2–4, 8, 10–12, 17, 18, 22]. These poorer outcomes may be defined as follows:

- Increased risk of mortality.
- Increased postoperative complications.
- Increased length of stay,
- Increased functional dependence or discharge destination being different from the original place the patient was admitted from.

Therefore, in this area, it is really difficult to give appropriate instruments for clinical choices. We should evaluate following elements:

- The degree of patient consciousness.
- The "quod vitam" prognosis, besides the acute disease for which the patient is actually observed (with particular reference to oncologic, cardiac, and pulmonary terminal diseases).
- The success rate of the procedure (in particular, regarding abdominal sepsis and bowel ischemia).
- The wish of patients and of their kins.

There have been some attempts to identify preoperative data helpful to determine the real impact associated with urgent intervention: globally, it is known that, in the last period of life, intensive treatments often prolong the suffering of the patient, and the hospitalization, even more in the ICU, worsens their quality of life and restricts the psychosocial well-being of the patient and his family [23].

2.2.2 Multidisciplinary Approach and Comprehensive Geriatric Assessment (CGA)

As demonstrated in other medical fields—such as cancer care—the role of multidisciplinary approach is mandatory for complex evaluations and decision-making.

Regarding elderly population and emergency surgery, the need of multidisciplinary team has started to be applied on trauma/hip fracture settings, including geriatric specialists in the overall work-up and treatment planning together with the surgeon, showing improvements in outcomes.

In multidisciplinary discussions, decisions should be shared among experienced professionals from different disciplines and should aim to consider the whole patient "journey" in hospital and all the potential adverse outcomes.

However, this can be very difficult to perform in the emergency setting, where it is essential to get the patient into the operating room as quickly as possible. Interestingly, Cooper et al. recently outlined the high burden of palliative care needs among older patients undergoing EGS and suggested that concurrent surgical and palliative care may improve the patient's quality of life and their end-of-life care [24].

A comprehensive geriatric assessment (CGA) is a multidimensional diagnostic and treatment process that addresses the medical, social, functional, and psychological needs of elderly patients to develop a coordinated and integrated plan to maximize their health care. CGA aims to identify those patients who are at greatest risk of complications to allow a better allocation of resources and a shared treatment plan [25]. Several specialists are involved in CGA, including elderly medicine consultants, physiotherapists, pyschogeriatricians, dieticians, and occasionally social workers. In addition, family and friends will be approached for information and support, and the need for community services established. With multidisciplinary support and targeted interventions, CGA has been shown to reduce length of stay, rates of institutionalization, and functional status in surgery such as orthopedics, oncology, and vascular surgery [16]. Although the majority of research has been conducted in the elective surgical setting, the CGA could also be applied to the emergency surgery where nonoperative versus operative surgical strategies should be considered [26].

From surgical point of view, CGA should be considered as a multidisciplinary and individualized emergency enhanced recovery program specifically designated for older patients, with similar targets as enhanced recovery after elective surgery program (ERAS) to improve intra- and postoperative course and reduce complications and adverse outcomes.

The CGA differs from a standard medical assessment for the following reasons:

1. It concentrates on frail older patients with complex problems.
2. It has an emphasis on functional status and quality of life.
3. It uses a multidisciplinary team.
4. It uses dedicated quantitative assessment scales.
5. It can vary in intensity from screening to a full diagnostic assessment.

A systematic review and meta-analysis of the use of CGA internationally showed that patients who received a CGA were more likely to be alive and in their own homes and less likely to be discharged in residential care compared with standard care (without the CGA) [25]. However, despite good evidence, the general surgical specialties have been slow to adopt this form of collaborative care with performance of a CGA.

Cost-effectiveness of a CGA has only been assessed in eight published articles. Seven out of eight articles were related to orthopedic patients and one was based on nonorthopedic trauma patients. However, all concluded that the addition of a CGA improved outcomes at a lower cost compared with usual care, making a

CGA performed in the perioperative period more economically viable when compared with usual care [27].

2.3 Screening and Assessment of Frailty in EGS

The concept of frailty, as properly described in this picture from a BJS review on geriatric patients and emergency surgery, results in a lack of resilience to any physiological insult that prevents recovery or achievement of the same functional level after the insult (Fig. 2.1) (Illustration from Desserud et al. [28]).

Preoperative frailty assessment is a well-established way to predict high risk and high resource use in treating the older surgical population. In detail, frailty has been increasingly recognized as a partially modifiable risk factor prior to elective general surgery and the effect of frailty on outcomes in elective surgical settings is quite well described in several cohort studies [29]; however, the association of frailty with outcomes and resource use after EGS is not established. This is due both to a lack of strong data on EGS procedures in elderly and to a lack of standardized definition of frailty itself [30].

2.3.1 Frailty and EGS

The association of frailty and in-hospital complications after EGS in older patients was examined in several studies showing a direct association between frailty and worse outcomes in EGS patients. When outcomes for elderly versus younger patients were compared, elderly had a significantly higher crude and adjusted risk for serious morbidity and mortality. Moreover, age and ASA score were not predictive of postoperative and major complications [11, 30–32]. These findings are consistent with a large database analysis of >35,000 older Americans who underwent emergent general surgery in which a modified frailty index (mFI) was deemed to be a superior predictor of 30-day mortality than ASA grading. As the modified frailty index increased, associ-

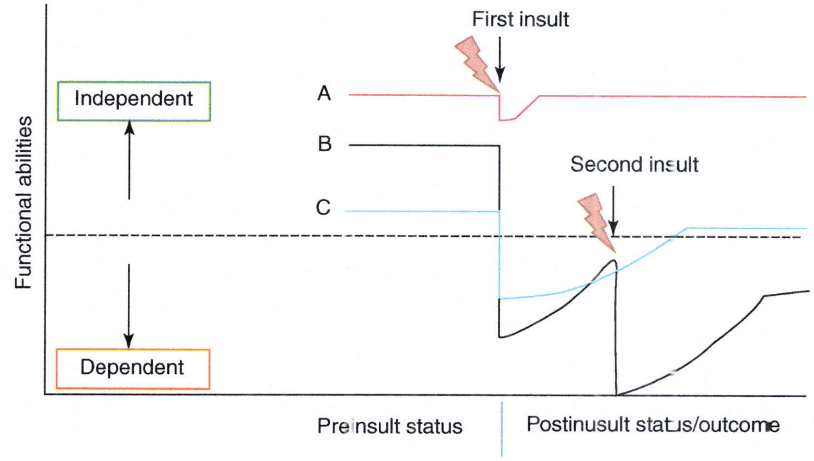

Fig. 2.1 Role of frailty on outcomes after a physiological insult. Patients may differ in physiological reserve and preinsult living status. Pathway A depicts independent living and a minor response to an insult (such as urinary tract infection or mild appendicitis) from which the patient recovers quickly to preinsult status and the same physiological reserve. In pathway B, the degree of independence is reduced and the insult (e.g., surgery for strangulated small bowel, or perforated peptic ulcer with abdominal sepsis) is more severe leading to dependence; if a second insult follows (such as postoperative pneumonia, cardiac event, or anastomotic leak) the chance of returning to the same preoperative level of function is decreased, and in the very frail may result in death. In pathway C, the return to independent existence is possible after an uneventful recovery (e.g., from emergency surgery for colonic cancer), with no effect on long-term independence [28]

ated increases occurred in wound infection, wound occurrence, any infection, any occurrence, and mortality [33].

A recent study, published in 2020, from Murphy et al. retrospectively analyzed a large cohort of elderly patients undergoing EGS procedures; preoperative mFI was determined for each patient and was used to determine the association with perioperative morbidity, mortality, and discharge destination. A total of 57,173 patients were enrolled and results were stratified according to type of operation performed. In this cohort, the most common operation of highly frail patients was colon resection (37%), compared with appendectomy (56%) in low/not frail patients. Among them, 25% of patients experienced any perioperative complication, and 22.2% experienced a serious complication with an overall 30-day mortality of 5.1%. Highly frail patients had a 30-day mortality of 19.0% across all kind of surgeries.

A stepwise relationship between severity of frailty and poor outcomes in patients undergoing the most common EGS operations has been clearly shown: frail patients were more likely to die and experience complications when controlling for multiple factors, including age. This relationship was present even in relatively straightforward and traditionally less morbid operations such as appendectomy and cholecystectomy. Authors hypothesized that this is due to the choice to pursue operations that are perceived by surgeons to be better tolerated compared with more invasive procedures such as colectomy. This study also showed that intermediate and high mFI were also inversely associated with discharge to home for each operation [34]. This fact is important not only for patient consent and managing expectations but also for health resource planning for patients undergoing EGS.

Taken together, these studies provided evidence that the use of frailty measurements may be superior to chronologic age in predicting outcomes and may provide added insight to postoperative hospital course in older patients who undergo EGS. Future studies are needed to prospectively evaluate objective measures of frailty to better inform patients and their families regarding risks, particularly nonoperative versus operative management.

2.3.2 Assessment of Frailty in EGS

As shown by literature analysis, predicting the risk of surgery for elderly patients can be very challenging, since age traditionally has demonstrated to be an imperfect indicator of patient's ability to tolerate an operation. Attempts have been made to create a risk stratification tool to estimate mortality specifically for elderly surgical patients, but many have not been validated externally and consequently have not been widely adopted. Due to the discrepant findings deriving from the use of different "Frailty Indexes", it is also evident that more research is needed to determine which frailty instrument is best suited for risk stratification in EGS [34, 35].

The five indicators of frailty defined as Fried index (weight loss, self-reported exhaustion, low energy expenditure, slow gait speed, and weak grip strength) may be measured easily in an elective setting. Application of the Fried index in the EGS setting has limitations because acute illness may preclude the ability to assess functional and physical performance measures or to perform specific activity questionnaires. Several scores exist to measure frailty in the elective setting, but none has been proven to be truly reliable in acute care surgical settings [36].

Attempts to adapt existing frailty indexes to elective and emergent surgical settings have produced a modified frailty index (mFI), which does not include a functional assessment and is, therefore, much suitable to be applied in EGS [37]. Several papers in literature showed that increasing mFI is associated with worse outcomes in patients undergoing elective operations, while the diagnostic accuracy of screening instruments for frailty in EGS is largely unknown [31].

In the United States, using the American College of Surgeons National Surgical Quality Improvement Program (NSQIP) database, a modified frailty index (mFI) was developed for patients over the age of 60 undergoing emergency general surgery and was found to be predictive of postoperative morbidity and mortality and better at predicting mortality than ASA-PS score or increasing age [33].

A retrospective study by Olufajo et al. examined records of patients aged over 70 years who had undergone EGS evaluated as a primary outcome 1-year mortality. Five clinical preoperative variables were found to be risk factors for a higher 1-year mortality. Out of the five, the most important were an acute kidney injury (AKI) preoperatively, ASA class, and a body mass index (BMI) of <18.5. Therefore, a geriatric emergency surgery mortality (GEM) score was created to predict 1-year mortality. The GEM is the first scoring system for emergency general surgery, elderly, and long-term mortality that has been created [35].

Many authors believe that the frailty scale with the most convincing data for use in emergency surgery and acute care is the Clinical Frailty Scale (CFS): this scale allows to simply collect information after clinical encounter with an older person and has been widely taken up as a judgment-based tool to screen for frailty and to broadly stratify degrees of fitness and frailty. In a recent review, focusing on elderly and EGS, CFS has been summarized and paired with Fried index (Table 2.1). Frailty is present if a score of greater than or equal to 4 is assigned. Despite its seemingly subjective appearance, the CFS has high inter-rater reliability and may be determined through simple proxy interview or chart review [38].

In one study, the diagnostic accuracy of six screening instruments for frailty was evaluated. The investigators compared the ability to predict outcome after emergency abdominal surgery. The screening instruments used were all developed

Table 2.1 Description of fried phenotype and clinical frailty scale

Fried phenotype	Clinical frailty scale
Weight loss: >10 lb. unintentionally in prior year	1. *Very fit:* people who are robust, very active, and motivated. These people commonly exercise regularly. They are among the fittest of their age
Grip strength: lowest 20% (by gender and body mass index)	2. *Well*: people who have no active disease symptoms but are less fit than those in category 1. Often, they exercise or are very active occasionally
Exhaustion: self-report	3. *Managing well*: people whose medical problems are well controlled but they are rarely active beyond walking
Slowness: 15-ft walking speed (by gender and height)	4. *Vulnerable*: although not dependent on others for daily help, symptoms often limit activities. A common complaint is being "slowed up" and/or being tired during the day
Low activity: kilocalories per week (men <383, women >270)	5. Mildly frail: these people often have more evident slowing and need help in high-order instrumental activities of daily living. Typically, this impairs shopping and walking outside alone, meal preparation and housework
	6. *Moderately frail*: people need help with all outside activities and with keeping house. Inside, they often have problems with stairs and need help with bathing and might need minimal help with dressing
	7. *Severely frail*: completely dependent for all personal care from whatever cause (physical or cognitive). Even so, they seem stable and not at high risk of dying (within approximately 6 months)
	8. *Very severely frail*: completely dependent, approaching the end of life. Typically, they could not recover from even a minor illness
	9. *Terminally ill*: approaching the end of life. This category applies to people with a life expectancy <6 months, who are not evidently frail
Frailty present if ≥3 characteristics present	*Frailty present if category ≥4*

Image from Aucoin S and McIsaac DI. Emergency general surgery in older adults: a review. Anesthesiology Clin.2019; 37:493–505 [38]

for elective surgery, except for the Triage Risk Screening Tool, which was developed for medical patients in the emergency room. The ability of these screening tools to predict postoperative morbidity and mortality varied, with sensitivity for mortality ranging from 52 to 85%. Among them, the Vulnerable Elderly Survey (VES-13) appeared to be the most accurate; nonetheless, four of the six screening tests independently predicted postoperative mortality [39].

Another study used scoring systems developed for intensive care medicine and elective surgery and analyzed whether they could predict mortality in the frail elderly patient needing emergency surgery. The scoring systems varied in terms of sensitivity and estimated mortality, but the Acute Physiology and Chronic Health Evaluation (APACHE) II system had a sensitivity of 96% in estimating postoperative mortality [40].

In conclusion, multiple scores have been assessed that might predict poor outcome after EGS. Many risk scores attempt to be too generic, and others are too disease specific. Thus, they either fail to take into account the complexity of the disease or fail to achieve good predictive values across variable populations. Indeed, further research is needed to help guide patient care and potentially improve outcomes.

2.4 Care Plan from Admission to Discharge

In caring for the elderly patient who needs emergency surgery, there are a number of considerations to implement in the decision-making process. Although the choice of treatment may not always be as straightforward as for younger, fitter patients, it is recommended to establish treatment goals early and in some cases the aim should be to preserve quality of life avoiding unnecessary and nonbeneficial treatment. Additional surgery and aggressive life-prolonging care, can in some cases, do more harm than good, and so tailoring the procedure by using a different risk–benefit ratio is necessary.

Last, but not least, it is absolutely necessary to include the patient, caregivers, and next of kin in the discussion to avoid unnecessary or futile treatments, and to prevent prolonged suffering and unnecessary procedures at the end of life [41]. Several reports about different emergency conditions support a tailored approach, even if in some situation it could result in controversial. For example, in acute cholecystitis, urgent cholecystectomy may still be the preferred choice even in elderly patients, if considered fit for surgery; however, percutaneous drainage may be just as efficient in relieving symptoms and might represent a definite treatment [42].

2.4.1 Clinical Assessment and Preoperative Optimization

Between emergent surgical conditions, acute abdomen remains a clinical challenge in the elderly patient. To distinguish which patients need surgery from nonsurgical abdominal illnesses can be difficult. Early diagnosis is essential, as delayed treatment can significantly worsen outcome, as demonstrated for perforated peptic ulcer and major bleedings.

Emergency surgery may often be performed as a lifesaving procedure, and delay to surgery can reduce overall outcome. It has been reported, in geriatric trauma patients, that outcomes might be more favorable if patients receive aggressive care during the initial phase of treatment [43].

In this phase, the utility of frailty assessment should extend beyond its role in preoperative risk stratification. In fact, the positive identification of degree of frailty in an elderly surgical patient could lead to implementation of interventions that may reduce morbidity and enhance functional recovery after surgery [9].

In addition to acute exacerbations of common comorbidities, such as heart failure or obstructive lung disease, many EGS patients have, or are at risk of, sepsis. Multivariable risk prediction models validated for EGS populations should be taken into account and consolidated guidelines (e.g., The 2018 Surviving Sepsis Campaign) should be considered to improve sepsis management, such as blood cultures, serum lactate measurement, and broad-spectrum antibiotic therapy [38]. Therefore, any patient optimization should be balanced against the risk of delaying urgent and necessary surgery. Nevertheless, in emergency setting, opportunities for preoperative optimization may be limited.

Since elderly patients poorly tolerate hypovolemia, it is wise to early treat shock and hypoperfusion, taking into account that some of these patients have reduced cardiovascular reserve and could suffer from occult heart failure. A goal-directed fluid therapy, proper monitoring of urinary output, and early use of vasopressors might be recommended to maintain a mean arterial pressure of 65 mm Hg or higher and at the same time to ensure renal perfusion and prevent renal failure. Elderly patients also have a higher prevalence of reduced pulmonary function; they may be at risk of pneumonia because of a reduced immune system and also have a higher risk of aspiration, either from an obstructed gastrointestinal tract or from cerebrovascular or neurological disease. Early measures should include ensuring a patent airway and relieving gastric contents by means of a nasogastric tube [38, 43].

2.4.2 Minimally Invasive Techniques in EGS in Elderly

The risk–benefit balance between traditional open surgery and minimally invasive techniques should be considered

individually after considering patient's frailty assessment and the range of therapeutic options available.

As an example, mortality from a bleeding peptic ulcer has decreased considerably with the advent of endoscopic and interventional radiologist options, whereas surgery for a bleeding ulcer in elderly, frail, and shocked patient carried a very high risk of death in the past [44].

Nowadays it is well accepted that laparoscopic surgery reduces surgical stress and improves recovery and there are now growing evidences that minimally invasive approach is safe in older surgical patients, as reported in a recent systematic review including subanalysis on over 70-years-old group of patients, leading to reduced postoperative pain, and subsequent reduction in postoperative complications such as pneumonia or venous thromboembolism, and reduced length of hospital stay [45]. Laparoscopic surgery is increasingly being considered also in the emergency setting, including for cholecystectomy, appendicectomy, perforated duodenal ulcers, washout and drain for diverticulitis, and abdominal exploration in suspected bowel ischemic disease [46].

Clearly the choice of this approach will depend on the experience of the emergency surgeon. However, it is likely that, as minimally invasive surgery continues to develop and further technological advances are made, older adults will be one of the main beneficiaries.

2.5 Outcomes After EGS in Elderly

2.5.1 Acute Postoperative Monitoring

After EGS procedures, observational evidence suggests that discharging elderly patients direct to the ward is associated with higher mortality than admission to the intensive care unit (ICU). In frail EGS patients, the relative impact of frailty on mortality was most pronounced for procedures with low baseline rates of ICU admission, such as acute appendectomies and cholecystectomies [27]. Therefore, clinicians should carefully consider the benefits of intensive monitored setting in vulnerable and acutely ill older EGS patients after surgery as suggested by guidelines, such as those provided by the American Geriatrics Society/American College of Surgeons [47].

2.5.2 Cognitive Impairment

Cognitive impairment is the decline in intellectual function and can be acute onset (delirium), chronic (dementia), or acute presentation on a chronic condition. Postoperative delirium is common but underdiagnosed in elderly surgical patients and delays rehabilitation. It occurs in 7–13% of patients after elective surgery, and up to 20% after EGS [48]. Delirium is characterized by disturbances of consciousness, disorientation, and perception abnormalities, alongside impaired thinking and speech that typically settles after several days. Unsurprisingly, several studies reported that development of delirium is not only associated with adverse postoperative outcomes such as significantly longer hospital stay and higher in-hospital mortality (compared to patients not showing cognitive impairment) but also functional decline, increased need of social support, and prolonged cognitive impairment even 1 year after surgery, which suggests that delirium may itself be a cause of dementia [48, 49].

The American Geriatrics Society recently suggested guidelines to improve prevention and treatment of delirium. Eight recommendations supported by strong evidence have been made, including the use of CGA/frailty assessment, early mobilization and walking, avoiding restraints, adequate nutrition, avoiding opioids for postoperative pain control, and optimal use of fluids and oxygen [50].

2.5.3 Loss of Independence and Recurrent Hospitalization

Elderly patients who undergo EGS may survive the initial treatment, but often suffer from long-term complications leading to higher frequency of rehospitalization after discharge from surgery [30].

Berian and colleagues reported that almost 80% of older people after EGS suffer a loss of independence, defined as a decrease in ability to perform daily living activities, need for a new mobility aid, or increase in care needs. This condition leads to at least 12–15% of elderly surgical patients discharged directly to a nursing home instead of returning to their homes [51].

In addition, patients with any grade of frailty experience higher frequency of recurrent hospitalization (four to six time more than not frail patients) in both elective and emergent surgical settings; this can be a devastating experience for both the patient and the family. Therefore, in discussions of preoperative risk with frail patients and their families, anesthesiologist and surgeons should highlight outcomes such as discharge disposition and possible loss of independence [52].

Five Things You Should know About the Burden of EGS in the Elderly Today

- Emergency surgery on elderly population represents a considerable workload in most health–care systems.
- EGS procedures lead to significant increase in morbidity and mortality rate in elderly and fragile patients.
- Identification of higher-risk patients through frailty assessment is essential to improve outcomes.
- The role of multidisciplinary approach is mandatory for complex evaluations and decision-making process.
- EGS in the geriatric patient needs a tailored approach to improve outcomes and avoid futile care. Overall evidences are still limited and further studies on the topic are needed.

References

1. Gale SC, Shafi S, Dombrovskiy VY, et al. The public health burden of emergency general surgery in the United States: a 10-year analysis of the Nationwide Inpatient Sample – 2001 to 2010. J Trauma Acute Care Surg. 2015;77:202–8.
2. Aggarrwal G, Pedel CJ, Quiney N. Emergency general surgery in older patients: where are we now? Curr Anesthesiol Rep. 2019;9:387–94.
3. Shah AA, Haider AH, Zogg CK, et al. National estimates of predictors of outcomes for emergency general surgery. J Trauma Acute Care Surg. 2015;78:482–90.
4. Scott JW, Olufajo OA, Brat GA, et al. Use of national burden to define operative emergency general surgery. JAMA Surg. 2016;151:e160480.
5. Ageing well: a global priority. Lancet. 2012;379(9823):1274.
6. Colby SL, Ortman JM. Projections of the size and composition of the US population: 2014 to 2060. Current population reports. Washington, DC: U.S. Census Bureau; 2015. p. 25e1143.

7. Kwok AC, Semel ME, Lipsitz SR, et al. The intensity and variation of surgical care at the end of life: a retrospective cohort study. Lancet. 2011;378:1408–13.
8. Revenig LM, Canter DJ, Taylor MD. Too frail for surgery? Initial results of a large multidisciplinary prospective study examining preoperative variables predictive of poor surgical outcomes. J Am Coll Surg. 2013;217:665–70.
9. Sandini M, Pinotti E, Persico I, et al. Systematic review and meta-analysis of frailty as a predictor of morbidity and mortality after major abdominal surgery: frailty metrics in major abdominal surgery. BJS Open. 2017;1:128–37.
10. Sheetz KH, Waits SA, Krell RW. Improving mortality following emergency surgery in older patients requires focus on complication rescue. Ann Surg. 2013;258:614–7.
11. Ingraham AM, Cohen ME, Raval MV, et al. Variation in quality of care after emergency general surgery procedures in the elderly. J Am Coll Surg. 2011;212:1039–48.
12. Shah AA, Haider AH, Riviello R, et al. Geriatric emergency general surgery: survival and outcomes in a low-middle income country. Surgery. 2015;158:562–9.
13. Wohlgemut JM, Ramsay G, Jansen JO. The changing face of emergency general surgery: a 20-year analysis of secular trends in demographics, diagnoses, operations and outcomes. Ann Surg. 2020;271(3):581–9.
14. Pofahl Deiner S, Westlake B, et al. Patterns of surgical care and complications in elderly adults. J Am Geriatr Soc. 2014;62:829–35.
15. Andersson RE. Short and long-term mortality after appendectomy in Sweden 1987 to 2006. Influence of appendectomy diagnosis, sex, age, co-morbidity, surgical method, hospital volume, and time period. A national population-based cohort study. World J Surg. 2013;37:974–81.
16. Vilches-Moraga A, Fox J. Geriatricians and the older emergency general surgical patient: proactive assessment and patient centred interventions. Salford-POPGS. Aging Clin Exp Res. 2018;30(3):277–82.
17. McGillicuddy EA, Schuster KM, Davis KA, et al. Factors predicting morbidity and mortality in emergency colorectal procedures in elderly patients. Arch Surg. 2009;144:1157–62.
18. Cooper Z, Scott JW, Rosenthal RA, et al. Emergency major abdominal surgical procedures in older adults: a systematic review of mortality and functional outcomes. J Am Geriatr Soc. 2015;63:2563–71.
19. Kuy S, Sosa JA, Roman SA, et al. Age matters: a study of clinical and economic outcomes following cholecystectomy in elderly Americans. Am J Surg. 2011;201:789–96.
20. Tran BK, Espolio Desbaillet Y, Groebli Y, et al. Abdominal pain among elderly patients in the emergency department. Rev Med Suisse. 2012;8:1548–52.
21. Reginelli A, Russo A, Pinto A, et al. The role of computed tomography in the preoperative assessment of gastrointestinal causes of acute abdomen in elderly patients. Int J Surg. 2014;12(Suppl 2):S181–6.
22. Lin HS, Watts JN, Peel NM, et al. Frailty and postoperative outcomes in older surgical patients: a systematic review. BMC Geriatr. 2016;16:157.
23. Cooper Z, Courtwright A, Karlage A, et al. Pitfalls in communication that lead to nonbeneficial emergency surgery in elderly patients with serious illness: description of the problem and elements of a solution. Ann Surg. 2014;260:949–57.
24. Cooper Z, Lilley EJ, Bollens-Lund E, et al. High burden of palliative care needs of older adults during emergency major abdominal surgery. J Am Geriatr Soc. 2018;66:2072–8.
25. Ellis G, Whitehead MA, O'Neill D, et al. Comprehensive geriatric assessment for older adults admitted to hospital. Cochrane Database Syst Rev. 2011;(7):CD006211.
26. Jay S, Whittaker P, Mcintosh J, et al. Can consultant geriatrician led comprehensive geriatric assessment in the emergency department reduce hospital admission rates? A systematic review. Age Ageing. 2017;46:366–72.
27. Eamer G, Saravana-Bawan B, van der Westhuizen B, et al. Economic evaluations of comprehensive geriatric assessment in surgical patients: a systematic review. J Surg Res. 2017;210:9–17.
28. Desserud KF, Veen T, Soreide K. Emergency general surgery in the geriatric patient. Br J Surg. 2016;103:e52–61.
29. Beggs T, Sepehri A, Szwajcer A, et al. Frailty and perioperative outcomes: a narrative review. Can J Anaesth. 2015;62:143–57.
30. McIsaac D, Moloo H, Bryson G, et al. The association of frailty with outcomes and resource use after emergency general surgery: a population-based cohort study. Anesth Analg. 2017;124:1653–61.
31. Parmar KL, Law J, Carter B, et al. Frailty in older patients undergoing emergency laparotomy. Ann Surg. 2021;273(4):709–18. https://doi.org/10.1097/SLA.0000000000003402.
32. Ward MAR, Alenazi A, Delisle M, et al. The impact of frailty on acute care general surgery patients. J Trauma Acute Care Surg. 2019;86:148–54.
33. Farhat JS, Velanovich V, Falvo AJ, et al. Are the frail destined to fail? Frailty index as predictor of surgical morbidity and mortality in the elderly. J Trauma Acute Care Surg. 2012;72:1526–30.
34. Murphy PB, Savage SA, Zarzaur BL, et al. Impact of patient frailty on morbidity and mortality after common emergency general surgery operations. J Surg Res. 2020;247:95–102
35. Olufajo OA, Reznor G, Lipsitz SR, et al. Preoperative assessment of surgical risk: creation of a scoring tool to estimate 1-year mortality after emergency abdominal surgery in the elderly patient. Am J Surg. 2017;213:771–7.
36. Fried LP, Tangen CM, Walston J, et al. Frailty in older adults: evidence for a phenotype. J Gerontol A Biol Sci Med Sci. 2001;56:146–57.

37. Rockwood K, Song X, MacKnight C, et al. A global clinical measure of fitness and frailty in elderly people. CMAJ. 2005;173:489–95.
38. Aucoin S, McIsaac DI, et al. Emergency general surgery in older adults: a review. Anesthesiol Clin. 2019;37:493–505.
39. Kenig J, Zychiewicz B, Olszewska U, et al. Six screening instruments for frailty in older patients qualified for emergency abdominal surgery. Arch Gerontol Geriatr. 2015;61:437–42.
40. Ozban M, Birsen O, Senel M. The analysis of scoring systems predicting mortality in geriatric emergency abdominal surgery. Ulus Travma Acil Cerrahi Derg. 2015;21:182–6.
41. Smith AK, Williams BA, Lo B. Discussing overall prognosis with the very elderly. N Engl J Med. 2011;365:2149–51.
42. Ni Q, Chen D, Xu R, et al. The efficacy of percutaneous transhepatic gallbladder drainage on acute cholecystitis in high-risk elderly patients based on the Tokyo guidelines: a retrospective case–control study. Medicine (Baltimore). 2015;94:e1442.
43. Jacobs DG, Plaisier BR, Barie PS, et al. Practice management guidelines for geriatric trauma: the EAST practice management guidelines work group. J Trauma. 2003;54:391–416.
44. Lu Y, Loffroy R, Lau JY, et al. Multidisciplinary management strategies for acute non-variceal upper gastrointestinal bleeding. Br J Surg. 2014;101:e34–50.
45. Moug SJ, McCarthy K, Coode-Bate J. Laparoscopic versus open surgery for colorectal cancer in the older person: a systematic review. Ann Med Surg (Lond). 2015;4:311–8.
46. Coccolini F, Trana C, Sartelli M, et al. Laparoscopic management of intraabdominal infections: systematic review of the literature. World J Gastrointest Surg. 2015;7:160–9.
47. Mohanty S, Rosenthal RA, Russell MM, et al. Optimal perioperative management of the geriatric patient: a best practices guideline from the American College of Surgeons NSQIP and the American Geriatrics Society. J Am Coll Surg. 2016;222:930–47.
48. Ansaloni L, Catena F, Chattat R, et al. Risk factors and incidence of postoperative delirium in elderly patients after elective and emergency surgery. Br J Surg. 2010;97:273–80.
49. Zaal IJ, Devlin JW, Peelen LM, et al. A systematic review of risk factors for delirium in the ICU. Crit Care Med. 2015;43:40–7.
50. American Geriatrics Society Expert Panel on Postoperative Delirium in Older Adults. American Geriatrics Society abstracted clinical practice guideline for postoperative delirium in older adults. J Am Geriatr Soc. 2015;63:142–50.
51. Berian J, Mohanty S, Ko CY, et al. Association of loss of independence with readmission and death after discharge in older patients after surgical procedures. JAMA Surg. 2016;151(9):e161689.
52. Robinson TN, Wu DS, Stiegmann GV, et al. Frailty predicts increased hospital and six-month healthcare cost following colorectal surgery in older adults. Am J Surg. 2011;202:511–4.

3 A Worldwide Overview of Emergency Laparoscopic Procedure in the Elderly

Giancarlo D'Ambrosio, Andrea Picchetto, Stefania La Rocca, Francesca De Laurentis, Laura Rossi, and Antonio Crucitti

3.1 Introduction

Since its rise in the 1980s′, laparoscopic surgery became the gold standard approach in the majority of abdominal elective procedures with improvement in oncologic and quality-of-life outcomes [1].

Despite its acknowledged advantages, laparoscopic procedures for emergency surgery are still considered too challenging and, therefore, not widely employed. Nielsen (2017) in a retrospective, multicentric study on 1139 emergency procedures reported a rate of 27% of laparoscopically completed operation, with a 63% rating of conversion to open surgery [2].

Agresta and colleagues (2017) reported in an Italian studies an increasing rate of abdominal emergency approached by laparoscopy during 4 years (24.74% in 2010 vs. 30.27% in 2014) [3].

Data from the UK National Emergency Laparotomy Audit (NELA) showed that in major general surgery emergencies, laparoscopy was employed in 13% of cases and completed in 7% [4].

In 2018, Pucher retrieved data, over a 30-month period, on 248 consecutive cases who underwent emergency surgery. In this studies, laparoscopic approach increased from 20 to 37% over the study period [5].

This low performance rate of laparoscopic procedures in the emergency setting sometimes could be related to intraoperative difficulties like peritonitis, abscess, or adhesions. Sometimes, instead, in low-volume centers, it can be difficult to plan a laparoscopic approach in emergency, especially in the night, because of logistic difficulties.

The worldwide share of people over 65 years is estimated to rise from 703 million in 2013 to over 1.5 billion in 2050. Furthermore, Italian people over 65 years represents 20% of total population and hospital costs are about 40%. (a) Currently, more than half of the operations in the USA are performed on 65 years and older patients. (b) Postoperative morbidity and mortality progressively increase with the age and emergency surgery is one of the most important factor related to these outcomes in elderly patients [6]. Watt reported in elderly patients who underwent emergency laparotomy a 30-day mortality of 22% and morbidity of 58%. Mortality risk in emergency laparotomies is up to eight times higher when compared with elective surgery [7]. Cocorullo and colleagues (2016) reported their

G. D'Ambrosio (✉) · A. Picchetto · S. La Rocca
F. De Laurentis · L. Rossi
General and Colorectal Surgery Division, Department of Cardiothoracic, Vascular Surgery and Organ Transplantation, Policlinico Umberto I University Hospital, Sapienza University of Rome, Rome, Italy
e-mail: giancarlo.dambrosio@uniroma1.it

A. Crucitti
General and Mininvasive Surgery, Ospedale Cristo Re, Rome, Italy

F. Agresta et al. (eds.), *Emergency laparoscopic surgery in the elderly and frail patient*,
https://doi.org/10.1007/978-3-030-79990-8_3

studies on 159 elderly patients who underwent emergency surgery. Laparoscopic approach was performed in 75 patients and open in 64 patients with a mortality rate of 0–7.7% versus 0–12.5%, respectively, related to the disease. Morbidity ranged between 0 and 12.9% in laparoscopic group and 0 and 19.4% in open group [8].

In a studies of Bàllesta López (2002) on 232 patients with a median age of 76 years who underwent various elective and emergency laparoscopic procedures, the overall morbidity and mortality rates were 10.8% and 3.4%, respectively [9].

The definition of elderly patients is still not clear in literature. Several criteria have been adopted to define "elderly patients" such as age, performance status, biological age, comorbidity, etc. According to Pisano, elderly patients can be defined as patients of an age older than 65 years. [10]

Frailty syndrome is a clinically recognizable increased vulnerability resulting from the age-associated accumulation of deficits [11].

As of today the definition of "frailty" is not clearly defined and there are no standardized criteria to correlate age and frailty.

The use of a specific frailty index (FI) can represent an evolving concept to establish the surgical risk in elderly patients.

Joseph (2016) employed the Rockwood FI in a prospective observational study of 220 consecutive elderly patients over 65 years who underwent emergency general surgery. In hospitals, complications in frail and nonfrail patients were 49% versus 27%, respectively. Moreover, frail patients have significantly longer hospital and ICU lengths of stay and higher mortality rate [11].

A lot of scoring systems were carried out in order to predict postoperative mortality (Vulnerable Elderly Survey, Charlson Age Comorbidity Index [CACI], and Charlson Co-Morbidity Index [CCI]), but none is universally adopted. The elderly patients may tolerate an operation, but they may not tolerate any subsequent complication. Thus, a planned risk-benefit balance evaluation should be considered individually.

Agresta and colleagues, published in 2020, the results of the FRAILSEL Italian multicenter prospective cohort study conducted on 1993 patients aged >65 years who underwent emergency abdominal surgery. Of these patients, 68.7% underwent open surgery (OS), whereas 31.3% underwent laparoscopic surgery (LS). The overall morbidity rate was 32.6% (36.2% OS vs. 22.1% LS, $p < 0.001$) and mortality rate 8.8% (11.2% OS vs. 2.2% LS, $p < 0.001$) [12].

In an Italian multicentric prospective cohort study conducted in elderly patients who underwent emergency abdominal surgery, the rate of surgical indications was as follows: cholecystectomy (71%), appendectomy (51.8%), perforated gastroduodenal ulcer repair (18.9%), adhesiolysis with or without small bowel resection (12.2%), large bowel resection (10.7%), and other procedures (20%) [12].

Here, we present a worldwide overview of data of the literature concerning the more frequent emergency surgical procedures performed in elderly patients.

3.2 Acute Calculous Cholecystitis (ACC)

In patients with gallstones, the incidence of ACC varies from 10 to 20%, and about 36% of cholecystectomies are performed for this reason.

In 90% of acute cholecystitis, the cause is cholelithiasis, remaining 10% is usually due to a wide range of conditions such as trauma, virus, recent surgery, multisystem organ failure, parenteral nutrition, AIDS, or ischemia. Laparoscopic cholecystectomy (LC) is nowadays the recommended surgical option to treat acute cholecystitis (AC). Available data show that early LC is superior to late or delayed LC in terms of outcome and cost. In literature, the optimal time to perform an early LC is 48–72 h [13].

Gutt in 2013 performed a randomized trial on 618 patients and showed that the LC performed within 24 h is safe [14].

Zafar in a retrospective review of prospective collected data conducted on 95.523 patients operated for AC concluded that "LC performed within

2 days yielded the best outcomes and lower costs." [15] Özkardeş (2014) in a prospective, randomized study conducted on 60 patients showed that early LC should be preferred in terms of hospital stay and low costs [16].

Since the rate of patients with gallstones increases with the age, it is reasonable to hypothesize a higher rate over 65 years and, thus, a higher rate of acute cholecystitis in the elderly.

While in young patients, early cholecystectomy is generally accepted as the standard treatment of acute cholecystitis, in elderly patients the better treatment remains controversial. Loozen (2017) performed a systematic review and meta-analysis of the literature regarding early cholecystectomy for AC in the elderly population. A total of 592 patients were selected, and cholecystectomy was performed laparoscopically in 316 patients (53%) while open in 276 patients (47%). Perioperative mortality ranged from 0 to 5% and perioperative complications from 4 to 31%. The rate of mortality and morbidity for emergency cholecystectomy for AC in nonelderly patients reported in previous studies are <1% and 15%, respectively [17].

The Tokyo guidelines have a guiding role in the diagnosis and treatment of acute cholecystitis, but a separate analysis was not performed for elderly patients [18].

In 2016, the World Society of Emergency Surgery (WSES) developed guidelines on ACC, but in only one statement the relationship between old age and surgery was analyzed [19]. Then, in 2019, the WSES and Italian Surgical Society for Elderly People (ESICG) published guidelines on ACC in the elderly population, which reported that no homogeneous criteria about the surgical approach of ACC in elderly are reported in the literature [10]. Some studies suggest that LC is feasible for the treatment of high-risk AC [19], while other studies suggested that percutaneous cholecystostomy (PC) plus delayed laparoscopic cholecystectomy could achieve better results [20, 21].

In elderly or critically ill patients, mortality rate of LC is very high (14–30%) [22, 23]. PC can be an alternative option in patients unfit for surgery due to their severe comorbidities [24].

CHOCOLATE study is a multicenter randomized trial performed to assess whether laparoscopic cholecystectomy is superior to percutaneous catheter drainage in elderly high-risk patients with AC. Acute cholecystitis was defined according to the Tokyo guidelines and the risk was based on the APACHE II score ≥7). This study showed that laparoscopic cholecystectomy is superior to percutaneous catheter drainage in terms of morbidity (12% and 65%, respectively), hospitalization (5 days and 9 days, respectively), and cost. Percutaneous drainage is still an appropriate treatment in patients with a strong contraindication to surgery, either as a bridge to surgery or as definitive treatment [25].

3.3 Acute Appendicitis

The incidence of acute appendicitis decreases with the age, settling in the elderly patients on a rate of 5–10%. Unfortunately, in these patients, the rate of complicated appendicitis (perforation and abscess) is very high (from 18 to 70%), and mortality is around 8% compared to 0–1% in younger patients [26].

The nonoperative management has been proposed in selected patients with uncomplicated appendicitis at imaging, who wish to avoid surgery, and who accept the risk of recurrence. No randomized study is reported in literature about the advantages of laparoscopic appendectomy (LApp) versus open appendectomy (OApp) in elderly patients. In 2013 Moazzez et al. reported that 75% of operation performed in USA on elderly patients with acute appendectomies were laparoscopic [27].

In a retrospective analysis on 257,484 patients, Ward (2014) reported better outcomes in laparoscopic group. Similar results were reported by Yehv (2012), Southgate (2012), and Wu (2017) [28–31].

2016 WSES Jerusalem guidelines for diagnosis and treatment of acute appendicitis do not contain any specific evaluation related to elderly patients. Just one statement reports: "laparoscopic offers clear advantages and should be preferred in obese patients, older patients and patients with comorbidity." [32] This recommendation is confirmed in the 2020 update of the WSES Jerusalem guidelines [33].

In 2019, the "SIFIPAC/WSES/SICG/SIMEU guidelines for diagnosis and treatment of acute appendicitis in the elderly" were published and are currently the only guidelines available in the literature. In the statement of these guidelines, the authors reported that in elderly patients with acute appendicitis, laparoscopic appendectomy reduces LOS, morbidity, and costs [26].

3.4 Colorectal Cancer (CRC)

More than 70% of CRCs are detected in elderly patients, and this number is expected to increase in the future. Approximately 30–40% of CRC patients present as an emergency. In elderly patients, a colonic resection is a high-risk procedure with a morbidity and mortality rate of 11–35% and 9–22%, respectively. The main indications to emergency surgery are large bowel obstruction (almost 80%) and perforation (approximately 20%). [34, 35]

The emergency setting usually precludes a preoperative multidisciplinary oncological discussion. Even in colorectal emergency surgery, frailty rather than chronological age is the most important risk factor for postoperative morbidity and mortality. Some studies conducted in older patients undergoing emergency abdominal surgery reported that sarcopenia is an independent factor associated with worse results [36].

Perforation seems to increase the risk of peritoneal carcinosis, but other studies do not support these data [37].

In elderly patients, postoperative complications seem to play a crucial role in survival. Weerink (2018) reported that among octogenarians postoperative complications (Clavien-Dindo grades 3 and 4) is the most predictive parameter for 5-year survival, according to the tumor stage [38]. In 16,847 cases reported by Lee (2019), about 75% of all emergency colorectal cancer surgery was performed with an open approach. Laparoscopic approach was feasible in about 20% of the emergency group compared to 43% in the elective group [39].

In a retrospective study by Costa (2019) on 123 patients, the rate of laparoscopic procedures was 12% in the elderly group [35].

An English study showed that, in the emergency setting of CRC, laparoscopic approach passed from 15% in 2010 to 30% in 2016 [39].

Laparoscopic approach for the colectomy is more feasible after decompression, which can be performed by endoscopic stenting or proximal stoma.

Data from literature showed better outcomes after colonic stenting as a bridge to surgery compared to emergency surgery (ESGE 2020, ESCO study, and CREST study) [40–42]. The success rate of colonic stent procedure is about 80–90% in high-volume centers.

3.5 Acute Left-Side Colonic Diverticulitis (ALCD)

Diverticulosis is a common illness after 40 years of age, affecting 5–10% of people in the fifth decade, 30% in the sixth, and 60% in the eighth decade of life. These patients have about 4% lifetime risk of developing acute left-side colonic diverticulitis, and 8–35% presented with perforated disease with abscess or peritonitis. The Hinchey classification is the most commonly used classification in international literature. In 2016, a CT-guided classification was proposed by WSES acute diverticulitis working group [43].

Up to 25% of patients hospitalized for ALCD may require urgent operation. In recent years, laparoscopic lavage and drainage have been proposed as an alternative to sigmoidectomy in patients with purulent peritonitis. The DILALA trial in 2014 [44], LADIES and SCANDIV trials in 2015 [45, 46], and the WSES 2020 update [47] failed to show a superiority of laparoscopic lavage versus colonic resection.

In patients with generalized peritonitis, Hartmann resection is still the procedure of choice. In a study of the American College of Surgeons on 1314 patients who underwent emergency surgery, Hartmann's procedure was performed in three-fourths of cases [48]. In a 2015 Australian study, Hartmann's procedure was the most common surgical procedure (72%), as in a Canadian study of 2014 (44%) [49, 50].

Laparoscopic sigmoidectomy with or without ileostomy is a feasible approach and can become the future gold standard in high-volume center with skilled colorectal surgeons.

In the literature, the prospective, randomized, clinical trials comparing primary anastomosis (PA) versus Hartmann's procedure (HP) [51–54], the WSES 2020 update [47] and a systematic review held by Halim in 2019 [55] suggested the safety of PA in patients with severe diverticular peritonitis (Hinchey III–IV), and provided additional evidences in favor of PA with a diverting stoma over HP.

The main limitation of these studies is the patients' recruitment due to insurmountable difficulties to draw up a study in emergency operation for a life-threatening condition.

A retrospective cohort study, published in 2019 Goldstone, reported data of 10,780 patients who underwent emergency colectomy for diverticulitis. Ninety-eight percent received HP and only 1.7% received PA with proximal diversion. Colorectal surgeons performed 6% of all operations. Postoperative mortality was 1.4 times greater among noncolorectal surgeons than among colorectal surgeons (7.5% vs. 5.3%) [56].

In 1999, EAES published the results of consensus conference on acute diverticulitis [57]. In 2019, the results of SAGES and EAES Diverticulitis Consensus Conference revision held during the SAGES 2018 and EAES congress 2018 were published. In SAGES/EAES guidelines, the modified Hinchey classification was utilized [58]. A wide consensus was achieved regarding these surgical issues:

Q 5.1: Patients with perforated diverticulitis with diffuse peritonitis (Hinchey III and IV) should undergone emergent surgical intervention.

Q 5.2: Laparoscopic sigmoid resection with or without stoma in the emergency setting has been shown to decrease overall complications compared to open resection.

Q 5.3: Hartmann's procedure is the preferred operation for hemodynamically unstable patients with perforated diverticulitis.

In a paper published on August 2019, Wexner underlined that "the most dramatic difference between 1999 and 2019 statements on diverticulitis, is the recommended role of minimally invasive approach. The difference between the documents attest to the ubiquitous acceptance of the advantages of laparoscopy realized during 20 years interval between publications." [59]

3.6 Small Bowel Obstruction

About 15% of patients who undergone a laparotomy will develop adhesions that lead to small bowel obstruction (SBO), which represents about 4% of all emergency admissions and 20 to 30% of them are managed with surgical intervention.

Laparoscopic Lysis of Adhesions (LLOA) for SBO was firstly reported by Clotteau in 1990 and Best in 1991 [60]. Since then, a lot of studies have reported the safety and low complications rate of LLOA in comparison to laparotomic adhesiolysis.

In Italian Consensus Conference Guidelines (2012), the authors recommended to perform an explorative laparoscopy in order to select the patients who can be benefited from a LLOA [61]. In a studies of Behman (2017), just 7.8% of patients had a laparoscopic procedure, but the annual rate increased over the study period from 4.3% in 2005 to 14.2% in 2014 [62]. In a retrospective study conducted by Pei (2016), the proportion of laparoscopic cases increased from 17.2% in 2006 to 28.7% in 2013 [63].

Several large population studies comparing laparoscopy and open surgery for SBO have reported a quicker recovery, a lower rate of mortality, and serious complications with laparoscopy [64–66].

Conversion to open during surgery for SBO is relatively common occurrence in about 30% of cases. Bowel resection and iatrogenic bowel injury account for one third of conversion. Conversion should not be considered a failure, but rather a good surgical judgment. In elderly patients, nonoperative management of SBO is particularly appealing, but the success rate ranges from 43 to 76%. In patients who underwent surgery, delayed approach for up to 5 days has been associated with increased mortality and morbidity.

To our knowledge, no prospective randomized trial in the elderly has been reported in the literature in order to compare advantages of laparoscopic approach to SBO. Despite the lack of prospective trial data, the steady increase in laparoscopic procedures could suggest the safety of this approach and the surgeons may consider the benefits of LLOA in their practice.

3.7 Perforated Peptic Ulcer

Peptic ulcer disease affects six million Americans every year. Across all ages, 2–14% of peptic ulcers result in perforation. Mortality ranges from 6 to 14%, but in elderly patients, it reaches the 41%. Morbidity is high, with rates ranging from 17 to 63% [67].

In 1989, Mouret performed the first laparoscopic PPU repair [68] and, in 2002, Lagoo proposed that laparoscopy should be routinely considered [69]. In 2016, Tan et al. published a meta-analysis of RCTs comparing laparoscopic versus open repair for PPU [70]. Five RCTs were included (549 patients), reporting a similar rate of laparoscopic repair (50.8%) versus open repair (49.2%). The results showed that laparoscopic repair had similar rates of overall postoperative complication, mortality, and reoperation to open repair. No significant differences were found in rates of leakage, abscess, ileus, and pneumonia. However, laparoscopic repair had lower surgical site infection, postoperative pain, and shorter nasogastric tube duration [70].

The LAMA trial enrolled 101 patients: 49 open approach and 52 laparoscopic procedures. The results showed that laparoscopic correction of PPU is safe, feasible, and causes less postoperative pain [71].

In 2010, Bertleff et al. published a review of the literature conducted on 56 papers [72]. These results support the 2006 EAES's statement that laparoscopy should be advocated as diagnostic and therapeutic tool [13]. No specific trials were conducted in the elderly patients, but a review of the literature reported that older ages and comorbidities are main risk factors. The authors stated that "surgeons that decide to apply laparoscopy must make a judicious cost-benefit assessment."[73]

Five Things You Should Know About

1. Laparoscopic approach in emergency is feasible in elderly patients and should not be denied based on age alone.
2. Postoperative complications are the main factor engraving on mortality; therefore, monitoring in postanesthesia intensive care unit is mandatory. A wide experience in laparoscopy is necessary to perform emergency surgery with good results.
3. Conversion must not be considered a failure in emergency laparoscopic surgery.
4. A specific risk stratification system (especially frailty detection) is necessary to help surgeons to tailor treatment.
5. Already in 1907, SMITH stated very eloquently that "because the patients are old, we must not consider that it is time for them to die. We must endeavour to prolong life and prolong it in comfort."

References

1. D'Ambrosio G, Picchetto A, Campo S, et al. Quality of life in patients with loco-regional rectal cancer after ELRR by TEM versus VLS TME after nChRT: long-term results. Surg Endosc. 2019;33(3):941–8.
2. Nielsen LBJ, Tengberg LT, Bay-Nielsen M. Laparoscopy in major abdominal emergency surgery seems to be a safe procedure. Dan Med J. 2017;64(5):A5370.
3. Agresta F, Campanile FC, Podda M, et al. Current status of laparoscopy for acute abdomen in Italy: a critical appraisal of 2012 clinical guidelines from two consecutive nationwide surveys with analysis of 271,323 cases over 5 years. Surg Endosc. 2017;31(4):1785–95.

4. Team NP. The second patient report of the National Emergency Laparotomy Audit. London: Royal College of Anaesthetists; 2016.
5. Pucher PH, Carter NC, Knight BC, Toh S, Tucker V, Mercer SJ. Impact of laparoscopic approach in emergency major abdominal surgery: single-centre analysis of 748 consecutive cases. Ann R Coll Surg Engl. 2018;100(4):279–84.
6. Turrentine FE, Wang H, Simpson VB, Jones RS. Surgical risk factors, morbidity, and mortality in elderly patients. J Am Coll Surg. 2006;203(6):865–77.
7. Watt DG, Wilson MS, Shapter OC, Patil P. 30-day and 1-year mortality in emergency general surgery laparotomies: an area of concern and need for improvement? Eur J Trauma Emerg Surg. 2015;41(4):369–74.
8. Cocorullo G, Falco N, Tutino R, et al. Open versus laparoscopic approach in the treatment of abdominal emergencies in elderly population. G Chir. 2016;37(3):108–12.
9. Bàllesta López C, Cid JA, Poves I, Bettónica C, Villegas L, Memon MA. Laparoscopic surgery in the elderly patient. Surg Endosc. 2003;17(2):333–7.
10. Pisano M, Ceresoli M, Cimbanassi S, et al. 2017 WSES and SICG guidelines on acute calcolous cholecystitis in elderly population. World J Emerg Surg. 2019;14:10.
11. Joseph B, Zangbar B, Pandit V, et al. Emergency general surgery in the elderly: too old or too frail? J Am Coll Surg. 2016;222(5):805–13.
12. Costa G, Fransvea P, Podda M, et al. The use of emergency laparoscopy for acute abdomen in the elderly: the FRAILESEL Italian Multicenter Prospective Cohort Study. Updat Surg. 2020;72(2):513–25.
13. Agresta F, Ansaloni L, Baiocchi GL, et al. Laparoscopic approach to acute abdomen from the Consensus Development Conference of the Società Italiana di Chirurgia Endoscopica e nuove tecnologie (SICE), Associazione Chirurghi Ospedalieri Italiani (ACOI), Società Italiana di Chirurgia (SIC), Società Italiana di Chirurgia d'Urgenza e del Trauma (SICUT), Società Italiana di Chirurgia nell'Ospedalità Privata (SICOP), and the European Association for Endoscopic Surgery (EAES). Surg Endosc. 2012;26(8):2134–64.
14. Gutt CN, Encke J, Köninger J, et al. Acute cholecystitis: early versus delayed cholecystectomy, a multicenter randomized trial (ACDC study, NCT00447304). Ann Surg. 2013;258(3):385–93.
15. Zafar SN, Obirieze A, Adesibikan B, Cornwell EE, Fullum TM, Tran DD. Optimal time for early laparoscopic cholecystectomy for acute cholecystitis. JAMA Surg. 2015;150(2):129–36.
16. Ozkardeş AB, Tokaç M, Dumlu EG, et al. Early versus delayed laparoscopic cholecystectomy for acute cholecystitis: a prospective, randomized study. Int Surg. 2014;99(1):56–61.
17. Loozen CS, van Ramshorst B, van Santvoort HC, Boerma D. Early cholecystectomy for acute cholecystitis in the elderly population: a systematic review and meta-analysis. Dig Surg. 2017;34(5):371–9.
18. Okamoto K, Suzuki K, Takada T, et al. Tokyo guidelines 2018: flowchart for the management of acute cholecystitis. J Hepatobiliary Pancreat Sci. 2018;25(1):55–72.
19. Ansaloni L, Pisano M, Coccolini F, et al. 2016 WSES guidelines on acute calculous cholecystitis. World J Emerg Surg. 2016;11:25.
20. Welschbillig-Meunier K, Pessaux P, Lebigot J, et al. Percutaneous cholecystostomy for high-risk patients with acute cholecystitis. Surg Endosc. 2005;19(9):1256–9.
21. Lin D, Wu S, Fan Y, Ke C. Comparison of laparoscopic cholecystectomy and delayed laparoscopic cholecystectomy in aged acute calculous cholecystitis: a cohort study. Surg Endosc. 2020;34(7):2994–3001.
22. Houghton PW, Jenkinson LR, Donaldson LA. Cholecystectomy in the elderly: a prospective study. Br J Surg. 1985;72(3):220–2.
23. Frazee RC, Nagorney DM, Mucha Jr P. Acute acalculous cholecystitis. Mayo Clinic Proceedings. 1989.
24. Søreide JA, Fjetland A, Desserud KF, Greve OJ, Fjetland L. Percutaneous cholecystostomy—an option in selected patients with acute cholecystitis. Medicine (Baltimore). 2020;99(19):e20101.
25. Loozen CS, van Santvoort HC, van Duijvendijk P, et al. Laparoscopic cholecystectomy versus percutaneous catheter drainage for acute cholecystitis in high risk patients (CHOCOLATE): multicentre randomised clinical trial. BMJ. 2018;363:k3965.
26. Fugazzola P, Ceresoli M, Agnoletti V, et al. The SIFIPAC/WSES/SICG/SIMEU guidelines for diagnosis and treatment of acute appendicitis in the elderly (2019 edition). World J Emerg Surg. 2020;15(1):19.
27. Moazzez A, Mason RJ, Katkhouda N. Thirty-day outcomes of laparoscopic versus open appendectomy in elderly using ACS/NSQIP database. Surg Endosc. 2013;27(4):1061–71.
28. Ward NT, Ramamoorthy SL, Chang DC, Parsons JK. Laparoscopic appendectomy is safer than open appendectomy in an elderly population. JSLS. 2014;18(3):e2014.00322.
29. Yeh CC, Wu SC, Liao CC, Su LT, Hsieh CH, Li TC. Laparoscopic appendectomy for acute appendicitis is more favorable for patients with comorbidities, the elderly, and those with complicated appendicitis: a nationwide population-based study. Surg Endosc. 2011;25(9):2932–42.
30. Southgate E, Vousden N, Karthikesalingam A, Markar SR, Black S, Zaidi A. Laparoscopic vs open appendectomy in older patients. Arch Surg. 2012;147(6):557–62.
31. Wu TC, Lu Q, Huang ZY, Liang XH. Efficacy of emergency laparoscopic appendectomy in treating complicated appendicitis for elderly patients. Saudi Med J. 2017;38(11):1108–12.
32. Di Saverio S, Birindelli A, Kelly MD, et al. WSES Jerusalem guidelines for diagnosis and treatment of acute appendicitis. World J Emerg Surg. 2016;11:34.
33. Di Saverio S, Podda M, De Simone B, et al. Diagnosis and treatment of acute appendicitis: 2020 update of

the WSES Jerusalem guidelines. World J Emerg Surg. 2020;15(1):27.

34. Pisano M, Zorcolo L, Merli C, et al. 2017 WSES guidelines on colon and rectal cancer emergencies: obstruction and perforation. World J Emerg Surg. 2018;13:36.
35. Costa G, Frezza B, Fransvea P, et al. Clinico-pathological features of colon cancer patients undergoing emergency surgery: a comparison between elderly and non-elderly patients. Open Med (Wars). 2019;14:726–34.
36. Zattoni D, Christoforidis D. How best to palliate and treat emergency conditions in geriatric patients with colorectal cancer. Eur J Surg Oncol. 2020;46(3):369–78.
37. Honoré C, Goéré D, Souadka A, Dumont F, Elias D. Definition of patients presenting a high risk of developing peritoneal carcinomatosis after curative surgery for colorectal cancer: a systematic review. Ann Surg Oncol. 2013;20(1):183–92.
38. Menegozzo CAM, Teixeira-Júnior F, Couto-Netto SDD, Martins-Júnior O, Bernini CO, Utiyama EM. Outcomes of elderly patients undergoing emergency surgery for complicated colorectal cancer: a retrospective cohort study. Clinics (Sao Paulo). 2019;74:e1074.
39. Lee CHA, Kong JCH, Heriot AG, Warrier S, Zalcberg J, Sitzler P. Short-term outcome of emergency colorectal cancer surgery: results from Bi-National Colorectal Cancer Audit. Int J Color Dis. 2019;34(1):63–9.
40. van Hooft JE, Veld JV, Arnold D, et al. Self-expandable metal stents for obstructing colonic and extracolonic cancer: European Society of Gastrointestinal Endoscopy (ESGE) guideline—update 2020. Endoscopy. 2020;52(5):389–407.
41. Arezzo A, Balague C, Targarona E, et al. Colonic stenting as a bridge to surgery versus emergency surgery for malignant colonic obstruction: results of a multicentre randomised controlled trial (ESCO trial). Surg Endosc. 2017;31(8):3297–305.
42. Hill J, Kay C, Morton D, Magill L, Handley K, RG G, CREST Trial Collaborative Group. CREST: Randomised phase III study of stenting as a bridge to surgery in obstructing colorectal cancer—Results of the UK ColoRectal Endoscopic Stenting Trial (CREST). J Clin Oncol. 2016;34.
43. Sartelli M, Catena F, Ansaloni L, et al. WSES guidelines for the management of acute left sided colonic diverticulitis in the emergency setting. World J Emerg Surg. 2016;11:37.
44. Thornell A, Angenete E, Gonzales E, et al. Treatment of acute diverticulitis laparoscopic lavage vs. resection (DILALA): study protocol for a randomised controlled trial. Trials. 2011;12:186.
45. Schultz JK, Yaqub S, Wallon C, et al. Laparoscopic lavage vs primary resection for acute perforated diverticulitis: the SCANDIV randomized clinical trial. JAMA. 2015;314(13):1364–75.
46. Vennix S, Musters GD, Mulder IM, et al. Laparoscopic peritoneal lavage or sigmoidectomy for perforated diverticulitis with purulent peritonitis: a multicentre, parallel-group, randomised, open-label trial. Lancet. 2015;386(10000):1269–77.
47. Sartelli M, Weber DG, Kluger Y, et al. 2020 update of the WSES guidelines for the management of acute colonic diverticulitis in the emergency setting. World J Emerg Surg. 2020;15(1):32.
48. Tadlock MD, Karamanos E, Skiada D, et al. Emergency surgery for acute diverticulitis: which operation? A National Surgical Quality Improvement Program study. J Trauma Acute Care Surg. 2013;74(6):1385–91; quiz 1610
49. Hong MK, Tomlin AM, Hayes IP, Skandarajah AR. Operative intervention rates for acute diverticulitis: a multicentre state-wide study. ANZ J Surg. 2015;85(10):734–8.
50. Li D, Baxter NN, McLeod RS, Moineddin R, Wilton AS, Nathens AB. Evolving practice patterns in the management of acute colonic diverticulitis: a population-based analysis. Dis Colon Rectum. 2014;57(12):1397–405.
51. Binda GA, Karas JR, Serventi A, et al. Primary anastomosis vs nonrestorative resection for perforated diverticulitis with peritonitis: a prematurely terminated randomized controlled trial. Color Dis. 2012;14(11):1403–10.
52. Oberkofler CE, Rickenbacher A, Raptis DA, et al. A multicenter randomized clinical trial of primary anastomosis or Hartmann's procedure for perforated left colonic diverticulitis with purulent or fecal peritonitis. Ann Surg. 2012;256(5):819–26; discussion 826–817
53. Bridoux V, Regimbeau JM, Ouaissi M, et al. Hartmann's procedure or primary anastomosis for generalized peritonitis due to perforated diverticulitis: a prospective multicenter randomized trial (DIVERTI). J Am Coll Surg. 2017;225(6):798–805.
54. Lambrichts DPV, Vennix S, Musters GD, et al. Hartmann's procedure versus sigmoidectomy with primary anastomosis for perforated diverticulitis with purulent or faecal peritonitis (LADIES): a multicentre, parallel-group, randomised, open-label, superiority trial. Lancet Gastroenterol Hepatol. 2019;4(8):599–610.
55. Halim H, Askari A, Nunn R, Hollingshead J. Primary resection anastomosis versus Hartmann's procedure in Hinchey III and IV diverticulitis. World J Emerg Surg. 2019;14:32.
56. Goldstone RN, Cauley CE, Chang DC, Kunitake H, Ricciardi R, Bordeianou L. The effect of surgical training and operative approach on outcomes in acute diverticulitis: should guidelines be revised? Dis Colon Rectum. 2019;62(1):71–8.
57. Köhler L, Sauerland S, Neugebauer E. Diagnosis and treatment of diverticular disease: results of a consensus development conference. The scientific Committee of the European Association for Endoscopic Surgery. Surg Endosc. 1999;13(4):430–6.
58. Francis NK, Sylla P, Abou-Khalil M, et al. EAES and SAGES 2018 consensus conference on acute diverticulitis management: evidence-based rec-

ommendations for clinical practice. Surg Endosc. 2019;33(9):2726–41.
59. Wexner SD, Talamini MA. EAES/SAGES consensus conference on acute diverticulitis: a paradigm shift in the management of acute diverticulitis. Surg Endosc. 2019;33(9):2724–5.
60. Clotteau JE, Premont M. [Occlusion by adhesions treated by celioscopic section]. Presse Med. 1990;19(25):1196.
61. Vettoretto N, Carrara A, Corradi A, et al. Laparoscopic adhesiolysis: consensus conference guidelines. Color Dis. 2012;14(5):e208–15.
62. Behman R, Nathens AB, Byrne JP, Mason S, Look Hong N, Karanicolas PJ. Laparoscopic surgery for adhesive small bowel obstruction is associated with a higher risk of bowel injury: a population-based analysis of 8584 patients. Ann Surg. 2017;266(3):489–98.
63. Pei KY, Asuzu D, Davis KA. Will laparoscopic lysis of adhesions become the standard of care? Evaluating trends and outcomes in laparoscopic management of small-bowel obstruction using the American College of Surgeons National Surgical Quality Improvement Project Database. Surg Endosc. 2017;31(5):2180–6.
64. Li MZ, Lian L, Xiao LB, Wu WH, He YL, Song XM. Laparoscopic versus open adhesiolysis in patients with adhesive small bowel obstruction: a systematic review and meta-analysis. Am J Surg. 2012;204(5):779–86.
65. O'Connor DB, Winter DC. The role of laparoscopy in the management of acute small-bowel obstruction: a review of over 2,000 cases. Surg Endosc. 2012;26(1):12–7.
66. Krielen P, Di Saverio S, Ten Broek R, et al. Laparoscopic versus open approach for adhesive small bowel obstruction, a systematic review and meta-analysis of short term outcomes. J Trauma Acute Care Surg. 2020;88(6):866–74.
67. Di Saverio S, Bassi M, Smerieri N, et al. Diagnosis and treatment of perforated or bleeding peptic ulcers: 2013 WSES position paper. World J Emerg Surg. 2014;9:45.
68. Mouret P, François Y, Vignal J, Barth X, Lombard-Platet R. Laparoscopic treatment of perforated peptic ulcer. Br J Surg. 1990;77(9):1006.
69. Lagoo S, McMahon RL, Kakihara M, Pappas TN, Eubanks S. The sixth decision regarding perforated duodenal ulcer. JSLS. 2002;6(4):359–68.
70. Tan S, Wu G, Zhuang Q, et al. Laparoscopic versus open repair for perforated peptic ulcer: a meta analysis of randomized controlled trials. Int J Surg. 2016;33(Pt A):124–32
71. Bertleff MJ, Halm JA, Bemelman WA, et al. Randomized clinical trial of laparoscopic versus open repair of the perforated peptic ulcer: the LAMA trial. World J Surg. 2009;33(7):1368–73.
72. Bertleff MJ, Lange JF. Laparoscopic correction of perforated peptic ulcer: first choice? A review of literature. Surg Endosc. 2010;24(6):1231–9

Appendix

Etzioni DA, Liu JH, Maggard MA, Ko CY. The aging population and its impact on the surgery workforce. Ann Surg. 2003;238:170–7.
ISTAT. Stime per l'anno 2016. 2017. http://www4.istat.it/it/anziani. Accessed 1 Apr 2019.
National Institute on Aging (NIA). 2018. https://www.nia.nih.gov. Accessed 22 May 2019.

4 The Economic Burden of Emergency Abdominal Surgery in the Elderly: What Is the Role of Laparoscopy?

Emidia Vagnoni

4.1 Introduction

In Western countries, an increasing life expectancy can be observed; in 2018, an EU resident who had survived to the age of 65 could expect to live, on average, a further 20 years. The highest levels of life expectancy at this age were recorded in a band of regions running from northern Spain through much of western and southern France and into northern and central parts of Italy [1]. In 2018, the life expectancy of a female newborn in the EU-27 was 83.7 years, which was 5.5 years higher than the corresponding figure for a newborn male (78.2 years). Female life expectancy was higher than male life expectancy in every region for which data are available. The same trend is observed when considering that the OECD health data referred to a broad group of Western countries [1]. According to the World Health Organization, people over 60 accounted for around 12% of world population in 2015, which was expected to increase to 22% in 2050. However, morbidity and mortality increase with the age.

In Italy, the life expectancy of a male newborn was 80.88 years in 2018 and 85.18 for a female (see Table 4.1).

With the current prospects of longevity, a considerable amount of resources will be required to the healthcare systems to deliver quality treatments and fulfill the demand for healthcare. This will result in a considerable burden for the countries, thus for the society.

In Italy, almost 900,000 surgical procedures are related to elderly patients out of about 2,000,000 in a year (2017 data). The same trends could be observed for the emergency surgery confirming Parker et al. [3] according to which approximately half of all emergency surgical procedures are performed in the elderly and the proportion is set to increase in future years as more of the population survive into their 70s. Studies have estimated that approximately 53% of all surgical procedures are performed on patients over the age of 65. Projections estimate that approximately half of the population over the age of 65 will require surgery once in their lives [4], while in Italy the population projections toward 2050 indicate the age-groups ≥65 would reach 34.1% of the entire population [5].

The surgery prevalence data in literature associated to the demographic clearly show how the conditions that require surgery increase as the population is aging. This adds consequences from both the patients' perspective and the society's perspective. More in-depth resources need to be allocated to the treatment of the elderly population considering both the

E. Vagnoni (✉)
Department of Economics and Management, University of Ferrara, Ferrara, Italy
e-mail: emidia.vagnoni@unife.it

F. Agresta et al. (eds.), *Emergency laparoscopic surgery in the elderly and frail patient*,
https://doi.org/10.1007/978-3-030-79990-8_4

Table 4.1 Life expectancy for males and females (Source: Istat data)

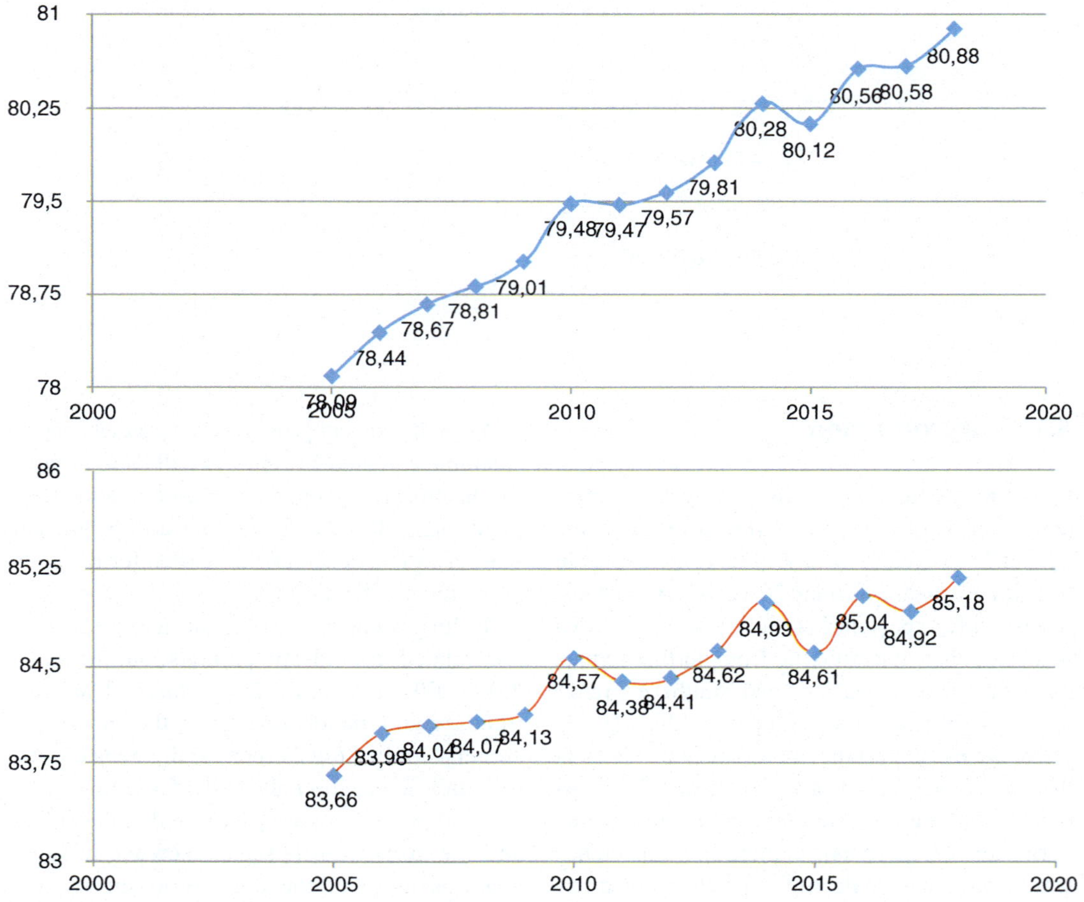

direct costs of surgery and the indirect costs linked to the consequences of surgery. In a time of increasing health care expenditure, there is growing concern pertaining to the financial sustainability of the current health care systems across the countries. According to a recent Organization for Economic Cooperation and Development (OECD) report, health care spending per capita in terms of GDP is increasing on average of 2.7% per year. This data emphasizes the importance of critically evaluating the delivery of both current and future interventions in order to ensure that resource allocation is cost-effective.

4.2 Emergency Surgery in the Elderly Patients

Many authors have addressed the topic of emergency surgery procedure in the elderly patients, and the literature has increased during last two decades. From long time, it has been acknowledged that elderly patients undergoing surgery might have worse outcomes. Depending on the context and on the clinical condition of patients, the poor outcomes can be appreciated in different ways. Ferrarese et al. [6] highlighted how the population aging implies new socio-sanitary problems, and less satisfactory results in terms of morbidity and mortality have been registered in the patients who underwent emergency surgery when compared with elective surgery; less satisfactory results were found also in terms of length of hospital stay and rehabilitation. Torrance et al. [7] focused on the increased risk of peri- or post-operative death, development of postoperative complications, and prolonged LOS.

An analysis of last decade literature on emergency surgery in the elderly, conducted on CINAHL, PubMed, and Medline databases, clearly confirms the need to adopt a dedicated strategy to emergency surgery in that vulnerable group of patients (Table 4.2). While some studies investigate the impact of age on surgery and post-operative results [9, 13], some others focus on the prediction of the outcomes. To this regard, the literature recognizes a key role of risk scoring [11, 13, 16] and of the timeliness of the surgery [14]. A stream of literature has addressed what organization and process the emergency surgery should follow when an elderly patient is considered; Andrew et al. [8] advocate the need to adopt

Table 4.2 Synthesis of the literature about emergency surgery in the elderly

Andrew et al. [8]	UK	Evidence has shown that there are specific strategies that hospitals and teams can develop to improve the care received by this vulnerable group. A paradigm shift is needed and change should be driven by expert MDTs that should include emergency physicians, geriatricians, anesthetists, critical care specialists, specialist nurses, therapists, and dieticians
Dowgiałło-Wnukiewicz et al. [9]	Poland	Huge impact of age on postoperative results
Søreide and Desserud [10]	Norway	Need for an ad hoc organization of emergency surgery to improve outcomes in the elderly
Anna et al. [11]	UK	Need to use risk scoring (P-POSSUM) in over 70 patients undergoing emergency laparotomy to predict outcomes
Campagna et al. [12]	Italy	Quick diagnosis and elective surgery as desirable to avoid those complications that occur in emergency surgery
Fukuda et al. [13]	Japan	Use of POSSUM disease scoring system to predict mortality in the elderly who undergo emergency abdominal surgery
Zeineb et al. [14]	Tunisia	In the elderly, the delay of surgery =24 h, the laparotomy procedure, and ICU stay are independent predictors of mortality
Maciej et al. [15]	Poland	Due to the existing additional disease in the elderly, the frailty syndrome, any surgical intervention should be minimally invasive. The discussion about therapy should be conducted by a team of specialists from a variety of medical fields
Shaheed et al. [16]	Canada	This study illustrates the importance of preventing an in-hospital complication in the elderly. ASA class is a robust tool that is predictive of mortality in the very elderly population and can be used to guide patient and family counseling in the emergency setting
Hwee et al. [17]	Singapore	The frailty assessment among elderly patients undergoing emergency abdominal surgery is a predictor for loss of functional independence at 1 year. Early recognition of this at-risk group could help with discharge planning and priority
McCann [18]	Ireland	This study provides important information to support a better process of informed consent for patients undergoing emergency abdominal surgery and help to improve the planning for a system of care that better meets the needs of older patients who present with an intra-abdominal emergency
Nishida [19]	Japan	Early cholecystectomy for patients with AC over 85 years of age was performed safely, and elderly patients with dementia had similar postoperative outcomes as compared with patients without dementia
Alessia et al. [20]	Italy	Laparoscopic cholecystectomy results to be safe and effective treatment for cholelitiasis and acute cholecystitis in ordinary and emergency setting, also in the elderly
Ferrarese et al. [6]	Italy	Laparoscopic cholecystectomy in our elderly patients represents a safe procedure to treat all cases of acute cholecystitis in an emergency setting
McComb et al. [21]	Canada	A pilot reconditioning program results show promise in helping offset declines in physical function in elderly patients following emergency abdominal surgery

a new paradigm to treat the elderly, focusing on a multidisciplinary team that would be able to better develop a treating pathway for the vulnerable patient. Aligned to the need to adopt a dedicated organization of emergency surgery is [10] in order to improve the outcome in the elderly patients.

The role of frailty has been widely recognized as a key pattern to consider when elderly undergoes emergency surgery. More recent studies [15, 17] recalled the need to adopt mini-invasive surgery procedures to avoid the loss of functional independence. Aligned with this, the laparoscopic procedure has been recognized as safe to treat some cases in the elderly [19, 6] and more specifically even over 80 patients. The literature is progressively evolving from considering aspects linked to the surgery process to a more broad approach to the elderly patients; thus, the physical function, the independence, and the planning of an approach to care that better meet the needs of the vulnerable have attracted the attention of further studies.

It clearly emerges how the emergency surgery in the elderly might bring to a variety of consequences in terms of loss of physical conditions, reduced level of autonomy and mobility, and cognitive abilities. Even if those consequences are not expressly addressed by the above-mentioned studies, they are highlighted among those conditions that need to be avoided adopting a different approach to the emergency surgery.

4.3 The Economic Burden

Although mortality and overall duration of hospital stay for these conditions has decreased overtime, the burden of emergency general surgery conditions remains substantial and continues to increase because of our aging population, with increasing numbers of comorbidities [22]. Ladhani et al. [23] studied a group of cases with diagnosis codes for acute appendicitis, acute cholecystitis, intestinal obstruction, incarcerated hernia, perforated viscus, and intestinal ischemia undergoing emergency surgery in a university trauma center in the USA. The median hospital duration of stay was 3.6 days and the median total charge was about 35.000 $, although the mean age of the studied population did not exceed 51.2. The study did not provide an analysis of costs by patients' age as the purpose was to compare surgeries approach. When elderly patients undergo abdominal emergency surgery, a variety of consequences can occur bringing to the need to deploy different activities both during the surgery and hospitalization and after discharge.

This would determine a variety of direct and indirect costs that could be observed, based on the components, on a short term and on a long term. As from economic discipline, direct costs usually represent the costs associated with medical resource utilization, which include the consumption of in-patient, out-patient, and pharmaceutical services within the health care delivery system. The term *indirect costs* has come to be defined as the expenses incurred from the cessation or reduction of work productivity as a result of the morbidity and mortality associated with a given disease. Indirect costs typically consist of work loss, worker replacement, and reduced productivity from illness and disease. These losses are typically valued from either societal, individual, or employer perspectives.

When addressing the economic evaluation of healthcare interventions, the direct costs are usually considered. This seems to be popular in most of the countries having a government funded healthcare system or even based on health insurance mechanisms; in these contexts, it is key to gather knowledge about the direct costs of healthcare treatments, procedures, services, to assess the ability of the funders to sustain or support the healthcare. The perspective of the payer or funder assumes great relevance at both the country level and the service providers' level. The recent budget constraint that many countries have experienced in the healthcare sector has emphasized the need to enhance the knowledge about how the scarce resources are allocated within the healthcare system. Considering the indirect costs would require to bridge a broader view; it might be the patient perspective or even the society's one. In this case, the cost components considered broaden to a greater context than the healthcare one. Thus, the loss of productivity of the patient or of his/her caregiver, the transport costs, the cost of products which are not covered by the healthcare system of the health insurance (such as supplements, to mention some) become key component of the overall cost of the disease. Undertaking costing studies which focus on the indirect cost needs the participation of the patient/caregiver to gather data and provide an estimation of the indirect costs. Therefore, most of the studies in literature rely on the direct costs only.

However, in Western countries, governments have deployed different models of welfare to protect people against the risks related to unemployment, parental responsibilities, healthcare, housing, old age, and social exclusion. Thus, governments provide fund to support the welfare regime. In this context, developing knowledge and awareness about the indirect costs incidence in the healthcare sector, and more in depth in the emergency surgery, becomes a key feature for both policy makers and service providers' top manager.

Treatment costs for emergency abdominal surgery in the elderly are determined by indirect and direct costs. The payer is responsible for the majority of the direct costs, such as the hospital charges. Indirect costs include patient workday losses, family workday losses, and caregiver costs to mention some of the components. Society absorbs the combination of these costs. In a value-based healthcare economy, cost of services should be supported by a concurrent benefit in clinical outcome.

Studies in the field of health economics [24] provide also a third component to consider when addressing the economic burden of an illness or a treatment that is the indirect psychological cost [25], sometime referred as the intangible costs. The intangible costs cannot be directly measured in monetary form. Intangible effects, such as pain, joy, or physical limitations, are often assessed using the patient's biopsychosocial quality of life after the major health event [26]; quality of life in this context includes physical health as well as social contacts and emotional health.

Most evaluations have a narrower perspective and focus on the relevant costs for the payer, but as argued by literature, all costs and benefits of interventions should be considered, no matter on whom they fall [27]. From long time, health economics studies have recognized how a broad perspective to address the economic evaluation of health interventions that considers the costs and the benefits for the different stakeholders is informative and contributes to a more effective decision-making.

4.4 Common Postsurgery Consequences for Elderly

Frailty is defined as a state of decline and vulnerability, characterized by weakness and a decrease in physiological reserve [28]; as a consequence, frail patients are unable to recover as quickly from a stressful event such as an illness or surgery. This has been found to be common in the elderly and it is thought to be due to an age-related decline in multiple organ systems [29]. Furthermore, the ability of elderly to recover after surgery is also linked to chronic diseases [30].

Considering the special conditions that make elderly a vulnerable category of patients, literature has demonstrated that frailty is associated with a significantly increased odds of postoperative mortality (OR 1.33–46.33) and morbidity (OR 1.24–3.36) [31]. Based on Khan et al. [32], those patients who fall in the category of frail also spend a longer time (median of 2.5 days longer) in hospital compared with fit patients, increasing healthcare costs and resource consumption. Frail patients have decreased physiological reserves and consequently, they are unable to recover as quickly from surgery. Thus, frailty is a risk factor of increased morbidity and mortality that is also associated with a longer time to discharge.

Fairchild et al. [33] identified the frailty risk factors associated to a group of 252 patients aged

65 years or older accessing a trauma center in USA (Table 4.3).

Adopting a broad definition of frailty, Fuertes-Guirò et al. [34] evaluated a group of patients (aged 65 or older, mean age 78.6), selected for emergency abdominal surgery, during the preoperative period considering four groups of predictors of the outcomes: physical, cognitive, functional, and social ones. Among the main risks factors studied by the authors: the nutritional status, the TLC values, the skeletal muscle mass, the cognitive status, the physical/functional status, and the social support (Table 4.4).

Based on the literature, the level of frailty of an elderly person provides valuable information for risk/benefit decision-making concerning the patient in situations in which there is little time to act, such as in the emergency surgery.

Fuertes-Guirò et al. [34] confirmed previous studies [35] about preoperative frailty in patients being linked with increased postoperative morbidity, thus with an increased consumption of resources and a considerable stressor to their psychological condition that may end out to further exacerbate their level of vulnerability [36].

Table 4.3 Frailty risk factors (adapted from [33])

Frailty risk factors	
Age	BMI
Sex	Activity of daily living (ADL)
Race	Hematocrit
Sarcopenia	Living situation
Altered cognition/ cognitive impairment (depression, delirium, disorientation unspecified, developmental delay ...)	Hospital complications (wound infection, urinary tract infection, pneumonia, bowel obstruction, skin breakdown...)
Weakness	Injury severity score
Charlson comorbidity index	

Table 4.4 Predictors of emergency abdominal surgery (Source: Fuertes-Guirò et al. [34])

Predictors of outcomes	
Physical factors	**Cognitive factors**
Nutritional status	Cognitive status (assessed based on the Pfeffer test)
TLC	
Skeletal muscular mass	
Functional status	**Social factors**
Level of dependency (Barthel index)	Level of social support (Duke UNC test)

Table 4.5 Consequences and morbidities associated to postoperative abdominal surgery in the elderly

Studies	Postoperative consequences and morbidity
Yingke et al. [37]	Longer length of hospital stay
Fuertes-Guirò et al. [34]	Access to ICU; loss of skeletal muscle mass; moderate and severe functional deficit; higher level of dependency; lower social support; higher mortality rate
Han et al. [38]	Postoperative complications in hospital [odds ratio: 16.59, 95% CI: 4.56–60.40, $P < 0.001$]
O'Neill et al. [39]	Delirium, sepsis, pro-longed hospital stay, postoperative re-admission
Lin et al. [40]	Mortality, complications, prolonged length of stay, functional decline and lower quality of life after surgery

Considering the recent (last 5 years) literature about abdominal surgery, elderly, and morbidities, researchers have addressed a variety of consequences from elderly undergoing emergency abdominal surgery (Table 4.5).

The above consequences of surgery in the elderly are associated to an increase of resources consumption within the services providers, but they determine further resources use from the relatives' and caregivers' perspective and from a social perspective, too. To this regard, a relevant impact of emergency abdominal surgery would require to take into account both the direct costs and the indirect and intangible ones.

4.5 The Surgery Procedure Innovation

Emergency surgery has become a major part of the day-to-day activities in most public hospitals [41, 42]. Organization and delivery of adequate emergency surgical services is challenged by financial constraints and fragmentation of surgical expertise to organ-, disease-, or procedure-specific subspecialties. Emergency surgery is an essential part of surgical services and cannot be neglected by health policy decision makers or put on a side by the demands of elective surgery.

Lee et al. [43] clearly state how the use of laparoscopic approach has spread to a variety of intervention since the first surgery was performed. As argued by Navez and Navez [44], laparoscopy has begun to be preferred for abdominal surgical emergencies in selected cases. In elective surgeries, the laparoscopic approach has rapidly spread to a variety of procedure and it has allowed at appreciating some benefits including reduced morbidity, postoperative pain, hospital length of stay (LOS), and time to resuming normal activities, likely also apply to appropriately selected emergency cases. Data provided by Eurostat with related to the European countries provides evidence of how the laparoscopic approach has progressively increased in a range of abdominal surgery procedures (Table 4.6).

Among the top 10 procedures, considering the cholecystectomy and the appendicectomy, all the countries show a very high rate of laparoscopic procedures. Generally, the benefits of laparoscopic are well appreciated as it allows a reduction of the resources consumption. The above-mentioned benefits might apply even to emergency surgery [45]. Based on Siletz et al. [46], patients undergoing open procedures, or laparoscopic procedures that were converted to open, were significantly less healthy and older than those who underwent laparoscopic procedures. Nevertheless, laparoscopic approach to emergency abdominal surgery is more and more used as literature reports benefits in a variety of settings [44, 47, 48]. Overall, laparoscopic surgery has allowed at identifying benefits in emergency abdominal interventions: postoperative pain, shorter LOS, less morbidity, shorter operative times than laparotomy procedure [49]. The effectiveness of the laparoscopic approach for the treatment of the colorrectal cancer in the very elderly is also stated by Roscio et al. (2016). The study conducted by Costa et al. [50] on a large Italian population of elderly undergoing emergency abdominal surgery demonstrated that emergency operations for acute abdomen in the elderly are mainly performed through open surgery, preventing these patients from the benefits of laparoscopic procedures. Considering these, laparoscopy can also be more cost-effective as concluded by Keller et al. [51].

However, literature is sometimes controversial. Ukkonen et al. [52] studied 430 patients whose mean age was 75.4, and beyond the innovation in surgery procedure, it was found that for elderly undergoing emergency abdominal surgery, it was still observed a relatively high morbidity and mortality as reported in earlier studies. The author also highlighted the role of the surgeons' skills against elderly as a relevant variable to be considered: "the results of emergency abdominal surgery vary not only between diagnostic groups but also by the surgical technique used. There were many surgeons who were highly experienced and some with less experience of emergency abdominal surgery on the elderly" (p. 2860). Devoto et al. [53] conducted a

Table 4.6 Laparoscopic surgery with regard to some of the top 10 procedures (Eurostat data 2018) per 100,000 inhabitants

	Cholecystectomy	Of which: laparoscopic cholecystectomy	Appendicectomy	Of which: laparoscopic appendectomy
Italy	184.7	162.7	68.0	44.4
The Netherland	159.0	149.4	95.5	78.4
The United Kingdom	135.6	126.1	87.3	69.8
Spain	165.7	144.4	105.4	63.8
France	193.3	178.4	107.5	91.3
Germany	239.9	198.8	149.5	125.3
Sweden	137.7	125.0	127.0	90.5

literature review to investigate the feasibility of laparoscopic colorectal resection in very elderly patients and whether there are benefits over open surgery for colorectal cancer. Considering that the patient's age has been demonstrated as an independent risk factor for mortality separate from comorbidity, across both elective and emergency admissions for open and laparoscopic surgery, advanced age should not be considered a contraindication to the laparoscopic approach. Studies converge on the need to undertake a robust preoperative assessment to provide accurate details to the surgeon to evaluate the risks and to adopt a multidisciplinary approach.

4.6 The Economic Impact of Emergency Abdominal Laparoscopic Surgery on the Elderly Patients

The technological innovation in surgery has clearly brought to benefits in terms of an increased cost-effective allocation of the scarce resources. Given the countries health budgets constraints, the surgeon decisions about the approach to adopt against a procedure have relevant effects in terms of direct costs' components.

Adkins et al. [54] analyzed the variable costs for surgical technique during elective laparoscopic cholecystectomy. The authors focus on operating room time and supply costs as the main cost component on which the surgeon should focus to increase the efficiency assuring the patient's safety. Furthermore, the length of stay deeply contributes to the cost of treatment of the patient.

Nakamura et al. [55] studied 80 patients aged 85 or older who were treated for colorectal cancer and concluded how laparoscopic surgery is associated with a variety of benefits, among them a shorter postoperative length of stay that results in an overall reduced LOS. Furthermore, literature [56] has associated better short-term outcomes in terms of postoperative complication an in-hospital mortality to laparoscopic resection against the open one. Aligned to the above studies is Cui et al. [57] that investigated the costs and clinical-efficacy of laparoscopic surgery against the laparotomy; a reduced postoperative pain, a reduced intraoperative blood loss, and a shorter hospital stay were observed with regard to laparotomy procedures. An improved quality of life and a reduction in the use of resources (a mean of 18.535€ for laparoscopy of over 80 aged patients against 22.832€ for laparotomy for the same group) are reported in the study by Mar et al. [58] with regard at any group of patients (even the elderly) undergoing laparoscopy, when compared to laparotomy, for colon cancer surgery. However, the authors highlight how the outcomes may be negatively affected by the mini invasive procedure in elderly patients. Thus, a clear decision needs to be taken well supported by data about the outcomes predictor factors.

It is not in the aim of this chapter to comprehensively compare the laparoscopic surgery against the laparotomy, as the literature about the topic has clearly shown the benefits associated to the laparoscopy. Table 4.7 synthesizes the different activities that contribute to reduce the economic burden of laparoscopic surgery; the latter provides an impact on a variety of stakeholders: the health provider, the surgeon, the health professionals in the multidisciplinary team to assess the elderly condition, the patient, the caregiver and relatives, and the home-care service, to mention some of them. Thus, a broad perspective to the economic evaluation is needed to include potential costs and benefits for all stakeholders. When undertaking an economic evaluation, the choice of perspective (the healthcare provider, the payer, the patient) is important. Elderly patients are often frail too and a variety of morbidities might develop when going through long hospitalization time; for this reason, the implication of the surgery approach in terms of indirect costs (called even social costs) and intangible costs should be considered.

The main argument for adopting a restrictive perspective is that the budget for the healthcare service is meant to be for improving health, thus

Table 4.7 Activities that contribute to assess the economic burden of emergency abdominal surgery in the elderly

	Direct costs	
Δ− LOS	Δ− cost of hospital staying	
Δ- postoperative complications	Δ− cost of treatment	
Δ+ supplies	Δ+ cost of supplies	
Δ− operation time	Δ− cost of the surgery theatre	
Δ+ unforeseen ICU admission (due to complications)	Δ+ cost of in-hospital staying	
	Cost drivers	**Indirect costs**
Δ− LOS	Δ+ preservation of the skeletal muscle mass Δ+ preservation of the functional deficit Δ− time to recovery	Δ− caregivers' cost (relatives' loss of productivity, for instance) Δ− postdischarge recovery in a social care institutions cost
		Intangible costs
Δ− LOS	Δ+ social support Δ+ quality of life	Δ+ Independence Δ− Stress

remaining with the provider's perspective. But alternatively, shouldn't the full social benefits of healthcare interventions be considered? In countries supporting strong welfare policies, funded by the general taxation (such as Italy, the UK, France), the healthcare organization should aim to provide benefits to families and carers as well as the patient.

The literature considered about emergency abdominal surgery in the elderly has reported both a high rate of complications and a relevant mortality rate. Therefore, the analysis of the economic burden requires an in depth analysis of the different types of complications and their consequences in terms of both resources consumption and indirect costs. Mortality rate cannot be ignored, of course. Given the above argument, some organizational changes need to be adopted to improve the performance of emergency abdominal surgery in the elderly, both in terms of costs and outcomes. An appropriate evaluation of the elderly patients is a key step that allows to select the surgery approach better consistent with the patient's physical, cognitive, social, functional predictors of the outcomes. Thus, a few actions might be adopted before the operation: prompt diagnosis, identification of frailty and prediction of risks, and consultation with a multidisciplinary team as determinants of the choice of the surgery approach.

4.7 Concluding Remarks

Given the increasing life expectancy of the population and more in details, the growing number of elderly aged 80 or older, the emergency abdominal surgery can be predicted as increasing and jointly with the volume of operations, the costs for both the National Health Service and the caregivers and the society. The technological innovation provides surgeons of new mini-invasive approaches that might reduce the length of staying and consequently the deterioration of the cognitive and physical conditions of elderly patients. While this type of benefits is like to be reached with regard to some abdominal surgery procedures, in most cases the literature provides evidences of high rate of in-hospital complications and high mortality rate for elderly undergoing emergency abdominal laparoscopic surgery. Hospital complications compromise the outcome and deeply affect the economic evaluation.

Considering the population target, the elderly, the need to broaden the perspective for the economic evaluation is aligned with many Western countries' policies. In the past, refusal to adopt a broader perspective has sometimes been justified because of data limitations, measurement difficulties, or limits in budgetary responsibilities. However, it is now time to overcome these practical difficulties and to think more broadly about the costs and benefits of healthcare interventions. Although literature is copious with regard to the analysis of the outcomes and their predicting factors, the economic evaluations associated to the emergency abdominal surgery in the elderly are still limited. Thus, as new guidelines are undertaken and technological innovation intervenes, the assessment of the economic burden should be developed to inform both health professionals' decision-making and healthcare system policymakers.

Five Things You Should Know About the Economic Burden of Emergency Abdominal Surgery in the Elderly Are As Follows

- The emergency abdominal surgery can be predicted as increasing, jointly with the volume of operations.
- The emergency surgery in the elderly might bring to a variety of consequences in terms of loss of physical conditions, reduced level of autonomy and mobility, and cognitive abilities.
- The elderlies going through emergency abdominal surgery are often affected by comorbidities and are frail patients.
- Both direct and direct costs for emergency abdominal surgery are expected to increase considering both the National Health Service and the caregivers' perspectives.
- Laparoscopy in emergency abdominal surgery brings to reduced LOS and consequences for the elderly; an appropriate evaluation of the elderly patients is key to select the surgery approach consistent with the patient's physical, cognitive, social, functional predictors of the outcomes.

References

1. Eurostat Statistics. Eurostat Regional Year book. 2020. https://ec.europa.eu/eurostat/web/products-eurostat-news/-/edn-20200930-1.
2. OECD. OECD health data. 2019. https://www.oecd.org/els/health-systems/health-data.htm
3. Parker MJ, Gurusamy K, Stoker M. Surgery in elderly patients. Curr Orthopaed. 2004;18(5):333–44.
4. Veering BT. Management of anaesthesia in elderly patients. Curr Opin Anaesthesiol. 1999;12(3):333–6.
5. Istat. Il future demografico del Paese. Statistiche Report; 2017.
6. Ferrarese A, Martino V, Nano M. Elective and emergency laparoscopic cholecystectomy in the elderly: early or delayed approach. BMC Geriatr. 2011;11:1–2.
7. Torrance ADW, Powell SL, Griffiths EA. Emergency surgery in the elderly: challenges and solutions. Open Access Emerg Med. 2015;7:55–68.
8. Andrew DWT, Susan LP, Ewen AG. Emergency surgery in the elderly: challenges and solutions. Open Access Emerg Med. 2015;7:55–68.
9. Dowgiałło-Wnukiewicz N, Kozera P, Lech P, Rymkiewicz P, Michalik M. Emergency surgery in older patients. Videosurgery and Other Miniinvasive Techniques. 2019;14(2):182.
10. Søreide K, Desserud KF. Emergency surgery in the elderly: the balance between function, frailty, fatality and futility. Scand Trauma Resusc Emerg Med. 2015;23(1):1–7.
11. Anna ES, Jenny ML, Robert C, et al. Emergency abdominal surgery in the elderly: can we predict mortality? World J Surg. 2016;41(2):402–9.
12. Compagna R, Rossi R, Fappiano F, Bianco T, Accurso A, Danzi M, Massa S, Aprea G, Amato B. Emergency groin hernia repair: implications in elderly. BMC Surgery. 2013;13(2):1–3.
13. Fukuda N, Wada J, Niki M, et al. Factors predicting mortality in emergency abdominal surgery in the elderly. World J Emerg Surg. 2012;7(1):12.
14. Zeineb M, Houssem F, Achref D, et al. Abdominal emergency surgery in the elderly: how to predict mortality? J Clin Diagn Res. 2018;12(3):16.
15. Maciej M, Natalia D-W, Paweł L, et al. Surgery of the elderly in emergency room mode. Is there a place for laparoscopy? Wideochir Inne Tech Maloinwazyjne. 2017;12(2):115–9.
16. Shaheed M, Judd P, Raj SP, et al. Predictors of in-hospital mortality and complications in very elderly patients undergoing emergency surgery. World J Emerg Surg. 2014;9(1):43.
17. Hwee LT, Shermain TXC, Nivedita, et al. Frailty and functional decline after emergency abdominal surgery in the elderly: a prospective cohort study. World J Emerg Surg. 2019;14(1):1–7.
18. McCann A, Sorensen J, Nally D, et al. Discharge outcomes among elderly patients undergoing emergency abdominal surgery: registry study of discharge data from Irish Public Hospitals. BMC Geriatr. 2020;20(1):72.
19. Nishida Y, Otagiri N, Yoshifuku S, et al. Dementia in elderly patients undergoing early cholecystectomy for acute cholecystitis: a retrospective observational study. BMC Surg. 2019;19(1):1–6.
20. Alessia GF, Mario S, Stefano E, et al. Elective and emergency laparoscopic cholecystectomy in the elderly: our experience. BMC Surg. 2013;13(2):21.
21. McComb A, Warkentin LM, McNeely ML, et al. Development of a reconditioning program for elderly abdominal surgery patients: the elder-friendly approaches to the surgical environment–bedside

reconditioning for functional improvements (ease-be fit) pilot study. World J Emerg Surg. 2018;13(1):1–6.

22. Ogola GO, Gale SC, Haider A, et al. The financial burden of emergency general surgery: national estimates 2010 to 2060. J Trauma Acute Care Surg. 2015;79:444–8.
23. Ladhani HA, Posillico SE, Zosa BM, Verbus EA, Brandt CP, Claridge JA. Efficiency of care and cost for common emergency general surgery conditions: Comparison by surgeon training and practice. Surgery. 2018;164(4):651—6. https://doi.org/10.1016/j.surg.2018.05.048.
24. Drummond MF, Schwartz JS, Jonsson B, Luce BR, Neumann PJ, Siebert Ü, et al. Key principles for the improved conduct of health technology assessments for resource allocation decisions. Int J Technol Assess Health Care. 2008;24:244–58.
25. Faulmuller N, Maslen H, Santoni de Sio F. The indirect psychological costs of cognitive enhancement. Am J Bioeth. 2013;13(7):45–7.
26. Schöffski O. Lebensqualität als Ergebnisparameter in gesundheitsökonomischen Studien. In: Schöffski O, Graf vd Schulenburg JM, editors. Gesundheitsökonomische Evaluationen. Berlin: Springer; 2007.
27. Drummond MF, Sculpher MJ, Torrance GW, et al. Methods for the economic evaluation of health care programmes. Oxford: Oxford University Press; 2005.
28. Clegg A, Young J, Iliffe S, et al. Frailty in elderly people. Lancet. 2013;381:752–62.
29. Aunan JR, Watson MM, Hagland HR, et al. Molecular and biological hallmarks of ageing. Br J Surg. 2016;103:e29–46.
30. Brown JC, Harhay MO, Harhay MN. The prognostic importance of frailty in cancer survivors. J Am Geriatr Soc. 2015;63:2538–43.
31. Velanovich V, Antoine H, Swartz A, et al. Accumulating deficits model of frailty and postoperative mortality and morbidity: its application to a national database. J Surg Res. 2013;183:104–10.
32. Khan SA, Chua HW, Hirubalan P, et al. Association between frailty, cerebral oxygenation and adverse post-operative outcomes in elderly patients undergoing non-cardiac surgery: an observational pilot study. Indian J Anaesth. 2016;60:102–7.
33. Fairchild B, Webb TP, Xiang Q, et al. Sarcopenia and frailty in elderly trauma patients. World J Surg. 2015;39(2):373–9.
34. Fuertes-Guiró F, Vitali-Erion E, Fernandez AR. Usefulness of the holistic context of frailty as a prognostic factor for the outcome of geriatric patients undergoing emergency abdominal surgery. European Surgery. 2019;51(5):261–70.
35. Makary MA, Segev DL, Pronovost PJ, et al. Frailty as a predictor of surgical outcomes in older patients. J Am Coll Surg. 2010;210:901–8.
36. Richardson K, Hopker J. One minute to assess frailty, but what should we do next? Anaesthesia. 2016;71(6):622–6.
37. Yingke H, Lydia WL, Ying H, et al. Assessment of predictive validity and feasibility of Edmonton Frail Scale in identifying postoperative complications among elderly patients: a prospective observational study. Sci Rep. 2020;10(1):1–10.
38. Han B, Li Q, Chen X. Frailty and postoperative complications in older Chinese adults undergoing major thoracic and abdominal surgery. Clin Interv Aging. 2019;14:947–57.
39. O'Neill BR, Batterham AM, Hollings-worth AC, et al. Do first impressions count? Frailty judged by initial clinical impression predicts medium-term mortality in vascular surgical patients. Anaesthesia. 2016;71:684–91.
40. Lin HS, Watts JN, Peel NM, et al. Frailty and post-operative outcomes in older surgical patients: a systematic review. BMC Geriatr. 2016;16:157.
41. Biffl WL, Mehler PS, Moore EE. Acute care surgery in the safety net hospital: maintaining referrals and optimizing outcomes. Scand J Surg. 2010;99:68–72.
42. Hsee L, Devaud M, Middleberg L, et al. Acute Surgical Unit at Auckland City Hospital: a descriptive analysis. ANZ J Surg. 2012;82:588–91.
43. Lee W-J, Chan C-P, Wang B-Y Recent advances in laparoscopic surgery. Asian J Endosc Surg. 2013;6(1):1–8.
44. Navez B, Navez J. Laparoscopy in the acute abdomen. Best Pract Res Clin Gastroenterol. 2014;28:3–17.
45. Agresta F, Ansaloni L, Baiocchi GL, et al. Laparoscopic approach to acute abdomen from the consensus development conference of the Societa Italiana di Chirurgia Endoscopicae nuove tecnologie (SICE), Associazione Chirurghi OspedalieriItaliani (ACOI), Societa Italiana di Chirurgia (SIC), Societa Ital-iana di Chirurgia d'Urgenza e del Trauma (SICUT), Societa Ital-iana di Chirurgia nell'Ospedalita Privata (SICOP), and the European Association for Endoscopic Surgery (EAES). Surg Endosc. 2012;26:2134–54.
46. Siletz A, Grotts J, Lewis C, et al. Comparative analysis of laparoscopic and open approaches in emergency abdominal surgery. Am Surg. 2017;83(10):1089–94.
47. Sangrasi AK, Talpu KA, Kella N, et al. Role of laparoscopyin peritonitis. Pak J Med Sci. 2013;29:1028–32.
48. Sartelli M, Viale P, Catena F, et al. 2013 WSES guidelines for management of intra-abdominal infections. World J Emerg Surg. 2013;8:3.
49. Di Saverio S. Emergency laparoscopy: a new emerging discipline for treating abdominal emergencies attempting to minimize costs and invasiveness and maximize outcomes and patients' comfort. J Trauma Acute Care Surg. 2014;77:338–50.
50. Costa G, Fransvea P, Podda M, et al. The use of emergency laparoscopy for acute abdomen in the elderly: the FRAILESEL Italian Multicenter Prospective Cohort Study. Updat Surg. 2020;72:513–25.
51. Keller DS, Pedraza R, Flores-Gonzalez JR, et al. The current status of emergent laparoscopic colectomy: a population-based study of clinical and financial outcomes. Surg Endosc. 2016;30:3321–6.
52. Ukkonen, Mika, et al. Emergency abdominal operations in the elderly: a multivariate regression analy-

sis of 430 consecutive patients with acute abdomen. World J Surg. 2015;39(12):2854–61.
53. Devoto L, Celentano V, Cohen R, et al. Colorectal cancer surgery in the very elderly patient: a systematic review of laparoscopic versus open colorectal resection. Int J Color Dis. 2017;32(9):1237–42.
54. Adkins HH, Hardacker TJ, Ceppa EP. Examining variation in cost based on surgeon choices for elective laparoscopic cholecystectomy. Surg Endosc. 2016;30(7):2679–84.
55. Nakamura T, Sato T, Miura H, et al. Feasibility and outcomes of surgical therapy in very elderly patients with colorectal cancer. Surg Laparosc Endosc Percutan Tech. 2014;24:85–8.
56. Chung KC, Lee KC, Chen HH, et al. Differential short-term outcomes of laparoscopic resection in colon and rectal cancer patients aged 80 and older: an analysis of Nationwide Inpatient Sample. Surg Endosc. 2021;35(2):872–83. https://doi.org/10.1007/s00464-020-07459-x.
57. Cui N, Liu J, Tan H. Comparison of laparoscopic surgery versus traditional laparotomy for the treatment of emergency patients. J Int Med Res. 2020;48(3):300060519889191. https://doi.org/10.1177/0300060519889191.
58. Mar J, Anton-Ladislao A, Ibarrondo O, Arrospide A, Lázaro S, Gonzalez N, Bare, M, Callejo D, Redondo M, Quintana J,M, Quintana López J, Mañas MB, Maximino RB, Eduardo Briones Pérez de la Blanca, Nerea Férnandez de LB, Eizaguirre CS, Antonio Escobar Martínez, Francisco Rivas Ruiz, Morales-Suárez-Varela MM, Blasco Amaro JA, Isabel Del Cura González, Inmaculada Arostegui Madariaga, Amaia Bilbao González, Nerea González Hernández, García-Gutiérrez S, Iratxe Lafuente Guerrero, Urko AL, Miren OC, Josune Martin Corral, Antón-Ladislao A, Torà N, Pont M, María Purificación Martínez dP, Totorikaguena AL, Ignacio Zabalza Estévez, José Errasti Alustiza, Gimeno García AZ, Santiago Lázaro Aramburu, Mercè Comas Serrano, Jose María Enríquez Navascues, Carlos Placer Galán, Perales A, Iñaki Urquidi Valmaña, Jose María Erro Azkárate, Lizarribar EC, Adelaida Lacasta Muñoa, Pep Peira Pibernat, Elena CC, Sotelo Gómez AI, Gómez-Abril S, Medina-Cano F, Alcaide J, Arturo Del Rey-Moreno, Manuel Jesús Alcántara, Campo R, Casalots A, Pericay C, Gil MJ, Pera M, Collera P, Espinàs JA, Martínez M, Espallargues M, Almazán C, Lindenbaum PD, Fernández-Cebrián JM, Rocío Anula Fernández Mayol Martínez JÁ, Ramón Cantero Cid, Héctor Guadalajara Labajo, Heras Garceau M, Damián García Olmo, Mariel Morey Montalvo. Cost-effectiveness analysis of laparoscopic versus open surgery in colon cancer. Surg Endosc. 2018;32(12):4912–22.

5 Goals of Care in Emergency Abdominal Surgery in the Elderly and Frail Patient

Antonino Agrusa, Giuseppe Di Buono,
Salvatore Buscemi, Francesco Saverio Latteri,
Antonio Giuseppe Biondi, and Giorgio Romano

5.1 Introduction

Elderly and frail patients are often those at highest risk during surgical procedures both in terms of intraoperative complications and postoperative outcome. At the same time, surgery in the elderly patient is increasingly frequent both in the elective and emergency setting due to the aging of population, the greater diffusion of mini-invasive surgery, enhanced recovery protocol, and the improvement in anesthesiologic management [1, 2].

5.2 Frailty Degree and Preoperative Predictive Factors: Evaluation of Surgical Patient

The identification of the elderly and frail patient is fundamental for the evaluation of the goals of care that can be achieved. The elderly patient has a complex clinical management because of the multiple comorbidities and the reduced functional reserve that compromises the ability to respond to stressors [3]. Based on the importance of these physiological changes related, but not strictly dependent on age, we can stratify the degree of frailty of the patient. In this concept plays a central role the impairment of interrelated systems that can have a negative synergistic effect on the patient such as the musculoskeletal system, nutritional status, and cognitive decline. In particular, the conditions of the musculoskeletal system and cognitive status, even if not directly related by the surgical procedure, are an expression of the ability of precoce mobilization and positive cooperation for postoperative recovery. The nutritional status is closely connected with the patient's metabolic and wound healing capacity [4]. The clinical manifestations that we can most commonly observe in these patients and which actually represent a critical point for the assessment of their degree of frailty are feeling of fatigue, weight loss, low levels of physical activity during daily life. Many studies have shown that the degree of frailty is a marker of increased risk of perioperative complications and mortality in patients undergoing surgery both in elective and emergency setting. Although numerous systems have been proposed for the stratification of these conditions, two are the most widespread and easy to apply, with some limitations even in emergency surgery: the Fried criteria and the

A. Agrusa (✉) · G. Di Buono · S. Buscemi
G. Romano
Department of Surgical, Oncological and Oral Sciences, University of Palermo, Palermo, Italy
e-mail: antonino.agrusa@unipa.it; giuseppe.dibuono@unipa.it; Salvatore.buscemi02@unipa.it; giorgio.romano@unipa.it

F. S. Latteri · A. G. Biondi
Department of General Surgery and Medical-Surgical Specialties, University of Catania, Catania, Italy
e-mail: saverio.latteri@unict.it; abiondi@unict.it

F. Agresta et al. (eds.), *Emergency laparoscopic surgery in the elderly and frail patient*,
https://doi.org/10.1007/978-3-030-79990-8_5

frailty index (FI). Fried's criteria take into account five different parameters such as grip strength, walking speed, level of physical activity, weight loss, and exhaustion and consider different cutoffs adjusting for gender, BMI, and standing height. The frailty index instead evaluates other variables such as the ability to perform daily activities with or without help, mental status (feel depressed, happy, lonely), and the presence of comorbidities (high blood pressure, heart attack, stroke, cancer, diabetes, chronic lung disease) [5]. The Fried index is very widespread in clinical practice because it is easy and quick to calculate and reproducible in different populations as it considers generic parameters [6]. These criteria are validated by several studies. The authors have shown that the Fried index allows to estimate the rate of postoperative complications which are 2–4 times more frequent in frail patients than in "nonfrailty" group. Similar results were obtained when we considered the overall 30-day mortality (8% in frail patients versus 1% in nonfrail patients). The same authors also considered the main conventional preoperative assessment scores (e.g., ASA score, Charlson weighted comorbidity index, and APACHE II) which, however, were unable to provide a significant predictive value in terms of postoperative outcome. From the analysis of the literature studies, despite the heterogeneity with respect to the surgical procedures performed, the patients considered, and the definition of frailty, in all cases exists a direct correlation between the degree of frailty and the worst postoperative outcomes in both elective and emergency setting. Other studies have used FI in patients undergoing enhanced recovery after surgery (ERAS) and therefore laparoscopic surgery. The rationale is due to the fact that the elderly and frail patients can benefit from the use of these protocols, but also in this case it has been shown that a greater degree of frailty is a predictor of a delayed discharge and higher readmission rate [7, 8]. A modified FI has been used recently by Akyar et al. [9] in a retrospective population study that considered over than 130,000 patients undergoing to emergency general surgery. In this study, modified FI was associated with an increased risk of mortality, unplanned reintubation, prolonged ventilation, pneumonia, and cardiac complications (myocardial infarction and cardiac arrest). Despite these significant results, most of the available studies are retrospective and this indicates that even the best known risk stratification tools are rarely used in urgency. On the basis of these difficulties in the elderly patient evaluation in emergency, it could be more useful the stratification of the degree of frailty through the assessment of the generalized reduction of muscle mass and strength. Sarcopenia is associated with musculoskeletal impairment, inability to mobilization, and increased mortality. The quantification of psoas muscle mass can be achieved with both CT scan and MRI due to their capacity to distinguish fat from other tissues. The evaluation is easy and does not require special image reconstruction software. Furthermore, thanks to its diffusion in clinical practice, CT scan is often used in the diagnostic phase even in an emergency setting and allows us to directly quantify the patient's degree of sarcopenia and therefore to estimate the risk of perioperative complications with considerable time savings compared to other tests for assessment of the patient's frailty [10]. Recent studies on the Caucasian population show that the mortality rate after emergency surgery is directly related to the density and total area of the psoas muscle evaluated by CT scan. Most of the authors take into consideration the cross sectional area of the psoas muscle (mm^2) and its density in terms of Hunsfiled units (HU) at the L4–L5 intervertebral disk space level bilaterally. A reduction of these parameters is associated with an increase of proteolytic enzymes and a lack in proteic synthesis [11].

Sarcopenia evaluated through the study of the psoas density is significantly related to the mortality of these patients to confirm that the quality rather than the quantity is associated with adverse events, poor outcome, and the degree of frailty of the patient himself. Considering that the classification of the frailty degree with Geriatric Complete Assessment (GCA) requires specific training and adequate time and can be difficult to perform in emergency, the possibility of using an objective and simple parameter such as the area and density of the psoas represents an important aid in the risk stratification of these patients. In the patients of Asiatic origin, these results must be validated from other studies because of the different body conformation, lifestyle, and cultural background [12].

5.3 What Kind of Procedure? Variables for Decision-Making Process

On the basis of these considerations, it emerges that the holistic assessment of the patient's frailty is essential to help the surgeon in the preoperative decision-making process and in the acquisition of informed consent. The surgeon can modify surgical technique (open vs laparoscopy) and the type of procedure in order to realize a "tailored" approach balancing the preoperative risks and the expected results. In oncology and emergency surgery, the treatment may differ from the standards expected for a young patient. For example, in oncologic elderly and frail patients with low rectal cancer, we can decide to carry out only a palliative procedure (placement of an endoscopic prosthesis or diverting ostomy) rather than a difficult rectal resection. In emergency surgery, we can choose a different approach: for example, elderly and frail patients with severe acute cholecystits underwent to percutaneous cholecystostomy or complicated groin hernia treated with anterior open approach with locoregional anesthesia [13, 14]. The better communication to the patient through the informed consent can also lead to a procedure that aims more at the postoperative quality of life than at the survival of the patient. This is because elderly patients often prefer to maintain a standard of quality of life that allows them to be independent at the expense of life expectancy. In this sense, the assessment of the patient frailty degree is fundamental to stratify the preoperative risk, to carry out a targeted surgical therapy and to optimize the postoperative management. The multidisciplinary preoperative evaluation process with risk assessment does not only represent a moment in which a possible operative strategy is evaluated, but also takes a key role in communication with the patient and his family. Contrary to what one might believe in the elderly patients in conditions of surgical emergency the time of clinical communication with informed consent to surgery must be an interactive discussion in order to arrive at shared choices that take into consideration not the best treatment ever but the best treatment for that patient. In these patients, the surgeon must realize a tailored treatment, shared by the full healthcare team and by the patients and their family members. Involving the patients and their family in decisions that concern them is not only a duty based on patient ethics and rights, but it also provides the opportunity to obtain a motivated patient who will respond in a better way to perioperative stress and a family environment prepared to take care of him earlier. The multidisciplinary team must carefully explain all phases of the therapeutic process from access to the operating room, to waking up, hospitalization, postoperative rehabilitation, and the times for oral food intake. Moreover, during the interview, we can recognize cognitive deficits that had not been previously noted. Therefore, the informed consent represents the last step in the patient's general assessment, and together with the other information collected previously, it allows us to define the best therapeutic management. The fact that this happens in concert with the patient and family members also adds a legal value, of recognized importance, to the scientific and ethical aspects [15, 16]. In emergency surgery, these concepts are further exasperated by the lack of prehabilitation. Therefore, the frail patients with reduced functional reserve and various comorbidities have not only a high risk of worsening their quality of life with loss of their functional independence, but also a higher mortality rate. The risk stratification systems most used in the world in emergency conditions (P-POSSUM and APACHE-2 score) do not provide for an adjustment for frailty. In clinical practice, many physicians use comorbidities, drugs assumption, disability, and cognitive impairment for the evaluation of elderly patients. The concept of frailty, instead, is independent of age and comorbidities and takes into account the physiological reserve of these patients, which makes it possible to distinguish, within elderly patients, those at low or high risk. As previously highlighted, the assessment of frailty is the only holistic approach that allows the identification of patients with limited functional capacity able to respond to stressors [17].

5.4 Goals of Care and Optimization of Therapeutic Management

The evidences described support the hypothesis that the degree of frailty and perioperative adverse events are closely associated as two independent variables. We must consider those factors that can improve the short- and long-term outcome of elderly and frail patients undergoing to emergency surgery. The management of these conditions is already complex per se because of the multiple comorbidities and the reduction of the functional reserve even in the elective surgery in which it is possible to optimize some preoperative parameters as much as possible in order to minimize the risk of specific postoperative complications. In emergency general surgery, the management becomes even more complex as the number of factors on which it is possible to act is reduced.

5.4.1 Preoperative Conditions

The identification of patients at higher risk is fundamental in the preoperative phase; however, in emergency surgery, it is almost never possible to provide a Complete Geriatric Assessment (CGA) and the stratification of the patient is committed to surgeon and anesthetist who, for their different role, will have to assume the responsibility of giving a tailored treatment. The crucial parameters in preoperative management, but which cannot be changed in emergency, are the cardio-respiratory reserve, the cognitive function, and pharmacological management for the prevention of postoperative delirium [18]. We have already mentioned the concept of prehabilitation with the possibility of increasing the functional reserve of these patients in order to reduce the risk of irreversible postoperative deficits and actually improve the postoperative outcome. The concept of prehabilitation is based on preoperative physiotherapy, on the nutritional status and on patient education. Unfortunately, all these conditions require long times and the active collaboration of family members; therefore, it is not possible to change these factors in conditions of emergency surgery. The early identification of the caregiver and his "training" allows an improvement in the home management of these patients, effectively favoring early discharge and postoperative rehabilitation. Only in part this recruitment and training can be carried out in emergency setting and in any case it has a considerable variability strictly related to the specific sociocultural conditions [19].

5.4.2 Intraoperative Management

In this phase, both surgical and anesthetic aspects are involved, on which it is possible to act in most cases. From a surgical point of view, it would be appropriate to perform a tailored surgery based on the patient and his risk assessment, the pathology, and the surgeon experience. In general, a mini-invasive/laparoscopic approach should be preferred in order to minimize surgical trauma; however, this type of procedure can lead to a considerable lengthening of operative time, an impairment of cardio-respiratory functional reserves, and an increase in intraoperative complications. Therefore, the choice must be made by the individual surgeon on the basis of his own experience and must take into account the preoperative evaluation of the patient and the specific pathology to be treated. Several studies have highlighted that while in elective surgery, the elderly and frail patient because of his difficult management is treated by a senior consultant surgeon and consultant anesthetist, this occurrence is less frequent in emergency. According to the World Health Organization (WHO) checklist for safe surgery, the presence of a consultant surgeon even during the preoperative briefing phases, and not only during surgical procedures, improves the outcome of these patients. Obviously, the degree of urgency and the possibility that waiting in unstable patients can significantly aggravate the clinical conditions must always be assessed. In elderly and frail patients, the general clinical conditions can change suddenly even during the execution of the surgery. The presence of an experienced surgeon in these cases seems to favor any changes in the surgical plan in order to obtain the best outcome for the patient (e.g., avoid making an anastomosis or temporarily use an open abdomen) [20]. Anesthesiologic management should regard particular attention to the fluid therapy administration and the prevention of hypothermia. Several studies have shown that in low/intermediate risk patients, the cardiac index (CI) can be maintained through the optimization of preload. The use of inotropes is only necessary in a small part of patients and in any case should be limited in high-risk patients with suspect reduced cardiac performance. The preoperative echocardiographic study of CI can be a valid option for patient stratification, but unfortunately it is almost never available in emergency setting. Another parameter to consider is the correct titration of drug therapy based on the patient age and on functional deficits in renal and hepatic metabolism. The prevention of deep vein thrombosis through compression devices and pharmacologic prophylaxis is also closely related to the anesthetic management. In fact, the risk of venous thromboembolism is increased in the elderly and frail patient due to possible comorbidities and the greater difficulty in early mobilization [3, 21, 22].

5.4.3 Postoperative Management

Postoperative management includes pain control through the use of patient-related analgesia systems or through titrated drug administration regardless of the patient's reported need. Pain control in the elderly and frail patient acts with a synergistic effect, not further reducing the functional reserve, improving rehabilitation, and promoting a collaborative mental status in the healing process. Early mobilization and rehabilitation should always be carried out in order to reduce functional and musculoskeletal decline which can aggravate the risk conditions of the frail patient. Recent studies show that rehabilitation in these patients would have a decisive role in reducing postoperative disability and related adverse events [23].

5.5 Complications in Frail and Elderly Patients

The elderly and frail patient can develop the same complications of a low-risk patient in qualitative terms, but with higher rate and strictly dependent on preoperative risk stratification. Instead a typical complication of frail and elderly patients is represented by postoperative delirium. Postoperative delirium and delayed postoperative neurocognitive disorders are among the most common postoperative complications in the elderly patients undergoing to emergency surgery. The risk of developing these complications increases with age. Postoperative delirium is often misunderstood, especially when it comes to hypoactive delirium which is the most frequent compared to the agitated and confused type of delirium, but can equally lead to a worse postoperative outcome with an increase in complications and mortality, and longer hospital stay. The most frequent causes are electrolyte disturbance, thyroid dysfunction, alcohol abuse, uncontrolled pain, infections, urinary retention, and constipation. The preoperative assessment of the cognitive function allows the identification of patients at high risk of postoperative delirium. In these patients, various strategies can be used to prevent the onset of this complication: correction of electrolytes, analgesic therapy, drug rationalization, and adequate information on the risk of delirium for both the patient and family members. The intra- and postoperative management includes the choice of the anesthetic technique and the drugs used both in qualitative and quantitative terms; ensure the presence of family members as much as possible; avoid isolation due to not use of glasses or hearing aids. The hospital environment should also be adapted with the presence of a clock, attention to the day/night cycle favoring rest and sleep. Several studies have shown that a 40% reduction in the onset of postoperative delirium can be achieved through some small attentions such as communication, assistance during oral food intake and early mobilization. The occurrence of perioperative complications is a predictive factor of poor outcome with a significant increase in mortality in the elderly and frail patient underwent to emergency surgery [24, 25]. This concept must be well explained to the patient but above all to family members. Theoretically, the possibility of carrying out a laparoscopic approach with reduced surgical trauma also decreases the risk of complications. These patients generally are able to get through the initial surgical treatment, but suffer from a greater rate of complications and comorbidities resulting in higher long-term mortality. A comprehensive geriatric assessment carried out by a multidisciplinary team can be useful to reduce length of hospital stay, Intensive Care Unit (ICU) admission, hospital re-admission, mortality, and costs. The multidisciplinary approach is quite widespread in trauma or orthopedics surgery, but it is still relatively little used in nontraumatic surgical emergencies. The fundamental concepts to be taken into consideration in these patients concern nutrition (about 80% of elderly patients are malnourished or at risk of malnutrition), early mobilization, and physiotherapy that promote the resumption of intestinal peristalsis and reduce complications such as deep vein thrombosis and respiratory infections [26, 27].

5.6 Conclusion

It is clear that the best therapeutic result in the elderly and frail patient can be obtained through multidisciplinary management of the problem. The multidisciplinary team must include different members such as surgeon, anesthetist, geriatrician, nurse, physiotherapist who work with each other in an integrated system. Only in this way is it possible to dismiss the individual vision and reach a holistic management of the elderly and frail patient. This therapeutic continuity does not end after discharge, but continues at home through the identification and training of the caregiver, favoring the final rehabilitation process. In conclusion, in the management of elderly and frail patients undergoing to emergency surgery, we can make a series of considerations that guide our decision-making process. First, correct diagnosis can be difficult because of the impaired cognitive and physical status of the patient or other clinical conditions and medications that mask signs and symptoms. Second, the choice of the treatment to be carried out, surgical or nonoperative, must be tailored to the patient and often is different from what would be done in a young fitter patient. Third, even if age is not a contraindication to surgery, the outcomes change. In elderly patients, it would be more appropriate to evaluate the best treatment to ensure a good quality of life, rather than performing surgical procedures aimed at ensuring the best results in terms of long-term survival. Finally, useless treatments should be avoided which would only have the effect of prolonging end-of-life suffering. To achieve these objectives, it is advisable to always put the patient at the center of the decision-making process, to adopt a holistic vision that includes not only the patient himself, but also his family and socio-cultural environment [28, 29].

Five Things You Should Know About Goal of Care in Emergency Abdominal Surgery in the Elderly and Frail Patient:

- The elderly and frail patients with emergent surgical pathology should be referred to an experienced general surgeon for the choice of operative or nonoperative treatment. Management should take place in accordance with a multidisciplinary team formed by anesthetist, radiologist, emergency physician, and geriatrician. The management protocol should include some fundamental points: appropriate antibiotic therapy, the need of a rapid radiological report (within 1 h), assessment of the patient's risk, and degree of frailty.
- Several scores can be used to obtain a comprehensive geriatric assessment (CGA). If it is

not able to carry out a CGA of the patient, it is possible to use other parameters such as the evaluation of sarcopenia by analyzing the cross sectional area and density of the psoas muscle with CT scan.

- The patients should be divided into three groups based on the severity of the disease: high-risk immediate surgery, high-risk nonimmediate surgery, and high-risk emergency nonoperative management.
- The correct management of elderly and frail patients should be carried out at three different levels. Preoperative conditions with evaluation of cardio-respiratory reserve, the cognitive function, and pharmacological management for the prevention of postoperative delirium and the identification of the caregiver. Intraoperative management: perform a tailored surgery based on the patient and his risk assessment, the pathology and the surgeon experience; anesthesiologic management should regard particular attention to the fluid therapy administration and the prevention of hypothermia. Postoperative management includes pain control early mobilization and rehabilitation with a synergistic effect, not further reducing the functional reserve, promoting a collaborative mental status in the healing process.
- Prevention of postoperative complication with particular attention to postoperative delirium and delayed postoperative neurocognitive disorders. These are among the most common postoperative complications in the elderly patients undergoing to emergency surgery. The occurrence of perioperative complications is a predictive factor of poor outcome with a significant increase in mortality in the elderly and frail patient underwent to emergency surgery.

References

1. Bergman H, Ferrucci L, Guralnik J, Hogan DB, Hummel S, Karunananthan S, et al. Frailty: an emerging research and clinical paradigm–issues and controversies. J Gerontol A Biol Sci Med Sci. 2007;62(7):731–7.
2. Makary MA, Segev DL, Pronovost PJ, Syin D, Bandeen-Roche K, Patel P, et al. Frailty as a predictor of surgical outcomes in older patients. J Am Coll Surg. 2010;210(6):901–8. https://doi.org/10.1016/j.jamcollsurg.2010.01.028.
3. Benes J, Giglio M, Brienza N, Michard F. The effects of goal-directed fluid therapy based on dynamic parameters on post-surgical outcome: a meta-analysis of randomized controlled trials. Crit Care. 2014;18(5):534. https://doi.org/10.1186/s13054-014-0584-z.
4. Farhat JS, Velanovich V, Falvo AJ, Horst HM, Swartz A, Patton JH, et al. Are the frail destined to fail? Frailty index as predictor of surgical morbidity and mortality in the elderly. J Trauma Acute Care Surg. 2012;72(6):1526–30; discussion 1530–1531. https://doi.org/10.1097/TA.0b013e3182542fab.
5. Searle SD, Mitnitski A, Gahbauer EA, Gill TM, Rockwood K. A standard procedure for creating a frailty index. BMC Geriatr. 2008;8(1):24. https://doi.org/10.1186/1471-2318-8-24.
6. Fried LP, Tangen CM, Walston J, Newman AB, Hirsch C, Gottdiener J, et al. Frailty in older adults: evidence for a phenotype. J Gerontol A Biol Sci Med Sci. 2001;56(3):M146–56.
7. Kenig J, Zychiewicz B, Olszewska U, Barczynski M, Nowak W. Six screening instruments for frailty in older patients qualified for emergency abdominal surgery. Arch Gerontol Geriatr. 2015;61:437–42.
8. Ozban M, Birsen O, Senel M, Ozden A, Kabay B. The analysis of scoring systems predicting mortality in geriatric emergency abdominal surgery. Ulus Travma Acil Cerrahi Derg. 2015;21:182–6.
9. Akyar S, Armenia SJ, Ratnani P, Merchant AM. The impact of frailty on postoperative cardiopulmonary complications in the emergency general surgery population. Surg J (N Y). 2018;4(2):e66–77. https://doi.org/10.1055/s-0038-1655756.
10. Trotter J, Johnston J, Ng A, Gatt M, MacFie J, McNaught C. Is sarcopenia a useful predictor of outcome in patients after emergency laparotomy? A study using the NELA database. Ann R Coll Surg Engl. 2018;100(5):377–81. https://doi.org/10.1308/rcsann.2017.0230.
11. Rangel EL, Rios-Diaz AJ, Uyeda JW, Castillo-Angeles M, Cooper Z, Olufajo OA, et al. Sarcopenia increases risk of long-term mortality in elderly patients undergoing emergency abdominal surgery. J Trauma Acute Care Surg. 2017;83(6):1179–86. https://doi.org/10.1097/TA.0000000000001657. Large sample size retrospective study that evaluates the short- and long-term outcomes and effects of sarcopenia.
12. Chen L-K, Liu L-K, Woo J, Assantachai P, Auyeung T-W, Bahyah KS, et al. Sarcopenia in Asia: consensus report of the Asian Working Group for Sarcopenia. J Am Med Dir Assoc. 2014;15(2):95–101. https://doi.org/10.1016/j.jamda.2013.11.025.
13. Cauley CE, Panizales MT, Reznor G, Haynes AB, Havens JM, Kelley E, et al. Outcomes after emergency abdominal surgery in patients with advanced cancer: opportunities to reduce complications and

improve palliative care. J Trauma Acute Care Surg. 2015;79(3):399–406. https://doi.org/10.1097/TA.0000000000000764.
14. Agrusa A, Romano G, Frazzetta G, Chianetta D, Sorce V, Di Buono G, Gulotta G. Role and outcomes of laparoscopic cholecystectomy in the elderly. Int J Surg. 2014;12(Suppl 2):S37–9. https://doi.org/10.1016/j.ijsu.2014.08.385. Epub 2014 Aug 23
15. Hogan KJ, Bratzke LC, Hogan KL. Informed consent and cognitive dysfunction after noncardiac surgery in the elderly. Anesth Analg. 2018;126(2):629–31. https://doi.org/10.1213/ANE.0000000000002689.
16. Giampieri M. Communication and informed consent in elderly people. Minerva Anestesiol. 2012;78(2):236–42. Epub 2011 Nov 18
17. Partridge JSL, Harari D, Martin FC, Dhesi JK. The impact of preoperative comprehensive geriatric assessment on postoperative outcomes in older patients undergoing scheduled surgery: a systematic review. Anaesthesia. 2014;69(Suppl 1):8–16. https://doi.org/10.1111/anae.12494.
18. American Geriatrics Society Expert Panel on Postoperative Delirium in Older Adults. Postoperative delirium in older adults: best practice statement from the American Geriatrics Society. J Am Coll Surg. 2015;220(2):136–148.e1. https://doi.org/10.1016/j.jamcollsurg.2014.10.019.
19. Hendrix CC, Bailey DE, Steinhauser KE, Olsen MK, Stechuchak KM, Lowman SG, et al. Effects of enhanced caregiver training program on cancer caregiver' s self-efficacy, preparedness, and psychological well-being. Support Care Cancer. 2016;24(1):327–36. https://doi.org/10.1007/s00520-015-2797-3.
20. The high-risk geenral surgical patient: raising the standard. A statement form the Royal College of Surgeon of England Working group on the peroperative care of the high-risk generale surgical patient. 2018.
21. Kozek-Langenecker S, Fenger-Eriksen C, Thienpont E, Barauskas G, ESAVTE Guidelines Task Force. European guidelines on perioperative venous thromboembolism prophylaxis: surgery in the elderly. Eur J Anaesthesiol. 2018;35(2):116–22. https://doi.org/10.1097/EJA.0000000000000705.
22. Shi S, Klotz U. Age-related changes in pharmacokinetics. Curr Drug Metab. 2011;12(7):601–10.
23. McIsaac DI, Jen T, Mookerji N, Patel A, Lalu MM. Interventions to improve the outcomes of frail people having surgery: a systematic review. PLoS One. 2017;12(12):e0190071. https://doi.org/10.1371/journal.pone.0190071.
24. Deiner S, Westlake B, Dutton RP. Patterns of surgical care and complications in elderly adults. J Am Geriatr Soc. 2014;62:829–35.
25. Merani S, Payne J, Padwal RS, Hudson D, Widder SL, Khadaroo RG. Predictors of in-hospital mortality and complications in very elderly patients undergoing emergency surgery. World J Emerg Surg. 2014;9:43.
26. Chow WB, Merkow RP, Cohen ME, Bilimoria KY, Ko CY. Association between postoperative complications and reoperation for patients undergoing geriatric surgery and the effect of reoperation on mortality. Am Surg. 2012;78:1137–42.
27. Kristjansson SR, Farinella E, Gaskell S, Audisio RA. Surgical risk and post-operative complications in older unfit cancer patients. Cancer Treat Rev. 2009;35:499–502.
28. Mangram AJ, Shifflette VK, Mitchell CD, Johnson VA, Lorenzo M, Truitt MS, et al. The creation of a geriatric trauma unit 'G-60'. Am Surg. 2011;77:1144–6.
29. Partridge JS, Harari D, Martin FC, Dhesi JK. The impact of pre-operative comprehensive geriatric assessment on postoperative outcomes in older patients undergoing scheduled surgery: a systematic review. Anaesthesia. 2014;69(Suppl 1):8–16.

Wound Healing in Elderly and Frail Patients

6

Valerio Caracino, Pietro Coletta, Piergaspare Palumbo, Simone Castiglioni, Diletta Frazzini, and Massimo Basti

After an acute damage to soft tissues, either of traumatic nature, referring to a pathology or as a consequence of surgical act, human body acts with a coordinated series of activities that take the name of "healing." This elaborate process involves the following phases: hemostasis, inflammation, proliferative phase, and tissue remodeling [1].

The first step is to stop the bleeding and achieve an adequate hemostasis by the formation of the platelet clot and local vasoconstriction. The destruction of the vascular micro-network and the high consumption of oxygen by the metabolically active cells within the wound, that will be the protagonists of the subsequent healing phases, lead to a hypoxic environment that characterizes the early stages of the healing process [2–4].

This leads to an increase in the expression of the hypoxia-inducible factor (HIF)-1, which regulates the transcription of multiple genes such as growth factors and cytokines, which are expressed by macrophages, keratinocytes, and fibroblasts. The synthesis of these genes guides the healing process through the subsequent steps of inflammation, angiogenesis, neovasculogenesis, and tissue remodeling [2–5].

Dendritic T-cells, neutrophils, and macrophages get involved in this substrate to start the inflammation phase with the activation of the complement cascade [6, 7].

The goal of the inflammation process is to sterilize the wound site killing any microbial organism present. The dendritic T-cells of the epidermis are specifically activated by the keratinocyte's damage and produce cytokines and chemokines that contribute to the infection control during the physiological healing process [3].

Peripheral neurons begin the production of neuropeptides such as the substance P (SP), neuropeptide Y (NPY), and others, promoting the inflammation phase. In the first 24 h, neutrophils occur releasing pro-inflammatory cytokines such as IL-1, IL-6, TNF-α, and producing metalloproteases (MMPs) which help lysing protein fragments [8].

Subsequently, the macrophages carry out their action as "scavengers" by removing all cellular debris and change the phenotype from M1 to M2 once completed their inflammatory action, to promote the healing process; this is required to switch from the inflammation to the proliferative phase. They are in charge of supplying growth

V. Caracino (✉) · S. Castiglioni · D. Frazzini
M. Basti
UOC Chirurgia generale e d'Urgenza, Ospedale Civile "Santo Spirito" Pescara, Pescara, Italy

P. Coletta
Clinica chirurgica generale e d'urgenza, AOU "Ospedali riuniti" Ancona, Ancona, Italy

P. Palumbo
Responsabile Day e Week surgery Policlinico Umberto I Università la Sapienza Roma, Rome, Italy
e-mail: piergaspare.palumbo@uniroma1.it

F. Agresta et al. (eds.), *Emergency laparoscopic surgery in the elderly and frail patient*,
https://doi.org/10.1007/978-3-030-79990-8_6

factors, establishing interactions with the extracellular matrix (ECM), and stimulating the migration of fibroblasts [3, 9, 10].

When the fibroblasts start the production of the platelet-derived growth factor (PDGF), transforming growth factor (TGF)-β, and the synthesis of a new ECM, the proliferation phase begins leading to the formation of granulation tissue. From this primitive and formless tissue, the neomyofibroblasts organize new collagen fibers that direct the scar and guide the neovascularization [11, 12]. Lastly, in the following months, the tissue remodeling starts; this is a process that takes a long time to mature and concludes with the formation of the definitive scar [11].

Many individual risk factors and systemic diseases such as stress, advanced age, hormonal imbalance, chronic infections, metabolic syndrome, and compromised nutritional and immunological status cause or contribute to chronic inflammation which consecutively delays and alters the physiological wound healing [13].

The healing of a surgical incision by primary intention is the ideal event that can occur: in this case, the surgeon guides the cicatrizing phases, obtaining adequate hemostasis, maintaining asepsis, and accosting the wound margins. However, the factors listed above can interfere with healing and lead to postoperative complications, especially in the elderly.

There is a strong correlation between the surgical wounds altered healing, sub-optimal clinical conditions, age, and the presence of comorbidities [14]. Normal blood microcirculation is essential for the healing of the surgical incision as it guarantees perfusion, cellular homeostasis and the sufficient oxygen, and other nutrients supplying, as well as normothermia and the response to inflammation. On the contrary, reduced microcirculation profoundly alters the supply of all these essential support elements [15].

There are many different aspects of the perioperative period to be checked and, if necessary, corrected for proper wound healing. Adequate oxygenation levels are indispensable for killing microbes; therefore, establishing an oxygen therapy [16] and ensuring correct respiratory dynamics with small incisions (less painful than bigger incisions) has an important beneficial effect on the prevention of wound infections. Furthermore, an adequate balance of fluid therapy by controlling inputs and outputs allows to avoid both hypovolemia (with consequent reduction in local perfusion) and the excessive administration of fluids (with consequent tissue edema) by altering cytokine homeostasis [16].

In wounds in which the oxygen supply is not adequately restored, the healing process is compromised, and this is the reason why it has been shown chronic wounds are ultimately hypoxic wounds. Systemic pathological conditions such as advanced age, cardiovascular diseases, obesity, and metabolic syndrome are frequently characterized by chronic hypoxic wounds. Under these conditions, there is a reduced expression of HIF-1, which further exacerbates the chronic feature of the wound and increases the susceptibility to the surgical site infections [2, 3, 17].

Elder patients are more susceptible to chronicization of the healing process, development of dehiscences, and wound infections [16, 18].

Wound hypoxia is typical in elderly and leads to prolonged tissue ischemia, due to microcirculation modifications in chronic vasculopathic patients which in turn is linked to diabetes and metabolic syndrome in a loop of cause–effect [19]; moreover, in the elderly the physiological processes of adhesion, cell migration, and production of cytokines are slowed down [9].

Advanced age is associated with a chronic inflammatory microenvironment, and consequently the switch from the initial inflammatory phase to the later proliferative one does not occur, or occurs with delay and/or in an altered way: the ECM is disrupted, there is no cell proliferation, metalloproteases are not inactivated, and angiogenesis is also impaired [14].

Good control of the inflammatory phase is compromised in the elderly. An evident delay in macrophage's arrival and in T-cell migration has been demonstrated, resulting in an altered healing process. In addition, it has been demonstrated an age-related reduced response to hypoxia, with a sharp decrease in the production of HIF-1, which alters all stages of inflammation, angiogenesis, neovasculogenesis, and tissue remodeling [14].

The switch from M1 to M2 macrophages phenotype is generally poorly regulated within chronic wounds. Therefore, chronic wounds, stopped at the late inflammatory phase of healing process, are blocked from starting the proliferative phase [8], and this occurs even more often in diabetic patients [20].

Malnutrition is an additional risk factor that impacts surgical wound healing and can result from a variety of nutritional stages which negatively affect physiological scarring [21].

Elder patients are also fragile from a nutritional point of view; malnutrition can be linked to chronic pathologies, pharmacological treatments, and psychological or social and economic factors. In the presence of a wound, the need for nutrients dramatically increases to cover the faster metabolism: the request for protein increases by 250% and calories by 50% [21].

Vitamin C and D and zinc are the most common micronutrient deficiencies found; the first two are actively involved in the healing process for the synthesis of collagen, while zinc deficiency predisposes to immunodeficiency and an increased susceptibility to infections [21].

The stress plays an important role in the emergency surgery, in particular in patients with an acute abdominal pathology interfering with the inflammatory and infective status that may have already exhausted the body's reserves. In those patients, there is no sufficient time for the compensation mechanisms to be properly activated, with a negative impact on cardiopulmonary and renal systems. This stress-induced increase of glucocorticoids and corticosteroid production leads to the inhibition of cicatrization process: inhibition of keratinocyte proliferation, increased permeability of the epidermal barrier, and suppression of growth factors [22]. The psychological stress, associated with significant comorbidities, increases the risk of complications such as the altered repair process and the increase in postoperative infections rate [23].

From the analysis of the pathophysiological processes of wound healing and the concept of the elderly patient as a fragile patient, characterized by a precarious balance and with a reduced ability of adapting to the acute morbid state and even more to an urgent surgical intervention, reflections on the utility of laparoscopic surgery in urgency arise. The reduction of surgical stress leads to a better wound healing. The use of minimal surgical accesses prevents the execution of extensive laparotomies often hesitating in a seroma or hematoma that leads to a healing delay or sometimes to complete dehiscences. A wound healing by second intention, occurring over months in an elderly patient, is the cause of a delayed discharge, an increase in the morbidity rate, and the healthcare-related costs [23].

6.1 Laparoscopy in the Elderly, Inflammatory Response, and Reduction of Complications in Emergency Surgery

The introduction of laparoscopy represented the most important technical revolution in general surgery in the last 100 years. It has made possible to perform increasingly complex surgical procedures without the need for the classic "large cut," burdened by numerous perioperative complications.

During the "pioneering" phase, some categories of patients, in particular, the obese, the elderly, patients with comorbidities, and those who had already undergone a laparotomy, represented a contraindication to the use of laparoscopy.

However, once standardized the technique and overcome the learning curve, it has been clarified that belonging to one of those categories represents at most a relative contraindication to the use of minimally invasive surgery. Moreover, patients belonging to those groups are those who benefit the most from a less invasive approach [24].

This cultural leap has been made possible by studies that have shown a lower impact of laparoscopy compared to large laparotomies on respiratory mechanics, on the recovery of gastrointestinal motility (with the possibility of resuming oral feeding from the first postoperative day), on systemic response to surgical stress (with reduction of pro-inflammatory cytokine production and immunosuppression) with reduction of perioperative complications in the face of equivalence from the point of view of outcomes (in particular, oncologic one) [25]. These advantages have been incorporated in the recommendations of the enhanced recovery after surgery (ERAS) working group, and minimally invasive surgery is one of the items constantly present in most of the protocols and recommendations developed [26].

Many studies, conducted in particular on patients undergoing interventions for neoplastic pathology in an emergency setting and in elective one, show a reduction in the production of pro-inflammatory cytokines in subjects operated with the minimally invasive technique when compared to those operated with the classical technique. It has been shown a reduction in the immunosuppression typical of the postoperative phase after laparotomy. The advantages of these evidences are theoretically superior in the elderly and/or fragile subjects operated under an emergency regime, but at the moment there is no conclusive study in this sub-group of patients [27].

The advantages of minimally invasive techniques are not limited to the interventions performed in the election setting, but there are numerous evidences that have demonstrated their feasibility and validity even in the emergency one. Laparoscopy is now considered the last diagnostic act and can often be used for surgical therapy in case of appendicitis, cholecystitis, perforations of gastro-duodenal ulcers or other hollow viscera, intestinal occlusions, etc. A separate chapter is the use of laparoscopy in abdominal trauma, especially in penetrating lesions in hemodynamically stable patients in whom there is suspicion or certainty of violation of the peritoneum [28].

If in the world about 10% of subjects are over 65 years old, in Italy this percentage is almost doubled and in 2050 it is expected that about one-third of the population will have passed this age. Elderly subjects are the most "frail" patients because they often suffer from one or more comorbidities, and they are also those who are more likely to need surgery in both elective and emergency regimes [29, 30].

The poor cardiopulmonary reserve typical of elderly, the increased PCO_2 and the reduction of venous return due to pneumoperitoneum, as well as the reduction of the diaphragm excursion and the extreme positions (in particular, the Trendelenburg one) are the most often pathophysiological variations observed in patients undergoing minimally invasive surgery, and therefore the anesthetist must be adequately trained in the management of such situations. In particular, for the correct anesthesiological management of these patients, the use of numerous invasive and non-invasive monitoring systems is needed with the expenditure of energy and resources in the phase preceding induction [31–34].

Mortality in patients undergoing urgent surgery grows steadily with increasing age, exceeding 20% in people over 70 and almost 45% in over 80; similar considerations are applicable to postoperative morbidity rates, which reach over 50% in over 65 [35, 36].

The use of laparoscopy in the treatment of surgical emergencies in elderly patients is a niche subject but of increasing interest because it aims to reduce the postoperative complications rate (especially medical ones) that impact so heavily on in-hospital mortality as well as on healthcare costs. In literature, patients over 65 years of age and with a history of chronic renal failure, diabetes, anemia, myocardial infarction, and heart failure have a higher mortality than controls; also the presence of systemic inflammatory response syndrome (SIRS), a history of malignant tumor, liver failure, the use of oral anticoagulant therapy, and the use of open surgery are associated with an increased risk of postoperative complications [37, 38].

The FRAILESEL study [39] conducted on about 2000 patients collected data from 36 Italian centers on patients over 65 undergoing urgent laparoscopy. The results are of enormous interest: first of all almost 70% of the subjects enrolled are ASA III or IV. The study demonstrated a statistically significant reduction in both mortality and morbidity in patients undergoing laparoscopic surgery (mort. 2.2%; morb. 22.1%) compared to those undergoing laparotomic surgery (mort. 11.2%; morb. 36.2%). Interestingly, converted patients have similar mortality and morbidity rates to those operated with an open access from the beginning.

The FRAILESEL study includes contraindications to laparoscopic surgery (or indications for conversion): patients who are unable to tolerate pneumoperitoneum and therefore those with severe respiratory and cardiac insufficiency. Relative contraindications are represented by the presence of extensive adhesion syndrome, abnormal intestinal dilation, severe sepsis (with hemodynamic instability), and lack of equipment/team expertise. Open surgery and conversion are negative prognostic factors in patients over 65 undergoing urgent surgery.

These considerations will have to guide us in the future in choosing the best surgical approach in relation to comorbidities and the availability of material and human resources in order to offer a treatment as tailored as possible to the patient, bearing in mind the evidence now available in the literature.

6.2 Minimally Invasive Surgery in the Elderly and Choice of the Correct Surgical Incision

Among the advantages of the minimally invasive approach, the reduced incidence of surgical site infection is one of the most important. This aspect is much more significant in frail patients and elderly ones which, since concomitant pathologies and metabolic alterations are often present, are particularly exposed to this complication.

Avoiding large laparotomies, even in emergency surgery, not only allows to reduce postoperative pain and ensure faster recovery but significantly reduces the risk of abdominal wall contamination and the subsequent risk of postoperative incisional hernias.

The surgical site infection represents in fact the most important risk factor in the development of incisional hernias; the contamination of laparotomies ranges from the simple parcel opening of the incisions with or without evident contamination, to arrive to complete dehiscences with evisceration, in association or not with the presence of visceral fistulas.

These sequelae, in addition to exposing the patient to potentially fatal septic complications, determine a troubled postoperative course, with a significant increase in the length of hospital stay and a consequent significant increase in healthcare-related costs. The same consequences occur in the case of the formation of incisional hernias which, in addition to significantly worsening the quality of life of patients, given their advanced age, often risk to remain a permanent sequela. The problem is even more serious when one considers that a good percentage of these patients suffer from chronic respiratory diseases, whose precarious balance can easily be damaged by the development of voluminous relapsing hernias.

Incisional hernias represent the most frequent complication in abdominal surgical procedures, with an incidence ranging from 10 to 25% in the various Western series, which in elderly patients can reach 38%, especially after urgent interventions for acute abdominal peritonitis [40].

Due to the high incidence of this pathology, over the last few years many studies have been conducted to verify which incision was to be preferred to minimize the risk of post-surgical hernia, both in open surgery and in laparoscopy, in emergency and in elective settings. Similarly, various authors tried to establish what was the optimal surgical technique for closing the abdominal wall, as well as the materials to be used, in order to allow a standardization of the technique.

At this time the studies present in the literature still have not provided definitive answers, presenting significant biases both in the methods of implementation (data collection, sample creation, definition of end points) and in the analysis of the results (duration of follow-up and postoperative diagnostic investigations).

However, some data emerged with a rather strong degree of evidence; in particular, most of the works in the literature agree that median laparotomies (i.e., the vertical trans and periumbilical incisions made through the linea alba), regardless of their size, are burdened by a significantly higher incidence of incisional hernias when compared to the transversal ones performed externally with respect to the linea alba (i.e., all those laparotomies performed laterally with respect to the anterior sheath of the rectus abdominis, transversely, by divaricating, and not sectioning the muscle fibers) [41].

These data are evident both in "open" surgery and in "minimally invasive" one, when we refer to the service incisions used to extract the surgical specimen (10.6% vs. 3.7%) [42].

This percentage is further lowered if we take into consideration the data related to incisional hernias on Pfannenstiel incision (suprapubic incision performed by transversally dissecting the cutaneous, subcutaneous, and anterior sheath of the rectum, and laterally spreading the muscle bundles with subsequent vertical incision of the peritoneum) which is as low as 0.9% [43].

The reason why there is a lower tendency to develop incisional hernia after this type of surgical incision is due to the lower tensile force exerted by the abdominal pressure on the muscle aponeurotic surfaces compared to that exerted in other quadrants of the abdomen (especially medial), and moreover it is affected to a minimal extent by the respiratory excursions of the diaphragm, which can significantly increase postoperative pain [44].

On the other hand, laparotomies performed along the midline or in the lateral quadrants of the abdomen, on the right as on the left side, are affected to a greater extent by the forces generated by abdominal pressure, especially in patients with a high body mass index (BMI). Furthermore, due to postoperative pain and the accessory respiratory function of the abdominal muscles, these incisions are associated with a reduction of the diaphragm and chest excursions, predisposing to the onset of lung infections.

In the event that the site of the incision used for the extraction of the surgical specimen coincides with the site of the ostomy, the risk of subsequent hernia increases considerably, so this site should be avoided when possible.

In this regard, especially in urgent cases, in the presence of contaminated operating fields, the use of wall protection devices is strongly recommended, in order to isolate the wall from contaminating material [45].

Similarly, antibiotic prophylaxis, aimed at reducing the bacterial load at the site of the surgical incision, as well as a targeted postoperative antibiotic treatment based on antibiogram, plays an important role in reducing the risk of septic sequelae.

As regards the surgical technique to be used in the phase of closing the abdomen, the data in the literature provide important information.

According to what was reported in most of the randomized trials [46], the preferred technique in order to minimize the risk of incisional hernia involves the closure of the aponeurotic plane by continuous suturing with close passages of the stitches (0.5 mm), avoiding piercing and subsequently necrotize the muscle fibers. The suture must be in monofilament with high elasticity and slow resorption time; the ratio between the total length of the suture and the length of the wall incision must be equal to or greater than a ratio of 4 to 1 (SST, small stiches).

The fascial closure by continuous suturing with stitches in monofilament 1 with rarer bites (between 0.5 mm and 1 cm) would be burdened by the incidence of incisional hernia from 2 to 4 times greater than the technique described above.

The limitation of these studies is represented by the short duration of the follow-up period (on average 12–24 months, while most of the studies have shown that the incidence of incisional hernias progressively increases starting from the third year from the execution of the surgical procedure) and the lack of uniformity in the diagnostic investigations used in the follow-up (from the simple physical examination to the ultrasound of the abdomen up to the computed tomography (CT) or magnetic resonance imaging (MRI) of the abdominal wall).

The studies about the prophylactic use of prosthetic material in the closure phase of laparotomies are very interesting. The investigations carried out up to now show a significant reduction in the incidence of incisional hernias through the application of light polypropylene nets in the preperitoneal plane, with subsequent anchoring of the same to the fascial plane by means of non-absorbable Prolene stitches after creating an overlap of 4 cm (PRIMA Trial). These results are further amplified by associating the use of the net with the small stitches technique [47].

The preventive use of prosthetic material is not associated with an increased incidence of surgical site infection and is associated with a mean prolongation of operating time of about 20 min.

Finally, the problem of the development of hernias on trocar site should not be neglected, but the real incidence of this situation is probably underestimated due to the scarce symptoms related to it.

Most of the studies agree on the need for fascial closure at the insertion site of 10–12 mm trocars; on the other hand, there are no reliable data on the real incidence of wall defects in the site of placement of the 5 and 8 mm trocars [48].

Five Things You Should Know About Wound Healing in the Elderly and Frail Patients

- The elderly constitute a special sub-class of patient, characterized by a peculiar physiology of cellular and inflammatory processes related to age, in which the effects produced by the comorbidities are added; every therapeutic act, including surgery, must take into consideration the physiopathological response of these patients.
- Laparoscopy, even in an emergency setting, has been shown to have a lower impact on the organism, both in terms of reduced alteration of the respiratory dynamics and speed of restoration of bowel motility and nutrition, and as regards the reduction of immunosuppression and the production of pro-inflammatory cytokines.
- Advanced age and the presence of multiple comorbid factors are not an absolute contraindication to minimally invasive techniques; this category of patients earns the greatest benefits from laparoscopy in terms of postoperative mortality and morbidity: 2.2% versus 11.2% mortality in patients treated with laparoscopy than with the open approach, 22.1% versus 36.2% in terms of morbidity.
- 38% of frail and elderly emergency patients operated for acute abdomen develop an incisional hernia due to the more or less extensive dehiscence of the aponeurotic plane, favored by the development of a surgical site infection, negatively affecting the quality of life and the onset of further comorbidities and overall health-related expenditure.
- Transverse and non-midline surgical incisions are to be preferred over median and longitudinal incisions; among the service incisions, Pfannenstiel is associated with fewer complication rate (incisional hernia rate of 0.9%). The fascial layer should be closed with close bites (0.5 mm) according to the small stitches technique, using continuous sutures with slow resorption monofilament material (2/0).

References

1. Gould L, et al. Chronic wound repair and healing in older adults: current status and future research. Wound Repair Regen. 2015;23(1):1–13.
2. Nauta TD, van Hinsbergh VWM, Koolwijk P. Hypoxic signaling during tissue repair and regenerative medicine. Int J Mol Sci. 2014;15(11):19791–815.
3. Williams RW, Mason LB, Bradshaws HH. Factors affecting wound healing. Surg Forum, 1950;410–7.
4. Hong WX, et al. The role of hypoxia-inducible factor in wound healing. Adv Wound Care. 2014;3(5):390–9.
5. Falanga V. Wound healing and its impairment in the diabetic foot. Lancet. 2005;366(9498):1736–43.
6. Cazander G, Jukema GN, Nibbering PH. Complement activation and inhibition in wound healing. Clin Dev Immunol. 2012;2012:534291.
7. Rafail S, et al. Complement deficiency promotes cutaneous wound healing in mice. J Immunol. 2015;194(3):1285–91.
8. Yussof SJM, Omar E, Pai DR, Sood S. Cellular events and biomarkers of wound healing. Indian J Plast Surg. 2012;45(2):220–8.
9. Koh TJ, DiPietro LA. Inflammation and wound healing: the role of the macrophage. Expert Rev Mol Med. 2011;13:e23.
10. Schultz GS, Wysocki A. Interactions between extracellular matrix and growth factors in wound healing. Wound Repair Regen. 2009;17(2):153–62.
11. Velnar T, Bailey T, Smrkolj V. The wound healing process: an overview of the cellular and molecular mechanisms. J Int Med Res. 2009;37(5):1528–42.
12. Werner S, Grose R. Regulation of wound healing by growth factors and cytokines. Physiol Rev. 2003;83(3):835–70.
13. Eming SA, Martin P, Tomic-Canic M. Wound repair and regeneration: mechanisms, signaling, and translation. Sci Transl Med. 2014;6(265):265sr6.
14. Stolzenburg-Veeser L, Golubnitschaja O. Mini-encyclopaedia of the wound healing—Opportunities for integrating multi-omic approaches into medical practice. J Proteomics. 2018;188:71–84.

15. Husmann M, Willenberg T, Keo HH, Spring S, Kalodiki E, Delis KT. Integrity of venoarteriolar reflex determines level of microvascular skin flow enhancement with intermittent pneumatic compression. J Vasc Surg. 2008;48(6):1509–13.
16. Bentov I, Reed MJ. Anesthesia, microcirculation, and wound repair in aging. Anesthesiology. 2014;120(3):760–72.
17. Ojeh N, Pastar I, Tomic-Canic M, Stojadinovic O. Stem cells in skin regeneration, wound healing, and their clinical applications. Int J Mol Sci. 2015;16(10):25476–501.
18. Martin P, Nunan R. Cellular and molecular mechanisms of repair in acute and chronic wound healing. Br J Dermatol. 2015;173(2):370–8.
19. Yang Y, et al. Compromised wound healing in ischemic type 2 diabetic rats. PLoS One. 2016;11(3):e0152068.
20. Pence BD, Woods JA. Exercise, obesity, and cutaneous wound healing: evidence from rodent and human studies. Adv Wound Care. 2014;3(1):71–9.
21. Molnar JA, Underdown MJ, Clark WA. Nutrition and chronic wounds. Adv Wound Care. 2014;3(11):663–81.
22. Chen Y, Lyga J. Brain-skin connection: stress, inflammation and skin aging. Inflamm Allergy Drug Targets. 2014;13(3):177–90.
23. de Luis A, Culebras JM, Aller R, Eiros-Bouza JM. Surgical infection and malnutrition. Nutr Hosp. 2014;30(3):509–13.
24. Scott MJ, Baldini G, Fearon KCH, Feldheiser A, Feldman LS, Gan TJ, Ljungqvist O, Lobo DN, Rockall TA, Schricker T, Carli F. Enhanced recovery after surgery (ERAS) for gastrointestinal surgery, part 1: pathophysiological considerations. Acta Anaesthesiol Scand. 2015;59(10):1212–3.
25. Caglià P, Tracia A, Buffone A, Amodeo L, Tracia L, Amodeo C, Veroux M. Physiopathology and clinical considerations of laparoscopic surgery in the elderly. Int J Surg. 2016;33(Suppl 1):S97–S102.
26. Gustafsson UO, Scott MJ, Schwenke W, Demartinesf N, Roulinf D, Francisg N, McNaughth CE, MacFieh J, Libermani AS, Soopj M, Hillk A, Kennedy RH, Lobom DN, Ljungqvisto FO. Guidelines for perioperative care in elective colonic surgery: Enhanced Recovery After Surgery (ERAS®) Society recommendations. Clin Nutr. 2012;31(6):783–800.
27. Xia X, Zhang Z, Xu J, Zhaoand G, Yu F. Comparison of postoperative lymphocytes and interleukins between laparoscopy-assisted and open radical gastrectomy for early gastric cancer. J Int Med Res. 2019;47(1):303–10.
28. Mandrioli M, Inaba K, Piccinini A, Biscardi A, Sartelli M, Agresta F, Catena F, Cirocchi R, Jovine E, Tugnoli G, Di Saverio S. Advances in laparoscopy for acute care surgery and trauma. World J Gastroenterol. 2016;22(2):668–80.
29. Istat: Stime per l'anno 2016. 2017.
30. United Nations, Department of Economic and Social Affairs, Population Division: World Population Ageing. (ST/ESA/SER.A/390). 2015.
31. Westerband A, Van De Water JM, Amzallag M, Lebowitz PW, Nwasokwa ON, Chardavoyne R, Abou-Taleb RA, Wang X, Wise L. Cardiovascular changes during laparoscopic cholecystectomy. Surg Gynecol Obstet. 1992;175:535–8.
32. Kelman GR, Swapp GH, Smith I, Benzie RJ, Gordon NL. Cardiac output and arterial blood-gas tension during laparoscopy. Br J Anaesth. 1972;44:1155–61.
33. Myre K, Buanes T, Smith G, Stokland O. Simultaneous hemodynamic and echocardiographic changes during abdominal gas insufflation. Surg Laparosc Endosc. 1997;7:415–9.
34. Feig BW, Berger DH, Dougherty TB, et al. Pharmacologic intervention can reestablish baseline hemodynamic parameters during laparoscopy. Surgery. 1994;116:733–41.
35. Gomes A, Rocha R, Marinho R, et al. Colorectal surgical mortality and morbidity in elderly patients: comparison of POSSUM, P-POSSUM, CR-POSSUM, and CR-BHOM. Int J Colorectal Dis. 2015;30(2):173–9.
36. Oliver CM, Walker E, Giannaris S, et al. Risk assessment tools validated for patients undergoing emergency laparotomy: a systematic review. Br J Anaesth. 115(6):849–60.
37. Ward NT, Ramamoorthy SL, Chang DC, Parsons JK. Laparoscopic appendectomy is safer than open appendectomy in an elderly population. JSLS. 2014;18(3):1–8.
38. Caglia P, Tracia A, Buffone A, Amodeo L, Tracia L, Amodeo C, Veroux M. Physiopathology and clinical considerations of laparoscopic surgery in the elderly. Int J Surg. 2016;33:S97–S102.
39. Costa G, Fransvea P, Podda M, Pisanu A, Carrano FM, Iossa A, Balducci G, Agresta F, the ERASO (Elderly Risk Assessment and Surgical Outcome) Collaborative Study Group. The use of emergency laparoscopy for acute abdomen in the elderly: the FRAILESEL Italian Multicenter Prospective Cohort. Updates Surg. 2020;72(2):513–25.
40. Lee L, Abou-Khalil M, Liberman S, Boutros M, Fried GM, Feldman LS. Incidence of incisional hernia in the specimen extraction site for laparoscopic colorectal surgery: systematic review and meta-analysis. Surg Endosc. 31(12):5083–93. https://doi.org/10.1007/s00464-017-5573-2.
41. Lee L, Mata J, Droeser RA, Kaneva P, Liberman S, Cherlebois P, Stein B, Fried GM, Feldman LS. Incisional hernia after midline versus transverse specimen extraction incision. Ann Surg. 2018;268(1):41–7.
42. Benlice C, Stocchi L, Costedio MM, Gorgun E, Kessler H. Impact of the specific extraction-site location on the risk of incisional hernia after laparoscopic colorectal resection. Dis Colon Rectum. 2016;59:743–50.
43. Orcutt ST, Balentine CJ, Marshall CL, Robinson CN, Anaya DA, Artinyan A, Awad SS, Berger DH, Albo D. Use of Pfannenstiel incision in minimally colorectal cancer surgery is associated with a lower

risk of wound complications. Tech Coloproctol. 2012;16:127–32.

44. Fabozzi M, Cirillo P, Corcione F. Surgical approach to right colon cancer: from open technique to robot. State of art. World J Gastrointest Surg. 2016;8(8):564–73.
45. Benlice C, Stocchi L, Sapci I, Gorgun E, Kessler H, Liska D, Steele SR, Delaney CP. Impact of the extraction-site location on wound infections after laparoscopic colorectal resection. Am J Surg. 2019;217(3):507–8.
46. Deerenberg EB, Harlaar JJ, Steyerberg EW, Lont HE, van Doorn HC, Heisterkamp J, Wijnhoven BP, Schouten WR, Cense HA, Stockmann HB, Berends FJ, Dijkhuizen FPH, Dwarkasing RS, Jairam AP, van Ramshorst GH, Kleinrensink GJ, Jeekel J, Lange JF. Small bites versus large bites for closure of abdominal midline incisions (STITCH): a double-blind, multicentre, randomised controller trial. Lancet. 2015;386(10000):1254–60.
47. Heger P, Feibt M, Krisam J, Klose C, Dorr-Harim C, Tenckhoff S, Buchler MW, Djener MK, Mihljevic AL. Hernia reduction fallowing laparotomy using small stitch abdominal wall closure with and without mesh augmentation (the HULC trial): study protocol for a randomized controller trial. Trials. 2019;20(1):738.
48. Harr JN, Juo Y-Y, Luka S, Agarwal S, Brody F, Obias V. Incisional and port-site hernias fallowing robotic colorectal surgery. Surg Endosc. 30(8) 3505–10. https://doi.org/10.1007/s00464-015-4639-2.

Part II

Surgery

Acute Cholecystitis

7

Fabio Cesare Campanile, Monica De Angelis, Elisabetta Santucci, and Ilaria Vecchioni

7.1 Introduction

Acute cholecystitis is found in 3–10% of all patients with abdominal pain [1, 2]. Gallstones cause more than 90% of acute cholecystitis [3, 4] because their prevalence increases with age, the disease is more common in the aged. About 50–70% of the acute cholecystitis occurs in elderly patients [5]. Life expectancy rises worldwide, and the challenges of diagnosis and treatment for acute cholecystitis in this population segment become more relevant every day.

Old age and frailty have crucial implications in the management of acute cholecystitis; higher prevalence of comorbidities, more frequent complications, and increased number of severe forms make the risk of severe consequences substantial. Retrospective studies have confirmed that surgery for acute cholecystitis is more lethal in the aged [6].

More than 50% of frail people are older than 70 years [7], and the literature on acute cholecystitis rarely analyzed separately the two aspects of chronological age and frailty; only a few series perform a subgroup or multivariate logistic regression analysis to distinguish age, comorbidity, and frailty; no study focuses on the frailty scores described in Chap. 1. One group even suggests defining the term *elderly* using immuno-inflammatory indices instead of a simple chronological age cut-off [8]. In this chapter, we will attempt to clarify the role of chronological age as an independent risk factor, but will use the term *elderly* or *aged* to indicate a population that is elderly and frail at the same time, unless differently specified.

7.2 Diagnosis

The clinical diagnosis of acute cholecystitis results from a combination of signs, symptoms, laboratory tests, and imaging. Every single diagnostic element has a limited predictive value [9–11]. Both the European Association for Endoscopic Surgery (EAES) and the Tokyo guidelines suggested sets of diagnostic criteria (Tables 7.1, 7.2, and 7.3) to improve the diagnosis accuracy [12–15] and the criteria do not vary for elderly or younger people. However, age-related changes influence many of those criteria and may challenge our diagnostic ability. A large retrospective study confirmed that older patients with acute abdominal pain were more often misdiagnosed than younger patients with similar conditions, both at the hospital admission and discharge [16].

F. C. Campanile (✉) · M. De Angelis · E. Santucci
I. Vecchioni
Division of Surgery, ASL Viterbo, Ospedale San Giovanni Decollato Andosilla, Civita Castellana, Italy

F. Agresta et al. (eds.), *Emergency laparoscopic surgery in the elderly and frail patient*,
https://doi.org/10.1007/978-3-030-79990-8_7

Table 7.1 EAES diagnostic criteria for acute cholecystitis

A. **Acute RUQ pain for more than 6 hours** AND **Ultrasound evidence of acute cholecystitis** (presence of gallstones with a thickened and edematous gallbladder wall, positive ultrasound Murphy's sign, and pericholecystic fluid collections)
B. **Acute RUQ pain for more than 6 hours** AND **Ultrasound evidence of gallstones** AND **One or more of the following:** 1. Temperature above 38 °C 2. WBC count greater than 10,000/mm^3 3. CRP higher than 10 mg/L

RUQ right upper abdominal quadrant, *CRP* C-reactive protein, *WBC* white blood cell

With kind permission from Springer Nature: Sauerland et al. (2006) Laparoscopy for abdominal emergency: Evidence-based guidelines of the European Association for Endoscopic Surgery. Surg Endosc 20(1):14–29. ©Springer Science + Business Media, Inc. 2005 [12, 13]

Table 7.2 TG13/TG18 diagnostic criteria for acute cholecystitis

A. Local signs of inflammation, etc. 1 Murphy's sign 2 RUQ mass/pain/tenderness
B. Systemic signs of inflammation, etc. 1. Fever 2. Elevated CRP 3. Elevated WBC count
C. Imaging findings Imaging findings characteristic of acute cholecystitis
Suspected diagnosis: One item in A + one item in B **Definite diagnosis: One item in A + one item in B + C**

RUQ right upper abdominal quadrant, *CRP* C-reactive protein, *WBC* white blood cell

With kind permission from John Wiley and Sons: Yokoe M, et al. (2018) Tokyo Guidelines 2018: diagnostic criteria and severity grading of acute cholecystitis (with videos). J Hepatobiliary Pancreat Sci 25(1):41–54. ©Japanese Society of Hepato-Biliary-Pancreatic Surgery and Springer 2018. Table 7.1 [14]. (modified)

7.2.1 History and Physical

Evaluating an acute condition in elderly patients takes more time and effort than in the general population. Many physiologic, pharmacologic, and psychological factors have to be considered, and the coexistence of multiple diseases makes the condition more complex. When we consider the age-related changes in the diagnostic criteria, we must be aware that most available data comes from low-evidence observational studies, often with conflicting results.

The most common symptom is the right upper quadrant abdominal pain; it is almost uniformly present in acute cholecystitis patients of all ages [17], and the elderly are not an exception: it is found in 73–98% of them [18, 19]. However, in the aged, the clinical picture is often misleadingly benign [20]. Experimental and clinical studies demonstrated a higher pain threshold with advancing age, but a lower tolerance to intense pain; this is probably due to neural and biochemical age-related differences [21]. Reduced pain perception has also been shown in several acute abdominal conditions [22, 23]; in acute cholecystitis, atypical presentations with reduced or even no pain are frequent [19].

The symptom's evaluation is also often difficult due to cognitive impairment or reduction in

Table 7.3 TG07 Imaging findings of acute cholecystitis

Ultrasonography findings Murphy sign (tenderness elicited by pressing the gallbladder with the ultrasound probe) enlarged gallbladder (long axis diameter > 8 cm, short axis diameter > 4 cm) incarcerated gallstone, debris echo, pericholecystic fluid collection Sonolucent layer in the gallbladder wall, striated intramural lucencies, and Doppler signals
Magnetic resonance imaging (MRI) findings Pericholecystic high signal Enlarged gallbladder Thickened gallbladder wall
Computed tomography (CT) findings Thickened gallbladder wall pericholecystic fluid collection Enlarged gallbladder Linear high-density areas in the pericholecystic fat tissue
Tc-HIDA scans Non-visualized gallbladder with normal uptake and excretion of radioactivity; Rim sign (augmentation of radioactivity around the gallbladder fossa)

With kind permission from John Wiley and Sons: Hirota M, et al. (2007) Diagnostic criteria and severity assessment of acute cholecystitis: Tokyo Guidelines. J Hepatobiliary Pancreat Sci 14:78–82. ©2007 Japanese Society of Hepatobiliary Pancreatic Surgery [15]. (modified)

the communication ability for visual or hearing loss. On the other side, an altered mental or cognitive status may be the consequence of an infection, particularly in geriatric patients [24], and be mistaken as pre-existent. All these factors may limit the possibility to collect a complete history. Also, older adults may underreport their condition, assuming it is due to aging or fearing to lose their autonomy with the hospitalization. For the same reason, they tend to present later in the course of their disease [16, 25].

If taking the history in an aged patient may be difficult, the physical examination is similarly challenging. Physiological age-related muscle atrophy may reduce the abdominal wall response, and peritoneal signs are milder in an older patient. Also, commonly used medications (pain killers, beta-blockers, anti-inflammatory and anticholinergic drugs) may alter the patient reaction to physical examination maneuvers or the disease itself. In a logistic regression analysis on a large cohort of patients with abdominal inflammatory conditions, signs such as rebound tenderness, guarding, and rectal tenderness were less common at higher ages [16]; Murphy's sign, one of the most important predictors of acute cholecystitis [9, 26], has only 48% sensitivity in older people [27]. We should not rely on the absence or mildness of peritoneal signs to rule out acute cholecystitis in an older patient.

7.2.2 Systemic Signs of Inflammation

Normal aging implies relevant changes in response to inflammatory stimuli, besides a higher baseline inflammatory condition.

Fever is one of the most significant signs in acute cholecystitis [28]; its sensitivity varies from 31 to 62% and its specificity from 37 to 74% [11, 29]. Studies comparing elderly and younger abdominal infection patients show that fever is often absent or low in the geriatric patients [25], and case series confirm that it is present in 36–74% of acute cholecystitis patients, but only 6.4–10% of them had a temperature higher than 38 °C [19, 30].

At least three comparative studies examined the differences in WBC between elderly and non-elderly patients: one of them showed a higher rate of leucocytosis in the elderly group (41.2 vs. 26.4%: $P = 0.005$) [31]; the other, significantly higher mean WBC [32, 33].

C-reactive protein (CRP) is also higher in the aged. In one study, the elderly patients were more likely to have elevated CRP (64.1 vs. 35.1%; $P < 0.01$) [31]; another study demonstrated significantly higher mean levels than in the younger patients (26.4 vs. 22.4; $P = 0.04$) [32].

The described differences in WBC and CRP could be due to the altered immunologic mechanisms or to the higher rate of severe cholecystitis in the aged: on one side, the activity and number of several white cell populations is modified, and elevated circulating levels of proinflammatory cytokines are found [34]; on the other, empyema of the gallbladder, gangrenous cholecystitis, or free gallbladder perforations are more common in the elderly [20, 28, 35–37].

7.3 Should We Operate on Elderly and Frail Patients?

Older people are commonly considered to carry a higher risk for surgery. A reduced life expectancy has also to be taken into consideration when we balance benefits and disadvantages of any surgical approach; and surgery in an acute condition implies additional risk. For these reasons, older patients are less likely to undergo a cholecystectomy for acute cholecystitis [38–40].

7.3.1 Does Advanced Age Increase the Risk for Surgery?

The reduced utilization of surgery for elderly and frail people largely derives from the perception of their increased surgical risk. The fear that the cure could be worse than the disease itself, coupled with a somewhat defensive attitude by the surgical teams, may end up with the denial of the best available therapeutic opportunity for this group of people.

A large Swedish nation-wide study analyzed the outcome of cholecystectomy: the mortality risk increased by age in each diagnostic group (chronic calculous, chronic acalculous, acute calculous, acute acalculous). The authors calculated a Standardized Mortality Ratios (SMR) using age-,gender-, and calendar year-specific expected survival estimates from the Swedish Death Register. In the acute calculous group, the SMR in octogenarians was 6.41 versus 1.75 in patients younger than 64. However, in their overall series, only 19.1% of the acute calculous cholecystitis patients had laparoscopic surgery. In the years 1995–99 the percentage was 35.5%, but only 17.7% of patients older than 70 [6].

On laparoscopic cholecystectomy only, focused a very recent systematic review and meta-analysis of 99 comparative studies and 326,517 patients: age above 65 resulted in a seven-fold increase in post-operative mortality of the overall cohort (ten-fold in patients ≥80 years old). The result was consistent even when stratified by the urgency of the procedure with higher rates in both elective (OR 13.34, CI 95% 2.07–85.92) and emergency (OR 5.54, CI 95% 1.96–15.70) surgery; this was true for all age cut-off subgroups (≥65, ≥70, ≥75, and ≥80 years). The elderly morbidity rate in elective (OR 2.46, CI 95% 1.63–3.71) and emergency (OR 1.98, CI 95% 1.33–2.94) laparoscopic surgery was also increased for all age cut-offs [41].

However, the large systematic review could not account for the coexistence of comorbidities in the cohort, and cannot clarify if age is an independent risk factor for morbidity and mortality. The issue is addressed in several other studies.

7.3.2 Is Age an Independent Risk Factor?

Is advanced age an independent risk predictor, due to a reduced physiological reserve, or the increased morbidity and mortality of the elderly patients are related to their more frequent and severe comorbidities? Most studies addressing the issues are observational, and their age groups are generally poorly comparable due to multiple confounding factors, the consistently higher presence of co-morbid conditions in the older patients in particular.

An extensive large cross-sectional analysis of the Health Care Utilization Project Nation-wide Inpatient Sample (1999–2006) compared elderly (65–79 and ≥80 years old) to younger (50–64 years old) cholecystectomy patients. The study did not perform a subgroup analysis for acute cholecystitis, but included admission urgency and comorbidity among the clinical covariates for the multivariate logistic regression. Age was an independent predictor of outcome; patients aged 65 to 79 had a greater than two-fold (OR = 2.31) and those 80 a six-fold (OR = 5.91) odds of death.[1] Elderly patients also had higher odds for complications [42].

In 2014, Nielsen et al. studied a large national cholecystectomy database and demonstrated that age is an independent prognostic predictor. Patients older than 80 had significantly worse mortality, even if they had a low anesthetic risk; they compared three age groups (>80 vs. 65–79 vs. 50–64) and found higher mortality in the ASA I and II subgroups (Odds Ratio 30.86 vs. 5.51 vs. 1), but their study included elective and emergency gallstone surgery [43].

In the same year, a large retrospective study on cholecystectomy in acute cholecystitis confirmed that octogenarians have significantly higher mortality (4% vs. 1%; $P = 0.038$) and morbidity (31% vs. 13%; $P < 0.001$). On the study multivariate analysis, age 80 years or greater was an independent risk factor for complications (Odds Ratio 2.5) [35].

Other large retrospective and population-based studies confirmed that advanced age is an independent predictor for morbidity and mortality in acute cholecystitis surgery [44, 45].

7.3.3 What Is the Risk of Not Operating?

Cholecystectomy for acute calculous cholecystitis carries a worse prognosis in elderly patients than in their younger counterparts and advanced

[1]After adjustment for time to surgery, gender, race, number of biliary diagnoses, type of procedure, admission urgency, comorbidities, year, hospital size, and hospital teaching status.

age is an independent risk factor. Still, we will not be able to make a decision about surgery for acute calculous cholecystitis in the aged, unless we compare those who had cholecystectomy to those who did not.

7.3.3.1 Mortality and Morbidity

In 2010, Riall et al. published a retrospective US-based study on 29,918 elderly acute cholecystitis patients, and showed that who did not receive surgery at the index admission had twice as high mortality as those who did. Their series included patients 66 years old or above, with a mean age of 77.7 ± 7.3 years.[2] Because this kind of data implies a high risk of selection bias (the healthier patients are commonly selected for surgery, and the sickest for conservative or delayed treatment), the authors used a multivariate Cox proportional hazard model, and confirmed that the patients in the non-surgical group were 56% more likely to die, even after adjustment for patient demographics and comorbidities.[3]

The study made clear that most US surgeons felt confident in offering cholecystectomy in an acute setting to elderly patients: 75% of the series had surgery on the first admission (71% laparoscopic), and only 25% was discharged without it [38].

The opposite is true in a recent UK based population-based cohort study by Wiggins et al.: in the analyzed series of 47,500 aged patients (≥80 years), only 7.5% received cholecystectomy; 89.7% was treated conservatively, and 2.8% had cholecystostomy. Despite the different treatment allocation, the study confirmed that lack of definitive surgery at the first admission was associated with a higher 1-year mortality rate (20.8 in the surgical group vs. 27.1% in the conservative and 35.5% in the cholecystostomy group). Again, the older and sicker patients were less likely to receive surgery, but the multivariate analysis confirmed that age was an independent mortality factor [45].

The UK study mortality in each subgroup was higher than in the above mentioned US series; however, we have to consider several differences in the studied populations. The much lower utilization of emergency cholecystectomy (in particular laparoscopic) in the UK is well known [46]; only a small fraction of the 3,539 cholecystectomies was laparoscopic; also, the UK series focused on octogenarians and included older patients (mean age 85 vs. 77.7), more males, but excluded those with common bile duct stones at the first admission.

7.3.3.2 Recurrence and Readmission

Another relevant aspect is the recurrence of biliary symptoms and the need for a new hospital admission after a non-operative or expectant decision.

The study by Riall demonstrated that lack of definitive therapy at the index admission was followed by a 38% gallstone-related readmission rate in the 2 years after discharge, against a 4% readmission rate in the surgical group patients ($P < 0.0001$). The subsequent cholecystectomy rate was 27% [38]. The readmission rate in Wiggins report is very similar; more than a half (55.2%) of conservatively treated patients needed a subsequent hospital admission during the study period.[4] After cholecystectomy at the index admission, 16.8% of the patients required emergency readmission; part of them for retained common bile duct stone or bile leak (1.3%); 2.1% required common bile duct reconstruction for a surgical injury [45].

A recent systematic review calculated a 19.7% pooled recurrence rate of gallstone-related disease during long term follow-up after conservative treatment for acute cholecystitis in elderly or high-risk patients. Most of the recurrences occurred within 2 years after the index admission [47].

---

[2] The 30-day, 1-year, and 2-year cumulative mortality rates were 2, 9, and 15.2% in surgical group; versus 5, 19.4, and 29.3% in the non-surgical group ($p < 0.0001$).

[3] Hazard Ratio = 1.56, 95% CI 1.47–1.65

[4] In 37.7% the readmission was due to a new episode of cholecystitis; they also reported 2.3% cholangitis, 6.8% obstructive jaundice, 6.5% biliary colic, and 1.9% pancreatitis.

7.4 Laparoscopic or Open Cholecystectomy in Advanced Age?

Laparoscopic cholecystectomy is the gold standard for the treatment of acute cholecystitis according to all the international guidelines [13, 48–50].

Several randomized and non-randomized studies show the superiority of laparoscopic cholecystectomy in the acute setting. A recent meta-analysis demonstrate a lower complication rate in laparoscopic than open surgery for acute cholecystitis [51]; the study, however, is not focused on elderly patients. On the other side, Antoniou et al., in a systematic review with meta-analysis, compared elderly patients and found that open cholecystectomy had two-fold morbidity and four-fold mortality than laparoscopic. However, their analysis (besides being limited by the low quality of the data) does not focus on acute cholecystitis.

Then, we are left with the original question: should we prefer laparoscopic or open cholecystectomy for elderly and frail patients for acute calculous cholecystitis?

7.4.1 Could Open Surgery Be Advantageous?

We know that older patients are more likely to undergo straight open cholecystectomy and have a laparoscopic procedure converted to open [43]. In Sect. 7.3.3.1, we have examined the diverse laparoscopic attitude in two different countries.

The large population-based research by Wiggins proved that laparoscopic cholecystectomy was associated with improved outcomes, with an 84% relative risk reduction in 30-day mortality compared to open surgery [45]. This confirms the results of previous observational studies that found that morbidity and mortality rates were either similar [52] or improved [53, 54] in laparoscopic over open cholecystectomy for acute cholecystitis in the elderly population, along with a reduction in hospital stay.

Laparoscopic cholecystectomy is better than open in the elderly for treating acute cholecystitis, probably for its reduced impact on this population's delicate physiological balance. Less surgical trauma, metabolic stress [55, 56], and immunosuppression [57, 58], improved postoperative cardiac [59] and respiratory function [55, 60] have been extensively shown in laparoscopic versus open cholecystectomy. The physiopathologic advantage is likely to be larger in the older patients, for which the impact of those factors is greater [61, 62].

7.5 Early or Delayed

A large amount of literature supports the use of "early" laparoscopic cholecystectomy for the treatment of acute calculous cholecystitis in the general population; the international guidelines analyze those data and agree that acute cholecystitis should be operated on as soon as possible after the onset of symptoms [13, 14, 48, 49].

Can we apply the same recommendation to the subset of the elderly patients, despite their higher morbidity and mortality in the acute setting? Should we consider deferring surgery to a more elective "delayed" situation?

7.5.1 Should we Delay Surgery in Elderly and Frail Patients?

The guidelines' panels examined several randomized controlled trials, meta-analyses, and large population-based studies. They differ in the exact definition of "early" (between 3 and 10 days) and "late" cholecystectomy, but support early surgery because it does not increase the complication and conversion rates, but reduce the total hospital length of stay.[5] Despite one of the meta-analysis warned about an increase in common bile duct injury in the delayed group (not statistically significant) [63], the recommendations are based on "soft" outcomes and do not

[5]A detailed description of their findings is outside the scope of this work; a more complete discussion about early and late surgical treatment in acute cholecystitis can be found in some of the mentioned guidelines [48, 49].

preclude that particular circumstances may suggest a different course of action.

Mortality in the aged is higher in an emergency than elective cholecystectomy in a Swedish population-based series [6]. A retrospective observational study by Lupinacci found higher mortality in aged patients if surgery was performed in an emergency rather than an elective setting [64]. However, these findings should not induce us to think that delaying surgical treatment is beneficial to the aged.

The two studies by Riall and Wiggins clarified that the lack of treatment at the index admission in the elderly is followed by worse medium term survival, and increased gallstone-related subsequent admission rate [38, 45].

A large population-based study included 10,304 acute cholecystectomy patients discharged without cholecystectomy. The authors performed an interesting subgroup analysis and found that the unadjusted probability of a gallstone-related event was inversely related to age; patients older than 80 had the lowest incidence of events across age groups, but still suffered from about 10% emergency room visit or hospital admission for biliary colic, recurrent cholecystitis, common bile duct stones, cholangitis, or pancreatitis, in the 6 weeks following the index episode (a commonly adopted interval for delayed cholecystectomy). The rate at 12 weeks was about 15% [65].

Other cohort studies directly compared early versus delayed surgery outcomes for acute calculous cholecystitis in the aged. As in the general population, morbidity, mortality, and conversion rates are similar for early and delayed cholecystectomy; hospital stay is longer for the latter [66–69]. In addition, recurrent cholecystitis, cholangitis, and pancreatitis are four times more frequent in the delayed than in the early group of a retrospective observational study [70].

7.6 Percutaneous Cholecystostomy

So far, we determined that aged persons with acute cholecystitis benefit from the same therapeutic indications as the general population, despite higher morbidity and mortality.

To avoid surgery for frail and elderly septic patients, alternative treatments have been introduced, such as the *percutaneous gallbladder drainage* (or *cholecystostomy*). Its rationale is to control the source of sepsis with a definitive or temporary procedure that improves the clinical conditions but avoids the general anesthesia and surgical stress.

The percutaneous drainage obtained a large visibility after the Tokyo guidelines recommended it not only for the *severe*, but also for a significant part of the *moderate* acute cholecystitis patients [50, 71].[6] Since then, the utilization of percutaneous drainage has been increasing worldwide [72, 73]. Other guidelines are more cautious about its use waiting for the results of the CHOCOLATE trial that has been published only very recently [74]. They limit the cholecystostomy indications only to patients that are unfit for surgery, after failure of the conservative therapy [13, 48, 49].

7.6.1 The Observational Studies

The practice of percutaneous gallbladder drainage has been endorsed by many poor quality case series that reported single groups' experience. They often concluded that the procedure has low short-term morbidity, mortality, and is "feasible and safe." In 2009, Winbladh et al. published a systematic review of the available literature and warned that, despite a reported high success rate (85.6%) and low mortality directly related to it, the procedure was associated with a 30-day mortality (15.4%) significantly higher than reported after early cholecystectomy in similar patients [75]. Therefore, the outcomes of the percutaneous drainage should be analyzed against those of the early surgical treatment.

Since then, several controlled studies have compared cholecystostomy to early laparoscopic cholecystectomy.

[6] The Tokyo guidelines classify as *severe* any cholecystitis with organ/system dysfunction (cardiovascular, respiratory, renal, hematologic, hepatic, neurological), and *moderate* any cholecystitis with elevated WBC count (>18,000/mm³), palpable tender mass, duration of complaints >72 h, or marked local inflammation [15].

An interesting small retrospective comparative study compared percutaneous cholecystostomy and emergency cholecystectomy in homogeneous groups by age and surgical risk (according to POSSUM, Charlson, APACHE II, and ASA scores). It found that in the cholecystostomy group the mortality rate was significantly higher (17.2% vs. nil); besides, one-third of the cholecystostomy patients had a failure of the percutaneous treatment, and cholecystectomy was necessary [76].

Stronger evidence is brought by three large retrospective cohort studies based on administrative databases. They are consistent in indicating that, even in this frail population, the percutaneous drainage is worse than emergency laparoscopic surgery in terms of mortality (from 1.45-fold to 34.22-fold in the diverse studies and examined subgroups) and readmission rates [72, 73, 77].

7.6.2 The Randomized Trials

In 2002, a randomized trial found that percutaneous gallbladder drainage was not better than conservative treatment in reducing mortality of 123 high-risk patients (APACHE II score ≥ 12) with acute cholecystitis.

The highest level of evidence on the topic is provided by the CHOCOLATE trial: a methodologically rigorous Dutch multicenter, randomized, superiority trial designed to assess if early laparoscopic cholecystectomy is superior to percutaneous catheter drainage in high-risk patients with acute calculous cholecystitis [74]. *Acute cholecystitis* was defined as in the Tokyo guidelines, and *high-risk* as an APACHE II score between 7 and 14. Patients with 15 or higher score were excluded because they were considered unfit for surgery and could not be randomized. The researchers expected to enroll 284 patients study, but the study had to be interrupted early for safety concerns about the adverse outcomes in the percutaneous drainage group a planned interim analysis showed a large and statistically significant difference in major complication (65% vs. 12%), reintervention (66% vs. 12%), and gallstone-related readmission rates (53% vs. 5%) in favor of the cholecystectomy group. At termination, 142 patients had been randomized. The mortality rate did not reach statistical significance; however, the cholecystostomy group had a three-fold mortality rate (6 vs. 3 patients; 9% vs. 3%) compared to the surgical group.[7] Emergency cholecystectomy was performed in 11 of the 68 patients (16%) assigned to the cholecystostomy group. Early surgery also reduced the use of healthcare resources and costs.

The trial provides strong evidence that early laparoscopic cholecystectomy is superior to percutaneous cholecystostomy to treat acute calculous cholecystitis in high-risk patients. Early emergency surgery should be the standard treatment even for this subset of patients, unless their condition is so severe to absolutely prevent the surgical option.

7.7 Is a Tailored Approach Possible?

Acute cholecystitis is a heterogeneous disease. Its clinical severity and prognosis are related not only to the local and systemic inflammation but also to the general conditions of the patients and their multiple interconnected risk factors.

The available research shows that definitive treatment by early laparoscopic cholecystectomy is the optimal available treatment not only for the general population, but also for elderly and frail patients affected by acute cholecystitis. The large population-based studies confirmed that early surgery offers the best cure for the elderly and frail population, but their series includes heterogeneous patients with different risk profiles. It might be argued that we could identify subgroups of patients that, for particular conditions or severity grade, may have a better chance of cure with an alternative treatment [78, 79]. An appropriate

[7] Two patients in each group died during the follow-up for unrelated causes (cancer or intestinal ischemia) and one (in the drainage group) for unknown cause. The remaining three deaths in the drainage group were due to cholecystitis related sepsis.

preoperative score or set of parameters could be of great help in tailoring the treatment to the individual patient's needs.

A few studies addressed the issue of risk stratification for acute cholecystitis. The ASA score has been used to determine the risk of morbidity in elderly high-risk patients [80, 81]. ASA, APACHE II, and POSSUM scores have been associated with morbidity and mortality in patients with perforated acute cholecystitis [82]. Some researchers proposed to use the Charlson Comorbidity Index (CCI) to help in identifying the best therapeutic option for higher risk patients [83, 84]. However, at present, we do not have a validated score with the granular prediction needed to play a significant role in the decision making for our frailer patients.

7.8 Conclusions

Elderly and frail people risk of death or complications as a consequence of acute cholecystitis is higher than in younger and healthier people. Their risks of a negative outcome after surgery are also higher than in the general population because of their coexistent pathological conditions, but also for the advanced age that is an independent risk factor.

Alternative treatments as percutaneous cholecystectomy have been proposed to reduce the risk, but they are associated with unacceptably high mortality and morbidity rate in the long term, and should be reserved for those patients clearly unsuitable for surgery. Delayed or conservative treatment has a worse outcome than emergency surgery.

To the best of our knowledge, early laparoscopic cholecystectomy remains the gold standard for the treatment of this acute condition in such a delicate segment of the population, despite the surgical risk being higher than in younger patients.

Five Things You Should Know About

- Age-related changes influence the diagnostic criteria and may challenge our diagnostic ability;
- Despite the increased risk, surgery is still the best option for elderly patients: mortality, morbidity, and readmission rate are higher in those who were not operated on;
- Laparoscopic cholecystectomy is better than open in the elderly for treating acute cholecystitis, probably for its reduced impact on this population's delicate physiological balance;
- As in the general population, early laparoscopic cholecystectomy is preferable to a delayed approach. Deferring surgery does not reduce the risk: morbidity, mortality, and conversion rates are similar for early and delayed cholecystectomy; hospital stay is longer for the latter;
- Percutaneous cholecystostomy is not an alternative to surgery and should be reserved for patients definitely unfit for surgery; it implies much higher morbidity and mortality.

References

1. Brewer BJ, Golden GT, Hitch DC, et al. Abdominal pain. An analysis of 1,000 consecutive cases in a university hospital emergency room. Am J Surg. 1976;131(2):219–23. https://doi.org/10.1016/0002-9610(76)90101-x.
2. Miettinen P, Pasanen P, Lahtinen J, Alhava E. Acute abdominal pain in adults. Ann Chir Gynaecol. 1996;85(1):5–9.
3. Reiss R, Deutsch AA. State of the art in the diagnosis and management of acute cholecystitis. Dig Dis. 1993;11(1):55–64. https://doi.org/10.1159/000171401.
4. Kimura Y, Takada T, Kawarada Y, et al. Definitions, pathophysiology, and epidemiology of acute cholangitis and cholecystitis: Tokyo guidelines. J Hepatobiliary Pancreat Surg. 2007;14(1):15–26. https://doi.org/10.1007/s00534-006-1152-y.
5. Borzellino G, de Manzoni G, Ricci F, et al. Emergency cholecystostomy and subsequent cholecystectomy for acute gallstone cholecystitis in the elderly. Br J Surg. 1999;86(12):1521–5. https://doi.org/10.1046/j.1365-2168.1999.01284.x.
6. Nilsson E, Fored CM, Granath F, Blomqvist P. Cholecystectomy in Sweden 1987-99: a nationwide study of mortality and preoperative admissions. Scand J Gastroenterol. 2005;40(12):1478–85. https://doi.org/10.1080/00365520510023972.
7. Velanovich V, Antoine H, Swartz A, et al. Accumulating deficits model of frailty and postoperative mortality and morbidity: its application to a

national database. J Surg Res. 2013;183(1):104–10. https://doi.org/10.1016/j.jss.2013.01.021.
8. Izumisawa Y, Morioka D, Fuse M, et al. Defining the term “elderly” in the field of surgery: a retrospective study regarding the changes in the Immunoinflammatory indices during the immediate perioperative period of the elective uncomplicated laparoscopic cholecystectomy. Surg Laparosc Endosc Percutan Tech. 2020;30(5):435–40. https://doi.org/10.1097/SLE.0000000000000803.
9. Trowbridge RL, Rutkowski NK, Shojania KG. Does this patient have acute cholecystitis? JAMA. 2003;289(1):80–6. https://doi.org/10.1001/jama.289.1.80.
10. Natesan S, Lee J, Volkamer H, Thoureen T. Evidence-based medicine approach to abdominal pain. Emerg Med Clin North Am. 2016;34(2):165–90. https://doi.org/10.1016/j.emc.2015.12.008.
11. Jain A, Mehta N, Secko M, et al. History, physical examination, laboratory testing, and emergency department ultrasonography for the diagnosis of acute cholecystitis. Acad Emerg Med. 2017;24(3):281–97. https://doi.org/10.1111/acem.13132.
12. Sauerland S, Agresta F, Bergamaschi R, et al. Laparoscopy for abdominal emergencies: evidence-based guidelines of the European Association for Endoscopic Surgery. Surg Endosc. 2006;20(1):14–29. https://doi.org/10.1007/s00464-0050564-0.
13. Agresta F, Ansaloni L, Baiocchi GL, et al. Laparoscopic approach to acute abdomen from the Consensus Development Conference of the Società Italiana di Chirurgia Endoscopica e nuove tecnologie (SICE), Associazione Chirurghi Ospedalieri Italiani (ACOI), Società Italiana di Chirurgia (SIC), Società Italiana di Chirurgia d'Urgenza e del Trauma (SICUT), Società Italiana di Chirurgia nell'Ospedalità Privata (SICOP), and the European Association for Endoscopic Surgery (EAES). Surg Endosc. 2012;26(8):2134–64. https://doi.org/10.1007/s00464-012-2331-3.
14. Yokoe M, Hata J, Takada T, et al. Tokyo guidelines 2018: diagnostic criteria and severity grading of acute cholecystitis (with videos). J Hepatobiliary Pancreat Sci. 2018;25(1):41–54. https://doi.org/10.1002/jhbp.515.
15. Hirota M, Takada T, Kawarada Y, et al. Diagnostic criteria and severity assessment of acute cholecystitis: Tokyo guidelines. J Hepatobiliary Pancreat Surg. 2007;14(1):78–82. https://doi.org/10.1007/s00534-006-1159-4.
16. Laurell H, Hansson LE, Gunnarsson U. Acute abdominal pain among elderly patients. Gerontology. 2006;52(6):339–44. https://doi.org/10.1159/000094982.
17. Lee SW, Chang CS, Lee TY, et al. The role of the Tokyo guidelines in the diagnosis of acute calculous cholecystitis. J Hepatobiliary Pancreat Sci. 2010;17(6):879–84. https://doi.org/10.1007/s00534-010-0289-x.
18. Kunin N, Letoquart JP, La Gamma A, et al. [Acute cholecystitis in the elderly]. J Chir (Paris). 1994;131(5):257–260.
19. Parker LJ, Vukov LF, Wollan PC. Emergency department evaluation of geriatric patients with acute cholecystitis. Acad Emerg Med. 1997;4(1):51–5. https://doi.org/10.1111/j.1553-2712.1997.tb03643.x.
20. Morrow DJ, Thompson J, Wilson SE. Acute cholecystitis in the elderly: a surgical emergency. Arch Surg. 1978;113(10):1149–52. https://doi.org/10.1001/archsurg.1978.01370220035006.
21. McCleane G. Pain perception in the elderly patient. Clin Geriatr Med. 2008;24(2):203–11. https://doi.org/10.1016/j.cger.2007.12.008.
22. Clinch D, Banerjee AK, Ostick G. Absence of abdominal pain in elderly patients with peptic ulcer. Age Ageing. 1984;13(2):120–3. https://doi.org/10.1093/ageing/13.2.120.
23. Paranjape C, Dalia S, Pan J, Horattas M. Appendicitis in the elderly: a change in the laparoscopic era. Surg Endosc. 2007;21(5):777–81. https://doi.org/10.1007/s00464-006-9097-4.
24. High KP, Bradley SF, Gravenstein S, et al. Clinical practice guideline for the evaluation of fever and infection in older adult residents of long-term care facilities: 2008 update by the Infectious Diseases Society of America. Clin Infect Dis. 2009;48(2):149–71.
25. Cooper GS, Shlaes DM, Salata RA. Intraabdominal infection: differences in presentation and outcome between younger patients and the elderly. Clin Infect Dis. 1994;19(1):146–8. https://doi.org/10.1093/clinids/19.1.146.
26. Yeh DD, Chang Y, Tabrizi MB, et al. Derivation and validation of a practical bedside score for the diagnosis of cholecystitis. Am J Emerg Med. 2019;37(1):61–6. https://doi.org/10.1016/j.ajem.2018.04.051.
27. Adedeji OA, McAdam WA. Murphy's sign, acute cholecystitis and elderly people. J R Coll Surg Edinb. 1996;41(2):88–9.
28. Borzellino G, Steccanella F, Mantovani W, Genna M. Predictive factors for the diagnosis of severe acute cholecystitis in an emergency setting. Surg Endosc. 2013;27(9):3388–95. https://doi.org/10.1007/s00464-013-2921-8.
29. Naidu K, Beenen E, Gananadha S, Mosse C. The yield of fever, inflammatory markers and ultrasound in the diagnosis of acute cholecystitis: a validation of the 2013 Tokyo guidelines. World J Surg. 2016;40(12):2892–7. https://doi.org/10.1007/s00268-016-3660-5.
30. McGillicuddy EA, Schuster KM, Brown E, et al. Acute cholecystitis in the elderly: use of computed tomography and correlation with ultrasonography. Am J Surg. 2011;202(5):524–7. https://doi.org/10.1016/j.amjsurg.2011.06.012.
31. Asiltürk Lülleci Z, Başyiğit S, Pirinççi Sapmaz F, et al. Comparison of ultrasonographic and laboratory findings of acute cholecystitis between elderly and non-elderly patients. Turk J Med Sci. 2016;46(5):1428–33. https://doi.org/10.3906/sag1507-13.

32. Ambe PC, Weber SA, Christ H, Wassenberg D. Primary cholecystectomy is feasible in elderly patients with acute cholecystitis. Aging Clin Exp Res. 2015;27(6):921–6. https://doi.org/10.1007/s40520-015-0361-0.
33. Demirkan A, Tanrıverdi AK, Çetinkaya A, et al. The effect of leucocytosis, gender difference, and ultrasound in the diagnosis of acute cholecystitis in the elderly population. Emerg Med Int. 2019;2019:6428340. https://doi.org/10.1155/2019/6428340.
34. Plackett TP, Boehmer ED, Faunce DE, Kovacs EJ. Aging and innate immune cells. J Leukoc Biol. 2004;76(2):291–9. https://doi.org/10.1189/jlb.1103592.
35. Nikfarjam M, Yeo D, Perini M, et al. Outcomes of cholecystectomy for treatment of acute cholecystitis in octogenarians. ANZ J Surg. 2014;84(12):943–8. https://doi.org/10.1111/ans.12313.
36. Bourikian S, Anand RJ, Aboutanos M, et al. Risk factors for acute gangrenous cholecystitis in emergency general surgery patients. Am J Surg. 2015;210(4):730–3. https://doi.org/10.1016/j.amjsurg.2015.05.003.
37. Fuks D, Duhaut P, Mauvais F, et al. A retrospective comparison of older and younger adults undergoing early laparoscopic cholecystectomy for mild to moderate calculous cholecystitis. J Am Geriatr Soc. 2015;63(5):1010–6. https://doi.org/10.1111/jgs.13330.
38. Riall TS, Zhang D, Townsend CM, et al. Failure to perform cholecystectomy for acute cholecystitis in elderly patients is associated with increased morbidity, mortality, and cost. J Am Coll Surg. 2010;210(5):668–77. https://doi.org/10.1016/j.jamcollsurg.2009.12.031.
39. Bergman S, Sourial N, Vedel I, et al. Gallstone disease in the elderly: are older patients managed differently? Surg Endosc. 2011;25(1):55–61. https://doi.org/10.1007/s00464-010-1128-5.
40. CholeS Study Group, West Midlands Research Collaborative. Population-based cohort study of variation in the use of emergency cholecystectomy for benign gallbladder diseases. Br J Surg. 2016;103(12):1716–26. https://doi.org/10.1002/bjs.10288.
41. Kamarajah SK, Karri S, Bundred JR, et al. Perioperative outcomes after laparoscopic cholecystectomy in elderly patients: a systematic review and meta-analysis. Surg Endosc. 2020;34(11):4727–40. https://doi.org/10.1007/s00464-020-07805-z.
42. Kuy S, Sosa JA, Roman SA, et al. Age matters: a study of clinical and economic outcomes following cholecystectomy in elderly Americans. Am J Surg. 2011;201(6):789–96. https://doi.org/10.1016/j.amjsurg.2010.04.018.
43. Nielsen LBJ, Harboe KM, Bardram L. Cholecystectomy for the elderly: no hesitation for otherwise healthy patients. Surg Endosc. 2014;28(1):171–7. https://doi.org/10.1007/s00464-013-3144-8.
44. McKay A, Katz A, Lipschitz J. A population-based analysis of the morbidity and mortality of gallbladder surgery in the elderly. Surg Endosc. 2013;27(7):2398–406. https://doi.org/10.1007/s00464-012-2746-x.
45. Wiggins T, Markar SR, Mackenzie H, et al. Evolution in the management of acute cholecystitis in the elderly: population-based cohort study. Surg Endosc. 2018;32(10):4078–86. https://doi.org/10.1007/s00464-018-6092-5.
46. Murray AC, Markar S, Mackenzie H, et al. An observational study of the timing of surgery, use of laparoscopy and outcomes for acute cholecystitis in the USA and UK. Surg Endosc. 2018;32(7):3055–63. https://doi.org/10.1007/s00464-0176016-9.
47. Loozen CS, Oor JE, van Ramshorst B, et al. Conservative treatment of acute cholecystitis: a systematic review and pooled analysis. Surg Endosc. 2017;31(2):504–15. https://doi.org/10.1007/s00464-016-5011-x.
48. Agresta F, Campanile FC, Vettoretto N, et al. Laparoscopic cholecystectomy: consensus conference-based guidelines. Langenbecks Arch Surg. 2015;400(4):429–53. https://doi.org/10.1007/s00423-015-1300-4.
49. Ansaloni L, Pisano M, Coccolini F, et al. 2016 WSES guidelines on acute calculous cholecystitis. World J Emerg Surg. 2016;11:25. https://doi.org/10.1186/s13017016-0082-5.
50. Okamoto K, Suzuki K, Takada T, et al. Tokyo guidelines 2018: flowchart for the management of acute cholecystitis. J Hepatobiliary Pancreat Sci. 2018;25(1):55–72. https://doi.org/10.1002/jhbp.516.
51. Coccolini F, Catena F, Pisano M, et al. Open versus laparoscopic cholecystectomy in acute cholecystitis. Systematic review and meta-analysis. Int J Surg. 2015;18:196–204. https://doi.org/10.1016/j.ijsu.2015.04.083.
52. Pessaux P, Regenet N, Tuech JJ, et al. Laparoscopic versus open cholecystectomy: a prospective comparative study in the elderly with acute cholecystitis. Surg Laparosc Endosc Percutan Tech. 2001;11(4):252–5.
53. Chau CH, Tang CN, Siu WT, et al. Laparoscopic cholecystectomy versus open cholecystectomy in elderly patients with acute cholecystitis: retrospective study. Hong Kong Med J. 2002;8(6):394–9.
54. Teixeira JA, Ribeiro C, Moreira LM, et al. [Laparoscopic cholecystectomy and open cholecystectomy in acute cholecystitis: critical analysis of 520 cases]. Acta Med Port. 2014;27(6):685–91.
55. Mealy K, Gallagher H, Barry M, et al. Physiological and metabolic responses to open and laparoscopic cholecystectomy. Br J Surg. 1992;79(10):1061–4. https://doi.org/10.1002/bjs.1800791024.
56. Luo K, Li JS, Li LT, et al. Operative stress response and energy metabolism after laparoscopic cholecystectomy compared to open surgery. World J Gastroenterol. 2003;9(4):847–50. https://doi.org/10.3748/wjg.v9.i4.847.
57. Sheen-Chen SM, Chen HS, Eng HL, et al. Systemic immune response after laparoscopic and open cho-

lecystectomy. World J Surg. 2002;26(12):1418–22. https://doi.org/10.1007/s00268-002-6388-3.
58. Boo YJ, Kim WB, Kim J, et al. Systemic immune response after open versus laparoscopic cholecystectomy in acute cholecystitis: a prospective randomized study. Scand J Clin Lab Invest. 2007;67(2):207–14. https://doi.org/10.1080/00365510601011585.
59. Wahba RW, Béïque F, Kleiman SJ. Cardiopulmonary function and laparoscopic cholecystectomy. Can J Anaesth. 1995;42(1):51–63. https://doi.org/10.1007/BF03010572.
60. Damiani G, Pinnarelli L, Sammarco A, et al. Postoperative pulmonary function in open versus laparoscopic cholecystectomy: a meta-analysis of the Tiffenau index. Dig Surg. 2008;25(1):1–7. https://doi.org/10.1159/000114193.
61. Zhao HQ, Liu HR, Xiao L, et al. Laparoscopic cholecystectomy in elderly patients: an evaluation of immunity. Aging Clin Exp Res. 2015;27(6):927–33. https://doi.org/10.1007/s40520-015-0363-y.
62. Fialho L, Cunha-E-Silva JA, Santa-Maria AF, et al. Comparative study of systemic early postoperative inflammatory response among elderly and nonelderly patients undergoing laparoscopic cholecystectomy. Rev Col Bras Cir. 2018;45(1):e1586. https://doi.org/10.1590/0100-6991e-20181586.
63. Gurusamy KS, Davidson C, Gluud C, Davidson BR. Early versus delayed laparoscopic cholecystectomy for people with acute cholecystitis. Cochrane Database Syst Rev. 2013;6:CD005440. https://doi.org/10.1002/14651858.CD005440.pub3.
64. Lupinacci RM, Nadal LR, Rego RE, et al. Surgical management of gallbladder disease in the very elderly: are we operating them at the right time? Eur J Gastroenterol Hepatol. 2013;25(3):380–4. https://doi.org/10.1097/MEG.0b013e32835b7124.
65. de Mestral C, Rotstein OD, Laupacis A, et al. A population-based analysis of the clinical course of 10,304 patients with acute cholecystitis, discharged without cholecystectomy. J Trauma Acute Care Surg. 2013;74(1):26–30; discussion 30–31. https://doi.org/10.1097/TA.0b013e3182788e4d.
66. Cheng Y, Leng J, Tan J, et al. Proper surgical technique approved for early laparoscopic cholecystectomy for non-critically ill elderly patients with acute cholecystitis. Hepatogastroenterology. 2013;60(124):688–91. https://doi.org/10.5754/hge121107.
67. Ferrarese AG, Solej M, Enrico S, et al. Elective and emergency laparoscopic cholecystectomy in the elderly: our experience. BMC Surg. 2013;13 Suppl 2:S21. https://doi.org/10.1186/1471-2482-13-S2-S21.
68. Haltmeier T, Benjamin E, Inaba K, et al. Early versus delayed same-admission laparoscopic cholecystectomy for acute cholecystitis in elderly patients with comorbidities. J Trauma Acute Care Surg. 2015;78(4):801–7. https://doi.org/10.1097/TA.0000000000000577.
69. Loozen CS, van Ramshorst B, van Santvoort HC, Boerma D. Early cholecystectomy for acute cholecystitis in the elderly population: a systematic review and meta-analysis. Dig Surg. 2017;34(5):371–9. https://doi.org/10.1159/000455241.
70. Cull JD, Velasco JM, Czubak A, et al. Management of acute cholecystitis: prevalence of percutaneous cholecystostomy and delayed cholecystectomy in the elderly. J Gastrointest Surg. 2014;18(2):328–33. https://doi.org/10.1007/s11605-0132341-z.
71. Yamashita Y, Takada T, Kawarada Y, et al. Surgical treatment of patients with acute cholecystitis: Tokyo guidelines. J Hepatobiliary Pancreat Surg. 2007;14(1):91–7. https://doi.org/10.1007/s00534-006-1161-x.
72. Lu P, Chan CL, Yang NP, et al. Outcome comparison between percutaneous cholecystostomy and cholecystectomy: a 10-year population-based analysis. BMC Surg. 2017;17(1):130. https://doi.org/10.1186/s12893-017-0327-6.
73. Hall BR, Armijo PR, Krause C, et al. Emergent cholecystectomy is superior to percutaneous cholecystostomy tube placement in critically ill patients with emergent calculous cholecystitis. Am J Surg. 2018;216(1):116–9. https://doi.org/10.1016/j.amjsurg.2017.11.002.
74. Loozen CS, van Santvoort HC, van Duijvendijk P, et al. Laparoscopic cholecystectomy versus percutaneous catheter drainage for acute cholecystitis in high risk patients (CHOCOLATE): multicentre randomised clinical trial. BMJ. 2018;363:k3965. https://doi.org/10.1136/bmj.k3965.
75. Winbladh A, Gullstrand P, Svanvik J, Sandström P. Systematic review of cholecystostomy as a treatment option in acute cholecystitis. HPB. 2009;11(3):183–93. https://doi.org/10.1111/j.1477-2574.2009.00052.x.
76. Rodríguez-Sanjuán J, Arruabarrena A, Sánchez-Moreno L, et al. Acute cholecystitis in high surgical risk patients: percutaneous cholecystostomy or emergency cholecystectomy? Am J Surg. 2012;204(1):54–9. https://doi.org/10.1016/j.amjsurg.2011.05.013.
77. de Mestral C, Gomez D, Haas B, et al. Cholecystostomy: a bridge to hospital discharge but not delayed cholecystectomy. J Trauma Acute Care Surg. 2013;74(1):175–9; discussion 179–180. https://doi.org/10.1097/TA.0b013e31827890e1.
78. Campanile FC, Catena F, Coccolini F, et al. The need for new "patient-related" guidelines for the treatment of acute cholecystitis. World J Emerg Surg. 2011;6(1):44. https://doi.org/10.1186/1749-7922-6-44.
79. Campanile FC, Pisano M, Coccolini F, et al. Acute cholecystitis: WSES position statement. World J Emerg Surg. 2014;9(1):58. https://doi.org/10.1186/1749-7922-9-58.
80. Yi NJ, Han HS, Min SK. The safety of a laparoscopic cholecystectomy in acute cholecystitis in high-risk patients older than sixty with stratification based on ASA score. Minim Invasive Ther

Allied Technol. 2006;15(3):159–64. https://doi.org/10.1080/13645700600760044.

81. Peker Y, Ünalp HR, Durak E, et al. Laparoscopic cholecystectomy in patients aged 80 years and older: an analysis of 111 patients. Surg Laparosc Endosc Percutan Tech. 2014;24(2):173–6. https://doi.org/10.1097/SLE.0b013e31828f6be4.
82. Ausania F, Guzman Suarez S, Alvarez Garcia H, et al. Gallbladder perforation: morbidity, mortality and preoperative risk prediction. Surg Endosc. 2015;29(4):955–60. https://doi.org/10.1007/s00464-014-3765-6.
83. Endo I, Takada T, Hwang TL, et al. Optimal treatment strategy for acute cholecystitis based on predictive factors: Japan-Taiwan multicenter cohort study. J Hepatobiliary Pancreat Sci. 2017;24(6):346–61. https://doi.org/10.1002/jhbp.456.
84. Bonaventura A, Leale I, Carbone F, et al. Pre-surgery age-adjusted Charlson comorbidity index is associated with worse outcomes in acute cholecystitis. Dig Liver Dis. 2019;51(6):858–63. https://doi.org/10.1016/j.dld.2018.10.002.

8 Cholangitis and Choledocholithiasis

Gennaro Perrone, Federica Gaiani, Andrea Morini, Mario Giuffrida, Gian Luigi de' Angelis, Fausto Catena, and Fabio Cesare Campanile

8.1 Introduction

Cholelithiasis is a highly prevalent disease in Western Countries, ranging from 7 to 15%; it varies in different ethnicities: much more prevalent in native Americans (60–70%) and Hispanics is less common in Asians and African Americans [1]. Between 5 and 30% of patients with cholelithiasis present with concomitant choledocholithiasis [2]. Acute cholangitis is often associated with cholelithiasis and its complications, mainly choledocholithiasis, as the obstruction of the biliary tree is most commonly caused by a gallstone, although it may be secondary to a neoplasm or extrinsic stricture. From 6 to 9% of patients admitted to the hospital with cholelithiasis are diagnosed with acute cholangitis [3].

G. Perrone · F. Catena
Emergency Surgery Unit, Parma University Hospital, Parma, Italy

F. Gaiani · G. L. de' Angelis
Gastroenterology and Endoscopy Unit, Parma University Hospital, Parma, Italy

A. Morini · M. Giuffrida
General Surgery Unit, Parma University Hospital, Parma, Italy

F. C. Campanile (✉)
Division of General Surgery, ASL VT - Ospedale San Giovanni Decollato - Andosilla, Civita Castellana, Italy

The prevalence of cholelithiasis increases with age in all populations and both sexes. As the population is aging in industrialized countries [4], the number of elderly patients referring to symptomatic gallstones is continuously increasing. Choledocholithiasis represents a greater proportion of gallstone in the elderly.

The management of cholelithiasis in the elderly population poses additional challenges compared to young patients. The elderly often present more comorbidities than younger patients [2]; old age is also associated with significant mortality, especially after complications such as acute cholangitis [5]. Moreover, older adults may develop symptoms gradually and rapidly deteriorate, resulting in delayed therapy and poor outcome [2, 4, 6]. Choledocholithiasis is likewise more frequent in the elderly: about 5–20% of patients with gallbladder disease at the time of cholecystectomy also have common bile duct stones, and their incidence increases with age [7].

Gallstone disease should always be thoroughly evaluated in elderly patients to recognize and timely treat its main complications, namely choledocholithiasis and acute cholangitis.

After minimally invasive surgery largely replaced open surgery, the management of these conditions in the elderly must be re-evaluated, and a new balance between risks and opportunities is necessary.

Emergency laparoscopic cholecystectomy has proven safe in elderly patients (see Chap. 7); in

F. Agresta et al. (eds.), *Emergency laparoscopic surgery in the elderly and frail patient*,
https://doi.org/10.1007/978-3-030-79990-8_8

this chapter, we will examine the peculiarities of choledocholithiasis and acute cholangitis, in the light of the newly available technical possibilities.

8.2 Choledocholithiasis

Choledocholithiasis occurs in about 5–20% of patients with gallbladder disease at the time of cholecystectomy, with the incidence increasing with age [7].

In the past, the increased risk associated with age and frailty often limited the therapeutic options for elderly patients with common bile duct stones. The development of laparoscopic and minimally invasive techniques and new technological solutions constitutes an opportunity for treatment in this frail population.

8.2.1 Diagnosis

The same diagnostic challenges described for the acute cholecystitis in the elderly is applied to other acute biliary conditions such as choledocholithiasis and cholangitis; we examined their details in Chap. 7. As for most acute abdominal conditions, the risk of erroneous or delayed diagnosis is high in aged patients [8], due to their clinical characteristics and age-related changes in the physiological responses to sepsis and inflammation.

As in acute cholecystitis, age may affect the disease's clinical presentation, and elderly adults with common bile duct stones often lack typical symptoms.

Common bile duct stones cause less significant symptoms in older individuals (>65). The occurrence of biliary colic is more predictive of choledocholithiasis in younger than older people, and its specificity reduces with age [9]. In the same study, cholangitis prevalence in individuals aged >65 with common bile duct (CBD) stones was higher, and jaundice less frequent. A milder and less specific clinical presentation has been related to a larger diameter of the biliary tree and reduced biliary pressure in the aged due to the weakness of the longitudinal muscle fibers [10].

In suspected choledocholithiasis, the first-level diagnostic exams include the measurement of liver transaminases, bilirubin, and transabdominal ultrasound. Ultrasound findings suggestive of choledocholithiasis include the dilation of the common bile duct >8 mm and the visualization of a bile duct stone. However, the serological liver function tests are less predictive in the elderly: transaminase and bilirubin are less likely elevated, but transabdominal ultrasound has a higher detection rate in older than younger patients with common bile stones [9]. The role of imaging is, therefore, particularly relevant in this population.

Second-level exams to confirm choledocholithiasis include magnetic resonance cholangiopancreatography (MRCP), with a sensitivity of>90% and specificity nearing 100%, and endoscopic ultrasound (EUS), whose sensitivity and specificity are approximately 95% and 97%, respectively [11].

8.2.2 Therapy

Endoscopic removal of common bile duct stones by Endoscopic Retrograde Cholangiopancreatography (ERCP) has been a first-line management strategy for choledocholithiasis for the past two decades. Reported success rates for removing CBD stones at ERCP have commonly ranged from 87 to 100%, with relatively low morbidity rates of about 5% [12]. ERCP is safely adopted in the elderly: its efficacy and safety have been recently assessed in octogenarians [13], and even in patients older than 90 [14].

Before the endoscopic procedure, an accurate history should always be taken, especially for elderly patients, as they are more and more frequently under polypharmacotherapy, possibly including antiplatelet and anticoagulant drugs.

Where available, the EUS-ERCP procedure has demonstrated to be a cost-effective and safe method also in elderly patients [15]; it allows to diagnose and treat choledocholithiasis during the same endoscopic session, avoiding the risks of diagnostic ERCP and shortening the waiting time for imaging procedures such as MRCP.

In elderly patients, the advent of the minimally invasive technique has allowed surgical treatment to become a valid alternative to ERCP [16–18]. Laparoscopic common bile duct exploration (LCBDE), with the improvement of minimally invasive surgery skills, has become safe and cost-effective [19–21]. In literature, several comparative studies (a Cochrane review and a meta-analysis [16, 17]) between LCBDE (*one-stage procedure*) and ERCP + following laparoscopic cholecystectomy (LC) (*two-stage procedure*), have shown that both are effective, with similar clinical outcomes, and higher costs associated with ERCP + cholecystectomy. LCBDE has a stone extraction success rate ranging from 85 to 95% [19, 22, 23] and avoids the potentially related ERCP-morbidity. For the elderly population, a possible role for LCBDE seems confirmed [16, 24–26].

Despite these data, in the elderly and general populations, ERCP + laparoscopic cholecystectomy is the most commonly used technique [16, 27, 28]. The LCBDE presents some technical steps requiring mini-invasive surgery skills and adequate instruments, which hinder its use [27]. Furthermore, in the elderly, the legacy of the high rate of complications from laparotomy has often led us to avoid surgery.

Laparoscopic exploration of the common bile duct is possible through two approaches: trans-cystic (via cystic duct) and trans-ductal (via choledochotomy). The technique and the indications do not change in the elderly population. In a recent meta-analysis of observational studies on laparoscopic common bile duct exploration, morbidity and mortality were higher in the elderly, but not significant [26].

In conclusion, both ERCP and LCBDE represent valid options; the choice must consider various factors, including local equipment and expertise [16, 29].

8.2.3 Is Cholecystectomy Necessary After CBD Clearance?

Most guidelines recommend cholecystectomy for all patients with ductal stones and concomitant cholelithiasis [30]. If ERCP is not followed by cholecystectomy, the risk of recurrent symptoms and gallstone-related complications is significantly higher [31, 32].

The question arises if such a recommendation applies to the elderly and frail patients. Can the increased surgical risk and shorter life expectancy justify to avoid surgery after the main bile obstruction has been resolved and an endoscopic sphincterotomy performed?

A large amount of literature scrutinized this wait-and-see policy. Two recent systematic reviews with meta-analysis of randomized clinical trials clarified that cholecystectomy is necessary, after ERCP, even in the elderly and frail patients. Cholecystectomy reduces the subsequent occurrence of pancreatitis, cholangitis, and biliary colic in this subset of patients. The wait-and-see policy was not associated with a significant improvement in mortality [32, 33].

8.3 Acute Cholangitis

Acute cholangitis is a life-threatening condition; its timely diagnosis and treatment are pivotal. The condition is more frequent and severe in the aged population. An extensive multi-center retrospective observational study in Japan and Taiwan showed that, in the unselected group of 6,433 patients, the mean age was 73 years, and two-thirds of them had multiple comorbidities (Charlson Comorbidity Index score of 5 or higher) [34].

Its etiology is most commonly related to common bile duct stones; other benign and malignant obstruction causes are possible. Sepsis and multiple organ dysfunction follow the interruption of the physiological barrier between the capillary bile ducts and the sinusoid, with bacterial invasion of the bloodstream.

Although mortality risk is high for any patient, acute cholangitis in the elderly may result in an extremely severe condition with a very poor prognosis. Old age is associated with significant mortality due to more frequent comorbidities, lower immune status, and declining general health.

In an aging global population with constantly emerging antibiotic-resistant strains, the acute cholangitis treatment is a continual challenge.

8.3.1 Diagnosis

The typical scenario of high fever for more than 24 h, jaundice, and abdominal pain, also called Charcot's triad, cannot confirm the diagnosis, being its sensitivity about 24%. This applies particularly to elderly patients, who typically develop symptoms gradually and often present acute exacerbations of the disease. A recent study about acute cholangitis patients older than 75 found Charcot's triad only in 4.2% of the study group [35].

The "Tokyo guidelines" established a set of diagnostic criteria, including the evaluation of systemic inflammation, cholestasis, and imaging (Table 8.1) [36, 37].

In Chap. 7, we discussed the consequences of age-related physiology changes and associated co-morbid conditions on the clinical evaluation and inflammatory parameters; in Sect. 8.2.1, we also learned that liver function tests, namely, transaminases and bilirubin, are less likely elevated in the older people. These changes directly impact the proposed diagnostic criteria; we must be aware of their influence and keep in mind that the delicate physiological balance of the older population is particularly demanding in acute cholangitis. For this reason, a correct grading of the disease severity is fundamental, as it impacts the elderly population's mortality.

The older age's relevance as a prognostic factor for acute cholangitis is stressed by its inclusion in the severity grading criteria defined by the Tokyo guidelines [37] (Table 8.2). Under these criteria,

Table 8.2 TG18 severity assessment criteria for acute cholangitis

Grade I (mild) acute cholangitis
"Grade I" acute cholangitis does not meet the criteria of "Grade III (severe)" or "Grade II (moderate)" acute cholangitis at initial diagnosis
Grade II (moderate) acute cholangitis
"Grade II" acute cholangitis is associated with any two of the following conditions:
1. Abnormal WBC count (>12,000/mm, <4000/mm)
2. High fever (≥39 °C)
3. Age (≥75 years old)
4. Hyperbilirubinemia (total bilirubin ≥5 mg/dL)
5. Hypoalbuminemia (<STD × 0.7)
Grade III (severe) acute cholangitis
"Grade III" acute cholangitis is defined as acute cholangitis that is associated with the onset of dysfunction at least in any one of the following organs/systems:
1. Cardiovascular dysfunction: hypotension requiring dopamine ≥5 lg/kg per min, or any dose of norepinephrine
2. Neurological dysfunction: disturbance of consciousness
3. Respiratory dysfunction: PaO/FiO ratio <300
4. Renal dysfunction: oliguria, serum creatinine >2.0 mg/dL
5. Hepatic dysfunction: PT-INR >1.5
6. Hematological dysfunction: platelet count <100,000/mm

With kind permission from John Wiley and Sons: Kiriyama S, Kozaka K, Takada T, et al. (2018) **Tokyo Guidelines 2018: diagnostic criteria and severity grading of acute cholangitis (with videos)**. J Hepatobiliary Pancreat Sci, 25:17–30 [36] © 2018 Japanese Society of Hepato-Biliary-Pancreatic Surgery

Table 8.1 TG18 diagnostic criteria for acute cholangitis

A.	Systemic inflammation	B.	Cholestasis	C.	Imaging
A-1.	Fever and/or shaking chills	B-1.	Jaundice	C-1.	Biliary dilatation
A-2.	Laboratory data: evidence of inflammatory response	B-2.	Laboratory data: abnormal liver function tests	C-2.	Evidence of the etiology on imaging (stricture, stone, stent, etc.)
Suspected diagnosis: one item in A + one item in either B or C					
Definite diagnosis: one item in A, one item in B, and one item in C					

With kind permission from John Wiley and Sons: Kiriyama S, Kozaka K, Takada T, et al. (2018) **Tokyo Guidelines 2018: diagnostic criteria and severity grading of acute cholangitis (with videos)**. J Hepatobiliary Pancreat Sci, 25:17–30 [36] © 2018 Japanese Society of Hepato-Biliary-Pancreatic Surgery patients aged >75 years presenting either fever >39 °C or one alteration of laboratory tests (albuminemia, bilirubin, or WBC count) can be defined as having moderate acute cholangitis. Severe cholangitis is characterized by the onset of organ dysfunction, to which old subjects are more prone.

8.3.2 Therapy

Hospital management of acute cholangitis is always recommended at all ages, as it is an emergent condition characterized by a rapid deterioration of clinical conditions due to sepsis.

Its treatment pillars are antibiotic therapy and biliary drainage; their therapeutic schemes and timing vary with the severity grade [38].

After resuscitation and diagnosis, antimicrobial agents should be administered as soon as the condition is suspected.

Empirical antibiotic therapy should be usually initiated until specific etiologic agents are isolated from blood or biliary cultures. Antibiotic therapy scheme is usually based on local susceptibility data and the knowledge of the most frequently isolated bacteria in biliary infections: *Escherichia coli* and *Enterobacteriaceae*. By the Tokyo guidelines [38], therapeutic schemes may be Penicillin-based, Cephalosporin-based, Carbapenem-based, Monobactam-based, or Fluoroquinolone-based. The combination of piperacillin and tazobactam is recommended for grade II–III cholangitis and healthcare-associated infections in the first group. In the second group, metronidazole is associated with cefazolin, ceftriaxone, or cefepime based on grade I–II or III cholangitis. Carbapenem-based therapy envisages the use of ertapenem, eventually substituted by imipenem/cilastatin, Meropenem, or doripenem only for grade III and hospital-associated biliary infections. For the last category, monobactam therapy may be advised, using aztreonam alone or in combination with metronidazole. Finally, fluoroquinolone-based therapy may be used only in the case of grade I and II cholangitis.

In the elderly, prescribing antimicrobials must consider all the possible co-morbid conditions and renal function in particular. With advanced age, the serum creatinine or creatinine-based calculations of the glomerular filtration rate could fail to accurately predict the excretory function due to the age-related muscle mass reduction; correct antibiotic prescription may be difficult.

Endoscopic transpapillary biliary drainage should be considered the first-line drainage procedure because of its less invasiveness and lower risk of adverse events than other drainage techniques [39]. ERCP is considered safe in the elderly and very elderly [40], also for cholangitis drainage [39]. The Tokyo guidelines recommend its use in acute cholangitis.

Percutaneous transhepatic cholangial drainage (PTCD) is an alternative drainage procedure in patients with an inaccessible papilla or when ERCP is not available [39].

Endoscopic transpapillary biliary drainage may be either external, by positioning endoscopic nasobiliary drainage (ENBD) or internal, using endoscopic biliary stenting (EBS). Both types of endoscopic biliary drainage can be performed in all forms of acute cholangitis [39].

If non-surgical drainage fails, surgical exploration of the common bile duct can be performed, even in the case of acute cholangitis. The surgical approach to CBD, as previously reported, can be obtained both laparoscopically (LCBDE) and open (OBCDE). Some authors showed that LCBDE is effective in rapidly improving the liver function in non-severe acute cholangitis patients [41–43]. A very recent study adopted it as an emergency primary procedure in elderly patients [44].

Therefore, urgent LCBDE (within 72 h of the onset of symptoms) may be a valid alternative drainage procedure in patients with non-severe acute cholangitis.

Five Things You Should Know About Cholangitis and Choledocholithiasis in the Elderly

- Choledocholithiasis and acute cholangitis are strictly related clinical conditions, common among the elderly, as their incidence increases with age.
- Especially in the case of aged patients, malignant causes of biliary obstruction should be ruled out.

- Among the elderly, prompt diagnosis and timely treatment of choledocholithiasis and acute cholangitis are crucial, as the outcome is negatively influenced by old age, comorbidities, and delayed treatment.
- Antimicrobial treatment and biliary drainage are the mainstays of acute cholangitis.
- Cholecystectomy is a crucial step in the treatment of acute cholangitis, sustained by choledocholithiasis. Even in the elderly patient, if a *two-stage procedure* (ERCP + LC) is performed, it is advisable to perform cholecystectomy within 72 h of the onset of symptoms.

References

1. Shaffer EA. Gallstone disease: epidemiology of gallbladder stone disease. Best Pract Res Clin Gastroenterol. 2006;20:981–96.
2. Nassar Y, Richter S. Management of complicated gallstones in the elderly: comparing surgical and non-surgical treatment options. Gastroenterol Rep. 2019;7:205–11.
3. Isayama H, Yasuda I, Tan D. Current strategies for endoscopic management of acute cholangitis. Dig Endosc. 2017;29(Suppl 2):70–7.
4. Agrusa A, Romano G, Frazzetta G, et al. Role and outcomes of laparoscopic cholecystectomy in the elderly. Int J Surg. 2014;12(Suppl 2):S37–9.
5. Agarwal N, Sharma BC, Sarin SK. Endoscopic management of acute cholangitis in elderly patients. World J Gastroenterol. 2006;12:6551–5.
6. Khashab MA, Tariq A, Tariq U, et al. Delayed and unsuccessful endoscopic retrograde cholangiopancreatography are associated with worse outcomes in patients with acute cholangitis. Clin Gastroenterol Hepatol. 2012;10:1157–61.
7. Collins C, Maguire D, Ireland A, et al. A prospective study of common bile duct calculi in patients undergoing laparoscopic cholecystectomy: natural history of choledocholithiasis revisited. Ann Surg. 2004;239:28–33.
8. Laurell H, Hansson L-E, Gunnarsson U. Acute abdominal pain among elderly patients. Gerontology. 2006;52(6):339–44.
9. Hu KC, Wang HY, Chang WH, et al. Clinical presentations of patients from different age cohorts with biliary tract stone diseases. J Gastroenterol Hepatol. 2014;29:1614–9.
10. Hu K-C, Chu C-H, Wang H-Y, et al. How does aging affect presentation and Management of Biliary Stones? J Am Geriatr Soc. 2016;64(11):2330–5. https://doi.org/10.1111/jgs.14481.
11. ASGE Standards of Practice Committee, Maple JT, Ikenberry SO, Anderson MA, et al. The role of endoscopy in the management of choledocholithiasis. Gastrointest Endosc. 2011;74:731–44.
12. Manes G, Paspatis G, Aabakken L, et al. Endoscopic management of common bile duct stones: European Society of Gastrointestinal Endoscopy (ESGE) guideline. Endoscopy. 2019;51:472–91.
13. Iida T, Kaneto H, Wagatsuma K, et al. Efficacy and safety of endoscopic procedures for common bile duct stones in patients aged 85 years or older: a retrospective study. PLoS One. 2018;13(1):e0190665. https://doi.org/10.1371/journal.pone.0190665.
14. Saito H, Koga T, Sakaguchi M, et al. Safety and efficacy of endoscopic removal of common bile duct stones in elderly patients ≥90 years of age. Intern Med. 2019;58(15):2125–32. https://doi.org/10.2169/internalmedicine.2546-18.
15. Narula VK, Fung EC, Overby DW, et al. Clinical spotlight review for the management of choledocholithiasis. Surg Endosc. 2020;34:1482–91.
16. Lee A, Min SK, Park JJ, et al. Laparoscopic common bile duct exploration for elderly patients: as a first treatment strategy for common bile duct stones. J Korean Surg Soc. 2011;81(2):128–33. https://doi.org/10.4174/jkss.2011.81.2.128.
17. Alexakis N, Connor S. Meta-analysis of one- vs. two-stage laparoscopic/endoscopic management of common bile duct stones. HPB (Oxford). 2012;14(4):254–9.
18. Dasari BV, Tan CJ, Gurusamy KS, Martin DJ, et al. Surgical versus endoscopic treatment of bile duct stones. Cochrane Database Syst Rev. 2013;9:CD003327.
19. Shojaiefard A, Esmaeilzadeh M, Ghafouri A, et al. Various techniques for the surgical treatment of common bile duct stones: a meta review. Gastroenterol Res Pract. 2009;2009:840208. https://doi.org/10.1155/2009/840208.
20. Clayton ESJ, Connor S, Alexakis N, et al. Meta-analysis of endoscopy and surgery versus surgery alone for common bile duct stones with the gallbladder in situ. Br J Surg. 2006;93(10):1185–91.
21. Poulose BK, Arbogast PG, Holzman MD. National analysis of in-hospital resource utilization in choledocholithiasis management using propensity scores. Surg Endosc. 2006;20(2):186–90.
22. Rojas-Ortega S, Arizpe-Bravo D, Marin Lopez ER, et al. Transcystic common bile duct exploration in the management of patients with choledocholithiasis. J Gastrointest Surg. 2003;7(4):492–6.
23. Thompson MH, Tranter SE. All-comers policy for laparoscopic exploration of the common bile duct. Br J Surg. 2002;89(12):1608–12.
24. Wu X, Huang Z-J, Zhong J-Y, et al. Laparoscopic common bile duct exploration with primary closure is safe for management of choledocholithiasis in elderly patients. Hepatobiliary Pancreat Dis Int. 2019;18(6):557–61.

25. Zheng C, Huang Y, Xie E, et al. Laparoscopic common bile duct exploration: a safe and definitive treatment for elderly patients. Surg Endosc. 2017;31(6):2541–7.
26. Zhu J, Tu S, Yang Z, et al. Laparoscopic common bile duct exploration for elderly patients with choledocholithiasis: a systematic review and meta-analysis. Surg Endosc. 2020;34(4):1522–33.
27. Shen F, Pawlik TM. Surgical management of choledocholithiasis: a disappearing skill. JAMA Surg. 2016;151(12):1130–1.
28. Wandling MW, Hungness ES, Pavey ES, et al. Nationwide assessment of trends in choledocholithiasis management in the United States from 1998 to 2013. JAMA Surg. 2016;151(12):1125–30.
29. Ansaloni L, Pisano M, Coccolini F, et al. WSES guidelines on acute calculous cholecystitis. World J Emerg Surg. 2016;11:25.
30. van Dijk AH, de Reuver PR, Besselink MG, et al. Assessment of available evidence in the management of gallbladder and bile duct stones: a systematic review of international guidelines. HPB. 2017;19(4):297–309.
31. McAlister VC, Davenport E, Renouf E. Cholecystectomy deferral in patients with endoscopic sphincterotomy. Cochrane Database Syst Rev. 2007;(4):CD006233.
32. Xu J, Yang C. Cholecystectomy outcomes after endoscopic sphincterotomy in patients with choledocholithiasis: a meta-analysis. BMC Gastroenterol. 2020;20(1):229.
33. Khan MA, Khan Z, Tombazzi CR, et al. Role of cholecystectomy after endoscopic sphincterotomy in the management of choledocholithiasis in high-risk patients: a systematic review and meta-analysis. J Clin Gastroenterol. 2018;52(7):579–89.
34. Gomi H, Takada T, Hwang TL, et al. Updated comprehensive epidemiology, microbiology, and outcomes among patients with acute cholangitis. J Hepatobiliary Pancreat Sci. 2017;24(6):310–8. https://doi.org/10.1002/jhbp.452.
35. Park CS, Jeong HS, Kim KB, et al. Urgent ERCP for acute cholangitis reduces mortality and hospital stay in elderly and very elderly patients. Hepatobiliary Pancreat Dis Int. 2016;15(6):619–25. https://doi.org/10.1016/s1499-3872(16)60130-3.
36. Kiriyama S, Kozaka K, Takada T, et al. Tokyo guidelines 2018: diagnostic criteria and severity grading of acute cholangitis (with videos). J Hepatobiliary Pancreat Sci. 2018;25:17–30.
37. Kiriyama S, Takada T, Strasberg SM, et al. New diagnostic criteria and severity assessment of acute cholangitis in revised Tokyo guidelines. J Hepatobiliary Pancreat Sci. 2012;19:548–56.
38. Gomi H, Solomkin JS, Schlossberg D, et al. Tokyo guidelines 2018: antimicrobial therapy for acute cholangitis and cholecystitis. J Hepatobiliary Pancreat Sci. 2018;25:3–16.
39. Mukai S, Itoi T, Baron TH, et al. Indications and techniques of biliary drainage for acute cholangitis in updated Tokyo guidelines 2018. J Hepatobiliary Pancreat Sci. 2017;24(10):537–49
40. Day LW, Lin L, Somsouk M. Adverse events in older patients undergoing ERCP: a systematic review and meta-analysis. Endosc Int Open. 2014;2(1):E28–36. https://doi.org/10.1055/s-0034-1365281.
41. Zhu B, Li D, Ren Y, et al. Early versus delayed laparoscopic common bile duct exploration for common bile duct stone-related nonsevere acute cholangitis. Sci Rep. 2015;5:11748. https://doi.org/10.1038/srep11748.
42. Gholipour C, Shalchi RA, Abassi M. Efficacy and safety of early laparoscopic common bile duct exploration as primary procedure in acute cholangitis caused by common bile duct stones. J Laparoendosc Adv Surg Tech A. 2007;17(5):634–8.
43. Atstupens K, Plaudis H, Fokins V, et al. Safe laparoscopic clearance of the common bile duct in emergently admitted patients with choledocholithiasis and cholangitis. Korean J Hepatobiliary Pancreat Surg. 2016;20(2):53–60.
44. Jia B, Jin Z, Han W, et al. Safety and efficacy of emergency laparoscopic common bile duct exploration in elderly patients with complicated acute cholangitis. Surg Endosc. 2020;34(3):1330–5.

Gallstone Ileus

9

Irnerio Angelo Muttillo, Federico Coccolini,
Biagio Picardi, Stefano Rossi,
Edoardo Maria Muttillo, and Ferdinando Agresta

9.1 Introduction and Epidemiology

Gallstone ileus is described as a mechanical obstruction resulting from the impaction of a large gallstone through the bilio-enteric fistula and is frequently preceded by an initial episode of acute cholecystitis. The inflammation and the compression of the gallstone cause erosion through the gallbladder wall, leading to the formation of a fistula between the gallbladder and the adjacent portion of the gastrointestinal (GI) tract, with further gallstone passage [1].

Gallstone ileus is a rare complication in patients with chronic cholelithiasis (0.3–1.5%) and is the etiology in 1–4% of ileus cases overall [2]. More frequently, it occurs in the elderly (late 70–80s) female patients: up to one quarter of nonstrangulated small bowel obstructions in elderly patients [1].

These patients suffer from several comorbid conditions increasing postoperative morbidity and mortality. *Halabi* et al. recently reported an average age from 60 to 84 years in American patients [2]. The most frequent fistula occurs between the gallbladder and the duodenum, due to their proximity [75–83%]. The stomach, small bowel, and the transverse portion of the colon may also be involved [3–5].

Rare cases of gallstone ileus after endoscopic retrograde cholangiopancreatography (ERCP) and endoscopic sphincterotomy (ES) and unsuccessful gallstone extraction are reported in the literature [6, 7].

The most common impaction site of the gallstone is the distal ileum and ileocecal valve (50–60.5%), jejunum (16–26%), duodenum (3.5–14.6%), and colon (3–4%) [1]. The incidence of gallstone ileus of the large bowel is higher, if patients have colonic stricture (inflammation or diverticulitis). Proximal obstruction (Bouveret's syndrome) of the gastric outlet or duodenum is rare (4%) [1, 5, 8].

The majority of gallstones smaller than 2–2.5 cm may pass spontaneously through a normal gastrointestinal tract and will be excreted in the stools [8].

The average size of obstructing gallstones is 4 cm [4]. *Nakao* et al. found that impacted gallstones ranged in size from 2 to 10 cm, with

I. A. Muttillo (✉) · B. Picardi · S. Rossi
Department of General and Emergency Surgery, Ospedale San Filippo Neri, Rome, Italy

F. Coccolini
General Emergency and Trauma Surgery, Pisa University Hospital, Pisa, Italy

E. M. Muttillo
Department of Surgical Sciences, Sapienza University of Rome, Rome, Italy

F. Agresta
Department of General Surgery, ULSS2 Trevigiana del veneto, Vittorio Veneto (TV), Italy

F. Agresta et al. (eds.), *Emergency laparoscopic surgery in the elderly and frail patient*,
https://doi.org/10.1007/978-3-030-79990-8_9

a mean size of 4.3 cm [3]. Gallstones larger than 5 cm are even more likely to become impacted [4, 5].

9.2 Clinical Presentation

Gallstone ileus is a mechanical digestive occlusion and therefore the site where the stone impacts will induce a variety of clinical scenarios. The presentation of gallstone ileus may be preceded by biliary symptoms, with rates between 27 and 80% of patients [6].

Acute cholecystitis may be present in 10–30% of the patients at the time of bowel obstruction. Biliary symptoms may be absent in up to one third of cases [5, 7].

Once the stone is in the intestinal lumen, it can obstruct any part of the gastrointestinal tract, but the most common place is the distal ileum.

The clinical signs and symptoms are often nonspecific, contributing to a delay in the diagnosis. Gallstone ileus may be manifested as acute, intermittent, or chronic episodes of gastrointestinal obstruction. Nausea, vomiting, abdominal pain, and distension are commonly present as signal of intermittent, partial, or complete obstruction. The intermittent nature of pain and vomiting of proximal gastrointestinal material is due to the "tumbling" gallstone advancement [5, 8].

Barnard's syndrome occurs when the stone obstructs the ileocecal valve [9].

Bouveret's syndrome is a rare type of gallstone obstruction which occurs when a gallstone lodges in the duodenal bulb causing gastric outlet obstruction [1, 10].

In Bouveret's syndrome, nausea and vomiting have been reported in 86% of the cases, while abdominal pain or discomfort is referred in 71% of the patients.

If the gallstone is not fully obstructing, the presentation will be of partial obstruction. Recent weight loss, anorexia, early satiety, and constipation may be referred. Bouveret's syndrome has also been reported to be preceded by upper gastrointestinal bleeding, secondary to duodenal erosion caused by the offending gallstone, with hematemesis and melena, in 15% and 7%, respectively [5, 11].

Fewer than 4.8% of all gallstone ileus patients present colonic obstruction secondary to a direct erosion into the large bowel (generally, the transverse colon) [1, 12].

Colonic diseases, such as the diverticular disease, that modify the normal structure of the intestinal wall, may increase the likelihood of a stone becoming impacted [13, 14].

Gallstone ileus usually affects women (70%) around 70–80 years old. Patients with acute gallstone ileus typically present in emergency with a sudden onset of abdominal pain, abdominal distention, nausea, and vomiting [1, 10].

Physical examination is usually nonspecific, contributing to a delay in the diagnosis. The patients are often acutely ill, with signs of dehydration, abdominal distension, and tenderness with high-pitched bowel sounds and obstructive jaundice. Fever, toxicity, and physical signs of peritonitis may be noted, if perforation of the intestinal wall had taken place [14].

In a review of 176 cases of gallstone, *Nakao* et al. reported abdominal pain at presentation in the majority of the patients (91.5%) with abdominal distension, vomiting, and fever in 84.7%, 59.7%, and 40.9% of all patients, respectively [3].

Subacute gallstone ileus differs from the acute form because the patients do not have stool passage but pass flatus (low-grade bowel obstruction).

Karewsky syndrome (chronic form) is characterized by intermittent episodes of pain caused by the passage of gallstones through the bowel, reaching complete obstruction in various stages [13].

Many of the patients with gallstone ileus are elderly people and suffer from a multitude of comorbidities, have poor general conditions, and have delayed diagnosis that leads to dehydration, shock, sepsis, or peritonitis.

In a systematic review of 38 cases of sigmoid gallstone ileus, *Farkas* et al. reported the age range of patients (between 65 and 94 years old), mean age of 81.1 years; as for the clinical symptoms, 74% of the patients presented abdominal pain, whereas 93% of the patients presented other obstructive symptoms of constipation (61%), vomiting (50%), and abdominal distension (26%) [14].

9.3 Diagnosis

Gallstone ileus does not have specific symptoms, but it is characterized by tumbling gallstone advancement with alternating aggravation and resolution of ileus [15].

The "tumbling phenomenon" may be the reason why the patient does not seek medical attention and admission is postponed. Patients usually present 4–8 days after the beginning of symptoms and the diagnosis is usually made 3–8 days after the onset of symptoms [10, 15].

Furthermore, many of them are elderly patients in poor general conditions, often with severe comorbidities. The delay in diagnosis involves dehydration, shock, sepsis, or peritonitis [16].

Therefore, the difficult clinical recognition of this particular kind of bowel obstruction, showing insidious onset and, often, underestimated in patients already affected by biliary colic, leads the diagnostic imaging (abdominal X-ray, computed tomography (CT), magnetic resonance imaging (MRI), ultrasonography (US)) to play a fundamental role in the management of these patients [17–19].

9.3.1 Abdominal X-ray

The classical abdominal X-ray presentation of gallstone ileus is the Rigler's triad that includes pneumobilia (also known as sign of Gotta-Mentschler), dilated small bowel loops with air-fluid levels, and a large calcified gallstone in the lumen of the small bowel.

At present, however, computed tomography (CT) is nearly ubiquitous and has 99% accuracy for diagnosing gallstone ileus. Typical CT findings include pneumobilia, dilated loops of small bowel with air-fluid levels consistent with small bowel obstruction, and the ectopic stone almost always radiologically visible.

Abdominal X-ray is an ideal imaging modality in the emergency setting. It is quick and technically easy and the radiation dose involved is 0.7 mSv. The sensitivity for the diagnosis of gallstone ileus ranges between 40 and 70%, and its positive predictive value reaches 80% in patients with high-grade intestinal obstruction [20–22]. In 1941, Rigler described his triad of radiological signs for gallstone ileus on X-ray: air within the biliary tree (pneumobilia), signs of small bowel obstruction, and ectopic radio-opaque gallstones [23].

The principal signs on abdominal X-ray are the same as any other bowel obstruction. If it involves the small bowel, it shows multiple loops of dilated small bowel with a few air in the large bowel and rectum, while in the case of colon, the large bowel is dilated and the same may sometimes also happen in the small bowel. In rare cases of Bouveret's syndrome (gastric outlet obstruction), the X-ray shows a prominent gastric shadow [22, 24]. On conventional radiography, the gallstones are difficult to visualize, with only 10–20% of stones containing enough calcium to be radio-opaque [25, 26].

Two other abdominal X-ray signs are described using oral contrast (either water-soluble contrast or barium): Forchet sign, when the contrast passes around a radiolucent calculus and Petren sign, when the contrast passes from bowel to gallbladder through a fistulous connection [19, 27].

In any case, oral or rectal contrast should not be routinely used in suspected gallstone ileus, because of the barium peritonitis (avoided by the use of water-soluble contrast) in case of perforation and vomiting in case of bowel obstruction.

9.3.2 Computed Tomography (CT)

Computed tomography (CT) is widely considered the investigation of choice in bowel obstruction, and, in general, in any other acute abdomen. CT scanning in emergency patients is relatively fast and more widely available [19, 23, 28–30]. The radiation dose involved is 10 mSv.

The advantage of CT scan is to provide finer anatomic details than X-ray like gallbladder anatomy, abnormal fistulous connections, small stones or even gallstone sludge in the gallbladder, biliary tree, or ectopic stones elsewhere in any tract of the GI system [31]. The diagnostic CT

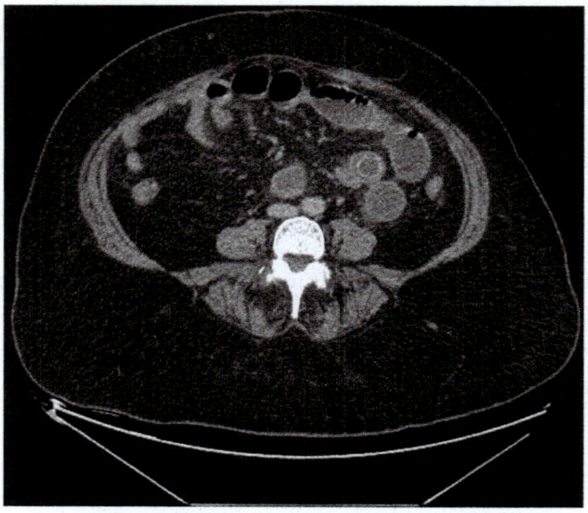

Fig. 9.1 Abdomen CT: small bowel obstruction and ectopic gallstone

criteria include: signs of intestinal obstruction, presence of ectopic gallstone, its size and exact location, abnormal gallbladder, direct visualization of the bilio-enteric fistula, and pneumobilia.

The diagnostic signs have been defined by *Yu* et al. in 2005 in a prospective study where 165 patients with acute small bowel obstruction were evaluated for gallstone ileus, with retrospective identification of three diagnostic criteria (Fig. 9.1) [32]:

1. small bowel obstruction;
2. ectopic gallstone, either rim-calcified or total-calcified;
3. abnormal gallbladder with complete air collection, presence of air-fluid level, or fluid accumulation with irregular wall.

Overall sensitivity, specificity, and accuracy were 93%, 100%, and 99%, respectively. Rigler's triad was detected only in 36% of cases.

In Bouveret's syndrome instead, the principal CT scan findings are obstruction due to a gastroduodenal mass, pneumobilia, or cholecystoduodenal fistula, pericholecystic inflammatory changes extending into the duodenum, thickened gallbladder wall, and a contracted gallbladder air in the gallbladder, filling defects due to one or more gallstones [30, 33].

Contrast-enhanced CT for gallstone ileus has a sensitivity of 90–93%, specificity of 100%, and accuracy of 99% in patients with acute small bowel obstruction and permits to define the cause and level of bowel obstruction, defining the size and structure of the ectopic stone [19, 23, 28–30].

CT contrast may be administered as intravenous (IV) or oral preparations. The oral contrast may be used to evaluate better the anatomy of the bowel and the presence of obstruction and may also visualize fistulous connections between the gallbladder and bowel through contrast accumulation within the gallbladder [30, 35]. The IV contrast is often preferred in an acute abdomen, enhancing the bowel as well as the other abdominal viscera and improving the diagnostic procedure. As well as in the abdominal X-ray, the excessive fluid intake in the form of oral contrast in bowel obstruction may aggravate the symptoms and pose risks of aspiration.

The CT scan defines precisely the type of gallstones, except for composite stones of calcium, cholesterol, and bile pigments, that may be missed on CT scanning due to isoattenuation relative to bile/fluid up to 25% of cases [17, 34–36].

There are also several reports of CT scanning underestimating the size of stones in gallstone ileus [37]. In summary, the identification of gallstones on CT scanning is complicated by variability in gallstone composition and structure [37]. Its applicability in this condition is highly dependent on a high index of suspicion and the competence of the observer.

9.3.3 Abdominal Ultrasonography

Abdominal ultrasonography (US) is the method of choice for the detection of gallstone disease, with efficacy greater than 95%. It is a noninvasive low-cost examination with no radiation exposure. However, it is rarely used for diagnostic purposes in patients with acute abdomen and, especially in cases of bowel obstruction, it is technically difficult because of the patient discomfort and gaseous/fluid distension of bowel [27, 38, 39].

Ultrasonography findings are absent in visualization of the gallbladder or presence of hyperechoic foci with posterior acoustic shadowing in the gallbladder bed, aerobilia, intralumen hyperechoic image with posterior acoustic shadowing (gallstone obstructing intestine lumen), and the image of intestine loop dilatation [32].

9.3.4 Magnetic Resonance Imaging (MRI)

Magnetic resonance imaging (MRI) is the gold-standard modality for visualizing the biliary tree. It can detect small gallstones or microcalculi (<3 mm diameter) missed on ultrasound scanning, or radiolucent and isoattenuating stones missed on conventional X-ray or CT scanning [17, 40]. The sensitivity in the diagnosis of gallstones is 97.7%, and it provides precise anatomical detail of the biliary tree [17].

Although MRI scanning can also demonstrate Rigler's triad in almost 100% of the cases compared to 77.8% with CT scanning, it is not so used in the acute setting, since it is less available and more time-consuming than CT.

A potential use could be in estimating the risk or tendency of chronic calculus gallbladder to produce a fistula into the bowel. In fact, MRI is able to demonstrate signs such as chronic calculus cholecystitis, large gallstones (>2 cm), gallbladder wall thinning, or loss of the fat line between the gallbladder and duodenum. Further evidence for its use is required [17].

9.3.5 Esophagogastroduodenoscopy

Also, the upper gastrointestinal endoscopy has a role in the diagnosis of gallstone ileus and can be used to confirm the diagnosis of impacted calculus and internal biliary fistulas.

In a review of 81 cases of esophagogastroduodenoscopy (EGDS), performed in Bouveret's syndrome, the gastroduodenal obstruction has been revealed in all of them, but gallstone visualization was possible only in 56 of the cases (69%). Among them, such gallstones were observed in the duodenal bulb in 51.8% of the cases, postbulbar duodenum in 28.6%, pylorus or prepylorus in 17.9%, and in one case the location has not been reported.

In 31% of the cases, the gallstone was not recognized because it was deeply hidden within the mucosa. When the gallstone cannot be visualized, the diagnosis should be strongly suspected when the observed mass is hard, convex, smooth, nonfriable, and nonfleshy, all characteristic of a gallstone.

For such cases, US and CT are the preferred noninvasive diagnostic tests to confirm the endoscopic diagnosis, identify the gastroduodenal anatomy, and find a cholecystoduodenal fistula [11].

9.4 Treatment

The main objective of the treatment of gallstone ileus remains the resolution of intestinal occlusion. However, the gold-standard treatment, such as the role of laparoscopy and endoscopy, is still widely debated.

Preoperatively, in order to manage the metabolic imbalance due to the occlusion through fluid therapy, antibiotic prophylaxis before the placement of a nasogastric tube is needed to stabilize the patient [41, 42].

At this point, the treatment depends on two fundamental aspects: the level of occlusion and the general condition of the patient [43, 44].

The site of occlusion remains a central aspect for endoscopic treatment, resolutive in pyloric/duodenal occlusion (Bouveret's syndrome) and colic occlusions [16].

However, these cases represent only 10–20% of the total cases, while the most frequent site of occlusion is the distal ileum (80–90%) [1, 6, 16].

The main risks of this treatment are represented by the fragmentation of the stones and its passage in the ileum, resulting in a new occlusive episode.

About the patient's conditions and comorbidities, these are fundamental in the choice of the best treatment for the patient.

In fact, enterolithotomy is the most commonly used procedure to solve occlusion, pro-

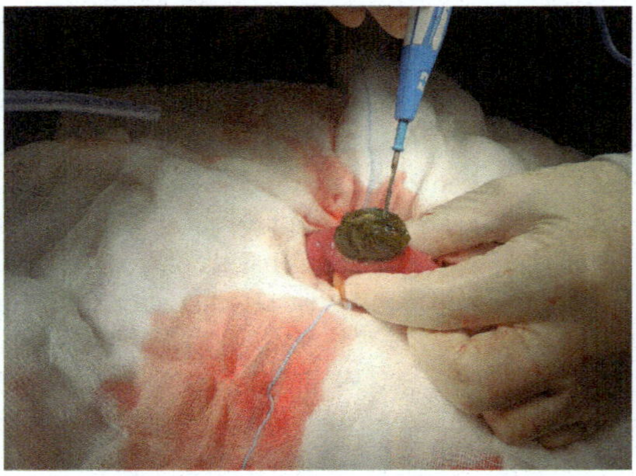

Fig. 9.2 Intraoperative view, enterolithotomy

vided there are no signs of intestinal ischemia (Fig. 9.2) [45].

After an exploratory laparotomy, the site of occlusion must be identified and through a longitudinal incision on the antimesenteric border proximal to the site of gallstone impaction, the gallstone is then extracted, avoiding the spread of enteric material in the peritoneal cavity.

A gently transverse suture of the enterotomy should be performed in order to avoid intestinal stenosis. If there are any signs of ischemia or perforation, bowel resection is necessary and consequent anastomosis (latero-lateral (L-L), termino-lateral (T-L), and termino-terminal (T-T)).

It is mandatory to avoid the presence of other stones in the intestinal lumen that must be promptly identified and extracted before the intestinal suture or any anastomosis [46].

This treatment is aimed at resolving the occlusion, without solving the cause of occlusion, the bilio-enteric fistula.

The curative treatment instead is represented by: enterolithotomy, fistula closure, and cholecystectomy. This procedure can be performed in one step (one stage procedure) or in two: enterolithotomy and delayed cholecystectomy and fistula closure (two stage procedures).

Treatment is still widely debated, and a gold standard for all patients is not yet clearly defined. In fact, the one stage procedures, although burdened by greater morbidity and mortality (11.7% mortality for enterolithotomy alone vs 16.9% for one stage procedures), allow to resolve the emergency and to avoid recurrence or exposure to complications [1].

Therefore, some authors show that the cholecystoenteric fistula not only exposes to the recurrence of gallstone ileus, but also exposes to episodes of cholangitis and an increased risk of carcinoma of the gallbladder [6, 16, 47].

However, it is necessary to point out that most patients with gallstone ileus are not eligible for one stage procedures, and that this is only applicable in selected cases, since most of these patients are elderly (>70 years), with comorbidity, and may present in septic shock (high-risk patient).

About laparoscopic treatment, this aspect is also widely debated, in fact minimally invasive surgery is becoming a feasible option even in emergency surgery.

However, some serious conditions such as hemodynamic instability or severe respiratory comorbidity remain absolute contraindications to laparoscopic access, also in this specific case, the excessive bowel dilatation became a contraindication especially in less experienced surgeons, due to the high risk of iatrogenic intestinal lesion [4, 48].

Therefore, the surgeon's expertise remains extremely important, especially in laparoscopic surgery, to select the best type of treatment. Currently, according to the literature, minimally invasive surgery is used only in 10% of gallstone ileus cases, with a high conversion rate, but at the same time offering better postoperative recovery [2, 49].

There are no differences in the literature between one and two stage procedures: *Tan* et al. in a retrospective study consisting of 19 patients treated in emergency for gallstone ileus (7 enterolithotomy alone and 12 one stage procedures) report an increased operating time of one stage procedures (178 min vs 70 min) but no differences in terms of morbidity [50]. *Riaz* et al. in a series of 10 patients, of whom 5 were treated with only enterolithotomy and 5 with one stage procedures, report that the choice was driven mainly by the clinical conditions of the patients, extremely different in the two groups [51].

The main complications are represented by acute renal insufficiency (30%), ileus (12.4%), wound infection (7%), and when an intestinal resection was necessary, anastomotic leak and intrabdominal abscesses have been reported.

Therefore, it could give rise to various scenarios that require different treatments (Fig. 9.3): pyloric or duodenal occlusion (Bouveret's syndrome) that could benefit from endoscopic treatment in selected cases, ileal occlusion in selected patients without contraindications to laparoscopy that could be treated with one stage laparoscopic procedures, ileal occlusion in a high-risk patient with contraindications to laparoscopy that will need enterolithotomy urgently and in some of these, delayed cholecystectomy and fistula closure.

Most authors in the literature agree that enterolithotomy alone is the safest procedure in high-risk patients, and some authors report spontaneous closures of bilio-enteric fistula, especially when the gallbladder has no stones and the cystic duct remains patent [2, 6, 16].

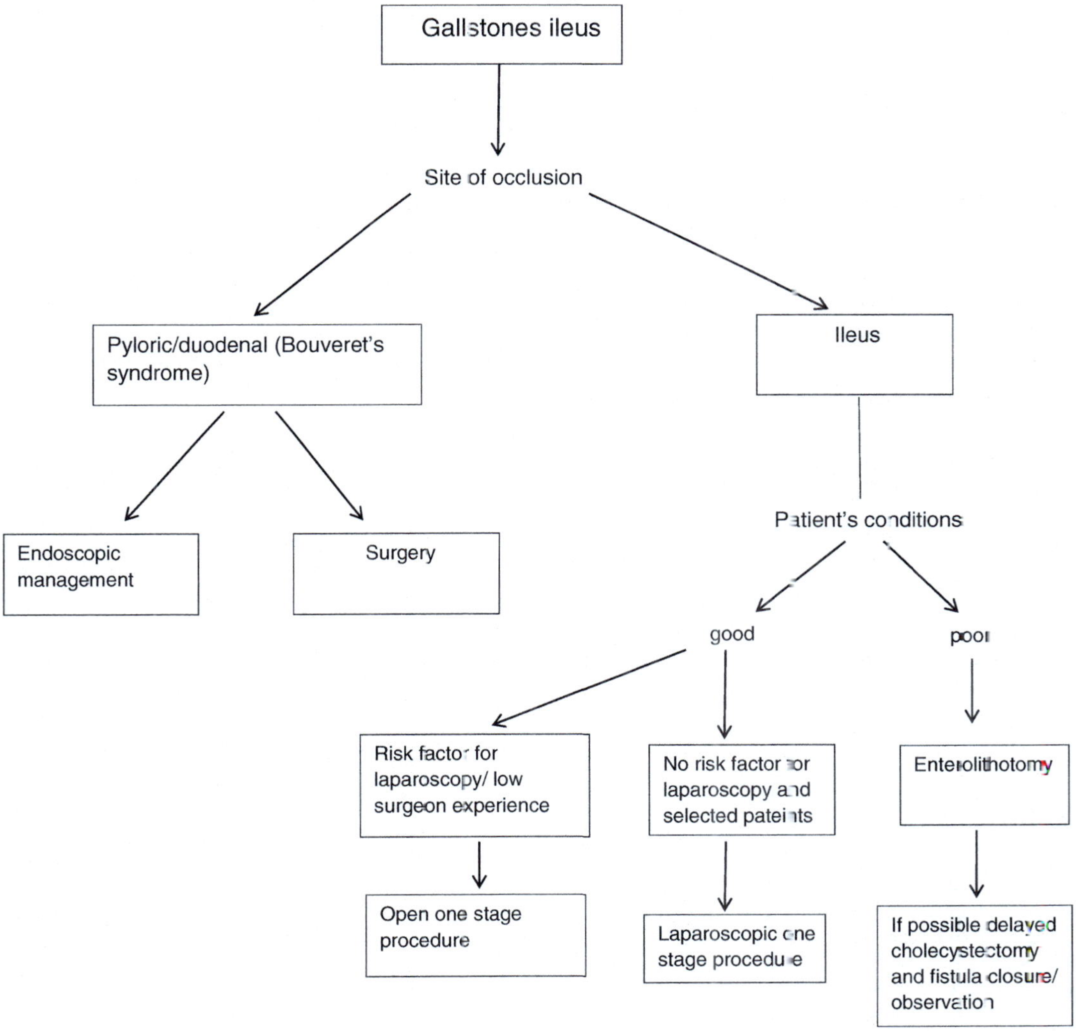

Fig. 9.3 Diagnostic algorithm for gallstone ileus

9.5 Conclusions

Gallstone ileus remains a rare and insidious complication of chronic cholelithiasis, which can occur with extremely severe clinical conditions and is associated with high mortality.

Therefore, the best treatment has to be decided promptly, considering the comorbidities of the patient. It remains difficult to find a gold standard, given the lack of studies in the literature and the differences in each case.

A prospective multicentric study about laparoscopic and endoscopic procedure could be useful.

Five Things You Should Know About Gallstone Ileus in the Elderly and Frail Patient

- Gallstone ileus is a rare complication of chronic cholelithiasis (0.3–1.5%), in the elderly people, it could be the cause of intestinal occlusion in 2–5% of the cases.
- Gallstone ileus patients have aspecific clinical presentations in emergency with abdominal pain, abdominal distention, nausea, and vomiting.
- CT scan represents the gold standard for diagnosis, showing Rigler's triad: pneumobilia, small bowel obstruction, and ectopic gallstone, usually in the right iliac fossa.
- The best surgical treatment is still debated: one stage procedure increases the rate of complications; while the two stage procedure exposes to a possible recurrence.
- Apollo endoscopic overstitch and robotic suture, in future, could be valid therapeutic alternatives in the treatment of bilio-enteric fistula.

References

1. Reisner RM, Cohen JR. Gallstone ileus: a review of 1001 reported cases. Am Surg. 1994;60(6):441–6.
2. Halabi WJ, Kang CY, Ketana N, Lafaro KJ, Nguyen VQ, Stamos MJ, et al. Surgery for gallstone ileus: a nationwide comparison of trends and outcomes. Ann Surg. 2014;259(2):329–35.
3. Nakao A, Okamoto Y, Sunami M, Fujita T, Tsuji T. The oldest patient with gallstone ileus: report of a case and review of 176 cases in Japan. Kurume Med J. 2008;55(1–2):29–33.
4. Ayantunde AA, Agrawal A. Gallstone ileus: Diagnosis and management. World J Surg. 2007;31(6):1292–7.
5. Masannat Y, Masannat Y, Shatnawei A. Gallstone ileus: a review. Mt Sinai J Med. 2006;73(8):1132–4.
6. Clavien PA, Richon J, Burgan S, Rohner A. Gallstone ileus. Br J Surg. 1990;77(7):737–42.
7. Ravikumar R, Williams JG. The operative management of gallstoine ileus. Ann R Coll Surg Engl. 2010;92(4):279–81.
8. Luu MB, Deziel DJ. Unusual complications of gallstones. Surg Clin North Am. 2014;94(2):377–94.
9. Williams NE, Gundara JS, Roser S, Samra JS. Disease spectrum and use of cholecystolithotomy in gallstone ileus. Hepatobiliary Pancreat Dis Int. 2012;11(5):553–7.
10. Abou-Saif A, Al-Kawas FH. Complications of gallstone disease: Mirizzi syndrome, cholecystocholedochal fistula, and gallstone ileus. Am J Gastroenterol. 2002;97(2):249–54.
11. Cappell MS, Davis M. Characterization of Bouveret's syndrome: a comprehensive review of 128 cases. Am J Gastroenterol. 2006;101(9):2139–46.
12. Ishikura H, Sakata A, Kimura S, Okitsu H, Ishikawa M, Ichimori T, et al. Gallstone ileus of the colon. Surgery. 2005;138(3):540–2.
13. Chang L, Chang M, Chang HM, Chang AI, Chang F. Clinical and radiological diagnosis of gallstone ileus: a mini review. Emerg Radiol. 2018;25(2):189–96.
14. Farkas N, Kaur V, Shanmuganandan A, Black J, Redon C, Frampton AE, et al. A systematic review of gallstone sigmoid ileus management. Ann Med Surg. 2018;27:32–9.
15. VanLandingham SB, Broders CW. Gallsone ileus. Surg Clin North Am. 1982;62(2):241–7.
16. Zaliekas J, Munson JL. Complications of gallstones: the Mirizzi syndrome, gallstone ileus, gallstone pancreatitis, complications of "lost" gallstones. Surg Clin N Am. 2008;88(6):1345–68.
17. Nuño-Guzmán CM. Gallstone ileus, clinical presentation, diagnostic and treatment approach. World J Gastrointest Surg. 2016;8(1):65–76.
18. Dai XZ, Li GQ, Zhang F, Wang XH, Zhang CY. Gallstone ileus: case report and literature review. World J Gastroenterol. 2013;19(33):5586–9.
19. Danzi M, Grimaldi L, Fabozzi M, Reggio S, Danzi R, Soscia E, et al. Usefulness of CT-scan in the diagnosis and therapeutic approach of gallstone ileus: report of two surgically treated cases. BMC Surg. 2013;13 Suppl 2(Suppl 2):S6.
20. Berger MY, Van Der Velden JJIM, Lijmer JG, De Kort H, Prins A, Bohnen AM. Abdominal symptoms: do they predict gallstones? A systematic review. Scand J Gastroenterol. 2000;35(1):70–6.
21. Ploneda-Valencia CF, Gallo-Morales M, Rinchon C, Navarro-Muñiz E, Bautista-López CA, de la Cerda-Trujillo LF, et al. Gallstone ileus: an overview of the literature. Rev Gastroenterol Mex. 2017;82(3):248–54.
22. Prasad RM, Weimer KM, Baskara A. Gallstone ileus presenting as intussusception: a case report. Int J Surg Case Rep. 2017;30:37–9.

23. Jackson PG, Raiji M. Evaluation and management of intestinal obstruction. Am Fam Physician. 2011;83(2):159–65.
24. Rigler LG, Borman CN, Noble JF. Gallstone obstruction: pathogenesis and roentgen manifestations. J Am Med Assoc. 1941;117:1753–9.
25. Shah SK, Walker PA, Fischer UM, Karanjawala BE, Khan SA. Bouveret syndrome. J Gastrointest Surg. 2013;17(9):1720–1.
26. Chuah PS, Curtis J, Misra N, Hikmat D, Chawla S. Pictorial review: the pearls and pitfalls of the radiological manifestations of gallstone ileus. Abdom Radiol. 2017;42:1169–75.
27. Bortoff GA, Chen MYM, Ott DJ, Wolfman NT, Routh WD. Gallbladder stones: imaging and intervention. Radiographics. 2000;20(3):751–66.
28. O'Brien JW, Webb LA, Evans L, Speakman C, Shaikh I. Gallstone ileus caused by cholecystocolonic fistula and gallstone impaction in the sigmoid colon: review of the literature and novel surgical treatment with trephine loop colostomy. Case Rep Gastroenterol. 2017;11, 95(1):–102.
29. Beuran M, Ivanov I, Venter MD. Gallstone ileus—clinical and therapeutic aspects. J Med Life. 2010;3(4):365–71.
30. Yu CY, Lin CC, Shyu RY, Hsieh CB, Wu HS, Tyan YS, et al. Value of CT in the diagnosis and management of gallstone ileus. World J Gastroenterol. 2005;11(14):2142–7.
31. Swift SE, Spencer JA. Gallstone ileus: CT findings. Clin Radiol. 1998;53(6):451–4.
32. Martín-Pérez J, Delgado-Plasencia L, Bravo-Gutiérrez A, Burillo-Putze G, Martínez-Riera A, Alarcó-Hernández A, et al. Gallstone ileus as a cause of acute abdomen. Importance of early diagnosis for surgical treatment. Cirugía Española (English Ed). 2013;91:485–9.
33. Koulaouzidis A, Moschos J. Bouveret's syndrome. Narrative review. Ann Hepatol. 2007;6, 89(2):–91.
34. Heger U, Sun H, Hinz U, Klaiber U, Tanaka M, Liu B, et al. Induction chemotherapy in pancreatic cancer: CA 19-9 may predict resectability and survival. HPB. 2020;22(2):224–32.
35. Furukawa A, Yamasaki M, Furuichi K, Yokoyama K, Nagata T, Takahashi M, et al. Helical CT in the diagnosis of small bowel obstruction. Radiographics. 2001;21(2):341–55.
36. Barakos JA, Ralls PW, Lapin SA, Johnson MB, Radin DR, Colletti PM, et al. Cholelithiasis: evaluation with CT. Radiology. 1987;162(2):415–8.
37. Gan S, Roy-Choudhury S, Agrawal S, Kumar H, Pallan A, Super P, et al. More than meets the eye: subtle but important CT findings in Bouveret's syndrome. Am J Roentgenol. 2008;191(1):182–5.
38. Warttig S, Ward S, Rogers G, McVeigh G, Evans ED, Dwerryhouse S, et al. Diagnosis and management of gallstone disease: summary of NICE guidance. BMJ (Online). 2014;349:g6241.
39. Calvo MM, Bujanda L, Heras I, Calderon A, Cabriada JL, Orive V, et al. Magnetic resonance cholangiography versus ultrasound in the evaluation of the gallbladder. J Clin Gastroenterol. 2002;34(3):233–6.
40. Liang X, Li W, Zhao B, Zhang L, Cheng Y. Comparative analysis of MDCT and MRI in diagnosing chronic gallstone perforation and ileus. Eur J Radiol. 2015;84(10):1835–42.
41. Yamauchi Y, Wakui N, Asai Y, Dan N, Takeda Y, Ueki N, et al. Gallstone ileus following endoscopic stone extraction. Case Rep Gastrointest Med. 2014;2014:271571.
42. Deitz DM, Standage BA, Pinson CW, McConnell DB, Krippaehne WW. Improving the outcome in gallstone ileus. Am J Surg. 1986 151(5):572–6.
43. Dumonceau JM, Devière J. Novel treatment options for Bouveret's syndrome: a comprehensive review of 61 cases of successful endoscopic treatment. Expert Rev Gastroenterol Hepatol. 2016;10(11):1245–55.
44. Warshaw AL, Bartlett MK. Choice of operation for gallstone intestinal obstruction. Ann Surg. 1966;164(6):1051–5.
45. Deckoff SL. Gallstone ileus; a report of 12 cases. Ann Surg. 1955;142(1):52–55.
46. Montgomery A. Laparoscope–guided enterolithotomy for gallstone ileus. Surg Laparosc Endosc. 1993;3(4):310–4.
47. Bossart PA, Patterson AH, Zintel HA. Carcinoma of the gallbladder. A report of seventy-six cases. Am J Surg. 1962;103:366–9.
48. Behrens C, Amson B. Laparoscopic management of multiple gallstone ileus. Surg Laparosc Endosc Percutaneous Tech. 2010;18(5):450–2.
49. Bircan HY, Koc B, Ozcelik U, Kemik O, Demirag A. Laparoscopic treatment of gallstone ileus. Clin Med Insights Case Rep. 2014;7:75–7.
50. Tan YM, Wong WK, Ooi LLPJ. A comparison of two surgical strategies for the emergency treatment of gallstone ileus. Singapore Med J. 2004;45(2):69–72.
51. Riaz N, Khan MR, Tayeb M. Gallstone ileus: retrospective review of a single centre's experience using two surgical procedures. Singapore Med J. 2008;49(8):624–6.

10 Acute Pancreatitis Management in Elderly/Frail Patients

Angelo Iossa and Gianfranco Silecchia

10.1 Introduction

Acute pancreatitis (AP) is a very unpredictable inflammatory disease with different outcomes [1–3] that may involve local tissues or systemic organs and tissues [4]. In the United States, >275,000 patients are hospitalized for AP annually with a cumulative cost of >$2.6 billion per year [5]. The global incidence of AP ranges from 5 to 30 cases per 100,000 inhabitants, and there is evidence that the incidence has been rising in recent years [6, 7]. Data from the Global Burden of Disease Study revealed a global incidence for acute pancreatitis of 5,210,000 patients in 2016, representing a 30% increase compared to 2006 [8]. In Europe, the incidence of acute pancreatitis ranged from 4.6 to 100 per 100,000 population. Incidence was the highest in eastern or northern Europe. The highest ratios of gallstone to alcohol etiologies were identified in southern Europe (Greece, Turkey, Italy, and Croatia), with the lowest ratios mainly in Eastern Europe (Latvia, Finland, Romania, Hungary, Russia, and Lithuania [9]). The most common age group is 30–40 years, and it occurs more in men than women, but it is worrying that several studies have suggested the incidence of AP in the elderly may be increasing [10, 11]. Causes include gallstones and alcohol abuse most frequently, while other causes include abdominal trauma, drugs, infections, hyperlipidemia, hypercalcemia, human immunodeficiency virus (HIV), neoplasms (e.g., ductal carcinoma, ampullary carcinoma, islet cell tumor, solid pseudotumor of the pancreas, sarcoma, lymphoma, cholangiocarcinoma, or metastatic tumor), and idiopathic [7]. The overall case fatality rate for AP is 5%; it may run a totally benign course in more than 80% of cases but in 10–20% it has a wildfire-like course which may proceed so fast as to reach a point of no return in short time [12]. Severity classification and diagnosis is made based on the Atlanta Classification (revised in 2012-RAC (revised Atlanta classification)) [13] or on the Determinant-based classification (DBC) [14] and are the following:

10.2 Revised Atlanta Classification (RAC)

Diagnosis Criteria (Two of the Following)

- Abdominal pain (acute onset of a persistent, severe, epigastric pain often radiating to the back)
- Serum lipase activity (or amylase) at least three times greater than the upper limit of normal

A. Iossa · G. Silecchia (✉)
Division of General Surgery and Bariatric Centre of Excellence, Department of Medical-Surgical Sciences and Biotechnologies, University of Rome "La Sapienza", Rome, Italy
e-mail: gianfranco.silecchia@uniroma1.it

F. Agresta et al. (eds.), *Emergency laparoscopic surgery in the elderly and frail patient*,
https://doi.org/10.1007/978-3-030-79990-8_10

- Characteristic findings of acute pancreatitis on CT scan or magnetic resonance imaging (MRI)

Severity Score

- *Mild acute pancreatitis:* No organ failure, local or systemic complications
- *Moderately severe acute pancreatitis:* Organ failure that resolves within 48 h and/or local or systemic complications without persistent organ failure
- *Severe acute pancreatitis:* Persistent organ failure >48 h
- *Interstitial edematous acute pancreatitis:* Acute inflammation of the pancreatic parenchyma and peripancreatic tissues, but without recognizable tissue necrosis
- *Necrotizing acute pancreatitis:* Inflammation associated with pancreatic parenchymal necrosis and/or peripancreatic necrosis; organ failure and systemic complications of acute pancreatitis. Respiratory: $PaO_2/FiO_2 \leq 300$; Cardiovascular: systolic blood pressure < 90 mm Hg (off inotropic support), not fluid responsive, or pH <7.3; Renal: serum creatinine ≥170 mmol/L
- *Local complications of acute pancreatitis:* Acute peripancreatic fluid collections, pancreatic pseudocysts, acute necrotic collections, walled-off pancreatic necrosis

DBC Criteria

- **Mild AP:** No organ failure AND No (peri) pancreatic necrosis
- **Moderate AP:** Transient organ failure AND/OR Sterile (peri)pancreatic necrosis
- **Severe AP:** Persistent organ failure OR Infected (peri)pancreatic necrosis
- **Critical AP:** Persistent organ failure AND Infected (peri)pancreatic necrosis

The disease is common among elderly (>65 years) who fall an easy prey to this disease due to comorbidities and compromised body systems [4]. There is increased diameter of common bile duct (CBD) in elderly, which makes them more susceptible to biliary pancreatitis and increased mortality with recurrent episodes [4]. Most scores have been established and the age it represents is usually a major negative prognostic factor. They include, based on patient demographics, clinical features, laboratory parameters, or imaging modalities, and are assessed on admission or within 48 h: Ranson criteria, Glasgow-Imrie score, Acute Physiology and Chronic Health Evaluation II (APACHE II), Simplified Acute Physiology Score (SAPS II), Bedside Index of Severity in Acute Pancreatitis (BISAP) score, and Japanese Severity Score (JSS). The severity with the relative mortality of largely used criteria is reported in the following table.

Criteria	Year	Parameters	Age (years)	Interpretation
Ranson	1974	For gallstones AP: 5 + 5 within 48 h For all the other causes: 5 + 6 within 48 h	**For gallstones AP: >70 (+1)** **For all the other causes: >55 (+1)**	Score ≥ 3: Severe pancreatitis likely. Mortality: Score 0–2: 2% mortality Score 3–4: 15% mortality Score 5–6: 40% mortality Score 7–8: 100% mortality
Glasgow-Imrie score	1978/modified in 1981	8 usually scored at admission and 48 h after	**>55 (+1)**	Score ≥ 3: severe pancreatitis likely Mortality similar to Ranson criteria

Criteria	Year	Parameters	Age (years)	Interpretation
APACHE II	1985	14 usually scored at admission and 48 h after	**<44 (0 point)** **45–54 (+2)** **55.64–(+3)** **65.74–(+5)** **>75 (+6)**	Score ≥ 9: severe pancreatitis likely Mortality: 0–4 points: 4% non-op, 1% post-op 5–9 points: 8% non-op, 3% post-op 10–14 points: 15% non-op, 7% post-op 15–19 points: 24% non-op, 12% post-op 20–24 points: 40% non-op, 30% post-op 25–29 points: 55% non-op, 35% post-op 30 to 34 points: Approx 73% both 35–100 points: 85% non-op, 88% post-op
SAPS II	1984	12 usually scored at admission and 48 h after	**<40 (0 point)** **40–59 (+7)** **60.69–(+12)** **70–74 (+15)** **75–79 (+16)**	Mortality predictive value similar to APACHE II
BISAP	2008	5 usually scored at admission and 48 h after	**>60 (+1)**	Score ≥ 3: severe pancreatitis likely Mortality: 0–2 points: <2% 3–5 points: >15%
JSS	2008	9 usually scored at admission and 48 h after	**>70 (+1)**	Score ≥ 3: severe pancreatitis likely Score ≥ 2: mild pancreatitis likely Mortality: Score < 3: 1.1%

Each score is considering the age > 45 years as a negative prognostic factor independently from the performing status. For example, the APACHE II score, worldwide used, adds two or six scores more in patients between 45 and 74 years and older than 75 years, respectively. Furthermore, the SAPS II adds +15 points in case of age older than 70 years. Similarly, the recently introduced score, BISAP, includes an age > 60 years as a severe negative factor affecting mortality and recovery time (score 1).

In the literature, some experience confirmed the age as the main factor affecting dramatically the mortality rate, [4] reporting in the elderly group (>55 years) an overall mortality of 19.11%, compared to a significantly low mortality 7.93 in the younger age group (<55 years) ($p < 0.001\%$). Similarly, Uomo et al. [15] retrospectively evaluating 439 patients admitted with a first episode of AP found that age older than 70 years was associated with necrotizing pancreatitis and increased mortality (25.8 vs. 7.8%). Patel et al. in 2019 evaluating the National Readmission Database including 184,763 AP admission with 41% elderly (>65 years), demonstrated an increased mortality (OR, 2.8; 95% CI: 2.2, 3.5) and severe acute pancreatitis (SAP) (OR, 1.2; 95% CI: 1.1, 1.3) incidence in that group [16]. The mechanisms underlying the increased severity of AP in elderly patients are not completely understood but can include the proinflammatory status in older people or organ-specific alterations [17] that may contribute to increased systemic inflammation and respiratory distress syndrome. Furthermore, there are reports of an increased cytokine production in elderly patients with sepsis, compared with younger people. In addition, the elderly tend to have more comorbidities which may add to the effect of several organ systems. Less reserve capacity for each organ system may account for a greater risk of failure in the elderly. Hard to define in the AP management the real and common definition of elderly that ranges from >45 years old to >65 years old (as indicated by the World Health Organization (WHO)-http://www.who.int/healthinfo/survey/ageingdefnolder/en/.6 June 2017), data that make hard-to-create recommendations on this people's subgroup. Furthermore, despite the age being included as a high = risk category, no specific treatment strategy has been recommended in elderly patients in all the available guidelines [17–19], such as prophylactic antibiotic use or intensive care unit (ICU) admission that should be preferred only in indicated cases (severe acute pancreatitis based on an APACHE II score greater than 8, C reactive protein (CRP) greater than 14,286 nmol/L (150 mg/L), or organ dysfunction for more than 48 h, despite adequate resuscitation, evidence of present or evolving organ dysfunction). Balance of deficiency, particularly Ca^{2+}, fast oral feeding restoration, strict parameters' monitoring, adequate fluid intake to reduce pancreatic microcirculation damage, and pain management do not differ by age and should be performed routinely [18–20].

Surgical treatment in AP management represents the choice in limited cases as: acute necrotic collections (ANCs) or walled-off pancreatic necrosis (WOPN) that failed the nonoperative treatment, gallstone in case of mild acute biliary pancreatitis without fluid collections, and pseudocysts symptomatic, infected, or increasing in size [18–20]. Typically, when these cases appear in fragile patients, a risk analysis should be performed to assess the risk of surgical approach. Based on the American Gastroenterological Association (AGA), National Institute for Health and Care Excellence (NICE), and World Society of Emergency Surgery (WSES) guidelines [18–20], all patients presenting with gallstone pancreatitis should be considered for cholecystectomy, as soon as possible in case of mild gallstone pancreatitis, when they are well enough to undergo surgery. In surgically unfit or frail elderly patients, ERCP with biliary sphincterotomy may be considered as definitive treatment, although the risks of sphincterotomy should be balanced against the risk of recurrent biliary events. As reported in a retrospective study published in 2019 by de la filia Morena [21] involving 247 patients unfit for surgery, in multivariate analysis, sphincterotomy showed a protective role for recurrence of pancreatitis (adjusted hazard ratio [HR]: 0.29, 95% CI: 0.08–0.92, $p = 0.037$) and for any gallstone-related event (HR 0.46, 95% CI: 0.21–0.98, $p = 0.043$). Regarding the other surgical cases, endoscopic management or step-up approaches [22–26] had to be preferred to an aggressive and early open surgical treatment to reduce potentially life-threatening complications.

Five Things You Should Know About AP in the Elderly

- Elderly patients represent a high-risk category for disease stage, hospital stay, and mortality.
- No specific medical treatment could reduce this risk.
- In case of gallstone AP, cholecystectomy should be performed, based on patient's risk.
- In case of patients unfit for cholecystectomy, ERCP with biliary sphincterotomy reduces the risk of recurrence.
- In case of other surgical complications (ANCs, WOPN, symptomatic pseudocysts), endoscopic or step-up approaches should be preferred.

References

1. Lund H, Tonnesen H, Tonnosen NH, Olsen O. Long term recurrence and death rates after acute pancreatitis. Scand J Gasteroenterol. 2006;41:234–8.
2. Voldov J, Tenner SM. Acute and chronic pancreatitis. Prim Care. 2001;28930:60728.
3. Stevens T, Paris MA, Walsh RM. Acute pancreatitis: Problems in adherence to the guidelines. Cleve Clin J Med. 2009;76(12):697–704. https://doi.org/10.3949/ccjm.76a09060.

4. Malik AM. Biliary pancreatitis. Deadly threat to the elderly. Is it a real threat? Int J Health Sci (Qassim). 2015;9(1):35–9. https://doi.org/10.12816/0024631.
5. Peery AF, Crockett SD, Barritt AS, et al. Burden of gastrointestinal, liver, and pancreatic diseases in the United States. Gastroenterology. 2015;149:1731–1741.e3.
6. Krishna SG, Kamboj AK, Hart PA, et al. The changing epidemiology of acute pancreatitis hospitalizations: a decade of trends and the impact of chronic pancreatitis. Pancreas. 2017;46:482–8.
7. Zilio MB, et al. A systematic review and meta-analysis of the aetiology of acute pancreatitis. HPB (Oxford). 2019;21(3):259–67. PMID: 30249509.
8. Vos T, Abajobir A, Abbafati C, Abbas K, Abate K, Abd-Allah F, et al. Global, regional, and national incidence, prevalence, and years lived with disability for 328 diseases and injuries for 195 countries, 1990–2016: a systematic analysis for the Global Burden of Disease Study 2016. Lancet. 2017;390:1211–59.
9. Roberts S, Morrison-Rees S, John A, Williams JG, Brown T, Samue DG. The incidence and aetiology of acute pancreatitis across Europe. Review. Pancreatology. 2017;17(2):155–65. https://doi.org/10.1016/j.pan.2017.01.005. Epub 2017 Jan 1.
10. Gloor Z, Ahmed Z, Uhi W, Buchler MW. Pancreatic disease in the elderly. Best Pract Res Clin Gastroenterol. 2002;16:159–70.
11. Somasekar K, Foulkes A, Morris-Stiff G, Hassn A. Acute pancreatitis in the elderly—can we perform better? Surgeon. 2011;9:305–8.
12. Crockett SD, Wani S, Gardner TB, Falck-Ytter Y, Barkun AN, American Gastroenterological Association Institute Clinical Guidelines Committee Collaborators. American Gastroenterological Association Institute guideline on initial management of acute pancreatitis review. Gastroenterology. 2018;154(4):1096–101. https://doi.org/10.1053/j.gastro.2018.01.032. Epub 2018 Feb 3. PMID: 29409760.
13. Banks PA, Bollen TL, Dervenis C, Gooszen HG, Johnson CD, Sarr MG, Tsiotos GG, Vege SS, Acute Pancreatitis Classification Working Group. Classification of acute pancreatitis—2012: revision of the Atlanta classification and definitions by international consensus. Gut. 2013;62(1):102–11. https://doi.org/10.1136/gutjnl-2012-302779. Epub 2012 Oct 25. PMID: 23100216.
14. Dellinger EP, Forsmark CE, Layer P, et al. Determinant-based classification of acute pancreatitis severity: an international multidisciplinary consultation. Ann Surg. 2012;256:875–80. https://doi.org/10.1097/SLA.0b013e318256f778.
15. Uomo G, Talamini G, Rabitti PG, Cataldi F, Cavallera RF. Influence of advanced age and related comorbidity on the course and outcome of acute pancreatitis. Ital J Gastroenterol Hepatol. 1998;30:616–21.
16. Patel K, Li F, Luthra A, Hinton A, Lara L, Groce R, Hosmer A, McCarthy ST, Strobel S, Conwell DL, Krishna SG. Acute biliary pancreatitis is associated with adverse outcomes in the elderly: a propensity score-matched analysis. J Clin Gastroenterol. 2019;53(7):e291–7. https://doi.org/10.1097/MCG.0000000000001108. PMID: 30157063.
17. Coelho AMM, Machado MCC, Sampietre SN, da Silva FP, Cunha JEM, D'Albuquerque LAC. Local and systemic effects of aging on acute pancreatitis. Pancreatology. 2019;19(5):638–45. https://doi.org/10.1016/j.pan.2019.06.005. Epub 2019 Jun 9. PMID: 31204259.
18. Greenberg JA, Hsu J, Bawazeer M, Marshall J, Friedrich JO, Nathens A, Coburn N, May GR, Pearsall E, McLeod RS. Clinical practice guideline: management of acute pancreatitis. Can J Surg. 2016;59(2):128–40. https://doi.org/10.1503/cjs.015015.
19. Leppäniemi A, Tolonen M, Tarasconi A, Segovia-Lohse H, Gamberini E, Kirkpatrick AW, Ball CG, Parry N, Sartelli M, Wolbrink D, van Goor H, Baiocchi G, Ansaloni L, Biffl W, Coccolini F, Di Saverio S, Kluger Y, Moore E, Catena F. 2019 WSES guidelines for the management of severe acute pancreatitis. World J Emerg Surg. 2019;14:27. https://doi.org/10.1186/s13017-019-0247-0. eCollection 2019.
20. Goodchild G, et al. Practical guide to the management of acute pancreatitis. Frontline Gastroenterol. 2019;10(3):292–9. Review.
21. de la Filia Molina IG, de Paredes AGG, Ortega AM, Carrasco NM, De Santiago ER, Aldehuelo RS, Olcina JRF, Martin JÁG, Duran SL, Sequeiros EV, Albillos A. Biliary sphincterotomy reduces the risk of acute gallstone pancreatitis recurrence in non-candidates for cholecystectomy. Dig Liver Dis. 2019;51(11):1567–73. https://doi.org/10.1016/j.dld.2019.05.007. PMID: 31151894.
22. Mehta V, Kumar R, Parkash S, Singla S, Singh A, Chaudhary J, Bains H. Role of percutaneous catheter drainage as primary treatment of necrotizing pancreatitis. Turk J Gastroenterol. 2019;30(2):184–7. https://doi.org/10.5152/tjg.2018.17542. PMID: 30457559 Free PMC article.
23. van Santvoort HC, Besselink MG, Bakker OJ, Hofker HS, Boermeester MA, Dejong CH, van Goor H, Schaapherder AF, van Eijck CH, Bollen TL, van Ramshorst B, Nieuwenhuijs VB, Timmer R, Laméris JS, Kruyt PM, Manusama ER, van der Harst E, van der Schelling GP, Karsten T, Hesselink EJ, van Laarhoven CJ, Rosman C, Bosscha K, de Wit RJ, Houdijk AP, van Leeuwen MS, Buskens E, Gooszen HG, Dutch Pancreatitis Study Group. A step-up approach or open necrosectomy for necrotizing pancreatitis. N Engl J Med. 2010;362(16):1491–502. https://doi.org/10.1056/NEJMoa0908821. PMID: 20410514 Free article. Clinical Trial
24. Baron TH, DiMaio CJ, Wang AY, Morgan KA. American Gastroenterological Association clinical practice update: management of pancreatic necrosis. Gastroenterology. 2020;158(1):67–75.e1. https://doi.org/10.1053/j.gastro.2019.07.064. Epub 2019 Aug 31. PMID: 31479658 Review.

25. van Brunschot S, van Grinsven J, Voermans RP, Bakker OJ, Besselink MG, Boermeester MA, Bollen TL, Bosscha K, Bouwense SA, Bruno MJ, Cappendijk VC, Consten EC, Dejong CH, Dijkgraaf MG, van Eijck CH, Erkelens GW, van Goor H, Hadithi M, Haveman JW, Hofker SH, Jansen JJ, Laméris JS, van Lienden KP, Manusama ER, Meijssen MA, Mulder CJ, Nieuwenhuis VB, Poley JW, de Ridder RJ, Rosman C, Schaapherder AF, Scheepers JJ, Schoon EJ, Seerden T, Spanier BW, Straathof JW, Timmer R, Venneman NG, Vleggaar FP, Witteman BJ, Gooszen HG, van Santvoort HC, Fockens P, Dutch Pancreatitis Study Group. Transluminal endoscopic step-up approach versus minimally invasive surgical step-up approach in patients with infected necrotising pancreatitis (TENSION trial): design and rationale of a randomised controlled multicenter trial [ISRCTN09186711]. BMC Gastroenterol. 2013;13:161. https://doi.org/10.1186/1471-230X-13-161. PMID: 24274589. Free PMC article. Clinical Trial.
26. Sion MK, Davis KA. Step-up approach for the management of pancreatic necrosis: a review of the literature. Trauma Surg Acute Care Open. 2019;4(1):e000308. https://doi.org/10.1136/tsaco-2019-000308. eCollection 2019.

Acute Appendicitis

11

Mauro Podda, Gaetano Poillucci, Chiara Gerardi,
Nicola Cillara, Leonardo Montemurro,
Giulia Russo, Massimo Carlini, and Adolfo Pisanu

11.1 Introduction

11.1.1 Acute Appendicitis in the Elderly: The Scale of the Problem

Acute appendicitis (AA) is one of the most common causes of acute abdominal pain in the Western world, with a reported lifetime incidence of 7%–15% [1].

Although 90% of cases occur in children and young adults, recent statistics have shown that AA currently accounts for 15% of all emergency room visits for acute abdominal pain in patients over 60 years of age, and appendectomy is actually the third most common reason for urgent abdominal surgery in geriatric patients [2, 3]. AA is burdened by rates of mortality of up to 8% among patients older than 65 years, compared to a rate ranging between 0 and 1% among young patients [4].

Elderly patients with suspected AA spend more time in the emergency department compared to younger patients because they have nonspecific symptoms or clinical findings and laboratory results: up to 25% of elderly patients with AA have no lower right quadrant (LRQ) pain and <25% present with fever >37.7 °C [5]. Moreover, geriatric patients present later in the course of their illness, with more than 85% of them presenting after 24 h of pain.

Atypical presentations may explain the possible difficulties in emergency department triage that, combined with the presence of comorbidities and general frailty, result in higher rates of perforation and higher mortality rate in elderly compared to younger patients [6]. While complicated AA with abscess, gangrene, or diffuse peritonitis is usually reported as high as 20% of cases in the overall population, the incidence of elderly patients diagnosed with complicated forms of AA varies between 40 and 70% [7–9].

Elderly patients with suspected AA show a higher risk of colonic and appendiceal cancer, compared to the general population. These aspects, considered all together, make AA in the elderly patient a separate clinical entity.

M. Podda (✉) · A. Pisanu
Department of Emergency Surgery, Policlinico Universitario "Duilio Casula", University of Cagliari, Cagliari, Italy

G. Poillucci
Department of General and Emergency Surgery, San Camillo Hospital, Rome, Italy

C. Gerardi
Center for Regulatory Policies, IRCCS Istituto di Ricerche Farmacologiche Mario Negri, Milan, Italy

N. Cillara
Department of Surgery, Santissima Trinità Hospital, Cagliari, Italy

L. Montemurro · G. Russo · M. Carlini
Department of General Surgery, Sant' Eugenio Hospital, Rome, Italy

F. Agresta et al. (eds.), *Emergency laparoscopic surgery in the elderly and frail patient*,
https://doi.org/10.1007/978-3-030-79990-8_11

11.1.2 Risk Factors for Perforation

The often atypical clinical presentation of AA in the elderly, and the delay in seeking medical help have been associated with delay in diagnosis and treatment resulting in higher morbidity and mortality rates compared to younger population. If, on the one hand, the prognosis of uncomplicated AA in both young and old age group is nearly equivalent, on the other, perforation worsens the perioperative condition dramatically, resulting in higher rates of adverse outcomes.

Omari et al. reported that, of all the risk factors studied, the patient's prehospital time delay was the most important risk factor for appendiceal perforation [8]. Further researches found that being of male sex was significantly related to perforation. A possible explanation for this fact is the elderly males' culture of reluctance to go to hospital [3].

Conversely, the perforation rate seems to be not dependent on the presence of comorbidities or in-hospital time delay [8].

11.1.3 Diagnostic Issues in Acute Appendicitis in the Elderly and Frail Patient

Geriatric patients admitted to the emergency department with acute abdominal pain require more aggressive workups, mainly for two reasons: geriatric patients discharged from the hospital who presented with abdominal pain will return in 10% of cases within 2 weeks for similar complaints, and of those who undergo surgery, 17% will die, with mortality approaching 40% for patients older than 80 years [10].

More than 30% of patients with AA in this age group are diagnosed after substantial delay in seeking medical attention. Moreover, only 50% of patients are correctly diagnosed on admission. This, added to the high incidence of frailty reaching almost 80% in elderly patients undergoing emergency abdominal surgery, obviously leads to poor outcomes [11]. Therefore, according to some authors, CT should be considered as the first-line option in the diagnostics of older patients with suspected AA [12].

In the general population, risk stratification of patients with suspected AA by clinical scoring systems could guide decision-making to reduce admissions, optimize the utility of diagnostic imaging, and prevent negative surgical explorations. Clinical scores alone seem sufficiently sensitive to identify low-risk patients and decrease the need for imaging and negative surgical explorations in patients with suspected AA [13].

Few studies evaluated the applicability of AA clinical scores in the elderly population. The retrospective study by Shchatsko et al. showed that the use of Alvarado score, with a cut-off value of 5, maintains reliability in older patients. According to the study data, Alvarado scores ranging from 5 to 10 should correspond to a high risk of AA in the elderly [14]. The study by Konan et al. showed an area under the curve of the Alvarado score for elderly patients of 96.9% with 100% negative and positive predictive values of the two cut-off points of 3 and 6 [15].

Contrast-enhanced CT scan is strongly recommended in all elderly patients with an Alvarado score ≥ 5 to confirm or exclude the diagnosis of AA [16].

Recent studies reported a high accuracy for unenhanced CT in the early diagnosis of acute abdominal pain in the emergency department and advocated its systematic use in elderly patients in order to avoid renal impairment or to expedite treatment and thus reduce morbidity or mortality, even before obtaining the serum creatinine [17]. However, the value of unenhanced CT scan in the differential diagnosis of AA in the elderly (i.e., acute diverticulitis, appendiceal tumors, perforated colon cancers, etc.) is limited.

Routine use of CT scan with intravenous contrast has been demonstrated to be associated with the highest sensitivity to confirm the diagnosis of AA [18]. A recent meta-analysis has failed to show a higher risk of contrast-induced acute renal failure in patients with chronic kidney disease [19].

11.1.4 Timing of Appendectomy

The theory hypothesizing that perforated AA might be a different disease entity from uncomplicated AA, rather than being the natural evolution of the disease, has some support in the recent meta-analysis by van Dijk et al., demonstrating that delaying appendectomy for up to 24 h after admission does not appear to be a risk factor for complicated AA, postoperative morbidity, or surgical-site infection (SSI) in the general population. Pooled adjusted odds ratios revealed no significantly higher risk for complicated AA when appendectomy was delayed for 7–12 or 13–24 h, and meta-analysis of unadjusted data supported these findings by yielding no increased risk for complicated AA or postoperative complications with a delay of 24–48 h [20].

Whether in-hospital surgical delay up to 24 h is safe also in elderly patients with uncomplicated AA is far to be established. However, realistically, perforation occurs earlier in the course of AA in patients aged >65 years when compared to younger patients, probably before hospital admission itself, thus suggesting that a correct diagnosis on admission is of particular relevance in these patients [21].

11.1.5 Laparoscopic Appendectomy

The use of LA for AA (especially in complicated cases) in older patients demonstrated to be a protective factor against the development of postoperative complications [7] (Figs. 11.1 and 11.2). Based on the results of a recent systematic review and meta-analysis showing that for elderly patients with AA, LA is associated with less postoperative mortality and complications, the World Society of Emergency Surgery (WSES) has recommended LA for elderly patients in the 2020 update of the Jerusalem guidelines for diagnosis and treatment of AA [13, 22].

In adults, LA is associated with less postoperative complications, less postoperative pain, and shorter return to activity. There is

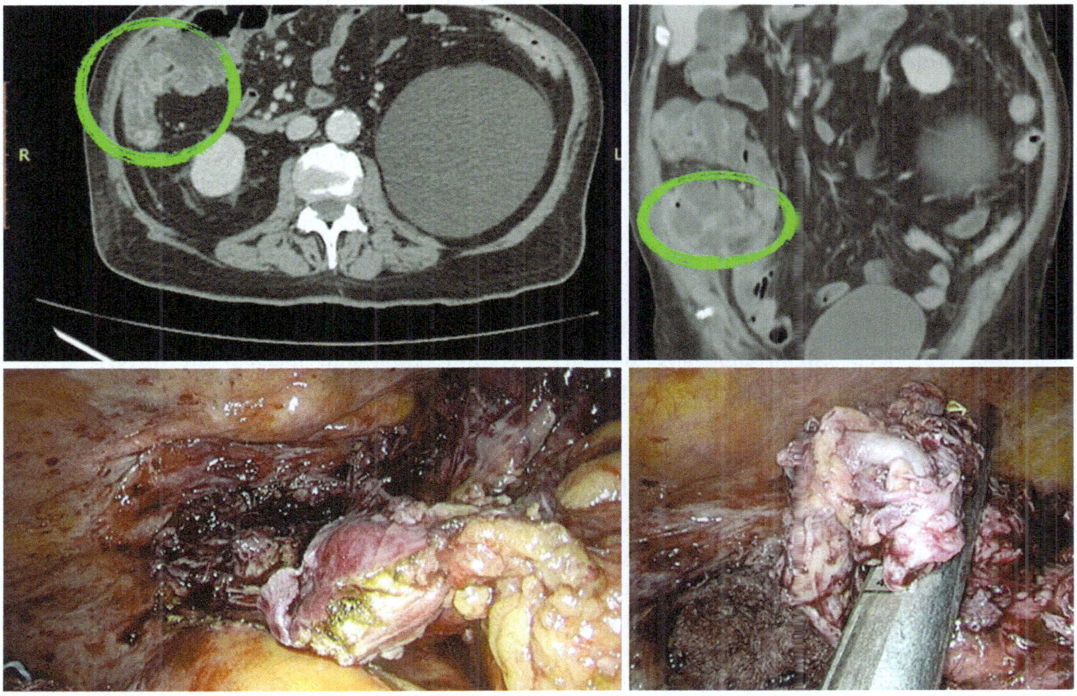

Fig. 11.1 Complicated acute appendicitis with large retroperitoneal abscess in an 85-year-old male patient. Laparoscopic approach: ileocecal resection with intracorporeal anastomosis

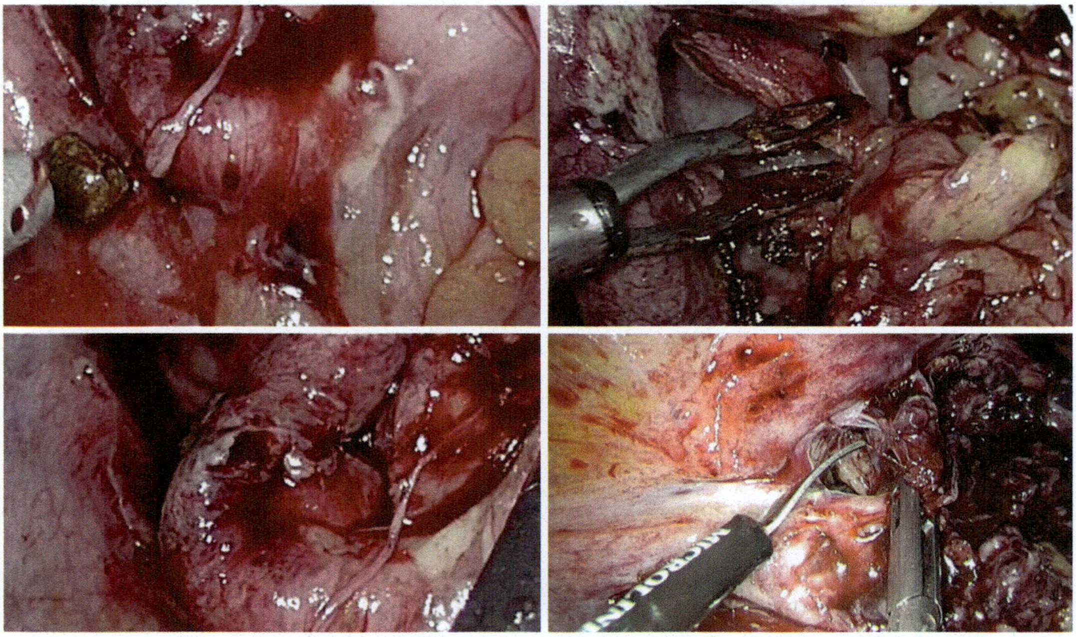

Fig. 11.2 Gangrenous acute appendicitis in elderly patients. Laparoscopic appendectomies

still a great amount of debate concerning postoperative intra-abdominal abscess following LA. Although a cumulative meta-analysis by Ukai et al. demonstrated that increased risk of intra-abdominal abscess following LA disappeared in studies published after 2001, the latest Cochrane review on the topic has shown increased risk of postoperative abscess following LA [23, 24].

In the elderly, LA is typically associated with faster recovery and a shorter length of hospitalization compared to open surgery, with all the benefits deriving in terms of reduction of pulmonary infections, deep vein thrombosis, pulmonary embolism, and physical and mental deconditioning related to prolonged hospitalization.

A trend toward increase in the use of LA for elderly patients has been reported since 2010 [25]. Previously, data from the 2007 Nationwide Inpatient Sample (NIS) showed that less than 50% of the patients older than 65 years underwent a LA in the USA compared with over 60% of the 40 to 64-year-old group. In 2013, Moazzez et al. reported that 75% of appendectomies performed on patients aged >65 years was laparoscopic in the USA. These data confirm that LA is becoming the gold standard approach even in older age group patients owing to the well-demonstrated benefits of laparoscopy [26].

Although conversion and re-intervention rates are greater among older patients, this aspect is not related to age but rather to the clinical stage of AA. In the recent meta-analysis by Wang et al., 12 studies with 126,237 elderly patients in the LA group and 213,201 patients in the open appendectomy group were analyzed. Postoperative mortality, as well as postoperative complications and surgical-site infections were reduced following LA. Intra-abdominal abscess rate was similar between LA and open appendectomy. Duration of surgery was longer following LA, while the length of hospital stay was shorter [22].

It is worth remarking that an experienced laparoscopic surgeon should operate on or take over when a resident is not able to move forward with the operation. This aspect is particularly important in older patients with delayed diagnosis and/or advanced disease.

11.1.5.1 Laparoscopic Appendectomy for Complicated Appendicitis with Phlegmon or Abscess

Appendiceal abscess has an incidence of approximately 3.8% in patients with perforated AA [21]. Generally, compared with younger populations, older patients are more often operated on when symptoms last longer than 48 hours and are more likely to develop complicated AA. The differences are observed already at the age of >40 years and are even more evident with older patients [12].

In the past, immediate surgery was associated with a higher morbidity if compared with conservative treatment, while the nonsurgical treatment of appendicular abscess or phlegmon was reported to succeed in over 90% of patients, with an overall risk of recurrence of 7.4% and only 19.7% of cases of abscess requiring percutaneous drainage [21].

Percutaneous drainage as an adjunct to antibiotics, if accessible, could be beneficial, although there is a lack of evidence for its use on a routine basis.

The meta-analysis by Similis et al. (including 16 retrospective studies and one nonrandomized prospective study for a total of 1572 patients, of whom 847 were treated with conservative treatment and 725 with appendectomy) revealed that conservative treatment was associated with significantly less overall complications (wound infections, abdominal/pelvic abscesses, ileus/bowel obstructions, and reoperations), if compared to immediate appendectomy [27].

However, in the general population, current evidence shows that LA in patients presenting with appendiceal abscess is preferable to nonoperative management (NOM) with antibiotics in the reduction of the length of hospital stay and need for readmissions, when laparoscopic expertise is available. The high-quality randomized controlled trial by Mentula et al. demonstrated that LA in experienced hands is a safe and feasible first-line treatment for appendiceal abscess, being related to fewer readmissions and fewer additional interventions than conservative treatment, with a comparable hospital stay. Patients in the laparoscopy group had a 10% risk of bowel resection and 13% risk of incomplete appendectomy. There were significantly fewer patients with unplanned readmissions following LA compared to NOM (3% versus 27%). Additional interventions were required in 7% of patients following LA (percutaneous drainage) and 30% of patients in the conservative group (appendectomy) [28].

However, in elderly patients with periappendiceal abscess and serious comorbidities, the use of NOM with percutaneous drainage, if accessible, is justified [16]. Such patients should undergo elective colonic screening and/or CT follow-up once the acute inflammatory phase has passed.

11.1.5.2 Technical Aspects

The standard technique for LA includes three incisions. Ports' size and position are variable in different practices. Once pneumoperitoneum is established with either a closed technique (Veress needle, direct trocar insertion—DTI) or an open Hasson's technique, further two ports are placed in order to obtain the proper triangulation: lower left quadrant (LLQ) and suprapubic, LLQ and lower right quadrant (LRQ), suprapubic and LRQ, or both ports in the suprapubic position.

Although recent studies provided level 1a evidence that single-incision LA (SILA) is as feasible, effective, and safe as the conventional three-port LA, high-level meta-analyses conducted in adults have not supported the application of SILA because of its significantly longer operative times and the higher doses of analgesia required compared with those for three-port LA [13].

The best available evidence suggests that peritoneal irrigation with normal saline during LA does not provide additional benefits compared with suction alone in terms of intra-abdominal abscess, surgical-site infection, and length of hospital stay, but it may prolong the operative time. The recent meta-analysis by Siotos et al., including more than 2500 patients from five studies, has shown that the use of irrigation, despite adding 7 min to the duration of the operation, overall did not demonstrate a significant decrease in intra-abdominal abscess [29].

There are no clinical advantages in the use of endostaplers over endoloops for stump closure in either simple or complicated AA, whereas polymeric clips may be the cheapest and easiest method (with shorter operative times) for stump closure in uncomplicated AA.

So, the use of endoloops/suture ligation or polymeric clips for stump closure in either uncomplicated or complicated AA is recommended, whereas endostaplers may be used when dealing with complicated cases depending on the intraoperative judgment of the surgeon and resources available [13].

The presence of an appendiceal mass, non-visualization of the appendix, delayed admission, and high C-reactive protein (CRP) level are predictive factors of extended bowel resection (ileocecectomy or right colectomy) during appendectomy [30]. A laparoscopic ileocecectomy or right colectomy with intracorporeal anastomosis can be safely performed in experienced hands, with either a three-port or a standard four-port technique, to guarantee the patient the best results in terms of reduction of SSI, less pain, and faster return to daily normal activity.

The updated 2019 Cochrane review on the use of intra-abdominal drains following appendectomy for complicated AA found that there was insufficient evidence to determine the effects of abdominal drainage on intraperitoneal abscess or for surgical-site infection. The increased risk of a 30-day overall complication rate in the drainage group was rated as very low-quality evidence, as well as the evidence that drainage increases hospital stay by 2.17 days compared to the no drainage group. Thus, there is no evidence for any clinical improvement by using abdominal drainage in patients undergoing appendectomy for complicated AA [31]. Low-quality studies have reported that routine drainage seems to cause more complications, higher length of hospital stay, and transit recovery time [32]. So, in adult patients, the use of drains after appendectomy for perforated AA and abscess/peritonitis should be discouraged.

11.1.6 Risk Factors Predictive for Postoperative Morbidity Following Appendectomy

Elderly patients have a higher risk for both mortality and morbidity following appendectomy. Morbidity rate is estimated to be around 70%, as compared to 1% in the general population [2].

Complications are three times more common following perforation (75% vs. 25%) than in nonperforated AA, while the mortality rate in elderly patients following perforated AA is reported between 2.3 and 10% [8]. Death is often related to septic complications compounded by the patient's comorbidities [33].

Higher adverse outcomes rates observed in the elderly population can be explained not only by delay in the appropriate diagnosis, more advanced disease, and operative technique, but also by a higher number of comorbidities, such as cognitive impairment and functional dependence, that might complicate the recovery.

Of all the risk factors for postoperative complications studied, the patient's prehospital time delay is the most important risk factor for appendiceal perforation [8].

Anemia and chronic renal insufficiency were also shown to be associated with poorer outcomes after appendectomy in the elderly [7]. Interestingly, age has not shown to be a predictor of adverse events.

Data from the American College of Surgeons National Surgical Quality Improvement Program (NSQIP) demonstrated that patients with decreased baseline physical status assessed by the American Society of Anesthesiologists (ASA) scoring system had the worst outcomes (1.5% mortality; 14% major complications) when an operation was delayed to hospital day 3. Logistic regression revealed higher ASA physical status class and open operations as the only predictors of major complications [34]. Since delayed diagnosis results in the development of complications following appendectomy in elderly patients, more efforts should be placed in improving both diagnostic and treatment patterns to improve clinical outcomes. It is important to emphasize that an appropriate patient selection is essential for achieving adequate outcomes in LA in the elderly. Laparoscopy may not be practicable in case of severe cardiovascular and respiratory impairment or in case of extensive adherences.

Moreover, significant physiological changes may occur in the elderly with additional concomitant illness such as diabetes, hypertension, ischemic heart disease, and chronic pulmonary disease during LA, especially during long operations. The pneumoperitoneum carries particular risk via carbon dioxide insufflation in elderly patients with reduced cardiopulmonary reserve, causing diaphragmatic splinting, reducing venous return and cardiac output, and predisposing the patient to myocardial infarction and basal atelectasis [35].

11.1.7 Nonoperative Treatment

Different randomized controlled trials and subsequent meta-analyses have suggested that NOM for AA is a safe and efficient alternative to the long-standing practice of immediately proceeding with an appendectomy on diagnosis, with respect to clinical outcomes such as symptoms relief, development of peritonitis, and return to work [36–39].

The safety and efficacy of antibiotics alone as primary treatment strategy in elderly patients with uncomplicated AA have not been fully assessed. A low-quality retrospective cohort study published in 2014 by Park et al. showed that patients aged >80 years with imaging-confirmed (CT 90.1%) AA and an appendiceal diameter ≤1 cm might benefit from NOM with antibiotics. In this study, only one patient of 26 years treated conservatively (4.8%) experienced an index admission antibiotic treatment failure, while, at the median follow-up period of 17 months, 5 patients (20%) experienced recurrence [40]. These data are equivalent to those reported by Podda et al., published in the Annals of Surgery in 2019, showing that NOM with antibiotics in the general population may fail during the primary hospitalization in about 8% of cases, and an additional 20% of patients might need a second hospitalization for recurrent AA [38].

However, due to the lack of high-quality evidence to date, it is unclear if NOM with antibiotics can be suggested as primary treatment to elderly patients with uncomplicated AA. The doubts in this sense may be associated with age-related risks and the difficulty in predicting the clinical course of AA in such patients.

A missing component in the evaluation of the safety profile of NOM has been the investigation and discussion of the possibility of missed malignancy, with particular regard to elderly patients. Generally, patients ≥40 years should undergo imaging investigation with CT scan in order to confirm the clinical suspicion of AA, especially when they are deemed to be candidates for NOM with antibiotics. In elderly patients, due to the rising rate of appendiceal neoplasms found at pathological examination following appendectomy for complicated AA, differential diagnosis between complicated and uncomplicated AA on CT scan is mandatory.

11.1.7.1 The Risk of Missing Appendiceal Tumors

Alarming rates of appendiceal neoplasms have been reported in patients presenting with appendiceal inflammatory masses varying from 10 to 29% [13].

Pathologically, obstruction of the appendiceal lumen is the usual cause of AA. In the elderly, this condition may also be due to a neoplasm, and AA can be its first manifestation.

Approximately 1% of patients in the general population who underwent appendectomy for possible AA was diagnosed with malignancy on pathology in the study by Lu et al. [41]

The distinction between complicated AA with abscess and uncomplicated AA is crucial. Several studies showed that the rates of appendiceal malignancies are much higher in complicated compared to uncomplicated cases. Teixeira et al. examined the rate of neoplasm in patients who presented with an appendiceal abscess or phlegmon and found the rate to vary between 10 and 29% [42]. Similarly, Furman et al. found that 29.4% of patients who underwent interval appendectomy for complicated AA had tumors discovered at the time of surgery [43]. These studies also found that the incidence of neoplasm found on interval appendectomy was higher for older patients, and such careful consideration of interval appendectomy has been suggested for patients over the age of 40.

Conversely, the incidence of colonic tumors in patients >40 years of age presenting with features of AA varies between 0.55 and 1.76% [44, 45]. This showed that colonic tumors present rarely with features of AA.

When counseling ≥40-year-old patients regarding operative vs NOM options for treatment of AA, the rising risk of a delayed or missed cancer diagnosis with increasing age must be discussed. A US retrospective cohort study on NSQIP appendectomy-targeted dataset from 2016 to 2017 enrolling a total of 21,069 patients with imaging-confirmed or imaging indeterminate AA who underwent appendectomy showed that increasing age had an increasing relationship with the odds of pathologic cancer diagnosis after appendectomy (age 50–59 OR 2.08; age 60–69 OR 2.89; age 70–79 OR 3.85; age ≥80 OR 5.32). The study also demonstrated that the preoperative imaging finding of indeterminate for AA was associated with significantly increased risk of finding appendiceal cancer on pathology [41].

11.1.7.2 Interval Appendectomy

The need for interval appendectomy after successful NOM for uncomplicated AA has been debated because the recurrence rate is very low. In case of complicated AA with abscess formation, the need for interval appendectomy after initial successful NOM has also been questioned, as the risk of recurrent AA is quite low between 5 and 20% [21].

The 2020 updated WSES Jerusalem Guidelines on AA recommended against routine interval appendectomy after NOM for complicated appendicitis only in young adults (<40 years old) and children, stating also that if the significant rate of neoplasms after periappendicular abscess will be validated by future studies, it would argue for routine interval appendectomy in this setting. Anyway, in adult patients ≥40 years with complicated AA treated nonoperatively, both colonic screening with colonoscopy and interval full-dose contrast-enhanced CT scan are recommended [13].

In the setting of increased gain for NOM of AA, the concern for missing early, resectable malignancies has increased. In the study performed by Mällinen et al. examining the outcomes of NOM of AA with associated periappendiceal abscess, the authors found a 20% neoplasm rate in enrolled patients [46]. So, although multi-institutional, high-quality studies to determine the indication to interval appendectomy in elderly patients are warranted, interval appendectomy and pathological examination of the appendix might be required in elderly patients to determine the underlying cause of appendiceal abscess.

Five Things You Should Know About Appendectomy in the Elderly and Frail Patient

- Acute appendicitis currently accounts for 15% of all emergency room visits for acute abdominal pain in patients over 60 years of age, and the incidence of elderly patients diagnosed with complicated forms of appendicitis varies between 40 and 70%.
- Geriatric patients admitted to the emergency department with acute abdominal pain require aggressive workups. CT scan is strongly recommended in all elderly patients with an Alvarado score ≥5 to confirm or exclude the diagnosis of acute appendicitis.
- Laparoscopic appendectomy in older patients demonstrated to be a protective factor against the development of postoperative complications, with all the benefits deriving in terms of reduction of pulmonary infections, deep vein thrombosis, pulmonary embolism, and physical and mental deconditioning related to prolonged hospitalization.
- When counseling elderly patients regarding operative vs NOM options for treatment of acute appendicitis, the rising risk of a delayed or missed cancer diagnosis must be discussed.
- Interval appendectomy and pathological examination of the appendix might be required in elderly patients to determine the underlying cause of appendiceal abscess.

References

1. Podda M, Cillara N, Di Saverio S. Appendicitis. Encyclopedia of Gastroenterology, II Edition. New York: Elsevier; 2020. pp. 164–176. https://doi.org/10.1016/B978-0-12-801238-3.66055-5.
2. Storm-Dickerson TL, Horattas MC. What have we learned over the past 20 years about appendicitis in the elderly? Am J Surg. 2003;185(3):198–201. https://doi.org/10.1016/s0002-9610(02)01390-9.
3. Sheu BF, Chiu TF, Chen JC, Tung MS, Chang MW, Young YR. Risk factors associated with perforated appendicitis in elderly patients presenting with signs and symptoms of acute appendicitis. ANZ J Surg. 2007;77(8):662–6. https://doi.org/10.1111/j.1445--2197.2007.04182.x.
4. Kotaluoto S, Ukkonen M, Pauniaho SL, Helminen M, Sand J, Rantanen T. Mortality related to appendectomy; a population based analysis over two decades in Finland. World J Surg. 2017;41(1):64–9. https://doi.org/10.1007/s00268-016-3688-6.
5. Clegg A, Young J, Iliffe S, Rikkert MO, Rockwood K. Frailty in elderly people [published correction appears in Lancet. 2013 Oct 19;382(9901):1328]. Lancet. 2013;381(9868):752–62. https://doi.org/10.1016/S0140-6736(12)62167-9.
6. Samaras N, Chevalley T, Samaras D, Gold G. Older patients in the emergency department: a review. Ann Emerg Med. 2010;56(3):261–9. https://doi.org/10.1016/j.annemergmed.2010.04.015.
7. Poillucci G, Podda M, Pisanu A, et al. Risk factors for postoperative morbidity following appendectomy in the elderly: a nationwide prospective cohort study [published online ahead of print, 2019 Jul 15]. Eur J Trauma Emerg Surg. 2019. https://doi.org/10.1007/s00068-019-01186-2.
8. Omari AH, Khammash MR, Qasaimeh GR, Shammari AK, Yaseen MK, Hammori SK. Acute appendicitis in the elderly: risk factors for perforation. World J Emerg Surg. 2014;9(1):6. https://doi.org/10.1186/1749-7922-9-6.
9. Segev L, Keidar A, Schrier I, Rayman S, Wasserberg N, Sadot E. Acute appendicitis in the elderly in the twenty-first century. J Gastrointest Surg. 2015;19(4):730–5. https://doi.org/10.1007/s11605-014-2716-9.
10. van Geloven AA, Biesheuvel TH, Luitse JS, Hoitsma HF, Obertop H. Hospital admissions of patients aged over 80 with acute abdominal complaints. Eur J Surg. 2000;166(11):866–71. https://doi.org/10.1080/110241500447254.
11. McComb A, Warkentin LM, McNeely ML, Khadaroo RG. Development of a reconditioning program for elderly abdominal surgery patients: the Elder-friendly Approaches to the Surgical Environment-BEdside reconditioning for Functional ImprovemenTs (EASE-BE FIT) pilot study. World J Emerg Surg. 2018;13:21. https://doi.org/10.1186/s13017-018-0180-7.
12. Lasek A, Pędziwiatr M, Kenig J, et al. The significant impact of age on the clinical outcomes of laparoscopic appendectomy: results from the polish laparoscopic appendectomy multicenter large cohort study. Medicine (Baltimore). 2018;97(50):e13621. https://doi.org/10.1097/MD.0000000000013621.
13. Di Saverio S, Podda M, De Simone B, et al. Diagnosis and treatment of acute appendicitis: 2020 update of the WSES Jerusalem guidelines. World J Emerg Surg. 2020;15(1):27. https://doi.org/10.1186/s13017-020-00306-3.
14. Shchatsko A, Brown R, Reid T, Adams S, Alger A, Charles A. The utility of the Alvarado score in the diagnosis of acute appendicitis in the elderly. Am Surg. 2017;83(7):793–8.
15. Konan A, Hayran M, Kılıç YA, Karakoç D, Kaynaroğlu V. Scoring systems in the diagnosis of acute appendicitis in the elderly. Ulus Travma Acil Cerrahi Derg. 2011;17(5):396–400.
16. Fugazzola P, Ceresoli M, Agnoletti V, et al. The SIFIPAC/WSES/SICG/SIMEU guidelines for diagnosis and treatment of acute appendicitis in the elderly (2019 edition). World J Emerg Surg. 2020 15(1) 19. https://doi.org/10.1186/s13017-020-00298-0.
17. Sala E, Watson CJ, Beadsmoore C, et al. A randomized, controlled trial of routine early abdominal computed tomography in patients presenting with non-specific acute abdominal pain. Clin Radiol. 2007;62(10):961–9. https://doi.org/10.1016/j.crad.2007.01.030.
18. Terasawa T, Blackmore CC, Bent S, Kohlwes RJ. Systematic review: computed tomography and ultrasonography to detect acute appendicitis in adults and adolescents. Ann Intern Med. 2004;141(7):537–46. https://doi.org/10.7326/0003-4819-141-7-200410050-00011.
19. Lee YC, Hsieh CC, Chang TT, Li CY. Contrast-induced acute kidney injury among patients with chronic kidney disease undergoing imaging studies: a meta-analysis. AJR Am J Roentgenol. 2019;213(4):728–35. https://doi.org/10.2214/AJR.19.21309.
20. van Dijk ST, van Dijk AH, Dijkgraaf MG, Boermeester MA. Meta-analysis of in-hospital delay before surgery as a risk factor for complications in patients with acute appendicitis. Br J Surg. 2018;105(8):933–45. https://doi.org/10.1002/bjs.10873.
21. Andersson RE, Petzold MG. Nonsurgical treatment of appendiceal abscess or phlegmon: a systematic review and meta-analysis. Ann Surg. 2007;246(5):741–8. https://doi.org/10.1097/SLA.0b013e31811f3f9f.
22. Wang D, Dong T, Shao Y, Gu T, Xu Y, Jiang Y. Laparoscopy versus open appendectomy for elderly patients, a meta-analysis and systematic review. BMC Surg. 2019;19(1):54. https://doi.org/10.1186/s12893-019-0515-7.
23. Ukai T, Shikata S, Takeda H, et al. Evidence of surgical outcomes fluctuates over time: results from a cumulative meta-analysis of laparoscopic versus open appendectomy for acute appendicitis. BMC Gastroenterol. 2016;16:37. https://doi.org/10.1186/s12876-016-0453-0.

24. Jaschinski T, Mosch CG, Eikermann M, Neugebauer EA, Sauerland S. Laparoscopic versus open surgery for suspected appendicitis. Cochrane Database Syst Rev. 2018;11(11):CD001546. https://doi.org/10.1002/14651858.CD001546.pub4.
25. Kim MJ, Fleming FJ, Gunzler DD, Messing S, Salloum RM, Monson JR. Laparoscopic appendectomy is safe and efficacious for the elderly: an analysis using the National Surgical Quality Improvement Project database. Surg Endosc. 2011;25(6):1802–7. https://doi.org/10.1007/s00464-010-1467-2.
26. Moazzez A, Mason RJ, Katkhouda N. Thirty-day outcomes of laparoscopic versus open appendectomy in elderly using ACS/NSQIP database. Surg Endosc. 2013;27(4):1061–71. https://doi.org/10.1007/s00464-012-2557-0.
27. Simillis C, Symeonides P, Shorthouse AJ, Tekkis PP. A meta-analysis comparing conservative treatment versus acute appendectomy for complicated appendicitis (abscess or phlegmon). Surgery. 2010;147(6):818–29. https://doi.org/10.1016/j.surg.2009.11.013.
28. Mentula P, Sammalkorpi H, Leppäniemi A. Laparoscopic surgery or conservative treatment for appendiceal abscess in adults? A randomized controlled trial. Ann Surg. 2015;262(2):237–42. https://doi.org/10.1097/SLA.0000000000001200.
29. Siotos C, Stergios K, Prasath V, et al. Irrigation versus suction in laparoscopic appendectomy for complicated appendicitis: a meta-analysis. J Surg Res. 2019;235:237–43. https://doi.org/10.1016/j.jss.2018.10.005.
30. Saida F, Matsumoto S, Kitano M. Preoperative predictor of extensive resection for acute appendicitis. Am J Surg. 2018;215(4):599–602. https://doi.org/10.1016/j.amjsurg.2017.06.033.
31. Li Z, Zhao L, Cheng Y, Cheng N, Deng Y. Abdominal drainage to prevent intra-peritoneal abscess after open appendectomy for complicated appendicitis. Cochrane Database Syst Rev. 2018;5(5):CD010168. https://doi.org/10.1002/14651858.CD010168.pub3.
32. Allemann P, Probst H, Demartines N, Schäfer M. Prevention of infectious complications after laparoscopic appendectomy for complicated acute appendicitis—the role of routine abdominal drainage. Langenbecks Arch Surg. 2011;396(1):63–8. https://doi.org/10.1007/s00423-010-0709-z.
33. Lee JF, Leow CK, Lau WY. Appendicitis in the elderly. Aust N Z J Surg. 2000;70(8):593–6. https://doi.org/10.1046/j.1440-1622.2000.01905.x.
34. Alore EA, Ward JL, Todd SR, et al. Population-level outcomes of early versus delayed appendectomy for acute appendicitis using the American College of Surgeons National Surgical Quality Improvement Program. J Surg Res. 2018;229:234–42. https://doi.org/10.1016/j.jss.2018.04.011.
35. Costa G, Fransvea P, Podda M, et al. The use of emergency laparoscopy for acute abdomen in the elderly: the FRAILESEL Italian multicenter prospective cohort study. Updates Surg. 2020;72(2):513–25. https://doi.org/10.1007/s13304-020-00726-5.
36. Vons C, Barry C, Maitre S, et al. Amoxicillin plus clavulanic acid versus appendicectomy for treatment of acute uncomplicated appendicitis: an open-label, non-inferiority, randomised controlled trial. Lancet. 2011;377(9777):1573–9. https://doi.org/10.1016/S0140-6736(11)60410-8.
37. Salminen P, Tuominen R, Paajanen H, et al. Five-year follow-up of antibiotic therapy for uncomplicated acute appendicitis in the APPAC randomized clinical trial [published correction appears in JAMA. 2018 Oct 23;320(16):1711]. JAMA. 2018;320(12):1259–65. https://doi.org/10.1001/jama.2018.13201.
38. Podda M, Gerardi C, Cillara N, et al. Antibiotic treatment and appendectomy for uncomplicated acute appendicitis in adults and children: a systematic review and meta-analysis. Ann Surg. 2019;270(6):1028–40. https://doi.org/10.1097/SLA.0000000000003225.
39. Harnoss JC, Zelienka I, Probst P, et al. Antibiotics versus surgical therapy for uncomplicated appendicitis: systematic review and meta-analysis of controlled trials (PROSPERO 2015: CRD42015016882). Ann Surg. 2017;265(5):889–900. https://doi.org/10.1097/SLA.0000000000002039.
40. Park HC, Kim MJ, Lee BH. Antibiotic therapy for appendicitis in patients aged ≥80 years. Am J Med. 2014;127(6):562–4. https://doi.org/10.1016/j.amjmed.2014.01.018.
41. Lu P, McCarty JC, Fields AC, et al. Risk of appendiceal cancer in patients undergoing appendectomy for appendicitis in the era of increasing nonoperative management. J Surg Oncol. 2019;120(3):452–9. https://doi.org/10.1002/jso.25608.
42. Teixeira FJR Jr, Couto Netto SDD, Akaishi EH, Utiyama EM, Menegozzo CAM, Rocha MC. Acute appendicitis, inflammatory appendiceal mass and the risk of a hidden malignant tumor: a systematic review of the literature. World J Emerg Surg. 2017;12:12. https://doi.org/10.1186/s13017-017-0122-9.
43. Furman MJ, Cahan M, Cohen P, Lambert LA. Increased risk of mucinous neoplasm of the appendix in adults undergoing interval appendectomy. JAMA Surg. 2013;148(8):703–6. https://doi.org/10.1001/jamasurg.2013.1212.
44. Khan SA, Khokhar HA, Nasr AR, Carton E. Incidence of right-sided colonic tumors (non-appendiceal) in patient's ≥40 years of age presenting with features of acute appendicitis. Int J Surg. 2013;11(4):301–4. https://doi.org/10.1016/j.ijsu.2013.02.004.
45. Lai HW, Loong CC, Tai LC, Wu CW, Lui WY. Incidence and odds ratio of appendicitis as first manifestation of colon cancer: a retrospective analysis of 1873 patients. J Gastroenterol Hepatol. 2006;21(11):1693–6. https://doi.org/10.1111/j.1440-1746.2006.04426.x.
46. Mällinen J, Rautio T, Grönroos J, et al. Risk of appendiceal neoplasm in periappendicular abscess in patients treated with interval appendectomy vs follow-up with magnetic resonance imaging: 1-year outcomes of the peri-appendicitis acuta randomized clinical trial. JAMA Surg. 2019;154(3):200–7. https://doi.org/10.1001/jamasurg.2018.4373.

Non-specific Abdominal Pain

12

Riccardo Brachet-Contul, Lorenzo Cinti, Mario Junior Nardi, Salvatore Condurro, Paolo Millo, and Daniele Marrelli

12.1 Definition and Epidemiology

Population ageing is a long-term trend that began several decades ago. Considering the age above 65 years as the critical indicator, in Italy, as well as in the USA, an increase from the current 18.2% to about 30% of population above 65 by 2050 [1, 2] has been estimated.

This trend results in a transformation of the age structure of the population and reflects an increasing demand of care needs [3]. The elderly's vulnerability is due to reduced or poor physiological reserve, and to the inability to respond to stressors such as acute diseases or invasive procedures like surgery as a direct consequence. This concept is defined with the term "frailty". It should be considered separately from ageing and comorbidity, even if frail patients are often aged and affected by multiple chronic diseases.

Frailty has been demonstrated to be an independent risk factor for poor outcomes: major complications, prolonged hospital stay and readmission. Furthermore, increased mortality rate in short- and long-term follow-up periods, and compromised return to functional status after surgery have been reported in elderly patients.

To date, there is no agreement on which score or scale should be used to measure frailty. Nevertheless, it is important to routinely assess frailty, especially in the emergency department.

Acute non-specific abdominal pain (NSAP) is defined as an abdominal pain lasting 7 days maximum, supported by unknown causes [4]. The non-specific pattern of symptoms related to wide conditions, ranging from self-limiting diseases to gastrointestinal (GI) malignancies, leads to uncertain diagnosis, increasing risk of error and negative surgical exploration [4].

NSAP is not only a common cause of admission to the emergency department, but it is actually increasing in incidence. According to the population ageing all over the globe, the burden of elderly patients with NSAP referring to the emergency departments has increased from 19 to 32% during the last 30 years [5].

Contrary to the younger population, in which there is gender discrepancy in epidemiology and aetiology among abdominal pain and NSAP, in elderly patients there are no differences based on gender, although a higher mortality rate among

R. Brachet-Contul (✉) · M. J. Nardi · S. Condurro · P. Millo
General and Emergency Surgery Unit, Umberto Parini Hospital, Aosta, Italy
e-mail: rbrachetcontul@ausl.vda.it

L. Cinti
Department of Surgical Sciences, University of Turin, Turin, Italy

D. Marrelli
Department of Surgical and Medical Sciences, Surgical and Oncological Unit, Policlinico Le Scotte, Siena, Italy

F. Agresta et al. (eds.), *Emergency laparoscopic surgery in the elderly and frail patient*,
https://doi.org/10.1007/978-3-030-79990-8_12

male patients within 3 months from the hospital admission has been reported [6].

In a global assessment of mortality in emergency surgical conditions [7], bowel obstruction, biliary disease, mesenteric ischaemia and appendicitis were the main abdominal causes of death. NSAP in elderly and frail patients can often hide these potential life-threatening pathologies.

The distribution of the diagnoses causing abdominal pain is different in elderly patients than in the general population. In particular, acute biliary disease (40% of missed NSAP) and bowel obstruction are more common in elderly than in younger patients [8] (Table 12.1).

The most common diagnoses for men with NSAP include biliary disease, urinary retention and constipation. For women, instead, biliary disease, urinary tract infection (UTI) and small bowel obstruction are more commonly diagnosed in elderly patients with NSAP.

With increasing age, important physiological changes occur: fever response to infection or inflammatory disease is less evident, and pain perception sensitiveness, as well as bowel and bladder continence, are less effective (nearly 45% of geriatric patients report taking five or more drugs which can mask symptoms and signs) [11].

The evaluation of abdominal pain in elderly patients must include the patient's history, clinical examination, laboratory tests, diagnostic imaging (US and especially CT) and a reliable classification of frailty.

Historically, laparoscopy has always played an important role both in the diagnosis and therapy of abdominal diseases, in particular for elderly patients, thanks to its mini-invasiveness. Nowadays, few data are reported in the literature on diagnostic laparoscopy in case of NSAP with regard to the adult population.

Table 12.1 The distribution of diagnoses causing abdominal pain was different in elderly patients than in the general population

	Elderly	Adult
NSAP	19–32%	30–40%
Cholecystitis	32%	3–10%
Appendicitis	15%	–
Diverticulitis	50–66%	2–10%
Small bowel obstruction	–	20%
Urinary (ex. UTI)	35%	10%

–: not reported; [5, 8–10]

12.2 Baseline Investigations

The process of obtaining a correct diagnosis begins when collecting the patient's clinical history. However, obtaining a detailed history could be challenging in elderly patients. Indeed, these patients are more like to have cognitive, functional and sensory impairments that limit their ability to communicate. Routine evaluation of cognitive and functional status may be time-consuming but, on the other hand, it helps to classify older patients properly.

It is important to distinguish para-physiological conditions, such as dementia, from acute confusional status such as delirium. Including caregiver and families in the diagnostic pathway may help to recall long and complex clinical history, multiple hospitalization and multidrug therapy. Laboratory tests may be useful for: a complete blood count to investigate leucocytosis, measurement of serum electrolytes, blood urea, amylase and bilirubin and inflammation markers.

12.3 Imaging

Diagnostic workup of patients presenting to the emergency department with acute abdominal pain usually includes sequential diagnostic imaging, such as abdominal ultrasound (US) and abdominal X-ray. Given the limited sensitivity of X-ray and US, abdominal computed tomography (CT) (Fig. 12.1) is often performed. CT has shown to provide a higher diagnostic accuracy than US (89% vs. 70%, $p < 0.001$) in patients with acute abdominal pain [12].

Sparing time is the main issue in older patients, as patients with abdominal pain have a twofold higher surgery rate [13] and a six- to eightfold higher mortality rate compared to younger adults [14]. Moreover, surgery delay has been underlined as a crucial morbidity and mortality fac-

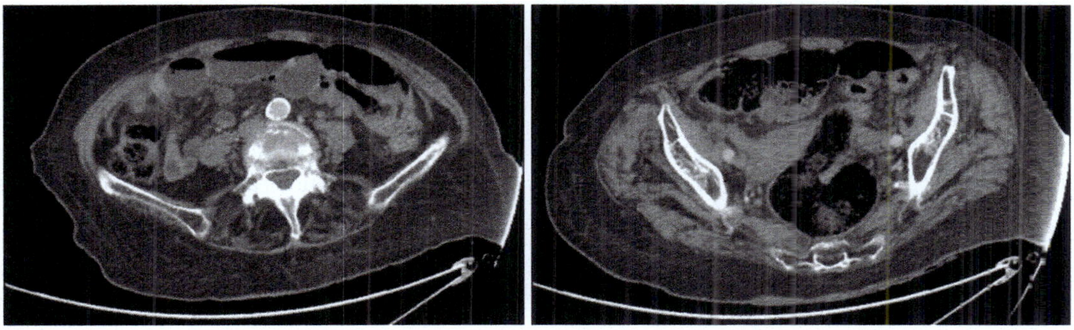

Fig. 12.1 Miss CC, 95-year-old, admitted to ED referring constipation and abdominal pain in right iliac fossa. No surgical history, multidrug therapy at home. At admission leucocytosis, diverticular disease was suspected by US, CT inconclusive. After 9 days of wait and see, the pain was resolved, but alvus still occluded. Diagnostic laparoscopy demonstrated internal hernia, in the right paracolic gutter. Adhesiolysis and defect repair were completed after mini-laparotomy. Discharged on postoperative day 9

tor in this population [15]. This is the reason why many authors have extended indication to CT scan in elderly patients, in order to shorten the time lag from the emergency department's assessment to surgery.

Abuse of the CT scan could cause exposure to radiation-induced cancer and kidney injury due to iodinated contrast medium. However, the former is a virtual problem for the older population because of the short expected lifespan. Contrary, the latter is a major concern, as it represents an independent risk factor for nephropathy [16].

Millet et al. [17] compared the current practice to systematic unenhanced CT scan in >75-year-old patients admitted to the emergency department with non-traumatic abdominal pain. Systematic unenhanced CT scan significantly improved the diagnostic accuracy (from 76.8 to 85%) and the decision-making process (from 88.5 to 95.8%) compared to current practice.

Unenhanced CT leads to a diagnosis of acute unsuspected causes of abdominal pain in 30% of patients, and to a change in the planned management in 37% of cases. Moreover, unenhanced CT leads to a reduction in the hospital admission rate.

Agarwal et al. [18] argued that enhanced CT adds additional information only in 5.3% of cases and prompts changes in the management strategy in 1.9% of cases, compared to unenhanced CT. Intravenous contrast administration allows a better discrimination only in focal diseases of solid organs and for vascular evaluation, as well as in the delineation of infectious, inflammatory and neoplastic conditions.

On the other hand, costs have to be paid in terms of slow emergency department throughput and time consumption. More important, the risk of allergic reactions following intravenous (IV) iodine contrast administration is 0.2–0.6% of cases, and the incidence of associated nephropathy is 2–7% (ACR Manual on Contrast Media). In addition, drinking a large amount of contrast, in case of oral administration, may be difficult for patients with severe pain or those with nausea and vomiting, increasing the risk for aspiration in these patients [12].

Salameh et al. concluded that contrast medium is not necessary, as unenhanced CT enables the radiologist and the clinician to accurately diagnose an acute abdominal process, especially in the elderly.

Furthermore, if the unenhanced CT should be considered inconclusive by the radiologist, contrast can be administered secondarily, in selected cases.

In conclusion, even though there are situations in which plain X-ray alone still represents an absolute indication to surgical exploration (ex. pneumoperitoneum), unenhanced CT scan may be the gold standard, particularly if performed early within the first hour from presentation [19].

12.4 Frailty Score

Frailty is a better predictor of mortality and morbidity than age alone [20, 21], and a reliable independent risk factor for adverse postoperative outcomes [22].

In association with ageing, frailty has proven to be an accurate predictor of perioperative morbidity and mortality. Up to date, there is a lack of consensus and no standardized and validated methods for assessment of frailty in the perioperative scenarios [23]. In the literature, more than 20 different tools have been reported to measure frailty [24]. Age > 75, polypharmacy, multi-morbidity, cognitive impairment and history of fall are the most significant predictors of frailty [21].

Frailty is a major contributing factor to outcomes in the older emergency surgical patient and it can help to classify patients, improve the whole diagnostic process, determine the proper management and enhance patient's care. Thus, a simple and reliable tool is needed to implement the decision-making process. Nowadays, Fried's frailty phenotype assessment tool [25] seems to be the most reliable and fastest method for preoperative assessment of frailty in the emergency department, as recommended by the American College of Surgeons and the American Geriatrics Society [26].

12.5 Management: Early Laparoscopy Versus Wait-and-See

The complexity of making a proper diagnosis in older patients stands by multiple factors, above all comorbidities, which can alter physical conditions and laboratory parameters, or paraphysiological changes in immune system.

Delirium, malaise and dizziness are not uncommon presentations of acute abdomen in elderly patients. Moreover, unspecific symptoms can last for days before admission because of cognitive issues, altered pain perception, high stoicism and transportation barriers. The importance of a rapid and correct diagnosis of an abdominal disease is crucial, although challenging, as it is associated with early treatment.

Early diagnosis and treatment of acute abdominal pain in the frail and comorbid elderly are the key elements for a clinical course characterized by minor complications and with a higher chance of rapid recovery [27].

As NSAP is an exclusion diagnosis based on clinical judgement, supplemented by first- and second-level investigations, it could be reasonable to observe patients over time, during which abdominal symptoms may become more specific or, in some cases, resolve spontaneously. Emergency abdominal surgery is usually reported in around 15–20% of cases and increasing with every decade of age beyond 50s, reaching 40–50% above 80s. As the prognosis may be unpredictable, ethical issue may be taken into account. It is important to set achievable goals with both patients and their families, avoiding unnecessary treatments that do not change life expectancy [7].

Morino et al. [28] reported that 49% of patients undergoing wait-and-see management avoided surgical procedures under general anaesthesia [29].

Among elderly patients discharged with NSAP, a definitive diagnosis is not achieved in 14.8% of cases at 2 weeks of follow-up [13]. Almost 28% of these patients describe their pain to remain the same, whereas 3.7% claim to be worse [30].

Literature is not univocal regarding readmission rates. At 3-month follow-up, 16% patients are readmitted to hospital [31], while 25% at 5 years still suffer from intermitting pain [32]. From the second admission, patients have a relatively high risk of being diagnosed with a somatic condition [31]. Early laparoscopy does not lead to a significant reduction in symptoms' recurrence at long-term follow-up [33].

As frailty is understood as poor recovery of homeostasis following stress, any surgical procedure could increase adverse outcomes. Changing in metabolism determines loss of the ability to regenerate, healing intestinal anastomosis or surgical wounds. Several risk factors were analysed by Duron et al. in their multicentric study on patients >65 years undergoing upper GI surgery: age above 85, emergency surgery and ASA class IV were three of the six items which contributed to increase the mortality risk [34]. Thus, when opting to operate on elderly patients, a minimally invasive operation could improve functioning and reduce pain and discomfort [35].

Laparoscopy is universally accepted to be less invasive and traumatic, and can allow at the same time both early diagnosis and definitive treatment. Diagnostic laparoscopy improves the diagnostic rate over 90% [33], allowing the inspection of the whole peritoneal cavity. The benefits of laparoscopy are relevant in elderly patients compared to adult ones, even if in poor conditions. The benefits are time related. Delayed approaches following wait-and-see strategies or concerns of being too aggressive can result in complications related to the disease or the further deterioration of general clinical conditions. Till the worst-case scenarios in which mini-invasive surgery is no longer useful or even contraindicated [36], mortality and morbidity increase and the prolonged hospital stay result in detrimental effects on functions [28].

Morino et al. agreed with Agresta on the importance to define the correct timing for laparoscopy. According to Morino, early laparoscopy should be performed within 12 h from admission to the emergency department [28]. Other authors argue that laparoscopy has the maximum advantage within 24–48 h.

Laparoscopic surgery is increasingly being considered in the emergency setting for cholecystectomy, appendectomy and perforated duodenal ulcers [37]. Despite the recognized advantages, laparoscopy adoption is still low in case of bowel involvement. Less than 17% of emergency colorectal resections for any cause are currently performed laparoscopically, of which less than 5% for cancer [38]. In addition, only 2.9% of small bowel resection are approached entirely laparoscopically [39].

The risk–benefit balance between open surgery and minimally invasive approaches should be considered on a case-by-case basis. Perioperative complications are a very strong predictor of poor outcomes in geriatric surgery [7]. When complications follow emergency laparotomy, the mortality rate is increased over threefold [7]. Nevertheless, conversion to open surgery does not have to be considered as a complication, or associated to an adverse intraoperative outcome, on the contrary it allows to choose the most appropriate surgical incision [36].

Laparoscopy in older patients guarantees better outcomes compared to laparotomy, in terms of overall morbidity (22.1 versus 36.2%, respectively). Conversion shows similar rates of complications compared to open. Similar advantages are seen in terms of mortality (2.2 versus 11.2%, respectively). Conversely, conversion has shown a higher mortality rate compared to laparoscopy (11.1 versus 2.2%) [40]. Costa et al. reported that these trends increase with age [40].

In addition, laparoscopy guarantees reduction in costs. Due to different countries' Health Systems' organizations, it is hard to assess the exact cost of the various procedures, investigations or hospital stay per day. Nevertheless, early laparoscopy improves the diagnostic rate and can be resolutive, thus reducing hospital stay, medications and painkiller consumption. Moreover, earlier patient recovery and return to work related with a minimally invasive surgery can lead to reduced social cost [35].

In summary, advantages of early laparoscopy in elderly patients are mainly related to the complete visualization of the peritoneal cavity, the immediate opportunity of treatment, the reduced hospital stay, its cost-effectiveness and the improved of quality life. Drawbacks are related to the insufficient visualization of the retroperitoneum and the insufflation of carbon dioxide [41].

12.6 Conclusions

So far, a scarce amount of evidence has been published about elderly frail patients and surgery. Despite the technological and technical development and the increased quality and duration of life, mortality following emergency surgery in elderly patients is still high. A multidisciplinary approach involving surgeons, geriatricians, radiologists, anaesthetists and other relevant specialties is important to achieve treatment goals, optimize care and evaluate the response through the pathway of care. To determine the proper early treatment, more attention should be paid to patient's selection. Frailty scores should be widely employed to identify a high-risk patient, especially in case of NSAP, although there is no agreement on which system or scale should be used to measure frailty in the emergency department. Even if laparoscopy has shown encouraging results in terms of diagnostic and therapeutic efficacy, it must be considered based on different local circumstances: well-trained laparoscopic surgeons must be present, and modern laparoscopes have to be available to allow a realistic view. Moreover, as usually emergency surgery happens during the night shift, surgeon's tiredness and reduced hospital services should be taken into account.

Five Things You Should Know About NSAP in the Elderly Patient

- NSAP is a frequent cause of admission to the emergency department, and it is growing, especially among elderly subjects.
- Unenhanced CT improves accuracy and management decision. Its indication should be extended to the emergency department for elderly patient to detect gastrointestinal and genito-urinary diseases. Contrast medium can be administered secondarily in selected cases.
- A standardized and validated method to assess frailty may help to classify patients, improve the whole diagnostic process and determine proper management.
- Early laparoscopy maintains both a diagnostic and a therapeutic role, reduces hospital stay, improves morbidity and mortality, is cost-effective and improves the quality of life. Risk and benefits have to be calculated on a case-by-case basis.
- A multidisciplinary approach involving surgeons, geriatricians, radiologists and anaesthetists is important to achieve treatment goals, optimize care and evaluate the results through the pathway of care.

References

1. Marois G, Bélanger A, Lutz W. Population aging, migration, and productivity in Europe. Proc Natl Acad Sci U S A. 2020;117(14):7690–5.
2. He W, Goodkind D, Kowal P. An aging world: 2015 International Population Reports. Aging (Albany, NY). 2016.
3. European Commission. Population structure and ageing. Eurostat [Internet]. 2015; (July 2019):1–10. http://ec.europa.eu/eurostat/statistics-explained/index.php/Population_structure_and_ageing.
4. Raheja SK, McDonald PJ, Taylor I. Non-specific abdominal pain—an expensive mystery. J R Soc Med. 1990;83(1):10–1.
5. Fagerström A, Paajanen P, Saarelainen H, Ahonen-Siirtola M, Ukkonen M, Miettinen P, et al. Non-specific abdominal pain remains as the most common reason for acute abdomen: 26-year retrospective audit in one emergency unit. Scand J Gastroenterol. 2017;52(10):1072–7.
6. Gardner RL, Almeida R, Maselli JH, Auerbach A. Does gender influence emergency department management and outcomes in geriatric abdominal pain? J Emerg Med. 2010;39(3):275–81.
7. Desserud KF, Veen T, Søreide K. Emergency general surgery in the geriatric patient. Br J Surg. 2016;103(2):e52–61.
8. Medford-Davis L, Park E, Shlamovitz G, Suliburk J, Meyer AND, Singh H. Diagnostic errors related to acute abdominal pain in the emergency department. Emerg Med J. 2016;33(4):253–9.
9. Matrana MR, Margolin DA. Epidemiology and pathophysiology of diverticular disease. Clin Colon Rectal Surg. 2009;22(3):141–6.
10. Medina M, Castillo-Pino E. An introduction to the epidemiology and burden of urinary tract infections. Ther Adv Urol. 2019;11:1756287219832172.
11. Magidson PD, Martinez JP. Abdominal pain in the geriatric patient. Emerg Med Clin North Am. 2016;34(3):559–74.
12. Salameh S, Antopolsky M, Simanovsky N, Arami E, Hiller N. Use of unenhanced abdominal computed tomography for assessment of acute non-traumatic abdominal pain in the emergency department. Isr Med Assoc J. 2019;21(3):208–12.
13. Lewis LM, Banet GA, Blanda M, Hustey FM, Meldon SW, Gerson LW. Etiology and clinical course of abdominal pain in senior patients: a prospective, multicenter study. J Gerontol A Biol Sci Med Sci. 2005;60(8):1071–6.
14. Van Geioven AAW, Biesheuvel TH, Luitse JSK, Hoitsma HFW, Obertop H. Hospital admissions of patients aged over 80 with acute abdominal complaints. Eur J Surg. 2000;166(11):866–71.

15. Arenal JJ, Bengoechea-Beeby M. Mortality associated with emergency abdominal surgery in the elderly. Can J Surg. 2003;46(2):111–6.
16. Hassen GW, Hwang A, Liu LL, Mualim F, Sembo T, Tu TJ, et al. Follow up for emergency department patients after intravenous contrast and risk of nephropathy. West J Emerg Med. 2014;15(3):276–81.
17. Millet I, Sebbane M, Molinari N, Pages-Bouic E, Curros-Doyon F, Riou B, et al. Systematic unenhanced CT for acute abdominal symptoms in the elderly patients improves both emergency department diagnosis and prompt clinical management. Eur Radiol [Internet]. 2017;27(2):868–77. https://doi.org/10.1007/s00330-016-4425-0.
18. Agarwal MD, Levenson RB, Siewert B, Camacho MA, Raptopoulos V. Limited added utility of performing follow-up contrast-enhanced CT in patients undergoing initial non-enhanced CT for evaluation of flank pain in the emergency department. Emerg Radiol. 2015;22(2):109–15.
19. Sala E, Watson CJE, Beadsmoore C, Groot-Wassink T, Fanshawe TR, Smith JC, et al. A randomized, controlled trial of routine early abdominal computed tomography in patients presenting with non-specific acute abdominal pain. Clin Radiol. 2007;62(10):961–9.
20. Ahmed N, Mandel R, Fain MJ. Frailty: an emerging geriatric syndrome. Am J Med. 2007;120(9):748–53.
21. Lin HS, Watts JN, Peel NM, Hubbard RE. Frailty and post-operative outcomes in older surgical patients: a systematic review. BMC Geriatr [Internet]. 2016;16(1). https://doi.org/10.1186/s12877-016-0329-8.
22. Richards SJG, Frizelle FA, Geddes JA, Eglinton TW, Hampton MB. Frailty in surgical patients. Int J Color Dis. 2018;33(12):1657–66.
23. Morley JE, Vellas B, Abellan van Kan G, Anker SD, Bauer JM, Bernabei R, et al. Frailty consensus: a call to action. J Am Med Dir Assoc. 2013;14(6):392–7.
24. de Vries NM, Staal JB, van Ravensberg CD, Hobbelen JSM, Olde Rikkert MGM, Nijhuis-van der Sanden MWG. Outcome instruments to measure frailty: a systematic review. Ageing Res Rev. 2011;10(1):104–14.
25. Fried LP, Tangen CM, Walston J, Newman AB, Hirsch C, Gottdiener J, et al. Frailty in older adults: evidence for a phenotype. J Gerontol A Biol Sci Med Sci. 2001;56(3):M146–56.
26. Chow WB, Rosenthal RA, Merkow RP, Ko CY, Esnaola NF. Optimal preoperative assessment of the geriatric surgical patient: a best practices guideline from the American college of surgeons national surgical quality improvement program and the American Geriatrics Society. J Am Coll Surg. 2012;215(4):453–66.
27. Lyon C, Clark DC. Diagnosis of acute abdominal pain in older patients. Am Fam Physician. 2006;74(9):1537–44.
28. Morino M, Pellegrino L, Castagna E, Farinella E, Mao P. Acute nonspecific abdominal pain: a randomized, controlled trial comparing early laparoscopy versus clinical observation. Ann Surg. 2006;244(6):881–6.
29. Decadt B, Sussman L, Lewis MPN, Secker A, Cohen L, Rogers C, et al. Randomized clinical trial of early laparoscopy in the management of acute non-specific abdominal pain. Br J Surg. 1999;86(11):1383–6.
30. Lukens TW, Emerman C, Effron D. The natural history and clinical findings in undifferentiated abdominal pain. Ann Emerg Med. 1993;22(4):690–6.
31. Ravn-Christensen C, Qvist N, Bay-Nielsen M, Bisgaard T. Pathology is common in subsequent visits after admission for non-specific abdominal pain. Dan Med J. 2019;66(7):1–5.
32. Banz VM, Sperisen O, de Moya M, Zimmermann H, Candinas D, Mougiakakou SG, et al. A 5-year follow up of patients discharged with non-specific abdominal pain: out of sight, out of mind? Intern Med J. 2012;42(4):395–401.
33. Morino M, Famiglietti F. Nonspecific abdominal pain. 2012.
34. Duron JJ, Duron E, Dugue T, Pujol J, Muscari F, Collet D, et al. Risk factors for mortality in major digestive surgery in the elderly: a multicenter prospective study. Ann Surg. 2011;254(2):375–82.
35. Michalik M, Dowgiałło-Wnukiewicz N, Lech P, Zacharz K. Surgery of the elderly in emergency room mode. Is there a place for laparoscopy? Wideochirurgia I Inne Tech Maloinwazyjne. 2017;12(2):115–9.
36. Agresta F, Mazzarolo G, Ciardo LF, Bedin N. The laparoscopic approach in abdominal emergencies: has the attitude changed? A single-center review of a 15-year experience. Surg Endosc Other Interv Tech. 2008;22(5):1255–62.
37. Rodríguez-Mañas L, Féart C, Mann G, Viña J, Chatterji S, Chodzko-Zajko W, et al. Searching for an operational definition of frailty: a Delphi method based consensus statement. The frailty operative definition-consensus conference project. J Gerontol A Biol Sci Med Sci. 2013;68(1):62–7.
38. Keller DS, Senagore AJ, Fitch K, Bochner A, Haas EM. A new perspective on the value of minimally invasive colorectal surgery—payer, provider, and patient benefits. Surg Endosc. 2017;31(7):2846–53.
39. Sharma R, Reddy S, Thoman D, Grotts J, Ferrigno L. Laparoscopic versus open bowel resection in emergency small bowel obstruction: analysis of the National Surgical Quality Improvement Program Database. J Laparoendosc Adv Surg Tech. 2015;25(8):625–30.
40. Costa G, Fransvea P, Podda M, Pisanu A, Carcano FM, Iossa A, et al. The use of emergency laparoscopy for acute abdomen in the elderly: the FRAILESEL Italian multicenter prospective cohort study. Updates Surg. 2020;72(2):513–25.
41. Domínguez LC, Sanabria A, Vega V, Osorio C. Early laparoscopy for the evaluation of nonspecific abdominal pain: a critical appraisal of the evidence. Surg Endosc. 2011;25(1):10–8.

13 Perforated Gastroduodenal Ulcer

Gabriele Anania, Alberto Campagnaro, Francesco Marchetti, Giuseppe Resta, and Roberto Cirocchi

13.1 Introduction

Peptic ulcer is a very common disease with a prevalence of 5–10% in the general population and an incidence of 0.1–0.3% per year [1, 2]. Complications of peptic ulcer include bleeding, perforation and obstruction. Perforation of peptic ulcer (PPU) is second in terms of frequency among the aforementioned complications, occurring in approximately 2–10% of patients hospitalized for peptic ulcer disease [3], and represents the most widespread surgical emergency worldwide, with a mortality of about 40% (almost five times greater than bleeding) [2, 4].

G. Anania (✉) · A. Campagnaro · F. Marchetti
Division of General Surgery, S. Anna University Hospital of Ferrara, Ferrara, Italy

Department of Medical Science, University of Ferrara, Ferrara, Italy
e-mail: gabriele.anania@unife.it; alberto.campagnaro@unife.it; francesco.marchetti@unife.it

G. Resta
Division of General Surgery, S. Anna University Hospital of Ferrara, Ferrara, Italy
e-mail: g.resta@ospfe.it

R. Cirocchi
Department of Surgical and Biomedical Sciences, University of Perugia, St. Mary's Hospital, Terni, Italy
e-mail: roberto.cirocchi@unipg.it

The incidence and mortality of these complications have decreased over the past 30 years thanks to the improvement of the patient's preoperative management, diagnostic techniques and surgical techniques. Today, these complications occur in about 10–20% of patients with peptic ulcer [2, 5, 6].

There are several different risk factors related to gastroduodenal peptic ulcer perforation [4]:

- NSAIDs, inhibitors of synthesis of prostaglandins, lead to increased production of gastric acids and reduced mucus secretion.
- Smoking inhibits secretion of bicarbonate and stimulates secretion of acid.
- Helicobacter Pylori: most common in low-income and middle-income countries
- Marginal ulcer after bariatric surgery: due to ischaemia of the anastomosis
- Drugs: due to vasoconstriction followed by ischaemia
- Zollinger-Ellison syndrome
- Steroids affects inflammatory cascade, including prostaglandin synthesis, and can blunt signs of peritonitis.
- Alcohol
- Chemotherapy with bevacizumab

In the elderly patients, we can identify a prevalence of perforated gastric ulcers due to the chronic use of steroids and NSAIDs, compared

F. Agresta et al. (eds.), *Emergency laparoscopic surgery in the elderly and frail patient*,
https://doi.org/10.1007/978-3-030-79990-8_13

to the typical duodenal form of the younger subject attributable to H. pylori infection. At the same time in the elderly patients, there is a greater correlation of perforation in the morning hours, probably linked to the circadian cycle of acid secretion in the stomach [7, 8]. About prevalent localization, prepyloric gastric ulcers are the most common, followed by those of the duodenal bulb [9]. The elective treatment involves surgical repair (simple suture repair) of the ulcer, but alternatives to traditional treatment are also possible. Laparoscopic repair is still relatively uncommon for perforated gastroduodenal ulcer: according to the multicentre Italian study 'FRAIESEL', only 20% of patients with PPU were treated laparoscopically [10].

Factors related to comorbidity, shock on admission, delayed surgery and post-operative infections have been associated with increased mortality and morbidity rates of up to 40% and 50%, respectively, for perforated peptic ulcer in the elderly [11].

13.2 Clinical Presentation and Diagnostic Procedures

PPU presents with sudden epigastric pain, which rapidly radiates to the whole abdomen. Characteristically, this symptom is usually referred to as stabbing, 'like a stab'. Usually, the patient lies still as even a deep breath aggravates the pain. Furthermore, some patients could show up in a shock status, with increasing heart rate and decreasing blood pressure and diuresis.

The classic presentation triad is abdominal pain, tachycardia and abdominal stiffness, although up to one-third of patients may not show typical signs of peritonism, particularly patients with covered perforation [4, 12]. On physical examination, a distended abdomen, tenderness on palpation, abdominal defence and positive Blumberg's sign can be found.

Laboratory markers are not diagnostic in the case of perforation but are useful in the differential diagnosis and for evaluating inflammation indexes. Indeed, laboratory tests show leucocytosis, increase of serum amylase and a finding of metabolic acidosis on blood gas analysis (decrease in pH, increase in lactates, decrease in bicarbonates and excess of bases). At the same time, a prompt blood culture is recommended before performing broad spectrum antibiotic prophylaxis.

Generally, PPU affects individuals with a story of peptic ulcer or gastro-oesophageal reflux disease, comprehending dyspepsia and epigastric pain with variable association with meals.

In elderly and frail patients, this disease may present with an unspecific or concealed behaviour, particularly in case of small perforations. Moreover, this subset of patients often carries comorbidities, capable of hiding classical clinical symptoms and signs (obesity, chronic therapy with steroids, diabetes mellitus, neurocognitive impairment, immune-suppression etc.), at least in the initial presentation [4, 12].

Some rare cases may present with the so-called 'Valentino syndrome', related to gastric fluid tracking down the retroperitoneum leading to chemical peritonitis in the right lower quadrant of the abdomen, which may be mistaken for appendicitis. Valentino syndrome should be suspected in patients who did not receive preoperative CT and with negative findings in laparotomy of right lower quadrant, revealing normal appendix [13].

It is indicated to delay imaging techniques in case the patient presents in critical conditions, such as septic status or haemodynamic instability (i.e. shock).

The final diagnosis can be assessed in case of X-ray or CT scan finding of free air below the diaphragm or inside the peritoneum (Fig. 13.1). Standing X-ray of thorax and abdomen should be preferred, though most of the patients might be unable to maintain the orthostatic position (e.g. peritonitis or any inability to keep the standing position), obligating to obtain a picture in lateral decubitus. However, in case this happens, the sensibility drops to 75%, leading to possible false-negative results because of the impossibility to detect the pneumoperitoneum. It is also possible to resort to US imaging, but its use is limited by two main factors: it is a highly operator dependent diagnostic method and generally patients are not adequately prepared in the emergency setting. Instead, computerized tomography (CT) scan of the abdomen is

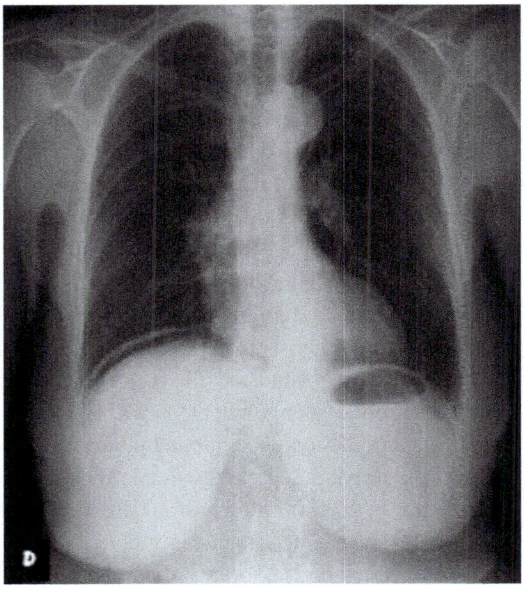

Fig. 13.1 Intraperitoneal gas under the diaphragm [14]

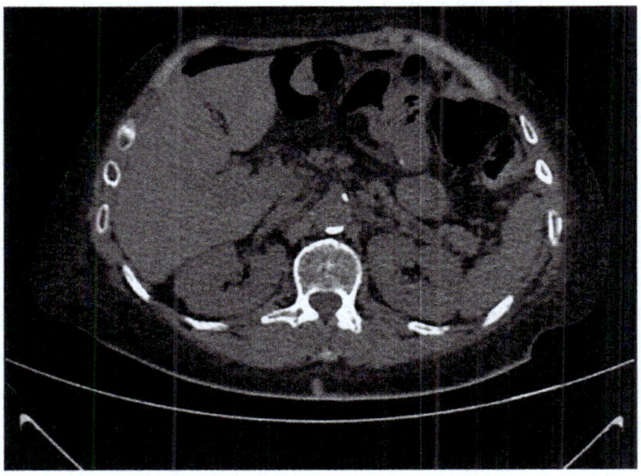

Fig. 13.2 CT scan with intraperitoneal air collection [15]

the gold standard method for diagnosis, with the 98% of sensitivity, being also useful for differential diagnosis of the abdominal clinical picture (Fig. 13.2). It is important to notice that the lack of free air in the imaging does not exclude the diagnosis of PPU, since up to 12% of patients affected by this condition do not show any particular finding at the CT scan; in case of strong suspect remaining, the execution of a triple contrast CT scan, with the administration of oral-water soluble contrast through nasal-gastric tube can implement the diagnostic sensitivity and specificity [4].

13.3 Management of the Patient

Among the main causes of death for patients with PPU there is sepsis, responsible for 40–50% of deaths [16]. For this reason, prevention, early detection and treatment of sepsis in these patients are fundamental, in order to reduce mortality and morbidity as much as possible. This objective can be achieved by systematically monitoring patients and treating them according to the guidelines of the Surviving Sepsis Campaign, in particular with fluid resuscitation, microbiological cultures, empirical broad-spectrum antibiotics and source control [17]. In addition to antibiotic therapy, based on IV antibiotics effective against intestinal flora (i.e. cefotetan or amikacin combined with clindamycin), in elderly, frail, immunocompromised patients with polycomorbidity and long stay in ICU, it is recommended to associate empirical therapy with antifungals (mainly azoles and echinocandins) [2]. The perioperative management based on these principles, if realized with multidisciplinary collaboration, allows a statistically significant reduction in mortality, also confirmed by a non-randomized clinical trial [18].

Older age, comorbidity and use of NSAIDs or steroids are conditions associated with mortality; shock upon admission, preoperative metabolic acidosis, tachycardia, acute renal failure, low serum albumin level, high ASA score and preoperative delay >24 h are also associated with poor prognosis [16].

Non-operative management (NOM) is an alternative, based on the potential advantage of avoiding surgery and its consequences, such as morbidity related to wound complications, postoperative adhesions, etc. It is based on the assumption that small perforations could seal thanks to omental adhesions, which would allow the healing without the need for surgery. This approach should be reserved for carefully selected cases, where the perforation is sealed, and this condition is confirmed with a water-soluble contrast study [2]. The measures taken include:

- Interruption of any type of feeding/oral administration (nil per OS, NPO)
- Positioning of nasogastric tube for decompression

- Fluid resuscitation
- Proton pump inhibitor and antisecretive therapy
- Intravenous administration of broad-spectrum antibiotics
- Endoscopic follow-up after 4–6 weeks [19]

Particular attention must be given to elderly patients, who, despite being those who would benefit most from a NOM, show a higher rate of failure of such management [20]. Therefore, it is necessary to consider the potential risk associated with the delay of surgical treatment following the adoption of this approach in the early stages.

It is important to remember that among the parameters mainly associated with mortality, there is the delay in surgery [19]. In fact, the surgical treatment is recommended as soon as possible, regardless of the time of day, since il was highligted an increase in mortality of up to 6% for each hour of delay, after the first 24 h [21–23].

Another possibility for patients with PPU is endoscopic treatment. Many techniques have been tested: use of endoscopic clips, subject to failure in case of the presence of fibrous tissue and subsequent loss of compliance of the wall [24, 25]; laparoscopic-endoscopic hybrid approach [26–28]; snaring of the omentum with pulling to close the perforation. However, most of these methods have not been standardized yet and their use, not being routine, has not been clinically validated on large patient cohorts.

In conclusion, the endoscopic option cannot be considered as a routine treatment, at least according to recent evidence [2].

Another clarification can be made about the surgical management of the perforation depending on the size. In fact, in case of perforation <2 cm, multiple retrospective studies highlighted that the gold standard is the direct suture of the perforation without omental patch, since the two procedures result in the same incidence of leakage and the same surgical outcome, at the expense of longer operative time for the omental patch technique [29]. Instead, in case of perforation >2 cm, the choice of the surgical procedure is led by the localization of the perforation itself. In case of gastric ulcer >2 cm, the malignant origin of the lesion must always be suspected, given that about 10–16% of large gastric perforations are caused by cancers [30]. In this case, it is recommended to perform gastric resection followed by reconstruction. On the other hand, surgical resection of perforated ulcers involving the ampullary region (e.g. Whipple procedure) is not recommended in patients with peritonitis, due to the high risk of post-operative complications. In fact, about 12% of this kind of ulcers treated with closure using omental patch result in leakage complications. In these cases, damage control surgery should be preferred [31, 32]: this type of surgery is indicated in patients showing severe conditions, such as septic shock, organ dysfunction, hypotension, coagulopathy or contamination of the abdominal cavity. Recommendations indicate not to perform the anastomosis in case of hypotension and haemodynamic instability, suggesting the placement of a temporary abdominal closure device and appropriately resuscitating the patient in the ICU. After that, the surgeon is allowed to return to the OR for re-exploration, restoration of continuity and closure of the abdominal wall once the patient is haemodynamically stable [33].

The elective treatment, in most cases, remains surgery [2]. Surgery is indicated in (Fig. 13.3):

According to a recent meta-analysis [34], there are no statistically significant differences in the majority of clinical outcomes between groups operated by Laparoscopic or Open technique for PPU. Furthermore, a lower incidence of post-operative pain and wound infections can be detected in the laparoscopic group. The substantial equivalence of the two methods highlighted in this study is important because it allows laparoscopy to be considered as a valid first choice,

In patients with perforated peptic ulcer with significant pneumoperitoneum or extraluminal contrast extravasation or signs of peritonitis, we recommend operative treatment (Strong recommendation based on low-quality evidences, 1C)

We recommend performing surgery as soon as possible, especially in patients with delayed presentation and patients older than 70 years old (strong recommendation based on moderate-quality evidences, 1B)

Fig. 13.3 Text copied from WSES Guidelines [2]

guaranteeing to the patients the advantages provided by this technique, in particular a reduction of post-operative functional recovery time and greater comfort for the patient.

In fact, according to this evidence, although the risk of bias in the assumptions made is not negligible, the laparoscopic approach seems to be a good or even better choice in haemodynamically stable patients, if the care setting and the skills of the surgical team allow it [2]. On the other hand, the risks associated with hypercapnia and pneumoperitoneum in patients with severe cardiopulmonary comorbidities or haemodynamic instability are too high [35], forcing in those cases to perform the open procedure.

13.4 Selection of Patients for Surgery

Abdominal emergency surgery is currently a highly debated problem in the elderly patient due to the progressive ageing of the world population. Estimates predict an increase in the over 65 population to a total of 1.5 billion in 2050. This phenomenon is very relevant for the resource management, given that currently 33% of this population is hospitalized and about 41% of healthcare-related costs are dedicated to it [10, 36, 37]. It is estimated that 21% of the population over 65 will require surgery and the most commonly involved clinical pictures are cholecystitis, incarcerated hernia, intestinal obstruction and gastroduodenal perforation [38–40].

The post-operative course is much more complicated in the elder than in the young patient, and there is a notable difference between the management of diseases requiring elective surgery, in which the patient can be carefully prepared with a correct management of comorbidities, and the emergency setting. In fact, the mortality of patients over 70 years old undergoing emergency surgery is 22%, with an increase to 44% in patients over 80. Therefore, studies were conducted in order to identify some parameters that can guide the choice of the most suitable care setting for these patients. One of the most recent studies regarding this topic is the FRAILESEL (Frailty and Emergency Surgery in the Elderly) [10] conducted and developed by ERASO (Elderly Risk Assessment And Surgical Outcome), ACOI (Italian Association of Hospital Surgeons), SIC (Italian Society of Surgery), SICUT (Italian Society of Emergency Surgery and Trauma), SICG (Italian Society of Geriatric Surgery), SICE (Italian Society of Endoscopic Surgery and new technologies), WSES (World Society of Emergency Surgery). This is a multicentre prospective cohort study that investigated the perioperative characteristics of patients over 65 who underwent emergency abdominal surgery between January 2017 and December 2017. The aim of the study was to identify the main factors involved in complications and mortality within 30 days, depending on the surgical pathologies investigated (mainly cholecystectomy, appendectomy, intestinal obstruction and perforated ulcer). The study found that patients with high creatinine and blood glucose levels, low haemoglobin levels (usually associated with oral anticoagulant therapy), respiratory failure, SIRS and history of cancer have a higher rate of post-operative complications (approximately 42.5%). Post-operative mortality, on the other hand, was increased in patients with high creatinine, high blood glucose levels and low haemoglobin values (approximately 20.8%). Conversely, a history of myocardial infarction and heart failure were factors independently associated with post-operative mortality rate.

Moreover, it emerged that only 31.3% of patients were operated through emergency laparoscopy. In fact, laparoscopy is associated with some risks due to CO_2 insufflation for the induction of pneumoperitoneum (with an even greater impact on the patient in the elder), leading to a reduction in cardiopulmonary capacity due to elevation of the diaphragm, reduction of venous return and of the cardiac output, predisposing the patient to myocardial infarction and basal atelectasis [41–43]. However, the literature indications suggest to choose the laparoscopic treatment, if possible, in stable patients with good cardiorespiratory conditions, and to reserve the Open technique only to those cases in which laparoscopy cannot be performed (severe sepsis, extensive adhesions etc.) given the high rate of complications and post-operative mortality [10].

Søreide et al. [4] highlighted some factors that can help identify patients with poor prognosis and increased risk of mortality, such as advanced age, comorbidities (acute or chronic kidney disease, COPD, diabetes, liver disease), delayed surgery after diagnosis, low serum albumin level and preoperative shock [4, 44–47]. A study by Patel et al. [47] confirms what emerges from the literature and also identifies scores that can be used to predict the risk of mortality in patients with PPU (ASA score, Boey score (Fig. 13.4) and PULP score (Fig. 13.5)). The evidence indicates that high PULP score and Boey score (Boey >1 and PULP >7) are related to higher mortality in patients with PPU, while ASA score does not provide useful information in this disease, even if it is one of the easiest scores to evaluate and calculate as well as one of the most popular. The only aspect still debated is that these scores have not been validated yet; therefore, particular attention is recommended in case they are used, with a particular regard on the population under study.

Risk Factors	Points
None of below	0
Pre-operative blood pressure <100mmHg	1
Delayed presentation >24h	2
Major comorbidity	3

Fig. 13.4 Boey's score [48]

13.5 Surgical Procedure

The laparoscopic surgical technique involves the same steps as the open technique: inspection, peritoneal washing, identification of the perforation, suturing of the same, possible omentopexy. The laparoscopic approach is preferred except in contraindicated cases. The patient is placed supine with legs open on the operating table and the first operator is in position between them. The monitor is positioned to the left of the patient. The first surgeon assistant holds the camera to

Risk Factors	Points
Age > 65 years	3
Serum creatinine > 1.47 mg/dl	2
Comorbid liver cirrhosis	2
Active comorbidity or AIDS	1
Concomitant use of steroids	1
Shock on admission	1
Time from perforation to admission >24h	1
ASA score 2	1
ASA score 3	3
ASA score 4	5
ASA score 5	7
TOTAL PULP score	**0-18**
Low risk of mortality (<25%)	0-7
High risk of mortality (>25%)	8-18

Fig. 13.5 PULP score [48]

the right of the patient and the surgical nurse positions himself to the left of the patient. The supine position with closed legs, preferred by some surgeons, requires a continuous movement of the first operator, especially in the phases of peritoneal washing. In the case of a patient positioned with legs closed, most surgeons perform the essential steps of the operation by positioning themselves to the left of the patient. In all cases, the patients are positioned in reverse Trendelenburg by 15/20° [49].

The pneumoperitoneum can be created with a Verres needle or with other methods that are more confident to the first operator. The position of the trocars changes according to the operator's habits. Most surgeons use the classic method with the optical trocar positioned on the midline 2/3 cm above the navel, depending on the patient's anthropometric characteristics and the position of the navel on the xipho-pubic line. A 30° laparoscope is inserted through this trocar. Having explored the abdomen and confirmed the diagnostic hypothesis of gastric or duodenal perforation, the remaining trocars are positioned. One trocar, 12 mm size, that is used like operator trocar, is positioned in the right hemiclavicular line, a couple of centimetres above the transverse umbilical line. Another one, 5 mm size, is positioned along the left hemiclavicular line at the same level of the previous one. If necessary, an additional 5 mm trocar may be useful in the epigastric region to insert the liver retractor. However, this 'classic' position of the trocars remains the best for the correct triangulation between laparoscope and other surgical instruments [50].

Once the site of the lesion has been identified, its diameter must be carefully evaluated, which must not exceed 2 cm [2]. In larger duodenal perforations, it will be necessary to change the programme and convert the procedure to open surgery. The surgical procedure is also contingent upon the position of the perforation. Perforations in the posterior wall of the stomach or along the lateral wall of the duodenal C require special skills. In these cases, if the surgeon does not have appropriate skills, it is advisable to convert the procedure because the protraction of operation increases the risk of post-operative complications. Typically, the conversion rate is reported between 8 and 29%. This variability mainly depends on the experience of the operators. The causes of conversion are to be referred to: skill of the surgeon, site and size of the lesion, characteristics of the lesion edges, inability to identify the lesion itself and finally the severity of peritoneal contamination. High risk of conversion occurs in these cases: septic shock, perforation event occurring more than 24 h from the time of treatment or suspicion of perforated carcinoma [51].

The suture of the lesion (raffia) should be performed with detached suture using absorbable braided suture or monofilament suture, in double layer. The suture procedure depends on both the surgeon's habits and the characteristics of the edges of the perforation depending on whether they are fibrous or brittle. The suture must be performed with an intracorporeal technique. If possible, an omentopexy is performed by placing an omentum patch over the raffia. In cases where the margins are pulled together easily and without tension, omentopexy can be avoided. At the end of the suture, a hydropneumatics test can be performed by blowing air. Some surgeons perform this test using methylene blue.

Once the raffia is completed, an abundant peritoneal wash is essential, using up to 5 L of saline solution, carefully tilting the patient in order to reach all the peritoneal recesses.

At the end, at least one drainage device is placed near the raffia. In the event of a recent event with little contamination, drainage device can be avoided after careful and abundant peritoneal lavage [52, 53].

13.6 ERAS Programme

Enhanced Recovery after Surgery (ERAS) programmes are evidence-based protocols designed to standardize and optimize perioperative care, allowing to limit the consequences of surgical trauma on physiological processes and organ function (inflammation, alteration in metabolism and endocrine system) following elective surgery [54].

The most recent evidence confirms that the ERAS protocols allow a reduction in post-operative complications, hospitalization and readmission rates even in an emergency regime [55].

These consist of 22 elements, shown in Fig. 13.6; in emergency surgery, some of them appear more important (peri and post-operative intravenous fluid management, preoperative carbohydrate treatment, non-NGT usage, early oral feeding and use of NSAIDs) [57], but further studies are needed to assess their primary importance. In some cases, the emergency setting does not allow to pursue some items (e.g. laparoscopic surgery, avoiding resection site drain and general anaesthetic ± epidural anaesthesia) in the best way [58].

In addition, there are measures that it is obviously not possible to obtain, such as cessation of smoking and alcohol consumption, starting from 4 weeks before surgery.

Elderly patients who undergo interventions in an emergency setting can also benefit from this approach [59]. In particular, measures can be taken to adapt these protocols to frail elderly patients affected by PPU: an RCT [60] confirms the feasibility and safety of this management, however, indicating the need to precisely standardize the procedures and confirm the evidence that emerges from that study.

Few Things You Should Know About Laparoscopy for Perforated Peptic Ulcer in the Elderly

- In elderly and frail patients, this disease may present with an unspecific or concealed behaviour, particularly in case of small perforations. Moreover, this subset of patients often carries comorbidities, capable of hiding classical clinical symptoms and signs, at least in the initial presentation.

ERAS items		
PREOPERATIVE	INTRAOPERATIVE	POSTOPERATIVE
• Preadmission counseling • Fluid and carbohydrate loading • No prolonged fasting • No/selective bowel preparation • Antibiotic prophylaxis • Thromboprophylaxis • No premedications	• Short-acting anesthetic agents • Mid-thoracic epidural anesthesia/analgesia • No drains • Avoidance of salt and water overload • Maintenance of normothermia (body warmer/warm IV fluids)	• Mid-thoracic epidural anesthesia/analgesia • No nasogastric tubes • Prevention of nausea and vomiting • Avoidance of salt and water overload • Early removal of catheter • Early oral nutrition • Non-opioid oral analgesia/NSAIDs • Early mobilization • Stimulation of gut motility • Aduit of compliance and outcomes

Fig. 13.6 ERAS items [56]

- Non-operative management could allow the healing without the need for surgery. Particular attention must be given to elderly patients, who, despite being those who would benefit most from a NOM, show a higher rate of failure. Therefore, it is necessary to consider the potential risk associated with the delay to surgery following the adoption of this approach in the early stages.
- Laparoscopic approach seems to be a good or even better choice than open surgery in haemodynamically stable patients, if the care setting and the skills of the surgical team allow it.
- Boey's score and PULP score may be used to predict the risk of mortality in patients with PPU, but they have not been validated yet.
- Elderly patients who undergo interventions in an emergency setting can benefit from ERAS protocol application.

References

1. Lanas A, Chan FKL. Peptic ulcer disease. Lancet. 2017;390(10094):613–24.
2. Tarasconi A, Coccolini F, Biffl WL, Tomasoni M, Ansaloni L, Picetti E, et al. Perforated and bleeding peptic ulcer: WSES guidelines. World J Emerg Surg. 2020;15:3.
3. Byrge N, Barton RG, Enniss TM, Nirula R. Laparoscopic versus open repair of perforated gastroduodenal ulcer: a National Surgical Quality Improvement Program analysis. Am J Surg. 2013;206(6):957–62; discussion 962–963.
4. Søreide K, Thorsen K, Harrison EM, Bingener J, Møller MH, Ohene-Yeboah M, et al. Perforated peptic ulcer. Lancet. 2015;386(10000):1288–98.
5. Bertleff MJOE, Lange JF. Perforated peptic ulcer disease: a review of history and treatment. Dig Surg. 2010;27(3):161–9.
6. Lau JY, Sung J, Hill C, Henderson C, Howden CW, Metz DC. Systematic review of the epidemiology of complicated peptic ulcer disease: incidence, recurrence, risk factors and mortality. Digestion. 2011;84(2):102–13.
7. Lanas A, Serrano P, Bajador E, Esteva F, Benito R, Sáinz R. Evidence of aspirin use in both upper and lower gastrointestinal perforation. Gastroenterology. 1997:112(3):683–9.
8. Ishikawa S, Inaba T, Mizuno M, Miyake Y, Okada H, Ishikawa H, et al. Characteristics of serious complicated gastroduodenal ulcers in Japan. Hepatogastroenterology. 2012;59(113):147–54.
9. Agaba EA, Klair T, Ikedilo O, Vemulapalli P. A 10-year review of surgical management of complicated peptic ulcer disease from a single center: is laparoscopic approach the future? Surg Laparosc Endosc Percutan Tech. 2016;26(5):385–90.
10. Costa G, Fransvea P, Podda M, Pisanu A, Carrano FM, Iossa A, et al. The use of emergency laparoscopy for acute abdomen in the elderly: the FRAILESEL Italian multicenter prospective cohort study. Updates Surg. 2020;72(2):513–25.
11. Møller MH, Larsson HJ, Rosenstock S, Jørgensen H, Johnsen SP, Madsen AH, et al. Quality-of-care initiative in patients treated surgically for perforated peptic ulcer. Br J Surg. 2013;100(4):543–52.
12. Lau JYW, Barkun A, Fan D, Kuipers EJ, Yang Y, Chan FKL. Challenges in the management of acute peptic ulcer bleeding. Lancet 2013;381(9882):2033–43.
13. Noussios G, Galanis N, Konstantinidis S, Mirelis C, Chatzis I, Katsourakis A. Valentino's syndrome (with retroperitoneal ulcer perforation): a rare clinico-anatomical entity. Am J Case Rep. 2020;21:e922647.
14. X-Ray imaging-AUSL Ferrara, Radiology Department, Delta Hospital, Lagosanto (FE).
15. CT scan-AUSL Ferrara, Radiology Department, Delta Hospital, Lagosanto (FE).
16. Møller MH, Adamsen S, Thomsen RW, Møller AM. Preoperative prognostic factors for mortality in peptic ulcer perforation: a systematic review. Scand J Gastroenterol. 2010;45(7–8):785–805.
17. Dellinger RP, Levy MM, Rhodes A, Annane D, Gerlach H, Opal SM, et al. Surviving sepsis campaign: international guidelines for management of severe sepsis and septic shock: 2012. Crit Care Med. 2013;41(2):580–637.
18. Møller MH, Adamsen S, Thomsen RW, Møller AM. Peptic ulcer perforation (PULP) trial group. Multicentre trial of a perioperative protocol to reduce mortality in patients with peptic ulcer perforation. Br J Surg. 2011;98(6):802–10.
19. Kavitt RT, Lipowska AM, Anyane-Yeboa A, Gralnek IM. Diagnosis and treatment of peptic ulcer disease. Am J Med. 2019;132(4):447–56.
20. Crofts TJ, Park KG, Steele RJ, Chung SS, Li AK. A randomized trial of nonoperative treatment for perforated peptic ulcer. N Engl J Med. 1989;320(15):970–3.
21. Boyd-Carson H, Doleman B, Cromwell D, Lockwood S, Williams JP, Tierney GM, et al. Delay in source control in perforated peptic ulcer leads to 6% increased risk of death per hour: a nationwide cohort study. World J Surg. 2020;44(3):869–75.
22. Buck DL, Vester-Andersen M, Møller MH. Danish clinical register of emergency surgery. Surgical delay is a critical determinant of survival in perforated peptic ulcer. Br J Surg. 2013;100(8):1045–9.
23. Surapaneni S, Rajkumar S, Vijaya Bhaskar Reddy A. The perforation-operation time interval; an important mortality indicator in peptic ulcer perforation. J Clin Diagn Res. 2013;7(5):880–2.

24. Katsinelos P, Beltsis A, Paroutoglou G, Galanis I, Tsolkas P, Mimidis K, et al. Endoclipping for gastric perforation after endoscopic polypectomy: an alternative treatment to avoid surgery. Surg Laparosc Endosc Percutan Tech. 2004;14(5):279–81.
25. Joshi MA, Gadhire M, Paranjpe AA. Treatment of duodenal peptic ulcer perforation by endoscopic clips: a novel approach. J Dig Endosc. 2017;8(1):24–6.
26. Malkov IS, Zaynutdinov AM, Veliyev NA, Tagirov MR, Merrell RC. Laparoscopic and endoscopic management of perforated duodenal ulcers. J Am Coll Surg. 2004;198(3):352–5.
27. Alvarado-Aparicio HA, Moreno-Portillo M. Multimedia article: management of duodenal ulcer perforation with combined laparoscopic and endoscopic methods. Surg Endosc. 2004;18(9):1394.
28. Bergström M, Arroyo Vázquez JA, Park P-O. Self-expandable metal stents as a new treatment option for perforated duodenal ulcer. Endoscopy. 2013;45(3):222–5.
29. Lin B-C, Liao C-H, Wang S-Y, Hwang T-L. Laparoscopic repair of perforated peptic ulcer: simple closure versus omentopexy. J Surg Res. 2017;220:341–5.
30. Ergul E, Gozetlik EO. Emergency spontaneous gastric perforations: ulcus versus cancer. Langenbecks Arch Surg. 2009;394(4):643–6.
31. Jani K, Saxena AK, Vaghasia R. Omental plugging for large-sized duodenal peptic perforations: a prospective randomized study of 100 patients. South Med J. 2006;99(5):467–71.
32. Di Saverio S, Bassi M, Smerieri N, Masetti M, Ferrara F, Fabbri C, et al. Diagnosis and treatment of perforated or bleeding peptic ulcers: 2013 WSES position paper. World J Emerg Surg. 2014;9:45.
33. Coccolini F, Montori G, Ceresoli M, Catena F, Moore EE, Ivatury R, et al. The role of open abdomen in non-trauma patient: WSES consensus paper. World J Emerg Surg. 2017;12:39.
34. Cirocchi R, Soreide K, Di Saverio S, Rossi E, Arezzo A, Zago M, et al. Meta-analysis of perioperative outcomes of acute laparoscopic versus open repair of perforated gastroduodenal ulcers. J Trauma Acute Care Surg. 2018;85(2):417–25.
35. Sharma KC, Brandstetter RD, Brensilver JM, Jung LD. Cardiopulmonary physiology and pathophysiology as a consequence of laparoscopic surgery. Chest. 1996;110(3):810–5.
36. Global Aging|National Institute on Aging [Internet]. [cited 2020 Oct 20]. https://www.nia.nih.gov/research/dbsr/global-aging
37. Indicatori demografici. 2017. 15.
38. Pisano M, Ceresoli M, Cimbanassi S, Gurusamy K, Coccolini F, Borzellino G, et al. 2017 WSES and SICG guidelines on acute calcolous cholecystitis in elderly population. World J Emerg Surg. 2019;14(1):10.
39. Poillucci G, Podda M, Pisanu A, Mortola L, Dalla Caneva P, Massa G, et al. Risk factors for postoperative morbidity following appendectomy in the elderly: a nationwide prospective cohort study. Eur J Trauma Emerg Surg. 2019.
40. Costa G, Tomassini F, Tierno SM, Venturini L, Frezza B, Cancrini G, et al. [Emergency colonic surgery: analysis of risk factors predicting morbidity and mortality]. Chir Ital. 2009;61(5–6):565–71.
41. On behalf of the Joined Italian Surgical Societies Working Group, Agresta F, Campanile FC, Podda M, Cillara N, Pernazza G, et al. Current status of laparoscopy for acute abdomen in Italy: a critical appraisal of 2012 clinical guidelines from two consecutive nationwide surveys with analysis of 271,323 cases over 5 years. Surg Endosc. 2017;31(4):1785–95.
42. Cocorullo G, Falco N, Tutino R, Fontana T, Scerrino G, Salamone G, et al. Open versus laparoscopic approach in the treatment of abdominal emergencies in elderly population. G Chir. 2016;37(3):108–12.
43. Cerdán Santacruz C, Frasson M, Flor-Lorente B, Ramos Rodríguez JL, Trallero Anoro M, Millán Scheiding M, et al. Laparoscopy may decrease morbidity and length of stay after elective colon cancer resection, especially in frail patients: results from an observational real-life study. Surg Endosc. 2017;31(12):5032–42.
44. Søreide K, Thorsen K, Søreide JA. Predicting outcomes in patients with perforated gastroduodenal ulcers: artificial neural network modelling indicates a highly complex disease. Eur J Trauma Emerg Surg. 2015;41(1):91–8.
45. Thorsen K, Søreide JA, Søreide K. What is the best predictor of mortality in perforated peptic ulcer disease? A population-based, multivariable regression analysis including three clinical scoring systems. J Gastrointest Surg. 2014;18(7):1261–8.
46. Thorsen K, Søreide JA, Søreide K. Scoring systems for outcome prediction in patients with perforated peptic ulcer. Scand J Trauma Resusc Emerg Med. 2013;21:25.
47. Patel S, Kalra D, Kacheriwala S, Shah M, Duttaroy D. Validation of prognostic scoring systems for predicting 30-day mortality in perforated peptic ulcer disease. Turk J Surg. 2019;35(4):252–8.
48. Nichakankitti N, Athigakunagorn J. The accuracy of prognostic scoring systems for post-operative morbidity and mortality in patients with perforated peptic ulcer. 2016.
49. Bertleff MJOE, Lange JF. Laparoscopic correction of perforated peptic ulcer: first choice? A review of literature. Surg Endosc. 2010;24(6):1231–9.
50. Bertleff MJOE, Halm JA, Bemelman WA, van der Ham AC, van der Harst E, Oei HI, et al. Randomized clinical trial of laparoscopic versus open repair of the perforated peptic ulcer: the LAMA trial. World J Surg. 2009;33(7):1368–73.
51. Siu WT, Leong HT, Law BKB, Chau CH, Li ACN, Fung KH, et al. Laparoscopic repair for perforated peptic ulcer: a randomized controlled trial. Ann Surg. 2002;235(3):313–9.

52. Søreide K, Thorsen K, Søreide JA. Strategies to improve the outcome of emergency surgery for perforated peptic ulcer: emergency surgery for perforated peptic ulcer. Br J Surg. 2014;101(1):e51–64.
53. Lau WY, Leung KL, Kwong KH, Davey IC, Robertson C, Dawson JJ, et al. A randomized study comparing laparoscopic versus open repair of perforated peptic ulcer using suture or sutureless technique. Ann Surg. 1996;224(2):131–8.
54. Kehlet H, Wilmore DW. Fast-track surgery. Br J Surg. 2005;92(1):3–4.
55. Hajibandeh S, Hajibandeh S, Bill V, Satyadas T. Meta-analysis of enhanced recovery after surgery (ERAS) protocols in emergency abdominal surgery. World J Surg. 2020;44(5):1336–48.
56. Varadhan KK, Lobo DN, Ljungqvist O. Enhanced recovery after surgery: the future of improving surgical care. 2010.
57. Paduraru M, Ponchietti L, Casas IM, Svenningsen P, Zago M. Enhanced recovery after emergency surgery: a systematic review. Bull Emerg Trauma. 2017;5(2):70–8.
58. Wisely JC, Barclay KL. Effects of an enhanced recovery after surgery programme on emergency surgical patients. ANZ J Surg. 2016;86(11):883–8.
59. Paduraru M, Ponchietti L, Casas IM, Svenningsen P, Pereira J, Landaluce-Olavarria A, et al. Enhanced recovery after surgery (ERAS)—the evidence in geriatric emergency surgery: a systematic review. Chir Buchar Rom. 2017;112(5):546–57.
60. Mohsina S, Shanmugam D, Sureshkumar S, Kundra P, Mahalakshmy T, Kate V. Adapted ERAS pathway vs. standard care in patients with perforated duodenal ulcer—a randomized controlled trial. J Gastrointest Surg. 2018;22(1):107–16.

Gastric Outlet Obstruction in the Elderly

14

Marcello Pisano, Corrado Gromo, Francesco Autuori, Antonio Lai, Federica Frongia, Giuseppe Esposito, Mauro Podda, and Francesco Balestra

14.1 Introduction

Gastric outlet obstruction (GOO) is a clinical syndrome secondary to an intrinsic or extrinsic mechanical obstruction of the distal one-third of the stomach and/or duodenum. GOO is caused by both benign and malignant diseases, but more commonly by advanced cancers of the upper segments of the digestive tracts [1].

The management of elderly patients with "malignant" GOO always implies a careful consideration of multiple clinical aspects such as the etiological diagnosis, cancer prognosis, and metabolic changes induced by digestive obstruction. The latter are able to break the precarious balance of associated comorbidity and pre-existing frailty. The resolution of symptoms and the improvement of the quality of remaining life are often the only therapeutic objectives in these patients and an effective communication between surgeon, patient, and family members is a fundamental support for understanding and sharing the palliative care proposed [2].

The correction of pathophysiological and metabolic alterations induced by high intestinal occlusion is the first fundamental step in the management of the elderly patient affected by GOO. Multidisciplinary management with the collaboration of geriatricians in the perioperative period will help in the prevention and treatment of the main postoperative complications of the geriatric age [3].

The restoration of food transit can be achieved with a surgical gastrojejunostomy (GJS) or endoscopic procedure with the use of self-expanding metal stent (SEMS). GJS appears to be associated with better results over time with the removal of symptoms for longer periods and should be reserved for patients with a better life expectancy [4].

Today, laparoscopic gastrojejunostomy (LGJS) is a feasible and safe alternative to open GJS. LGJS and technical variants, such as laparoscopic stomach partitioning gastrojejunostomy (LSP-GJS), have confirmed the long-term benefits of surgical

M. Pisano (✉) · A. Lai
General Surgery Unit, Department of Surgery, St. Marcellino Hospital Muravera, ASSL Cagliari-ATS Sardegna, Sardinia, Italy

C. Gromo
Digestive Endoscopy Service, Department of Surgery, St. Marcellino Hospital Muravera, ASSL Cagliari-ATS Sardegna, Sardinia, Italy

F. Autuori
General Surgery Unit, Department of Surgery, St. Trinità Hospital Cagliari, ASSL Cagliari-ATS Sardegna, Sardinia, Italy

F. Frongia · G. Esposito · M. Podda
Department of Emergency Surgery, Cagliari University Hospital, Azienda Ospedaliero-Universitaria, Cagliari, Italy

F. Balestra
General Surgery Unit, Department of Surgery, St. Francesco Hospital Nuoro, ASSL Nuoro-ATS Sardegna, Sardinia, Italy

F. Agresta et al. (eds.), *Emergency laparoscopic surgery in the elderly and frail patient*
https://doi.org/10.1007/978-3-030-79990-8_14

palliation and aim to counteract the increased risk of unfavorable perioperative outcomes for patients undergoing palliative surgery for GOO [5–7].

14.2 Pathogenesis

GOO is a clinical syndrome which today is caused more commonly by malignant diseases in advanced stages of the upper digestive tract, and less frequently by benign diseases [1].

Peptic ulcer has historically been the primary cause of GOO. The introduction of antacid therapy and the discovery of the pathogenetic role and therapy of Helicobacter Pylori infection have led to a reduction in the prevalence of peptic ulcerative disease. Today, the etiopathogenesis has shifted mainly toward gastric and pancreatic tumors, both in the Western world and developing countries [8, 9].

Age is a recognized risk factor for the onset and treatment of gastric and pancreatic tumors [10, 11].

The incidence of both types of cancers increases with age, and 80% of patients with pancreatic cancer have a metastatic or locally advanced tumor which is found inoperable at diagnosis [12, 13].

These epidemiological data justify the reason why the diagnosis of GOO in the elderly should be considered a real warning bell for advanced cancer of the upper GI tract, and, until proven otherwise, a malignant tumor should always be suspected [14, 15].

Furthermore, considering the survival improvement of modern palliative chemoradiotherapy, an increasing number of patients with pancreatic cancer will develop GOO [16].

Other rarer malignant tumors such as those of the duodenum, GIST, NET, lymphomas, and metastatic tumors are also described as causing GOO [17].

Benign diseases responsible for GOO in adults are several and rare, but only few have prevalence in the elderly. Peptic ulcer disease (PUD) with a combination of edema, pyloric spasms, and sclerosis is the main cause of benign GOO [15]. In the elderly, there is still a high prevalence of infection with Helicobacter Pylori that together with the increased use of NSAIDs and pluri-pharmacological therapies (oral steroids, anticoagulants, serotonin reuptake inhibitors) contribute to increasing the risk of PUD and its complications in this patient population. However, other complications such as bleeding and perforations are more common than obstructive complications [18].

The rare Bouveret syndrome is mainly found in elderly female patients with a long clinical history of cholelithiasis [19]. The elongation and laxity of the ligamentous structures of the stomach are at the base of the main mechanism that leads to the torsion of the stomach in the gastric volvulus in both its axial and mesenteroaxial organ variants [20]. The prevalence of paraesophageal hernia and the physiological weakening of the ligaments in the elderly explain the increased incidence of gastric volvulus in this patient population. A complete torsion of >180 leads to GOO framework, ischemia, and necrosis of the gastric wall, representing a surgical emergency with high mortality rates [21].

14.3 Presentation and Workup

Nausea, an early sense of satiety, and vomiting are the key symptoms of GOO, present in over 90% of patients [22]. Vomiting is characteristically not biliary in pre-duodenal obstructions and foods ingested many hours before can be recognized. Repeated vomiting is debilitating and the patient can have a real "fear of food" which leads to progressive weight loss and malnutrition. Chronic epigastric pain is characteristic of peptic ulcer but equally frequent in OGG secondary to advanced gastric and/or pancreatic cancer.

A clinical picture of acute onset is found in multiple benign GOO causes, such as lithiasic obstruction in Bouveret syndrome, obstruction by phytobezoar or by migration of devices such as nutritional probes or mesh.

Borchart's clinical triad, acute epigastric pain radiated to the chest, dry retching, and inability to advance the nasogastric tube, are pathognomonic of acute gastric volvulus (organ-axial) [23].

Clinical examination highlights signs of dehydration and associated malnutrition, meteoric distention of the epigastric region, or palpable swelling. The presence of cholestatic jaundice associated with the symptoms of GOO suggests an advanced pancreatic-biliary malignancy [24].

The maneuver of the "Hippocratic succussion" carried out several hours after a meal can evoke a gurgling noise which indicates the pathological delayed emptying of the stomach [25].

The typical metabolic alteration of high digestive obstructions is hypochloremic-hypokalemic metabolic alkalosis. Mental confusion and hypocalcemic tetany are rare signs of the most serious forms [26].

All patients with GOO should undergo instrumental investigations to confirm the clinical diagnosis and define the etiology. In emergency setting, CT scan is the first-line imaging modality for evaluating quickly patients with GOO. CT scan shows gastric distention with retained stomach contents and identifies the most common and rarest causes of malignant GOO [27] (Fig. 14.1).

Short strictures without abnormal thickening or signs of penetrating ulcer are visible in GOO secondary to PUD [28]. Ectopic gallstone in the distal stomach or duodenum and pneumobilia are the features of Bouveret syndrome. Phytobezoar is also easily visualized by CT [29].

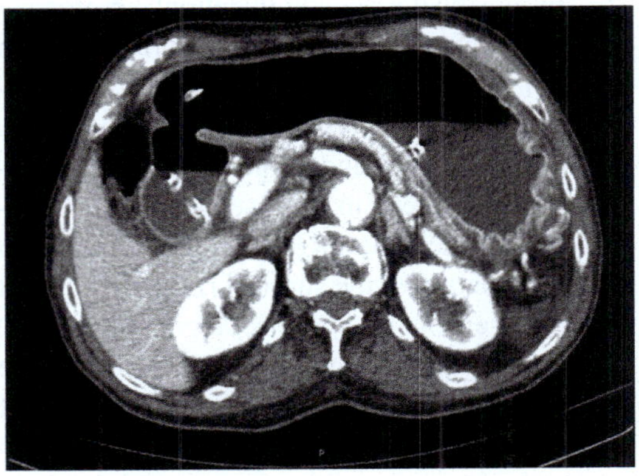

Fig. 14.1 An 87-year-old male patient reaches clinical observation with malnutrition and dehydration after recurrent episodes of vomiting occurred in the last few weeks. CT shows gastric ectasia (**a**) and irregular thickening of the third portion of the duodenum. Endoscopic biopsy was indicative of a duodenum adenocarcinoma. The patient was referred to palliative surgery. Intraoperatively, a solid mass in the third and fourth part of the duodenum was identified and open GJS performed. The patient survived for 24 months

Following radiologic evaluation, upper endoscopy with direct biopsy is performed to reach a definitive diagnosis [30]. Instead, for extraluminal masses, additional ultrasound fine-needle biopsy endoscopy is useful, where necessary [31].

Nasogastric aspiration is recommended to reduce the risk of inhalation during endoscopy or prior to administration of water-soluble contrast media during the CT scan.

14.4 Goals of Palliative Intervention: Endoscopic and Surgical Management

GOO is a frequent clinical expression of locally advanced and/or metastatic malignant neoplasia. The surgeon is often faced with a clinical scenario in which he will have to communicate to the patient and his family members the diagnosis of an inoperable malignant tumor and propose to them exclusively palliative care that will aim at removing the symptoms and improving the quality of residual life [32]. Advanced age, pre-existing co-morbidities, and precarious nutritional status will also expose the patient to a greater risk of postoperative complications, long hospitalization, and mortality [33]. Within this context, doctor-patient communication plays a key role in the management of palliative care [34]. The dynamic interaction between surgeon, patient, and family members is crucial in the decision-making process that will lead to the customization of the therapeutic choice. Unfortunately, the renunciation of surgical treatment can be experienced by the patient with distress and resignation and, especially in these circumstances, an effective and empathic communication has the important function of helping the patient and his family members to understand the decisions taken [35].

The palliative therapy of the "malignant" GOO includes two options: endoscopy (endoscopic stenting) and surgery (gastrojejunostomy).

The choice of the therapeutic option will depend on multiple factors, such as the type of tumor and its extent, patient's performance status, quality and life expectancy, patient's personal choices (e.g., refusal of surgery) [36]. Even randomized prospective studies highlight this last aspect of real daily clinical practice. In the SUSTENT trial, almost 50% of patients refused the proposed surgical option [37].

Higher performance status score (WHO 3–4), obstructive jaundice, weight loss (>10%), metastatic disease, and pancreatic tumors are considered the main negative prognostic factors, which condition the survival of patients with "malignant" GOO [38–40].

When the surgical risk is high and life expectancy is low, endoscopic palliation is the gold standard treatment in terms of efficacy and safety [41].

The use of Self Expanding Metal Stents (SEMS) has undisputed advantages such as a rapid recovery of oral nutrition, short hospital stay, fewer medical complications, and the possibility of offering palliative treatment even to patients with poor performance status and not fit for surgery [42, 43]. Technical success is almost always guaranteed, and the rapid resumption of oral nutrition with resolution of symptoms is obtainable in over 85% of patients [44, 45].

Uncovered stents are those generally used for palliative treatment of "malignant" GOO, since they are less prone to migration, are more flexible, can be used in the presence of bile stents, but the tumor can grow between the metal meshes causing obstruction. Covered stents (C-SEMS) conceptually have a lower obstructive risk but can be easily dislocated and impair their operation [46].

Comparative studies between SEMS and C-SEMS show no significant differences in efficacy and safety [47]. Good knowledge of the limits and advantages of different types of stents, together with the clinical-prognostic framework, will allow a reasoned and personalized choice for each individual patient [48].

A new endoscopic technique, EUS-guided gastroenterostomy (EUS-GE) has recently been introduced in the clinical practice in highly specialized centers [49]. The digestive bypass is realized with different EUS-guided techniques, inserting Lumen Apposing Metal Stent (LAMS) between the gastric lumen and the jejunal lumen downstream from the obstruction.

Conceptually, EUS-GE offers the possibility of overcoming the limits of traditional methods, reducing the risk of obstruction of the stent, and avoiding the perioperative morbidity of surgical bypass [50]. Although preliminary data in terms of safety and efficacy are comforting, they are still insufficient to propose it routinely as an alternative technique [51].

Surgical GJS is the traditional procedure for treating malignant GOO. Despite the extensive use of SEMS favored by higher short-term results, GJS maintains its therapeutic validity [52]. Clinical success is guaranteed and lasting in almost all cases. Surgical palliation should be preferred in patients with better performance status, those with better cancer prognosis and life expectancy of more than 2 months [53].

14.5 Perioperative Care

Elderly and frail patients are exposed to a higher risk of postoperative complications, prolonged hospitalization, readmission, and mortality within 30 days of both elective and emergency surgery [54]. An effective collaboration with geriatrics should be promoted and implemented in the perioperative management of these patients. The geriatrician will help the surgeon and the entire team in the evaluation of the surgical risk, will support the management of pharmacological therapies, prevention, clinical framing, and therapies of the most common "non-surgical" complications of the elderly [55].

The perioperative management of the elderly patient with GOO is focused on the correction of pathophysiological alterations induced by upper digestive obstruction. Repeated vomiting causes dehydration and alteration of the acid-base balance (metabolic alkalosis hypochloremic hypokalemia). The volemic correction should be performed with isotonic solutions and should include sequentially the correction of potassium deficiency. The placement of a nasogastric tube decompresses the stomach and reduces the risk of inhalation, especially during induction. Gastric decompression reduces the ischemic suffering of the mucosa and accelerates the recovery of muscle tone.

Weight loss and malnutrition are common in patients with "malignant" GOO. An adequate perioperative nutritional support must be guaranteed in patients who are malnourished or with a high nutritional risk [56]. Total parental nutrition is an obligatory choice in case GOO obstruction is complete. If the stenosis is passable by a gastroscope with the introduction of a nose tube, preoperative EN is also feasible, safe, and effective [57].

The use of metoclopramide is to be avoided to control nausea and vomiting, because of the risk of adverse neurological effects. The use of Ondansentron, with precautions (Q-T elongation), is preferable in patients with arrhythmogenic heart disease and electrolytic alterations. The use of PPI should be preferred to histamine receptor inhibitors due potentially deliriogenic effect [58]. The use of NSAIDs, such as Ketorolac, can increase the risk of gastric bleeding and kidney failure and should be avoided. Acetaminophen is the first drug to be tried, if not contraindicated, whereas opioids should be used with caution and at low doses [59, 60].

Dehydration and electrolytic and acid-basic balance alterations are recognized as factors precipitating delirium in hospitalized patients [61]. Early recognition of GOO metabolic changes and their timely correction are therefore also essential for the prevention of postoperative delirium [62].

14.6 Surgery

Open gastrojejunostomy (OGJS) has been the standard approach for these patients for a long time. However, due to the poor general condition of these patients, postoperative morbidity and delayed gastric emptying are still the principal limits of surgical GJS [63].

Laparoscopic gastrojejunostomy (LGJS) is a safe and less invasive surgical procedure and GOO patients can also benefit from the advantages of minimally invasive surgery with a lower risk of delayed gastric emptying and faster resumption of oral nutrition than with open surgery [6, 64, 65]. LGDS is commonly performed in antecolic position, with the use of an endoscopic stapler and manual suture of enterotomy [6, 65].

It is unclear whether the laparoscopic technique alone can help reduce the risk of delayed gastric emptying, but many experiences show that when laparoscopy is combined with the use of stomach partitioning gastrojejunostomy (SP-GJS) (modified Devin's technique), the short-term functional results are favorable [7, 66]. Even with a laparoscopic approach, the already known functional validity of the open SP-GJS is confirmed [67, 68].

In addition, good functional results allow, when indicated, rapid access to medical oncology and do not preclude the possibility of subsequent resective surgery [7].

Matsumoto and others described the first laparoscopic approach for SP-GJS in 2005. The stomach is only partially divided upstream of the obstruction, leaving a communication of 2–3 cm along the small curve between the distal segment and the proximal segment. Therefore, the proximal part of the stomach is anastomosed with proximal jejunum (Fig. 14.2). This method promotes rapid stomach emptying and minimized contact between food and the tumor, reduced bleeding from tumors, and also allows endoscopic examination through the tunnel in the lesser curvature of the stomach [69].

14.7 Laparoscopic Stomach Partitioning Gastrojejunostomy: Step-by-Step Technique

Under general anesthesia, the patient is placed in reverse Trendelenburg with the legs apart, while the surgeon is positioned between the legs of the patient as for supramesocolic surgery

After performing the pneumoperitoneum with open technique, four trocars are placed. The optic

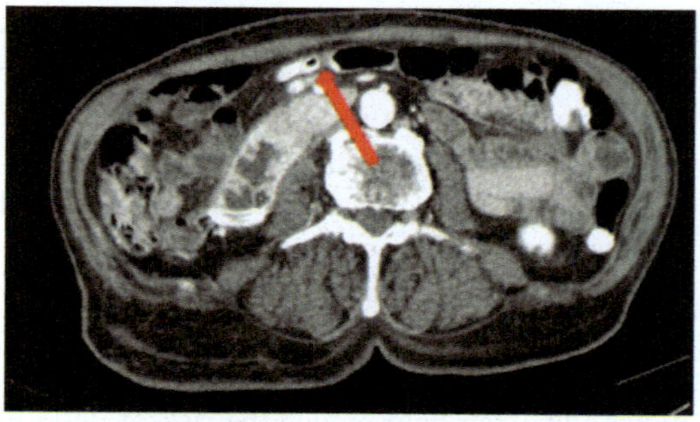

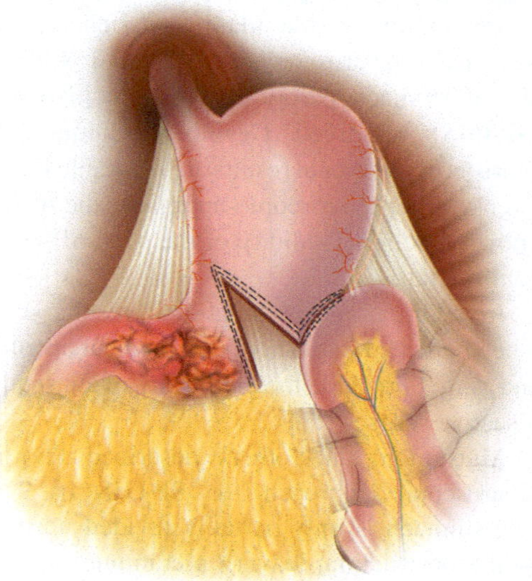

Fig. 14.2 Stomach partitioning gastrojejunostomy (modified Devine's technique)

trocar in the umbilical region, two working trocars (10–12 mm trocars) are placed paramedian right and left and a 5-mm trocar is placed in the subxiphoid area for retraction of the left hepatic lobe.

The gastrocolic ligament is opened starting adjacent to the large gastric curvature, a few inches cranially at a suitable distance from the tumor. The section of the gastrocolic ligament is performed with advanced high-energy devices able to perform hemostasis and cutting.

The back wall of the stomach is explored in order to verify the point of the future GJ. A big size gastric tube (30–33 Fr) is introduced and positioned along the small curve up to the neoplastic stenosis.

With a 60-mm endoscopic linear stapler, the stomach is then dissected, from the greater curvature up to about 2–3 cm from the lesser curvature, leaving the correct space for the passage of the tube previously positioned (Fig. 14.2).

Then, an antiperistaltic GJ anastomosis is fashioned between the first jejunal loop, measured at about 20–30 cm from the ligament of Treitz and the posterior wall of the stomach in its proximal portion, always using a 45-mm endoscopic mechanical stapler. The reconstruction is antecolic (Fig. 14.3).

The procedure ends with the closure of the incisional site of the stomach and jejunum with manual suturing. A single or double layer with continuous barbed suture is performed (Fig. 14.4). The placement of an intra-abdominal drainage is not necessary and can be avoided.

An X-ray study of the upper gastrointestinal tract with water-soluble contrast should be carried out in the second postoperative day, in order to assess the gastric emptying and the absence of leak. This allows the early removal of the nasogastric tube and the start of progressive oral feeding.

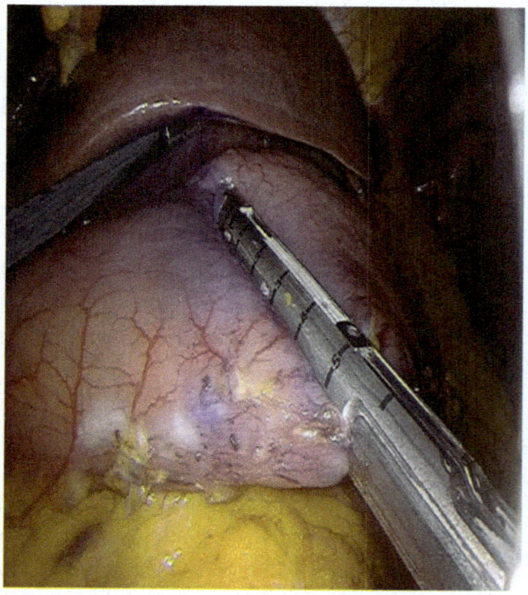

Fig. 14.3 The stomach is partitioned through mechanical linear stapler (60 mm) from the greater curvature toward the lesser curvature. The presence of a big size gastric tube ensures a small conduit between the two gastric chambers

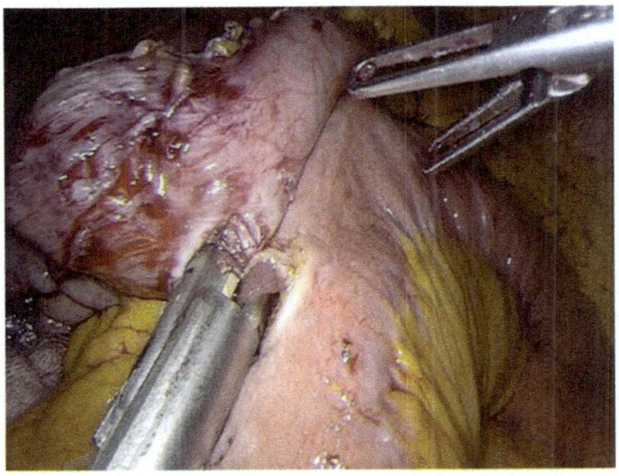

Fig. 14.4 Antecolic antiperistaltics anastomosis GJ along the posterior gastric curvature is performed using a 45-mm endoscopic mechanical stapler

14.8 GOO for Acute Gastric Volvolus: A Surgical Emergency

Acute gastric volvulus is a rare life-threatening condition characterized by an abnormal rotation of the stomach of more than 180° along one of its axes. It can begin suddenly with acute abdominal symptoms and rapidly evolve to a state of hemodynamic instability that suggests severe complications such as massive bleeding or necrosis and gastric perforation of the stomach. In the presence of complications, the mortality rate is 30–50%. Early diagnosis and treatment are the key to management, and vital to prevent life-threatening complications. About 40% of patients with gastric volvulus have an acute onset of symptoms and gastric strangulation is more common in axial volvulus organ and in the presence of a paraesophageal hernia [70].

Diagnosis of gastric volvulus can be difficult for clinicians as it is a rare entity, often presenting with variable, nonspecific clinical scenarios, which requires a high level of diagnostic guesswork and differential diagnosis with other causes of acute abdomen and chest pain. The clinical presentation of acute gastric volvulus is classically described by a Borchardt's triad and is composed of severe acute epigastric pain, vomiting followed by nonproductive retching, and the difficulty or inability to pass a nasogastric tube. This triad occurs in up to 70% of patients who have acute organoaxial volvulus [23].

Chest and abdominal X-ray are a good starting point for patients with acute abdominal pain presenting to the emergency department. Upper gastrointestinal X-ray with a water-soluble contrast medium (e.g., gastrografin) study is useful, but not always available in emergency settings. CT scan is the gold standard for immediate diagnostic framing and the planning of therapeutic management of acute gastric volvulus. CT scan identifies the volvulus, distinguishes its type, and detects predisposing factors and other abnormalities associated with complicated gastric volvulus (absence of parietal contrast enhancement, gastric pneumatosis, and pneumoperitoneum) [71, 72].

The initial management of acute gastric volvulus in every patient is gastric decompression with nasogastric tube. Immediate surgery can be avoided by most patients through the use of gastric decompression, allowing them to undergo planned definitive treatment after completing diagnostic evaluation and medical/anesthetic risk assessment. Endoscopy can be used to assist the placement of a nasogastric tube and simultaneously assess the viability of the gastric mucosa.

Endoscopy in elderly and frail patients with high surgical risk is considered the first therapeutic option. The treatment consists of decompression and de-rotation of the stomach, and the placement of two percutaneous gastrostomy tubes to perform a gastropexy, during which the stomach is fixed to the abdominal wall [73].

Emergency surgical intervention is required if gastric decompression is unsuccessful via nasogastric tube or endoscopic techniques and obviously when necrosis, gastric perforation, shock, and sepsis are present.

The principal aims of surgical operation for a patient with an acute gastric volvulus are: immediate reduction and de-rotation of the stomach, prevention of recurrence, and repairing any predisposing factors such as simultaneous paraesophageal hernia, if present. Gastrectomy is required for necrosis or perforation of the stomach.

Open surgery is generally performed. In recent years, some centers have proposed that acute gastric volvulus can be managed in emergency settings, in the early stages, with a laparoscopic approach when the patient is hemodynamically stable, and ischemic and perforative complications are not present [21, 74, 75].

All the stages of the open surgical intervention for gastric volvulus can be accomplished by laparoscopic surgery [76]. However, in emergency cases with high-risk elderly patients unable to tolerate prolonged surgery, the sole reduction of volvulus and anterior gastropexy without correcting hiatal defect is a viable option, and in many cases, the definitive solution [21, 70, 77].

The laparoscopic repair of the diaphragmatic defect requires complex and time-consuming surgical procedures and should be performed by surgeons with advanced laparoscopic skills (Fig. 14.5).

Once the volvulus is reduced and the stomach is in its normal anatomic position, an anterior gastropexy (AGP) can be performed with a laparoscopic direct suture of the stomach to the diaphragm and abdominal wall, preferably with multiple non-absorbable stitches (every 3 cm) along the greater curvature and prepyloric region of the stomach (Fig. 14.6).

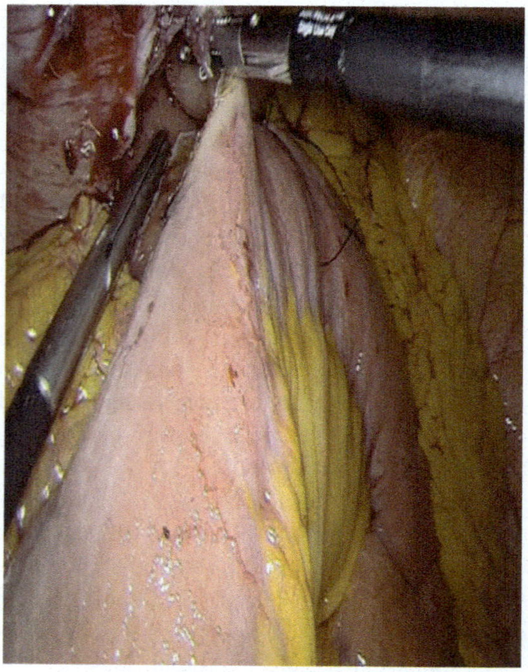

Fig. 14.5 Entero-gastrostomy is closed with a single or double layer using a continuous barbed suture

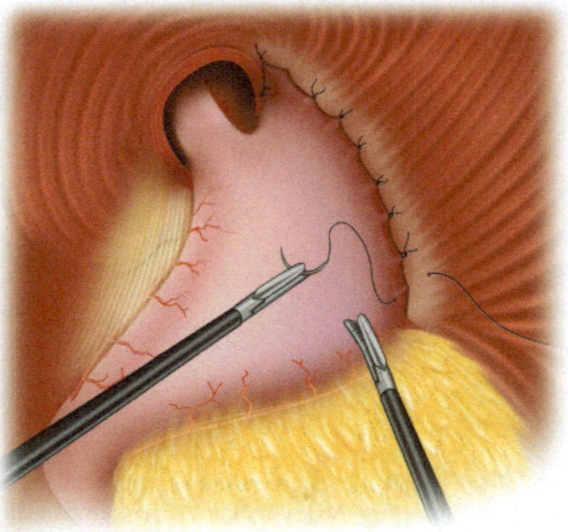

Fig. 14.6 Laparoscopic anterior gastropexy: multiple points fix fundus and greater curvature to diaphragm and anterior parietal peritoneum

Multiple anchor points can reduce the risk of volvulus recurrence and gastrostomy is unnecessary. A gastrostomy tube should be placed only selectively: when the sutured gastropexy is technically challenging, or in those patients who are at high risk of being unable to feed by mouth [78].

14.9 Conclusion

Palliation of GOO in elderly patients may be challenging, and multidisciplinary teamwork is often needed to evaluate the best therapeutic strategy, taking into account acute metabolic alterations, the patient's performance status, life expectancy, surgical risks, and, importantly, patient's preferences. In this scenario, the endoscopist may offer effective minimal invasive approaches, but surgical gastrojejunostomy is still the best therapeutic option for patients fit for surgery and with longer term life expectancy.

Nowadays, laparoscopic surgery represents a valid technical option. It reduces the trauma related to surgery, offering a safe and effective alternative surgical palliation. The LGP-GJS technique can ensure better functional results than conventional GJS.

Even in emergency situations such as in acute gastric volvulus, laparoscopic approach could be proposed in selected patients. After gastric de-rotation and repositioning of the stomach in its anatomical position, the laparoscopic anterior gastropexy alone without diaphragmatic repair can be considered a strategic, quick, and definitive treatment in elderly and frail patients.

Five Things You Should Know About Gastric Outlet Obstruction in the Elderly

- GOO in the elderly is a common expression of a metastatic or locally advanced oncological disease. Usually, palliative care represents the only possible treatment.
- Oncological disease, malnutrition, and GOO-induced acute metabolic alterations worsen the condition of frailty of the elderly patient. Synergistic collaboration with geriatricians is desirable in the perioperative period to counteract the increased risk of postoperative complications of these patients.
- The restoration of food transit and the improvement of the residual quality of life are the therapeutic goals of endoscopic and surgical palliative care. Surgical palliation with gastrojejunostomy (GJS) should be reserved for patients who are fit for surgery and those with longer life expectancy.
- Laparoscopic GJS is a feasible, safe, and effective surgical option. Laparoscopic stomach partitioning gastrojejunostomy (LSP-GJS) appears to offer better functional outcomes, but further research is needed to confirm this finding.
- In the emergency scenario of acute gastric volvulus in elderly patients with high surgical risk, the sole reduction of the volvulus and anterior laparoscopic gastropexy without correcting hiatal defect is a viable and definitive therapeutic option.

References

1. Khullar SK, DiSario JA. Gastric outlet obstruction. Gastrointest Endosc Clin N Am. 1996;6(3):585–603.
2. Potz BA, Miner TJ. Surgical palliation of gastric outlet obstruction in advanced malignancy. World J Gastrointest Surg. 2016;8(8):545–55. https://doi.org/10.4240/wjgs.v8.i8.545. PMID: 27648158; PMCID: PMC5003933.
3. Colburn JL, Mohanty S, Burton JR. Surgical guidelines for perioperative management of older adults: what geriatricians need to know. J Am Geriatr Soc. 2017;65:1339–46.
4. Upchurch E, Ragusa M, Cirocchi R. Stent placement versus surgical palliation for adults with malignant gastric outlet obstruction. Cochrane Database Syst Rev. 2018;(5):CD012506. https://doi.org/10.1002/14651858.CD012506.pub2.
5. Min SH, Son SY, Jung DH, et al. Laparoscopic gastrojejunostomy versus duodenal stenting in unresectable gastric cancer with gastric outlet obstruction. Ann Surg Treat Res. 2017;93(3):130–6. https://doi.org/10.4174/astr.2017.93.3.130.
6. Choi YB. Laparoscopic gatrojejunostomy for palliation of gastric outlet obstruction in unresectable gastric cancer. Surg Endosc. 2002;16(11):1620–6. https://doi.org/10.1007/s00464-002-0010-5. Epub 2002 Jun 20. PMID: 12073005.
7. Tanaka T, Suda K, Satoh S, Kawamura Y, Inaba K, Ishida Y, Uyama I. Effectiveness of laparoscopic stomach-partitioning gastrojejunostomy for patients with gastric outlet obstruction caused by advanced gastric cancer. Surg Endosc. 2017;31(1):359–67. https://doi.org/10.1007/s00464-016-4980-0. Epub 2016 Jun 10. PMID: 27287913.
8. Shone DN, Nikoomanesh P, Smith-Meek MM, Bender JS. Malignancy is the most common cause of gastric outlet obstruction in the era of H2 blockers. Am J Gastroenterol. 1995;90:1769–70.
9. Jaka H, Mchembe MD, Rambau PF, Chalya PL. Gastric outlet obstruction at Bugando Medical Centre in Northwestern Tanzania: a prospective review of 184 cases. BMC Surg. 2013;13:41. https://doi.org/10.1186/1471-2482-13-41. PMID 24067148; PMCID: PMC3849005.
10. Saif MW, Makrilia N, Zalonis A, Merikas M, Syrigos K. Gastric cancer in the elderly: an overview. Eur J Surg Oncol. 2010;36(8):709–17.
11. Riall TS. What is the effect of age on pancreatic resection? Adv Surg. 2009;43:233–49. https://doi.org/10.1016/j.yasu.2009.02.004.
12. Forman D, Burley VJ. Gastric cancer: global pattern of the disease and an overview of environmental risk factors. Best Pract Res Clin Gastroenterol. 2006;20(4):633–49.
13. Higuera O, Ghanem I, Nasimi R, Prieto I, Koren L, Feliu J. Management of pancreatic cancer in the

elderly. World J Gastroenterol. 2016;22(2):764–75. https://doi.org/10.3748/wjg.v22.i2.764. PMID: 26811623; PMCID: PMC4716075.
14. Johnson CD. Gastric outlet obstruction malignant until proved otherwise. Am J Gastroenterol. 1995;90(10):1740. PMID: 7572886.
15. Koop AH, Palmer WC, Stancampiano FF. Gastric outlet obstruction: a red flag, potentially manageable. Cleve Clin J Med. 2019;86(5):345–53. https://doi.org/10.3949/ccjm.86a.18035. PMID: 31066665.
16. Shah A, Fehmi A, Savides TJ. Increased rates of duodenal obstruction in pancreatic cancer patients receiving modern medical management. Dig Dis Sci. 2014;59(9):2294–8. https://doi.org/10.1007/s10620-014-3170-y. Epub 2014 Apr 30. PMID: 24781163.
17. Schulz C, Schütte K, Malfertheiner P. Rare neoplasia of the stomach. Gastrointest tumors. 2015;2(2):52–60. https://doi.org/10.1159/000435899. Epub 2015 Aug 7. PMID: 26674659; PMCID: PMC4668797.
18. Dumic I, Nordin T, Jecmenica M, Stojkovic Lalosevic M, Milosavljevic T, Milovanovic T. Gastrointestinal tract disorders in older age. Can J Gastroenterol Hepatol. 2019;2019:6757524. https://doi.org/10.1155/2019/6757524. PMID: 30792972; PMCID: PMC6354172.
19. Cappell M, Davis M. Characterization of Bouveret's syndrome: a comprehensive review of 128 cases. Am J Gastroenterol. 2006;101(9):2139–46.
20. Rodriguez-Garcia HA, Wright AS, Yates RB. Managing obstructive gastric volvulus: challenges and solutions. Open Access Surg. 2017;10:15–24. https://doi.org/10.2147/OAS.S91357.
21. Light D, Links D, Griffin M. The threatened stomach: management of the acute gastric volvulus. Surg Endosc. 2016;30(5):1847–52. https://doi.org/10.1007/s00464-015-4425-1. Epub 2015 Aug 15. PMID: 26275540.
22. Tringali A, Didden P, Repici A, et al. Endoscopic treatment of malignant gastric and duodenal strictures: a prospective, multicenter study. Gastrointest Endosc. 2014;79(1):66–75. https://doi.org/10.1016/j.gie.2013.06.032.
23. Borchardt M. Zun pathologie and therapy des magnevolvulus. Arch klin Chir. 1904;74:243–8.
24. Lillemoe KD. Palliative therapy for pancreatic cancer. Surg Oncol Clin N Am. 1998;7(1):199–216.
25. Provenzale L. Manuale di Semeiotica Chirurgica 1983 XX 732–761 Edizioni Luigi Pozzi 1983 Roma.
26. Ahmad J, Thomson S, Taylor M, Scoffield J. A reminder of the classical biochemical sequelae of adult gastric outlet obstruction. BMJ Case Rep. 2011;2011:bcr0520102978. https://doi.org/10.1136/bcr.05.2010.2978. PMID: 22714599; PMCID: PMC3066630.
27. Guniganti P, Bradenham CH, Raptis C, Menias CO, Mellnick VM. CT of gastric emergencies. Radiographics. 2015;35(7):1909–21. https://doi.org/10.1148/rg.2015150062. PMID: 26562229.
28. Tonolini M, Ierardi AM, Bracchi E, Magistrelli P, Vella A, Carrafiello G. Non-perforated peptic ulcer disease: multidetector CT findings, complications, and differential diagnosis. Insights Imaging. 2017;8(5):455–69. https://doi.org/10.1007/s13244-017-0562-5.
29. Zulfiqar M, Shetty A, Shetty V, Menias C. Computed tomography imaging of non-neoplastic and neoplastic benign gastric disease. Curr Probl Diagn Radiol. 2019;48(1):75–96. https://doi.org/10.1067/j.cpradiol.2017.12.004. Epub 2018 Jan 11. PMID: 29449042.
30. ASGE Standards of Practice Committee, Fukami N, Anderson MA, Khan K, Harrison ME, Appalaneni V, Ben-Menachem T, Decker GA, Fanelli RD, Fisher L, Ikenberry SO, Jain R, Jue TL, Krinsky ML, Maple JT, Sharaf RN, Dominitz JA. The role of endoscopy in gastroduodenal obstruction and gastroparesis. Gastrointest Endosc. 2011;74:13–21. https://doi.org/10.1016/j.gie.2010.12.003.
31. Valero M, Robles-Medranda C. Endoscopic ultrasound in oncology: an update of clinical applications in the gastrointestinal tract. World J Gastrointest Endosc. 2017;9(6):243–54. https://doi.org/10.4253/wjge.v9.i6.243. PMID: 28690767; PMCID: PMC5483416.
32. Miner TJ. Communication skill in palliative surgery: skill and effort are key. Surg Clin N Am. 2011;91:355–66.
33. Turrentine FE, Wang H, Simpson VB, Jones RS. Surgical risk factors, morbidity, and mortality in elderly patients. J Am Coll Surg. 2006;203(6):865–77. https://doi.org/10.1016/j.jamcollsurg.2006.08.026. PMID: 17116555.
34. Bradley CT, Brasel KJ. Core competencies in palliative care for surgeons: interpersonal communication skills. Am J Hosp Palliat Med. 2008;24(6):499–507.
35. Mner TJ. Communication as a core skill of palliative surgical care. Anesthesiol Clin. 2012;30:47–58.
36. Potz BA, Miner TJ. Surgical palliation of gastric outlet obstruction in advanced malignancy. World J Gastroinet Surg. 2016;8(8):545–55.
37. Jeurnink SM, Steyerberg EW, van Hooft JE, et al. Surgical gastrojejunostomy or endoscopic stent placement for the palliation of malignant gastric outlet obstruction (SUSTENT study): a multicenter randomized trial. Gastrointest Endosc. 2010;71(3):490–9. https://doi.org/10.1016/j.gie.2009.09.042.
38. Jeurnink SM, Steyerberg EW, Vleggaar FP, van Eijck CH, van Hooft JE, Schwartz MP, Kuipers EJ, Siersema PD, Dutch SUSTENT Study Group. Predictors of survival in patients with malignant gastric outlet obstruction: a patient-oriented decision approach for palliative treatment. Dig Liver Dis. 2011;43:548–52. https://doi.org/10.1016/j.dld.2011.01.017. Epub 2011 Mar 4. PMID: 21376680.
39. Park JK, Yoon YB, Kim YT, Ryu JK, Yoon WJ, Lee SH. Survival and prognostic factors of unresectable pancreatic cancer. J Clin Gastroenterol. 2008;42:86–91. https://doi.org/10.1097/01.mcg.0000225657.30803.9d. PMID: 18097296.
40. Bednarsch J, Czigany Z, Heise D, Zimmermann H, Boecker J, Ulmer TF, Neumann UP, Klink C. Influ-

ence of peritoneal carcinomatosis on perioperative outcome in palliative gastric bypass for malignant gastric outlet obstruction—a retrospective cohort study. World J Surg Oncol. 2020;18(1):25. https://doi.org/10.1186/s12957-020-1803-5. PMID: 32005250; PMCID: PMC6995201.
41. Graber I, Dumas R, Filoche B, et al.; Société Française d'Endoscopie Digestive (SFED). The efficacy and safety of duodenal stenting: a prospective multicenter study. Endoscopy. 2007;39:784–7.
42. Uemura S, Iwashita T, Iwata K, Mukai T, Osada S, Sekino T, et al. Endoscopic duodenal stent versus surgical gastrojejunostomy for gastric outlet obstruction in patients with advanced pancreatic cancer. Pancreatology. 2018;18(5):601–7.
43. Zheng B, Wang X, Ma B, Tian J, Jiang L, Yang K. Endoscopic stenting versus gastrojejunostomy for palliation of malignant gastric outlet obstruction. Dig Endosc. 2012;24:71–8.
44. Tringali A, Didden P, Repici A, Spaander M, Bourke MJ, Williams SJ, Spicak J, Drastich P, Mutignani M, Perri V, Roy A, Johnston K, Costamagna G. Endoscopic treatment of malignant gastric and duodenal strictures: a prospective, multicenter study. Gastrointest Endosc. 2014;79(1):66–75.
45. Canena JM, Lagos AC, Marques IN, Patrocínio SD, Tomé MG, Liberato MA, Romão CM, Coutinho AP, Veiga PM, Neves BC, Além HD, Gonçalves JA. Oral intake throughout the patients' lives after palliative metallic stent placement for malignant gastroduodenal obstruction: a retrospective multicentre study. Eur J Gastroenterol Hepatol. 2012;24(7):747–55. https://doi.org/10.1097/MEG.0b013e328353d9d3. PMID: 22522142.
46. Kim SG, Yang CH. Upper gastrointestinal stent. Clin Endosc. 2012;45(4):386–91.
47. Yang Z, Wu Q, Wang F, Ye X, Qi X, Fan D. A systematic review and meta-analysis of randomized trials and prospective studies comparing covered and bare self-expandable metal stents for the treatment of malignant obstruction in the digestive tract. Int J Med Sci. 2013;10(7):825–35. https://doi.org/10.7150/ijms.5969.
48. Tringalia A, Giannettia A, Adler DG. Endoscopic management of gastric outlet obstruction disease. Ann Gastroenterol. 2019;32(4):330–7.
49. Khashab MA, Kumbhari V, Grimm IS, Ngamruengphong S, Aguila G, El Zein M, Kalloo AN, Baron TH. EUS-guided gastroenterostomy: the first U.S. clinical experience (with video). Gastrointest Endosc. 2015;82(5):932–8. https://doi.org/10.1016/j.gie.2015.06.017. Epub 2015 Jul 26. PMID: 26215646.
50. Irani S, Baron TH, Itoi T, Khashab MA. Endoscopic gastroenterostomy: techniques and review. Curr Opin Gastroenterol. 2017;33(5):320–9. https://doi.org/10.1097/MOG.0000000000000389. PMID: 28767501.
51. Iqbal U, Khara HS, Hu Y, Kumar V, Tufail K, Confer B, Diehl DL. EUS-guided gastroenterostomy for the management of gastric outlet obstruction: a systematic review and meta-analysis. Endosc Ultrasound. 2020;9(1):16–23. https://doi.org/10.4103/eus.eus_70_19. PMID: 31898587; PMCID: PMC7038736.
52. Endoscopic stenting for gastric outlet obstruction in patients with unresectable antro pyloric cancer. Systematic review of the literature and final results of a prospective study. The point of view of a surgical group. Am J Surg. 2013;206(2):210–217. https://doi.org/10.1016/j.amjsurg.2012.08.018.
53. Miyazaki Y, Takiguchi S, Takahashi T, Kurokawa Y, Makino T, Yamasaki M, Nakajima K, Mori M, Doki Y. Treatment of gastric outlet obstruction that result from unresectable gastric cancer: current evidence. World J Gastrointest Endosc. 2016;8(3):165–72.
54. Parmar KL, Law J, Carter B, Hewitt J, Boyle JM, Casey P, Maitra I, Farrell IS, Pearce L, Moug SJ, ELF Study Group. Frailty in older patients undergoing emergency laparotomy: results from the UK Observational Emergency Laparotomy and Frailty (ELF) Study. Ann Surg. 2021;273(4):709–18. https://doi.org/10.1097/SLA.0000000000003402. Epub ahead of print. PMID: 31188201.
55. Mohanty S, Roshental RA, Russell MM, et al. Optimal perioperative management of the geriatric patient: a best practices guideline from the American College of Surgeons NSQIP and the American Geriatrics Society. J Am Coll Surg. 2006;222(5):930–47.
56. Arved Weimanna A, Bragab M, Carlic F, Higashiguchid T, Hübnere M, Klekf S, Lavianog A, Ljungqvisth O, Loboi DN, Martindalej R, Waitzbergk DL, Bischoffl SC, Singerm P. ESPEN guideline: clinical nutrition in surgery. Clin Nutr. 2017;36:623–50.
57. Chen ZH, Lin SY, Dai QB, Hua J, Chen SQ. The effects of pre-operative enteral nutrition from nasal feeding tubes on gastric outlet obstruction. Nutrients. 2017;9(4):373. https://doi.org/10.3390/nu9040373. PMID: 28394302; PMCID: PMC5409712.
58. Fujii S, Tanimukai H, Kashiwagi Y. Comparison and analysis of delirium induced by histamine h(2) receptor antagonists and proton pump inhibitors in cancer patients. Case Rep Oncol. 2012;5(2):409–12. https://doi.org/10.1159/000341873. Epub 2012 Jul 31. PMID: 22949902; PMCID: PMC3433017.
59. Mohanty S, Rosenthal RA, Russell MM, Neuman MD, Ko CY, Esnaola NF. Optimal perioperative management of the geriatric patient: a best practices guideline from the American College of Surgeons NSQIP and the American Geriatrics Society. J Am Coll Surg. 2016;222(5):930–47. https://doi.org/10.1016/j.jamcollsurg.2015.12.026.
60. American Geriatrics Society 2019 Updated AGS Beers Criteria® for Potentially Inappropriate Medication Use in Older Adults. Panel., 2019 American Geriatrics Society Beers Criteria® Update Expert. By the 2019 American Geriatrics Society Beers Criteria® Update Expert Panel. American Geriatrics Society 2019 Updated AGS Beers Criteria® fo J Am Geriatr Soc. 2019;67(4):674–694. https://doi.org/10.1111/jgs.1.

61. Marcantonio ER. Delirium in hospitalized older adults. N Engl J Med. 2017;377(15):1456–66. https://doi.org/10.1056/NEJMcp1605501. PMID: 29020579; PMCID: PMC5706782.
62. American Geriatrics Society Expert Panel on Postoperative Delirium in Older Adults. Postoperative delirium in older adults: best practice statement from the American Geriatrics Society. J Am Coll Surg. 2015;220(2):136–48.e1. https://doi.org/10.1016/j.jamcollsurg.2014.10.019. Epub 2014 Nov 14. PMID: 25535170.
63. Kung SP, Lui WY, P'eng FK. An analysis of the possible factors contributing to the delayed return of gastric emptying after gastrojejunostomy. Surg Today. 1995;25(10):911–5. https://doi.org/10.1007/BF00311758. PMID: 8574059.
64. Ojima T, Nakamori M, Nakamura M, Katsuda M, Hayata K, Yamaue H. Laparoscopic gastrojejunostomy for patients with unresectable gastric cancer with gastric outlet obstruction. J Gastrointest Surg. 2017;21(8):1220–5. https://doi.org/10.1007/s11605-017-3387-0.
65. Navarra G, Musolino C, Venneri A, De Marco ML, Bartolotta M. Palliative antecolic isoperistaltic gastrojejunostomy: a randomized controlled trial comparing open and laparoscopic approaches. Surg Endosc. 2006;20:1831–4. [PMID: 17063298]. https://doi.org/10.1007/s0046.
66. Eguchi H, Yada K, Shibata K, Matsumoto T, Etoh T, Yasuda K, Inomata M, Shiraishi N, Ohta M, Kitano S. Laparoscopic stomach-partitioning gastrojejunostomy is an effective palliative procedure to improve quality of life in patients with malignant gastroduodenal outlet obstruction. Asian J Endosc Surg. 2012;5(4):153–6. https://doi.org/10.1111/j.1758-5910.2012.00151.
67. Kumagai K, Rouvelas I, Ernberg A, Persson S, Analatos A, Mariosa D, Lindblad M, Nilsson M, Ye W, Lundell L, Tsai JA. A systematic review and meta-analysis comparing partial stomach partitioning gastrojejunostomy versus conventional gastrojejunostomy for malignant gastroduodenal obstruction. Arch Surg. 2016;401(6):777–85. https://doi.org/10.1007/s00423-016-1470-8. Epub 2016 Jun 23. PMID: 27339200.
68. Lorusso D, Giliberti A, Bianco M, Lantone G, Leandro G. Stomach-partitioning gastrojejunostomy is better than conventional gastrojejunostomy in palliative care of gastric outlet obstruction for gastric or pancreatic cancer: a meta-analysis. J Gastrointest Oncol. 2019;10(2):283–91. https://doi.org/10.21037/jgo.2018.10.10. PMID: 31032096; PMCID: PMC6465492.
69. Matsumoto T, Izumi K, Shiromizu A, Shibata K, Ohta M, Kitano S. Laparoscopic gastric partitioning gastrojejunostomy for an unresectable duodenal malignant tumor. J Minim Access Surg. 2005;1(3):129–32. https://doi.org/10.4103/0972-9941.18997. PMID: 21188010; PMCI.
70. García RM, Tomás NP, Del Pozo CD, Tarragón AV, Mas EM, Juan RT, Abad MM. Tratamiento del vólvulo gástrico agudo mediante abordaje laparoscópico [Laparoscopic treatment of acute gastric volvulus]. Cir Esp. 2013;91(3):189–93. https://doi.org/10.1016/j.ciresp.2012.03.011. Epub 2012 May 22. PMID: 22624957.
71. Millet I, Orliac C, Alili C, Guillon F, Taourel P. Computed tomography findings of acute gastric volvulus. Eur Radiol. 2014;24(12):3115–22. https://doi.org/10.1007/s00330-014-3319-2. Epub 2014 Oct 4. PMID: 25278244.
72. Verde F, Hawasli H, Johnson PT, Fishman EK. Gastric volvulus: unraveling the diagnosis with MPRs. Emerg Radiol. 2019;26(2):221–5. https://doi.org/10.1007/s10140-019-01669-0. Epub 2019 Jan 14. PMID: 30644001.
73. Eckhauser ML, Ferron JP. The use of dual percutaneous endoscopic gastrostomy (DPEG) in the management of chronic intermittent gastric volvulus. Gastrointest Endosc. 1985;31(5):340–2. https://doi.org/10.1016/s0016-5107(85)72221-3. PMID: 4043688.
74. Teague WJ, Ackroyd R, Watson DI, Devitt PG. Changing patterns in the management of gastric volvulus over 14 years. Br J Surg. 2000;87(3):358–61. https://doi.org/10.1046/j.1365-2168.2000.01385.x. PMID: 10718808.
75. Palanivelu C, Rangarajan M, Shetty AR, et al. Laparoscopic suture gastropexy for gastric volvulus: a report of 14 cases. Surg Endosc. 2007;21:863–6. https://doi.org/10.1007/s00464-006-9089-4.
76. Channer LT, Squires GT, Price PD. Laparoscopic repair of gastric volvulus. JSLS. 2000;4(3):225–30.
77. Naim HJ, Smith R, Gorecki PJ. Emergent laparoscopic reduction of acute gastric volvulus with anterior gastropexy. Surg Laparosc Endosc Percutan Tech. 2003;13(6):389–91. https://doi.org/10.1097/00129689-200312000-00009. PMID: 14712102.
78. Yates RB, Hinojosa MW, Wright AS, Pellegrini CA, Oelschlager BK. Laparoscopic gastropexy relieves symptoms of obstructed gastric volvulus in high operative risk patients. Am J Surg. 2015;209(5):875–80; discussion 880. Epub 2015 Feb 19. PMID: 25754844. https://doi.org/10.1016/j.amjsurg.2014.12.024.

15 Obstructing Colorectal Tumor

Alberto Arezzo, Giacomo Lo Secco,
Giovanni Distefano, Edoardo Forcignanò,
and Mario Morino

15.1 Introduction

Despite the progressive improvement of screening programs, colorectal cancer (CRC) is still a major cause of morbidity and mortality worldwide. It represents the third most common cancer affecting men and the second affecting women. The median age of patients at the time of diagnosis is 73 years. In up to 10% [1] of cases, the first clinical presentation is bowel obstruction. This is more common in the left colonic segments, due to the smaller size of the lumen, so that 75% of obstructing tumors are located distal to the splenic flexure [2–4].

Colonic obstruction represents a surgical emergency, and the patient can present with acute abdominal pain, distension of the abdomen, failure of passage of the flatus and stools, or with a chronic history of pain and progressive change in bowel habits. Nausea and vomiting are more common in right colon obstructions [5]. Late diagnosed cases can show with sepsis and multiple organ failure (MOF). Perforation can occur as a consequence of colonic obstruction, more frequently at the point of obstruction (70% of cases), likely due to local tumor invasion or inflammatory reaction rather than in the proximal dilated colon [6, 7].

Patients with chronic obstruction can experience several days of reduced oral intake and vomiting, with signs of dehydration, alteration of hydro-electrolytic balance, or even abdominal compartment syndrome [6]. In case of elderly and frail patients, the emergency resection represents a very high-risk procedure. A tailored treatment decision should be based on the intent of surgery, curative or palliative, the risk profile of the patient, the degree of obstruction, and the resources available. Initial decompression of the distended colon, either by performing a stoma or by placement of a self-expandable metal stent (SEMS), can be a safe option. Once the obstruction is treated, the interval before elective surgery is useful for accurate preoperative staging, multidisciplinary evaluation, improvement of the patient's conditions, and to organize an experienced surgical team.

15.2 Diagnostic Workup and Initial Care

The most common symptoms are the failure of passage of flatus and/or stools associated with abdominal distension. Abdominal examination shows tenderness, abdominal distension, and hyperactive or, at a later stage, absent bowel sounds [4]. Routine laboratory exams

A. Arezzo (✉) · G. Lo Secco · G. Distefano
E. Forcignanò · M. Morino
Department of Surgical Sciences, University of Torino, Turin, Italy
e-mail: alberto.arezzo@unito.it

F. Agresta et al. (eds.), *Emergency laparoscopic surgery in the elderly and frail patient*,
https://doi.org/10.1007/978-3-030-79990-8_15

are mandatory as they can show the presence of chronic anemia, electrolyte alteration, metabolic abnormalities like elevated blood urea nitrogen, and metabolic alkalosis. The first-line radiologic evaluation includes the abdominal X-ray which can highlight the presence of air-fluid levels, confirming the intestinal obstruction, and potentially free intra-abdominal air in case of simultaneous perforation [8]. Although the presence of free air leads to surgical exploration, CT scan examination is recommended when available [4]. Hemodynamically, stable patients without radiologic signs of perforation should undergo CT scan with contrast, due to its high sensitivity and specificity in detecting CRC [9]. Moreover, CT scan can identify multifocal disease, metastatic tumor, ascites or carcinomatosis, and, in up to 10% of patients, synchronous tumors, which can influence further surgical decision [10]. For this reason, it is recommended to extend the CT exam to the chest after diagnosis, so to have a complete staging of the disease. Lower endoscopic exam (sigmoidoscopy, colonoscopy) is not routinely performed but can be useful in those patients, particularly those having chronic symptoms, in whom CT scan cannot exclude an inflammatory obstruction (diverticulitis or autoimmune disease), so to confirm the diagnosis and, when indicated, to assess the feasibility of SEMS placement with both curative or palliative intent [11, 12].

Whatever the location of the obstruction, and no matter the staging, the patient affected by CRC obstruction is initially managed with supportive care which includes gastric decompression, in case of nausea or vomiting, and intravenous fluid therapy with correction of electrolyte abnormalities [13].

15.3 Right-Sided Malignant Colonic Obstruction

Right-sided malignant colonic obstruction is generally due to a more advanced neoplasm, as obstruction can occur only at a later stage, due to the different caliber of the bowel compared to the left side. Often these patients are affected by a severe anemia and iron deficiency, due to chronic blood loss. Right-sided tumors are more frequently invading near organs and are associated with suspected involvement of lymph nodes or synchronous metastases, as well as peritoneal carcinomatosis [14].

Nevertheless, an emergency resection is more frequently performed in right-sided compared to left-sided obstructing tumor. In fact, right-sided lesions can be safely treated by segmental resection with direct ileo-colic anastomosis, mainly because the right colonic segments are easier to dissect and because the small bowel mobility allows the surgeon to perform the anastomosis without the need of additional dissection with an optimal blood supply [4].

In case of proximal malignant colonic obstruction, a right colectomy with primary anastomosis should be considered based on patient's general condition. In an emergency scenario, laparoscopic surgery for intestinal obstruction has had a modest spread due to the difficulty to reach an adequate working space. Moreover, emergency laparoscopic surgery can be performed only by experienced and skilled surgeons [15]. A lateral ileostomy protecting a primary anastomosis should be considered in particularly frail patients. Unstable patients should better receive a terminal ileostomy than a primary anastomosis [16].

As an alternative to emergent colectomy, recent retrospective studies indicate that endoscopic stent decompression of obstructing right-sided colon cancers can be safely and effectively performed, with an increased rate of elective laparoscopic resections without affecting long-term oncologic outcomes [17]. A recent systematic review showed a lower mortality and morbidity rate and a lower risk of anastomotic leak after stent bridge to surgery (SBTS) compared to emergency surgery (ES), but the included studies were small and their quality is low [18]. Therefore, recently, ESGE guidelines opened to SBTS in case of malignant obstruction of the right colon. SBTS could be considered an alternative to emergency surgery, especially in elderly and frail patients [19].

Nevertheless, it is our opinion that alternatives to emergency resections have not been studied because right colectomy with primary ileo-colic anastomosis is a safe and feasible procedure, it represents the option of choice in obstructing right colonic tumor, despite the fact that patients are usually older and with a more advanced loco-regional disease [4].

15.4 Left-Sided Malignant Colonic Obstruction

The most appropriate treatment for the left CRC obstruction is still controversial. The choice depends on many different factors: the general condition of the patient, the experience of the surgical team, the resources available in the hospital.

There are three possible solution for upfront surgery: Hartmann's resection, segmental resection, and primary anastomosis with or without diverting stoma, subtotal colectomy with ileo-rectal anastomosis.

15.4.1 Hartmann's Procedure

Hartmann's procedure consists of a sigmoid/left colectomy, with closure of the anorectal stump and formation of an end colostomy. It was first described by Henri Hartmann in 1923 for the treatment of a malignant lesion in the recto-sigmoid tract [20]. The procedure is quick, effective, and safe, in fact it remains one of the most common procedures in emergency surgery for the left colon. Future restoration of the intestinal continuity is possible, but it occurs in less than half of the patients who undergo Hartmann's procedure, due to the difficulty of the procedure and the high rate of postoperative complications, in patients who are often already not in optimal general conditions for age and comorbidities [21]. Hereby, according to the guidelines of the World Society of Emergency Surgery (WSES), Hartmann's procedure should be reserved for those patients at high risk for surgery or in case of simultaneous perforation [4].

15.4.2 Resection and Primary Anastomosis

Primary resection and anastomosis consist of resection of the colon affected by the obstructing neoplasm followed by the anastomosis of the proximal (descending colon) and distal (rectal stump) tracts, usually in the emergency setting, completed with a diverting stoma. An intraoperative colon washing could also be performed to make the diversions more effective, but it appears unnecessary [22]. There have always been doubts about the potential anastomotic leak caused by fecal load and sepsis but in recent years, there has been a growing trend toward resection in one stage, because primary anastomosis could avoid a second major operation and it appears to be safe especially for fit patients. The WSES guidelines recommend primary resection and anastomosis as the preferred surgical treatment for simple malignant obstruction in hemodynamically stable patients in the absence of risk factor [4].

15.4.3 Subtotal Colectomy

Subtotal colectomy with ileo-rectal anastomosis is an alternative to segmental colectomy. It is proposed to overcome the problem related to the unprepared and dilated colon and consequently to avoid a stoma formation. Nevertheless, this is a difficult procedure requiring a long operating time and linked to a reduced quality of life, due to poor functional results. In fact, the well-known SCOTIA trial first compared in a multicentric randomized trial, subtotal colectomy and segmental resection and primary anastomosis following intraoperative irrigation for the management of malignant left-sided colonic obstruction [23]. Whereas hospital mortality and complication rates did not differ significantly, 4 months after operation increased bowel frequency (three or more bowel movements per day) was significantly more common in the subtotal colectomy group, concluding that segmental resection following intraoperative irrigation is the preferred option except when the obstruction caused an ischemia of the right colon or a cecal perforation, or in the rare case in which a synchronous right colon cancer is present [4].

15.5 Bridging Strategies

In the last years, several authors compared bridge to surgery techniques (BTS) with the emergency resection. This is more relevant in frail and elderly patients, in whom gaining time before major surgery may be crucial to rebalance the clinical conditions. Moreover, by allowing a higher rate of elective left colectomy, this reduces the risk, on the one side, of a permanent stoma while on the other the risk of a bad quality of life for a discomfortable incidence of bowel movements.

The most common BTS strategies are performing a diverting stoma or placing a self-expandable metal stent.

15.5.1 Self-Expanding Metal Stent SEMS

As an alternative to emergency surgery, self-expanding metal stents (SEMS) could be inserted endoscopically with the intent of solving the acute obstruction, this way transforming an emergency surgical case into an elective one. Although SEMS can be placed along the entire colon, the majority of studies on colon stenting focused on left-sided obstruction. Colonic stents are generally well tolerated when positioned above 5 cm above the anal verge with their distal margin. Therefore, low rectal obstructive carcinoma is also usually not treated by stent placement in order to avoid tenesmus, rectal pain, fecal incontinence, and stent migration [24]. In view of the above statements, most of the following descriptions refer to stenting left-sided colon obstruction.

The use of one or more enemas, in distal obstruction, before the insertion of the endoscope, is recommended in order to facilitate the procedure [19]. Antibiotic prophylaxis in obstructed patients is generally not recommended, since the risk of bacteremia is very low after stent placement, as reported by a prospective study [25], in which only 6.8% of patients developed positive blood cultures after the procedure with no clinical relevance.

The only real contraindication to stent placement, in obstructive diseases, is represented by intestinal perforation, assessed by radiological findings of free intra-abdominal gas. In all randomized studies published in the literature, uncovered metal stents were used. Although covered stents can also be used as a bridge to surgery, uncovered stents are preferred because they have a lower migration rate, complications that could lead to emergency surgical treatment [19]. The use of covered stents is currently object of a randomized trial (ISRCTN54834267) in order to verify if this may reduce the risk of perforation, which occurs during or after colonic stenting and is considered responsible of severe worsening of the prognosis [26].

Although considered a procedure at relatively low risk, with a mortality rate of less than 4%, the placement of a SEMS for colonic obstructions can be associated with various complications that occur in 20–30% of patients in the case series, with higher rates reported in randomized studies, taking into account both early and late complications [27]. Perforation is the most serious complication, which occurs in about 7% of patients, which is associated with a high mortality rate [28]. When perforation occurs, emergency surgery is usually required, although some microperforations which could occur in up to 14% of patients [29] can be treated with just antibiotic therapy [30].

The clinical and technical success reaches about 80% in emergency setting. Emergency surgery is indicated in case of complications, or technical or clinical failure, respectively, as incorrect positioning of the stent and failure to resolve the obstruction symptoms. If relief from obstruction is obtained, elective surgery is scheduled based on the patient's clinical condition; an interval of about 15 days is suggested that this interval is optimal for alleviating the obstruction, stabilizing the patient's clinical condition, reducing the risk of anastomotic leak, and still allowing a higher number of laparoscopic resection [31].

The use of SBTS has gained popularity again recently, after the presentation of two large randomized clinical trials: the ESCO [32] and the CREST studies [26]. The ESCO study reported lower median operating time in the SBTS group compared to the ES group, a higher number of colorectal resections performed laparoscopically, a higher rate of primary anastomosis, a higher number of lymph nodes collected and yet a 100% R0 resection rate [31]. Similarly, but supported by an even larger number of participants, the CReST trial demonstrated that SBTS reduced stoma formation without a detrimental effect on the 3-year survival. Postoperative mortality, length of hospital stay, critical care usage, and quality of life were not different between the two treatment groups. These data confirmed what already shown by a meta-analysis of only RCTs [12] on SBTS approach provides a significantly lower rate of overall adverse events within 60 days of the intervention with no significant difference in short-term mortality compared to emergency surgery.

Nevertheless, after the publication of the Stent-in-2 trial [12, 31], criticism had been raised regarding the possible risk of stent worsening the prognosis of patients affected by curative malignant obstruction. Indeed, several retrospective studies had reported that mechanical compression on neoplastic lesion performed by SEMS could be responsible to spread tumor cells [33–36]. This pushed the ESGE in their guidelines published in 2014 [37] to exclude the possibility of SBTS in potentially curable patients. The new data available allowed to restore this option as declared in the NCCN 2019 guidelines and more recently in the ESGE 2020 guidelines [19]. Here, it is reported, "ESGE recommends stenting as a bridge to surgery to be discussed, within a shared decision-making process, as a treatment option in patients with potentially curable left-sided colon cancer as an alternative to emergency surgery. This discussion should include the following factors: availability of required stenting expertise, risk of stent-related perforation, higher recurrence rates, similar overall survival and postoperative mortality, lower overall complication rates and permanent stoma rates, higher proportion of laparoscopic one-stage surgery procedures, and technical and clinical failure rates of stenting."

It is reasonable to believe that SBTS strategy could be the approach of choice for elderly and frail patients, for whom the lower risk of complications and the lower stoma rate may be more important than a potentially higher risk of recurrence. Furthermore, the ESCO trial [32] demonstrated a laparoscopic approach, much more tolerable in frail and elderly individuals, was attempted in no patient in the ES group and in 23 (42.6%) patients in the SBTS group ($P < 0.00001$), in 17 (31.5%) of whom resection was completed laparoscopically and by conversion to open surgery in 6.

15.5.2 Decompressing Stoma

The primary aim of colonic decompressing stoma (DS) and delayed resection is to reduce postoperative mortality. This technique, consisting of the construction of a stoma proximal to the obstruction, to obtain a decompression of the colon, gained popularity after the ban of the SBTS strategy. In a recent population-based study comparing DS with emergency resection (ER) for left-sided obstructive colon cancer using propensity score matching, more laparoscopic resections were performed (56.8% vs. 9.2%, $P < 0.001$) and more primary anastomoses were constructed (88.5% vs. 40.7%, $P < 0.001$) after DS [38]. Most importantly, DS resulted in significantly lower 90-day mortality compared to ER (1.7% vs. 7.2%, $P = 0.006$), and this effect could be mainly attributed to the subgroup of patients over 70 years (3.5% vs. 13.7%, $P = 0.027$). Patients treated with DS as bridge to surgery had better 3-year overall survival (79.4% vs. 73.3%, hazard ratio 0.36, 95% confidence interval 0.20–0.65) and fewer permanent stomas (23.4% vs. 42.4%, $P < 0.001$).

Objectively, the risk of mortality reported in this study is similar to what can be expected from primary elective colon cancer surgery, and much better even compared to what found in the meta-analysis by Amelung et al. (OR 0.77) [39]. Of relevant clinical implication is that the reduction in mortality and the improved survival are particularly observed in elderly patients (>70 years old). Similarly cannot be said for frail patients, as the impact in individuals ASA 1–2 and ASA 3–4 was comparable which was attributed to a less accurate assessment of the ASA class in the emergency setting [40].

Usually, it is wrongly assumed that stoma closure always needs an additional intervention. On the contrary, the continuity of the bowel can already be restored during resection in one-third of patients (2-stage) [41]. In fact, the construction of a DS close to the tumor location enables resection of the tumor and stoma site in one segment, this way avoiding a second anastomosis. A clear benefit of the construction of a DS is its low surgical complexity in the emergency setting.

With the limits of a propensity score matching and the possible residual confounding, the study presented by Veld [38] revealed that bowel decompression by a stoma is able to transform a high-risk acute surgery into minimally invasive resections with bowel restoration in a substantial proportion of patients.

15.5.3 Stent as a Bridge to Elective Surgery Versus Diverting Stoma as a Bridge to Surgery

Acute decompression, after colon obstruction, can be achieved either by placing an endoscopic stenting or by creating a derivative stoma. They are both a bridge for surgical approaches that convert an emergency into an elective case, restoring intestinal transit and stabilizing the patient's condition before elective resection performed by dedicated colorectal surgeons. So far, only a few retrospective studies have compared these two techniques. Amelung et al. report a lower rate of temporary stoma, number of surgeries, and long-term complications in patients initially treated with SEMS, while there was no significant difference between stoma and stent as a bridge to surgery with regard to morbidity and mortality rates, hospital stay, and, above all, disease-free and overall survival [42]. On the contrary, Mege et al., while reporting better short-term results for the SBTS approach, showed a higher overall median survival in the derivative stoma group compared to SBTS (123.6 vs. 58.5 months, $p = 0.046$), although no difference was observed regarding the median disease-free survival (54.1 vs. 53.6 months, $p = 0.646$) [43]. The difference in the overall survival between the studies could be explained by the different rate in stent-related perforation (1.9% Amelung et al., 11% Mege et al.). SEMS might be considered an alternative for DS based on a previously published comparison of these two bridging strategies from our group, provided that the lesion is considered eligible for stenting, sufficient stenting experience is available, and patients are well informed [44, 45]. SEMS as BTS results in the lowest risk of having a stoma at any time during treatment [44]. Therefore, it is important to perform endoscopic stenting only in high volume centers with expert operators in order to reduce the risk of stent-related colonic perforation. A derivative stoma could be a viable alternative to overcome acute obstruction, especially in those circumstances where the skilled operator is unavailable or patients are not suitable candidates for colonic stenting, as recommended by the ESGE guidelines [19]. Nevertheless, it requires at least a further surgical procedure and is often considered as a three-step procedure: construction of the stoma, subsequent resection, and finally restoration of intestinal continuity at a third time. According to the WSES guidelines, it should be reserved for highly hemodynamically unstable patients and for those patients who are not suitable for the surgical procedure on general anesthesia [4].

Prospective clinical trials comparing these two techniques are now needed.

15.6 Palliative Treatment

In case of uncurable obstructing neoplasm for the presence of distant metastases or carcinomatosis, palliation of the obstruction and bowel decompression may be obtained either by a transverse or descending loop colostomy or by endoscopic stenting. Placement of cecostomy tube is an alternative for gastrointestinal decompression, but this option is rarely used because of issues with ongoing care of the tube, which frequently obstructs [46]. Nevertheless, for patients with a short life expectancy who are high-risk surgical candidates, cecostomy may still be a reasonable option (right- or left-sided lesions). The procedure is performed using local anesthetic in an interventional suite or operating room using fluoroscopic guidance. In patients' fit-for-surgery in a palliative setting, ESGE strongly recommends that colonic stenting is a better option if the lesion is accessible and providing that an appropriately experienced endoscopist is available to perform the procedure [19].

Stenting resulted in shorter hospital stay when compared to decompressing stoma in the palliative setting (OR 0.50, 95% CI 0.26–0.97, $P = 0.04$) [47]. Surgical stoma formation was significantly lower after palliative colonic stenting compared with emergency surgery. In an RCT by Young et al. [48], the surgery group had significantly reduced quality of life if compared with the stent group from baseline to 1 and 2 weeks ($P = 0.001$ and $P = 0.012$, respectively), and from baseline to 12 months. ESGE recommends chemotherapy as a safe treatment in patients who have undergone palliative colonic stenting [19].

Five Things You Should Know About Obstructing Colorectal Cancer in the Elderly and Frail Patients

- CT scan is essential to diagnose and stage an obstructing colorectal cancer; lower endoscopy is not usually performed in an acute scenario unless to evaluate the possibility of stenting.
- Although colonic stenting is feasible, right obstructing colonic tumor is usually managed by an emergency resection, rarely protected by a diverting ileostomy.
- The correct management of a left obstructing colorectal cancer is still controversial, with the different emergency surgical resection techniques proposed all affected by important drawbacks.
- In left obstructing colorectal cancer, bridging strategies should be considered, especially in elderly and frail patients, including stenting as a bridge to surgery or decompressing stoma.
- In a palliative scenario, stenting is strongly recommended if the neoplasm is endoscopically accessible and if an experienced endoscopist is available.

References

1. Jullumstro E, Wibe A, Lydersen S, et al. Colon cancer incidence, presentation, treatment and outcomes over 25 years. Color Dis. 2011;13(5):512–8.
2. Biondo S. Large bowel obstruction: predictive factors for postoperative mortality. Dis Colon Rectum. 2004;47(11):1889–97.
3. Chen TM, Huang YT. Outcome of colon cancer initially presenting as colon perforation and obstruction. World J Surg Oncol. 2017;15(1):164.
4. Pisano M. 2017 WSES guidelines on colon and rectal cancer emergencies: obstruction and perforation. World J Emerg Surg. 2018;13:36.
5. Sule AZ. Adult large bowel obstruction: a review of clinical experience. Ann Afr Med. 2011;10(1):45–50.
6. Aliev SA. Surgical correction of the intraabdominal hypertension in patients with colon cancer. Kirurgiia. 2012;11:45–52.
7. Mitchell ED. Risk factors for emergency presentation with lung and colorectal cancers: a systematic review. BMJ. 2015;5(4):e006965.
8. Tanis PJ. Resection of obstructive left-sided colon cancer at a national level: a prospective analysis of short-term outcomes in 1,816 patients. Dig Surg. 2015;32(5):317–24.
9. Frager D. Prospective evaluation of colonic obstruction with computed tomography. Abdom Imaging. 1998;23(2):141–6.
10. Dalal KM. Management of patients with malignant bowel obstruction and stage IV colorectal cancer. J Palliat Med. 2011;14(7):822–8.
11. Hennekinne-Mucci S. Emergency subtotal/total colectomy in the management of obstructed left colon carcinoma. Int J Color Dis. 2006;21(6):538–41.
12. Arezzo A. Stent as bridge to surgery for left-sided malignant colonic obstruction reduces adverse events and stoma rate compared with emergency surgery: results of a systematic review and meta-analysis of randomized controlled trials. Gastrointest Endosc. 2017;86(3):416–26.
13. Markogiannakis H. Acute mechanical bowel obstruction: clinical presentation, etiology, management and outcome. World J Gastroenterol. 2007;13(3):432–7.
14. Mege D. Right-sided vs. left-sided obstructing colonic cancer: results of a multicenter study of the French Surgical Association in 2325 patients and literature review. Int J Color Dis. 2019;34(6):1021–32.

15. Cirocchi R. Laparoscopic versus open colectomy for obstructing right colon cancer: a systematic review and meta-analysis. J Visc Surg. 2017;154(6):387–99.
16. Ji WB, Kwak JM, Kang DW, et al. Clinical benefits and oncologic equivalence of self-expandable metallic stent insertion for right-sided malignant colonic obstruction. Surg Endosc. 2017;31(1):153–8.
17. Kye BH, Lee YS, Cho HM, et al. Comparison of long-term outcomes between emergency surgery and bridge to surgery for malignant obstruction in right-sided colon cancer: a multicenter retrospective study. Ann Surg Oncol. 2016;23(6):1867–74.
18. Amelung FJ. Emergency resection versus bridge to surgery with stenting in patients with acute right-sided colonic obstruction: a systematic review focusing on mortality and morbidity rates. Int J Colorectal Dis. 2015;30(9):1147–55.
19. Van Hooft J. Self-expandable metal stents for obstructing colonic and extracolonic cancer: European Society of Gastrointestinal Endoscopy (ESGE) guideline—update 2020. Endoscopy. 2020;52(5):389–407.
20. Hartmann H. Note sur un procede nouveau d'extirpation des cancers de la partie terminale due colon. Bull Mem Soc Chir Paris. 1923.
21. Van de Wall BJM. Conventional and laparoscopic reversal of the Hartmann procedure: a review of literature. J Gastrointest Surg. 2010;14(4):743–52.
22. Nyam DC. Colonic decompression without on-table irrigation for obstructing left-sided colorectal tumours. Br J Surg. 1996;83(6):786–7.
23. Single-stage treatment for malignant left-sided colonic obstruction: a prospective randomized clinical trial comparing subtotal colectomy with segmental resection following intraoperative irrigation. The SCOTIA Study Group. Subtotal colectomy versus on-table irrigation and anastomosis. Br J Surg. 1995;82(12):1622–7.
24. Sager J. Role of colonic stents in the management of colorectal cancers. World J Gastrointest Endosc. 2016;8(4):198–204.
25. Chun YJ. Prospective assessment of risk of bacteremia following colorectal stent placement. Dig Dis Sci. 2012;57(4):1045–9.
26. Hill J. The CReST2 Trial: Are uncovered or covered stents more effective in relieving bowel obstruction in people with colorectal cancer.
27. Takahashi G. Oncological assessment of stent placement for obstructive colorectal cancer from circulating cell-free DNA and circulating tumor DNA dynamics. Ann Surg Oncol. 2018;25(3):737–44.
28. Van Hansema EE. Perforation in colorectal stenting: a meta-analysis and a search for risk factors. Gastrointest Endosc. 2014;79(6):970–82.e7.
29. Allievi N. Endoscopic stenting as bridge to surgery versus emergency resection for left-sided malignant colorectal obstruction: an updated meta-analysis. Int J Surg Oncol. 2017;2017:2863272.
30. Repici A. WallFlex colonic stent placement for management of malignant colonic obstruction: a prospective study at two centers. Gastrointest Endosc. 2008;67(1):77–84.
31. Arezzo A. Colonic stenting as a bridge to surgery versus emergency surgery for malignant colonic obstruction: results of a multicentre randomised controlled trial (ESCO trial). Surg Endosc. 2017;31(8): 3297–305.
32. Arezzo A. Long-term oncologic results after stenting as a bridge to surgery versus emergency surgery for malignant left-sided colonic obstruction: a multicenter randomized controlled trial (ESCO trial). Ann Surg. 2020;272(5):703–8.
33. Mashar M. Uncovered versus covered stent in management of large bowel obstruction due to colorectal malignancy: a systematic review and meta-analysis. Int J Color Dis. 2019;34(5):773–85.
34. Amelung FJ. A population-based analysis of three treatment modalities for malignant obstruction of the proximal colon: acute resection versus stent or stoma as a bridge to surgery. Ann Surg Oncol. 2016;23(11):3660–8.
35. Amelung FJ. Self-expandable metal stent placement versus emergency resection for malignant proximal colon obstructions. Surg Endosc. 2017;31(11):4532–41.
36. Malgras B. Insertion of a stent in obstructive colon cancer can induce a metastatic process in an experimental murine model. Ann Surg Oncol. 2015;22 Suppl 3:S1475–80.
37. Van Hooft J, Self-expandable metal stents for obstructing colonic and extracolonic cancer: European Society of Gastrointestinal Endoscopy (ESGE) Clinical Guideline 2014 Nov;46(11):990–1053;
38. Veld JV. Decompressing stoma a s bridge to elective surgery is an effective strategy for left-sided obstructive colon cancer: a national propensity-score matched study. Ann Surg. 2020;272(5):738–43.
39. Amelung FJ. Acute resection versus bridge to surgery with diverting colostomy for patients with acute malignant left sided colonic obstruction: systematic review and meta-analysis. Surg Oncol. 2015;24(4):313–21.
40. Hyder JA. Risk prediction accuracy differs for emergency versus elective cases in the ACS-NSQIP. Ann Surg. 2016;264(6):959–65.
41. Veld JV. Changes in management of left-sided obstructive colon cancer: national practice and guideline implementation. J Natl Compr Cancer Netw. 2019;17(12):1512–20.
42. Amelung FJ. Deviating colostomy construction versus stent placement as bridge to surgery for malignant left-sided colonic obstruction. Surg Endosc. 2016;30(12):5345–55.
43. Mege D. What is the best option between primary diverting stoma or endoscopic stent as a bridge to surgery with a curative intent for obstructed left colon cancer? Results from a propensity score analysis of the French Surgical Association multicenter cohort of 518 patients. Ann Surg Oncol. 2019;26(3): 756–64.

44. Veld JV. Comparison of decompressing stoma vs stent as a bridge to surgery for left-sided obstructive colon cancer. JAMA Surg. 2020;155(3):206–15.
45. Wrenn SM. Patient perceptions and quality of life after colon and rectal surgery: what do patients really want? Dis Colon Rectum. 2018;61(8):971–8.
46. Perrier G. Cecostomy is a useful surgical procedure study of 113 colonic obstructions caused by cancer. Dis Colon Rectum. 2000;43(1):50–4.
47. Abelson JS. Long-term postprocedural outcomes of palliative emergency stenting vs stoma in malignant large-bowel obstruction. JAMA Surg. 2017;152(5):429–35.
48. Young CJ. Improving quality of life for people with incurable large-bowel obstruction: randomized control trial of colonic stent insertion. Dis Colon Rectum. 2015;58(9):838–49.

Acute Diverticulitis

16

Monica Ortenzi, Sophie Williams, Amyn Haji,
Roberto Ghiselli, and Mario Guerrieri

16.1 Epidemiology in Elderly People

Diverticular disease (DD), and the complications that derive from it, constitute an increasing burden on Western healthcare systems. Previous reports state that this condition accounts for over 300,000 hospital admissions, 1.5 million inpatient care days and $2.4 billion in direct costs annually in the United States [1–3]. In the Western population, DD is characteristically located in the left colon; right-sided DD exists commonly in Asian populations and is considered distinct, principally due to genetic predispositions [4, 5]. DD is typical of industrialized countries and is regarded as a consequence of socioeconomic development and the associated dietary changes [6–8].

The risk of acquiring DD increases uniformly with age. Post-mortem studies have demonstrated the prevalence of colonic diverticula in those under 30 years to be between 1 and 2% [9, 10], whereas the reported prevalence of 40% of people aged over 60 years and 50–70% in patients over 80 years [6–8, 11, 12].

M. Ortenzi (✉) · R. Ghiselli · M. Guerrieri
Department of Clinica Chirurgica Generale e d'urgenza, Università Politecnica delle Marche, Ancona, Italy

S. Williams · A. Haji
Department of Colorectal Surgery, King's College Hospital NHS Foundation Trust, London, UK

This is particularly relevant, as age significantly influences the management of DD and may affect future treatment choices, in both elective and emergency settings.

Although the majority of those with DD are asymptomatic, approximately 25% will experience an episode of acute diverticulitis; of these, 15% will develop other significant and often serious complications such as abscess, fistula, or perforation [2, 9, 10, 13, 14].

It is likely that, given the aging population the number of patients with symptomatic DD will continue to increase and, with it, the incidence of complications [1, 15].

There is, however a lack of consensus across the literature. A 2013 retrospective study found that each additional year of age following detection of diverticulosis conveys a 2.4% lower risk of developing diverticulitis (hazard ratio, 0.976; 95% confidence interval, 0.958–0.994) [1].

The lifetime risk of developing diverticulitis is traditionally cited as 10–25% in patients with uncomplicated diverticulosis [15–17]. This figure is widely quoted throughout the literature [1, 15–22] and largely cites a review paper, published by Parks [16] in 1975. This article, however, refers to studies from the mid-twentieth century and includes references dating as far back as 1937 [23, 24]. Additionally, these studies were conducted prior to population-based screening colonoscopies. Therefore, it is impossible to accurately discern the population prevalence of diverticulosis,

F. Agresta et al. (eds.), *Emergency laparoscopic surgery in the elderly and frail patient*,
https://doi.org/10.1007/978-3-030-79990-8_16

and accordingly, the true incidence of acute diverticulitis. There are few modern studies investigating the progression from diverticulosis to acute diverticulitis, with most focusing on repeated attacks after an index event [21, 25–27]. The results suggest that the traditionally cited 10–25% incidence rate may be an overestimate.

Patients over 80 years may also have different clinical presentations. Indeed, the presence of abdominal pain and fever in patients ≥80 years is reported as significantly less than those <80 years. Furthermore, there is a higher rate of associated bleeding and atypical symptoms in this group, including syncope and fatigue resulting in a major cause of emergency department referral [28]. A further analysis comparing clinical outcomes in patients ≥80 years and <80 years, revealed that heart failure, dyspnoea and the absence of abdominal pain at presentation were independent predictors of poor outcome. This is concurrent with other studies which report reduced pain in elderly patients in the emergency department, which may be linked to a greater capacity to endure, or more frequently, a reduced capacity to report pain [29]. Dementia is, in addition, independently related to poorer outcomes. These factors could influence patient management as well as negatively influence the true incidence of diverticulitis in the elderly [28].

16.2 Surgery in Diverticulitis

Over the past decade, the management of diverticulitis has changed and the differentiation between complicated and uncomplicated diverticulitis has become the major factor directing treatment. Some key guidelines [30–42] have been updated and now recommend outpatient treatment for afebrile clinically stable cases of uncomplicated diverticulitis with no additional reason for admission (Table 16.1) [44–46].

Complicated diverticulitis may be an indication for surgery, however, this definition varies in the literature and encompasses a broad spectrum of disease presentation, ranging from small pericolic

Table 16.1 Current guidelines for the management of diverticular disease

Region	Year	Society abbreviation	Society	Authors
Diverticular disease				
Poland	2015	PSG/PSS	Polish Society of Gastroenterology/ Polish Society of Surgery	Pietrzak et al. [32]
Italy	2015	SICCR	Italian Society of Colon and Rectal Surgery	Binda et al. [33]
USA	2014	ASCRS	American Society of Colon and Rectal Surgeons	Feingold et al. [34]
Germany	2014	DGVS/DGAV	German Society for Gastroenterology, Digestive and Metabolic Diseases with Endoscopy Section	Leifeld et al., Kruis [35, 36]
Denmark	2012	DCCG	Danish Colorectal Cancer Group	Andersen et al. [37]
Acute left-sided diverticulitis				
World	2020	WSES	World Society of Emergency Surgery	Sartelli et al. [38, 43]
USA	2015	AGA	American Gastroenterological Association	Stollman and Raskin [17]
The Netherlands	2013	NSS	The Netherlands Society of Surgery	Andeweg et al. [43]
USA		AAFP	American Academy of Family Physicians	Wilkins et al. [39]
Surgical management				
Europe	2012	EAES	The European Association for Endoscopic Surgery	Agresta et al. [40]
GB, Ireland	2011	ACPGBI	The Association of Coloproctology of Great Britain and Ireland	Fozard et al. [41]

abscesses to perforation with generalized peritonitis and sepsis, as well as late complications, including fistula and stricture formation (Fig. 16.1).

Traditionally, the most commonly used grading system describing complicated diverticulitis severity is the Hinchey classification (Table 16.2) [47–49].

In several studies the Hinchey severuty has been found to directly correlate to an increased risk of either recurrence and complications [50–52]. To further evaluate this relationship, Ambrosetti et al. developed a CT-based severity grade and correlated this retrospectively with patient outcomes (Table 16.3) [52].

Due, in part, to a lack of quality trials providing evidence of an optimal treatment strategy, there is no universal practice for the management of complicated diverticulitis [44].

Table 16.3 Diverticulitis classification according to CT findings

CT classification by Ambrosetti et al. [51]	
Moderate diverticulitis	Localized sigmoid wall thickening (<5 mm)
	Pericolic fat stranding
Severe diverticulitis	Abscess
	Extraluminal air
	Extraluminal contrast

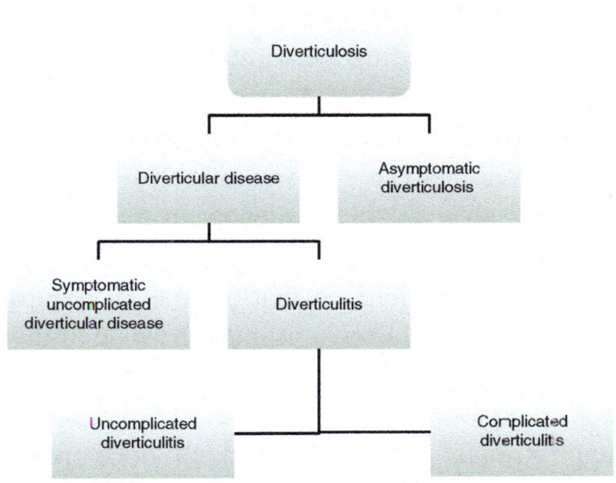

Diverticulosis: asymptomatic presence of mucosal and submucosal herniations due to defects in weaker areas of the muscolar wall of the colon

Diverticular disease: a wide spectrum disease including diverticular bleeding and diverticulitis

Symptomatic uncomplicated diverticular disease (SUDD): subtype of diverticular disease in which there are persistent, recurrent abdominal symptoms without signs of overt diverticulitis.

Diverticulitis: diverticula become acutely inflamed, most likely due to obstruction of the neck by faecal matter leading to bacterial overgrowth.

Uncomplicated diverticulitis: diverticulitis without perforation, abscess, bleeding, fistula, peritonitis or stenosis.

Complicated diverticulitis: diverticulitis with complicating features such as perforation, abscess, bleeding, fistula, peritonitis or stenosis; it may be localised or lead to infection of the peritoneal cavity; stricture obstruction or bleeding may be evident.

Fig. 16.1 Terminology used in diverticular disease (adapted from You et al. [31])

Table 16.2 Hinchey classification of acute diverticulitis and its subsequent modifications

Diverticulitis classification					
Hinchey classification [38, 43]		Modified Hinchey classification by Sher et al. [39]		Modified Hinchey classification by Wasary et al. [40]	
				0	Mild clinical diverticulitis
I	Pericolic abscess or phlegmon	I	Pericolic abscess	Ia	Confined pericolic inflammation or phlegmon
				Ib	Pericolic or mesocolic abscess
II	Pelvic, intra-abdominal or retroperitoneal abscess	IIa	Distant abscess amendable to percutaneous drainage	II	Pelvic, distant intra-abdominal or retroperitoneal abscess
		IIb	Complex abscess associated with fistula		
III	Generalized purulent peritonitis	III	Generalized purulent peritonitis	III	Generalized purulent peritonitis
IV	Generalized faecal peritonitis	IV	Faecal peritonitis	IV	Generalized faecal peritonitis

This debate not only relates to the indications and timing for surgery, but also to the optimal surgical technique [53, 54].

For several years, elective colonic resection has been recommended for patients presenting with a second episode of diverticulitis [55] owing to a high probability of recurrent attacks with reduced probability of response to medical treatment [15, 56–58]. More recent studies have questioned these indications, primarily because the long-term risk of relapse is relatively low [59–62].

The use of urgent colectomy for primary diverticulitis in both young and elderly patients [63] carries substantial morbidity, which could explain the reduction in its use in recent years, from 71 to 55% in 2015 [15, 64].

Increasingly, conservative approaches, including image-guided drainage for diverticular abscess and laparoscopic lavage for purulent peritonitis, have gained favour over colonic resection [63].

Recurrent episodes of uncomplicated diverticulitis do not lead to failure of conservative treatment or to increased risk of poor outcomes if patients develop complicated diverticulitis [37, 64–66]; and, notably, long-term risks of emergency surgery, stoma formation and mortality are low [64, 67, 68].

To date, several national guidelines suggest that indications for elective surgery must be decided on a case-by-case basis, dependent on patient's wishes, anaesthetic risk and consideration of the impact of recurrent episodes on quality of life [2, 29, 42, 63, 69, 70].

16.3 Impact of Age over Treatment

Despite several published and revised guidelines [15, 27, 48, 71] over the past decade, the role of age in the treatment of diverticulitis remains unclear [64].

An estimated 15–20% of patients admitted with complicated or uncomplicated diverticulitis will require surgical intervention during their initial admission [2, 6, 72]. Over 50% of those with complicated diverticulitis are likely to undergo surgery [73].

However, when age and age-related co-morbidities significantly increase perioperative risks, the use of surgery as first-line treatment even in emergency settings is questioned and there is an argument for conservative approaches [74, 75].

Furthermore, there is a general belief that diverticulitis may be more severe in patients under 50 years in terms of greater recurrence and complication rates [56, 76]. Early studies from 1970s and 1980s demonstrated that patients under 50 years were more likely to experience recurrent episodes with up to 88% requiring emergency surgery for diverticulitis-related complications including perforation and abdominal abscesses [56, 76, 77]. More recent studies, however, are not concurrent with this hypothesis [64].

A meta-analysis performed in 2013 [64] summarized all available evidence on the course of diverticulitis in patients over and under 50 years. The authors concluded that the risk of requiring urgent surgery during a primary episode of diverticulitis was equal in both age groups (pooled RR, 0.99; 95% CI, 0.74–1.32) and estimated at approximately 20%. The risk of developing at least one diverticulitis recurrence after a conservatively treated primary episode appeared significantly higher among patients younger than 50 years (pooled RR, 1.73; 95% CI, 1.40–2.13) with an estimated cumulative risk of 30% compared with 17.3% in older patients. Patients younger than 50 years also more frequently required urgent surgery during a subsequent recurrent episode (pooled RR, 1.46; 95% CI, 1.29–1.66). The estimated cumulative risk, in this case, was 7.3% in younger patients and 4.9% in the older group. Although low-quality data demonstrate that older patients more frequently present with fistulae and abscess [14, 78, 79], the equal risk of requiring urgent surgery suggested a similar disease course in both age groups [64]. Given this conclusion, the author stated that patients should not be treated differently only on an age basis.

Notably, an Italian national survey on 174,436 hospitalizations for acute diverticulitis noticed a different disease course with respect to age, noting a significant increase of in-hospital mortality in elderly patients, especially among women, and during the index hospitalization [80].

However, despite the importance of defining clinical outcomes in older patients, there are few studies with limited data and contrasting results present in the literature [29, 81–86].

The major, somewhat anticipated finding in the existing literature, is that age is an independent predictor of post-operative mortality and major complications.

A retrospective analysis of 2264 patients who underwent emergency surgery for diverticulitis described the impact of age on post-operative outcomes. In this review, patients aged 65–79 years have a fourfold greater odds of post-operative death, increasing to ten-fold in those >80 years, compared with non-elderly patients. Conversely, the effect of advanced age on post-operative morbidity was less striking, with a 1.5-fold increase in the odds of developing complications in the elderly, compared with younger patients. The analysis concludes that advancing age should be considered an independent risk factor associated with 30-day post-operative mortality [84].

Another report specifically addressing post-operative outcomes in patients over 80 years confirmed this hypothesis [87]. Here, mortality rate was higher in the oldest patients (0.5% in <80 years group vs. 2.5% in ≥80 years group; $p = 0.002$). Similarly, the cumulative endpoint death or major complications occurred only in 3.1% of younger patients and up to 10.1% of ≥80 years AD ($p < 0.001$).

The effect of age could be further pronounced in the emergency setting when morbidity risk is expected to be higher and time to evaluate operative risks is limited [88–91].

Two studies, aimed to assess the risk factors for mortality in emergency surgery [53, 54], concluded that age ≥80 years, together with corticosteroid therapy, ASA score >3, Hinchey IV, high creatinine level, poor nutrition, recent radiotherapy, loss of autonomy, ascites and dyspnoea were independent risk factors for mortality [78].

These findings indicate that age does indeed matter and is a significant factor influencing post-operative outcomes, therefore should be considered in the decision-making process for diverticulitis treatment in the urgent setting. In this group, it is essential to take steps in both prevention and early detection of major complications.

However, it is unclear whether the increased mortality in this group is due to the decreased physiologic ability to recover from surgery and infection, or to withstand post-operative complications or whether mortality is attributable to pre-existing co-morbidities that negatively influence the already reduced physiological functions in geriatric patients [90]

16.4 Technical Considerations

16.4.1 Approach to Surgery: Laparoscopy or Laparotomy?

When surgery is the chosen treatment modality, debates continue to exist with regard to both the technical approach into the abdominal cavity and choice of resection.

Following the first report of laparoscopic colectomy in 1991 [92] it was proposed for treatment of DD in elective and emergency settings following several reports demonstrating its feasibility [56, 78, 93–100]. Currently the advantages of laparoscopy over laparotomy in the elective setting are well established [37, 96, 97, 101–103], and despite a lack of universal concordance, generally, a laparoscopic approach conveys improved patient outcomes [30, 104].

In the emergency setting, however, the role of laparoscopy is incompletely evaluated [56, 105].

The 2009 EAES guidelines stated that in Hinchey I and II patients, the laparoscopic approach is not the first choice, however, it may be justified if no gross abnormalities are found during diagnostic laparoscopy. There were no indications for laparoscopic resections in Hinchey III and Hinchey IV patients [79].

In less than a decade, with advancing technology and experience, the surgical scenario has changed [106]. Several studies have been published aiming to identify significant differences between laparoscopy and laparotomy in complicated diverticulitis. These studies reach the same conclusions, namely demonstrating the feasibility of laparoscopy in the management of complicated diverticulitis, despite different enrolment criteria [107–113].

In 2013, a study compared >1000 patients undergoing open (94%) and laparoscopic (6%) Hartmann's procedure (HP) [110]. After adjustment with a propensity score, laparoscopy and open surgery produced the same post-operative results. However, the main drawback of this study was that the Hinchey grades were unknown. Other studies found the laparoscopic approach feasible, but the division of Hinchey grades between groups was either different (more Hinchey I/II in laparoscopic group) or unknown [87].

Recent data derived in parallel to the LADIES Trial DIVA arm showed laparoscopic sigmoid colectomy as superior to open for perforated diverticulitis in terms of post-operative morbidity and LoS [114].

Another meta-analysis exploring the role of emergency laparoscopic colectomy concluded that laparoscopy improves post-operative complication rates (RR, 0.62; 95% CI, 0.49–0.80) and LoS (MD, 6.53; 95% CI= 2.99-16.05). Conversely, laparoscopy did not improve other clinical outcomes, including rate of primary anastomosis, operating time, re-operation rate and 30-day mortality [115].

However, robust data on the laparoscopy for perforated diverticulitis are lacking. Indications for laparoscopy remain unclear and this approach is not widely accepted for Hinchey grades III or IV. However, increasing scientific evidence suggests that laparoscopy may lead to significant benefits over open surgery in cases of acute, perforated diverticulitis, and in case of Hinchey IV diverticulitis, it has been demonstrated not only to be feasible, but in some cases, easier than in Hinchey II or III diverticulitis, where typically an abscess involves the surrounding viscera and retroperitoneum [115].

Current guidelines and systematic reviews stress the importance of two major factors that should determine use of laparoscopy in the emergency setting: appropriate patient selection and surgeons' expertise [87].

Despite the proven feasibility of laparoscopy, even in the urgent setting [88, 116–119], the approach remains infrequently performed, reported as 3.4–6% of all procedures [56, 119, 120].

Age is undoubtedly a significant, yet somewhat overlooked factor in surgical decision making. It is well established that the emergency laparotomy coveys a high mortality rate (up to 21.4%) in people over 70 years and poorer still in octogenarians with a reported 44% mortality rate and over 50% in the presence of co-morbidity and perioperative conditions including sepsis [87, 121, 122].

Nevertheless, some authors emphasize suspected risks linked to laparoscopy, including carbon dioxide insufflation in elderly patients with reduced cardiopulmonary reserve, leading to diaphragmatic splinting, reduced venous return and cardiac output, predisposing patients to myocardial infarction and basal atelectasis [87].

Several studies have demonstrated that laparoscopic cholecystectomy can be safely applied to the elderly and that results are favourable compared with open cholecystectomy; the authors concluded that laparoscopic outcomes in other conditions requiring urgent surgery, including sigmoid colon resection for diverticulitis, should be investigated [123].

The FRAILESEL study, which aimed to analyse clinical data, management strategies and short-term outcomes of emergency surgery for the acute abdomen in the elderly, found that emergency laparoscopic colorectal resections were technically feasible and demonstrated improved post-operative outcomes and reduced length of stay (LoS) as compared to open surgery [88].

Another review found only two articles focused on laparoscopic colorectal outcomes in patients over 70 years. There was no statistically significant difference in conversion rate or morbidity; and the authors suggested that laparoscopic colectomy for diverticulitis can be applied safely in older patients with fewer complications, less pain and a shorter LoS than patients treated by laparotomy [124].

Emergency laparoscopy, however, has not been widely adopted in the elderly, and therefore, the potential benefits of mini-invasive procedures are prevented. Little is known about the reasons for avoiding emergency laparoscopy in this group, however, choices may be influenced by poorer patient condition or a lack of expertise during night-time or weekend shifts when emergency surgery is often performed. Patient selection may play a significant role in outcome differences, as more complex patients are more likely to undergo open intervention, which may skew results in favour of laparoscopic surgery. Additionally, laparoscopy may be not practical in patients with cardiovascular and respiratory impairment, or in those where laparoscopy is unlikely to be successful, such as extensive adhesions, marked small bowel dilatation, severe sepsis and obstructing colorectal cancers. Therefore, availability of experienced laparoscopic surgeons and theatre staff is imperative, arguably more so than in younger patients [87]. Indeed, laparoscopic sigmoid resection for acute complicated diverticulitis is a feasible approach with potential to become the future gold standard [124, 125].

16.4.2 Colonic Resection: One-Stage or Two-Stage Procedure?

Increasingly, conservative approaches for complicated diverticulitis are advocated, including interventional radiology for abscesses and laparoscopic lavage for purulent peritonitis. In earlier years, the debate around technique was based on the level of proximal and distal resection, level of vascular ligation [126] and the use of synchronous anastomosis [127].

Surgical options for acute diverticulitis include a simple colostomy formation, sigmoid resection with end colostomy (HP) and colonic resection with primary anastomosis (PRA) with or without diverting loop ileostomy (PRA ± I) (Table 16.3) [30, 128, 129].

HP, either open or laparoscopic, has been the standard treatment for complicated sigmoid diverticulitis [115, 130, 131]. Despite being the primary choice, mortality rate is between 2.6 and 7.3% [131], with high associated morbidity and low subsequent colostomy closure rate [66, 132].

In the National Surgical Quality Improvement Program Study of the American College of Surgeons [133], 1314 patients underwent emergency surgery for acute diverticulitis with 75% undergoing HP and PRA ± I performed in the remaining 25%. This study confirmed HP as the most commonly selected operation in the United States for surgical treatment of diverticulitis. However, these findings may mirror a lack of surgeon experience and timing of emergency procedures over nights or weekend shifts precluding use of laparoscopy [124, 125].

A systematic review published in 2014 demonstrated a minor preference for PRA ± I compared with HP, but only when performed by experienced surgeons [134]. Some randomized controlled trials demonstrated a small improvement in stoma reversal rate for patients undergoing PRA ± I but only in subsets where operator experience was high [134]. American guidelines recommend a two-stage procedure: HP or PRA and diverting protective ostomy [135, 136], where loop ileostomy is almost always used. In view of these findings, the American Society of Colon Rectal Surgeons (ASCRS) recommended that the decision for PRA with or without an ileostomy should be decided on a case-by-case basis.

In general, PRA with ileostomy is recommended by American guidelines for patients with peritonitis; however, it should be based on factors including haemodynamic instability, acidosis, acute organ failure and co-morbidities, in conjunction with surgeon expertise. It is generally accepted that HP has more clinical value in patients' haemodynamic instability, older or multi-co-morbid [30, 31, 80, 137, 138].

In these patients, the ASCRS and the World Society of Emergency Surgery recommended sigmoid colectomy with end colostomy or HP [31, 38, 43].

Similarly, the 2019 EAES consensus stated that in Hinchey III diverticulitis, PRA with proximal diversion has similar mortality, lower morbidity and lower stoma rate at 12 months compared to HP with reversal. The derived recommendation thereafter was to consider PRA and proximal diversion over HP in patients with Hinchey III/IV diverticulitis in the appropriate clinical setting, whereas HP appeared to be the preferred operation for haemodynamically unstable patients with perforated diverticulitis. In unstable patients, damage control strategies including resection without anastomosis and temporary abdominal closure with re-look laparotomy should also be considered [108].

The same conclusions were reached in the LADIES trial where authors concluded that in haemodynamically stable, immunocompetent patients under 85 years, PRA ± I is preferable to HP as a treatment for perforated diverticulitis (Hinchey III or Hinchey IV disease) (Table 16.4) [114].

However, a gold standard technique does not exist. In sigmoid colonic perforation, PRA ± I could be the ideal operation [139, 141], but a case-by-case choice of the procedure is recommended in current clinical practice [85, 140, 142].

16.4.3 Laparoscopic Peritoneal Lavage

The 2009, EAES guidelines proposed laparoscopic peritoneal lavage (LPL) for localized abscesses [79]. LPL has now been proposed as an alternative strategy for patients with peritonitis in order to control contamination and bridge patients to an elective PRA [106, 143–145].

Given this premise, it could be argued that this procedure constitutes an appealing option in elderly patients, serving to delay a definitive resection, which may be performed in a more controlled, elective setting.

In the literature, LPL has been advocated in Hinchey III diverticulitis, as well as Hinchey I and II diverticulitis, after failure of medical treatment [146, 147]. The first non-randomized series showed promising results [64, 86, 142, 143, 148–154], namely a reduced LoS and similar morbidity. Before 2015, six systematic reviews were published [143, 154–158]. There were no RCTs and most series were retrospective.

Since 2015, three RCTs [114, 150, 159] and three meta-analyses [87, 160, 161] have been published.

In the LADIES trial, the LOLA group aimed to compare LPL with HP in Hinchey III diverticulitis. The 30-day mortality was comparable as were primary endpoints (OR = 1.28; 95% CI, 0.54–3.03; $p = 0.52$), 1-year mortality (8.9% vs. 14.3%; $p = 0.43$) and QoL. However, the trial was prematurely terminated because of an increased rate of adverse events in the LPL group after the inclusion of 90 patients in 42 centres [114]. The Scandinavian diverticulitis trial randomized LPL and colectomy in Hinchey III diverticulitis. The primary endpoint was 90-day morbidity, which was comparable between groups (LPL 30.7% vs. colectomy 26%; $p = 0.53$). Secondary endpoints, including operative time, reduced in the LPL group ($p < 0.001$), 90-day mortality (LPL 13.9% vs. colectomy 11.5%; $p = 0.67$) and QoL and LoS, both of which were comparable. However, the 90-day re-operation rate (20.3% vs. 5.7%; $p = 0.01$) and rate of secondary peritonitis (12% vs. 0%; $p = 0.03$) had poorer results in the LPL group. Hence, authors did not recommend LPL. At 1 year, morbidity and mortality were comparable between groups. However, LPL was associated with more severe sepsis and more

Table 16.4 Randomized controlled trials (RCTs) and meta-analyses assessing the use of primary anastomoses in Hinchey III/IV diverticulitis adapted from Beyer et al. [86]

Authors	Year	Groups	Mean age	Hinchey grade	Primary endpoints	Results	Conclusions
Binda et al. [62] *RCT*	2012	PRA ($n = 34$) HP ($n = 56$)	**PRA** 63.5 ± 2.2 **HP** 65.7 ± 1.8	**PRA** Hinchey III = 30 Hinchey IV = 4 **HP** Hinchey III = 45 Hinchey IV = 11	Adverse events	**Morbidity** 35% versus 46% ($p = 0.38$) **Mortality** 3% versus 11% ($p = 0.25$)	No conclusions because prematurely terminated
Oberkofler et al. [139] *RCT*	2012	PRA ($n = 32$) HP ($n = 30$)	**PRA** 72 (60–83) **HP** 74 (61–81)	**PRA** Hinchey III = 24 Hinchey IV = 8 **HP** Hinchey III = 23 Hinchey IV = 7	Cumulative Morbidity	**Morbidity** 84% versus 80% ($p = 0.81$) **Mortality** 9% versus 13% ($p = 0.70$) **CR rate PRAI > HP** 90% versus 57% ($p = 0.005$)	Strong evidence favouring PA with protective ileostomy over HP in the treatment of acute left-sided colonic perforation with generalized peritonitis
Constantinides et al. [140] *Meta-analysis*	2006	**PRA** 57% **HP** 43% 15 studies 963 patients		I–IV	Mortality	**Mortality in Hinchey > II** 14.1% versus 14.4% OR = 0.81(95% CI, 0.36–2.01); **Wound abscess** OR = 0.42 **Deep sepsis** OR = 0.43	Patients selected for PRA have a lower mortality than those treated by HP in the emergency setting and comparable mortality under conditions of generalized peritonitis (Hinchey >II)
Cirocchi et al. [115] *Meta-analysis*	2013	**PRA versus HP** 14 studies 1041 patients		III/IV	Mortality	**Mortality** OR = 0.38 (95% CI, 0.17–0.85), $p = 0.02$ **Length of stay** $p < 0.001$ **Re-operation rate** $p = 0.30$	Marked heterogeneity between; the advantages in the group of PRA in terms of lower mortality rate and post-operative stay should be interpreted with caution because of several limitations

unscheduled operations. Finally, there were fewer stomas at 1 year in the LPL group (14% vs. 42%; $p < 0.001$) compared with 73.5% in the HP group and only 26.5% PRA ± I [150].

The third RCT, randomizing Hinchey III diverticulitis for LPL or HP, was the DILALA trial [142, 149, 151].

The primary endpoint was 1-year re-operation rate, including elective sigmoid colectomies after LPL and continuity restoration after HP. This primary endpoint was significantly higher after HP (28% vs. 63%; $p = 0.004$) [149]. The secondary endpoint, short-term morbidity was comparable between groups as was the short-term re-operation rate ($p = 0.63$) [142]. At 1 year, morbidity, mortality and QoL were comparable, whereas cumulative LoS was reduced after LPL (risk ratio = 0.65; 95% CI, 0.45–0.94; $p = 0.047$) [142]. However, in this trial, HP was always performed in resection cases. Secondly, most re-operations consisted of elective continuity restoration in the HP group (84%), whereas LPL group re-operations were largely unplanned.

On the basis of these RCTs, two meta-analyses were published to asses LPL [2, 106]. The main finding of the first meta-analysis was a lower rate of 1-year re-operation after LPL (risk ratio = 0.54; 95% CI, 0.38–0.76). However, this was not clearly defined in the original publication rate of the LOLA trial, and the drawbacks in the DILALA trial are explained above. Moreover, this meta-analysis did not use heterogeneity tests and was based on just three trials with different designs [161]. The second meta-analysis found no differences in terms of mortality or major morbidity [106].

However, LPL was associated with an increased risk of post-operative abscess and percutaneous drainage (OR = 4.12; 95% CI, 1.89–8.98; $p = 0.0004$ and OR = 5.41; 95% CI, 1.62–18.12; $p = 0.006$).

As for LPL failure, co-morbidities, as well as an elevation of the C-reactive protein or of the Mannheim peritonitis index [152], and ASA score >2 [106] were reported as a major risk factors, whereas age >65 years (OR = 4.1; $p < 0.001$) and the presence of a chronic disease, namely a rheumatologic disease (OR = 7.3; $p < 0.05$) or chronic renal disease (OR = 8; $p < 0.001$) were found to be independent risk factors for post-operative mortality [100].

In conclusion, there is insufficient clinical evidence to support the safety and efficacy of LPL as an alternative to colonic resection, regardless of patient age, and therefore, all guidelines discourage the use of lavage in purulent or faecal peritonitis (Table 16.5) [30, 31, 35, 115].

There is yet more controversy when advanced age is specifically considered. Where some authors propose the use of LPL as a safe and feasible alternative in elderly people [158], others report that age and immunosuppression were predictive factors for repeat intervention [160]. Overall, these findings highlight the challenges in surgical decision making in the treatment of complicated diverticulitis in elderly patients.

Five Things You Should Know About Acute Diverticulitis in the Elderly and Frail Patient

- Since diverticulosis is an age-related condition, the incidence of complicated diverticulitis is expected to rise.
- Aging and the related co-morbidities play a key role in post-operative outcomes.
- Laparoscopy has been proven to be feasible and safe in complicated diverticulitis even in urgent settings.
- There is a substantial lack of data, but laparoscopic PRA could be the best choice in complicated diverticulitis, including in the elderly.
- Clinical evidence supporting the safety and efficacy of LPL as an alternative to colonic resection, regardless of patient age, is insufficient and all guidelines discourage the use of lavage in purulent or faecal peritonitis.

Table 16.5 Randomized controlled trials assessing laparoscopic peritoneal lavage in acute diverticulitis adapted from Beyer et al. [87]

Authors	Year	Groups	Hinchey grade	Primary endpoints	Results	Conclusions
Vennix et al. [114] *LADIES trial* *RCT*	2015	**LOLA group** **LPL** ($n = 47$) **Sigmoidectomy** ($n = 43$)	III	**Composite endpoint** 1-year major morbidity + mortality	**Morbidity** 39% versus 19% ($p = 0.043$) **Composite score** LPL 67% versus 60% ($p = 0.52$) **Mortality** 9% versus 14% ($p = 0.43$)	Early discontinuation for increased short-term LPL is not superior to sigmoidectomy for the treatment of purulent perforated diverticulitis
Schultz et al. [148] *SCANDIV trial* *RCT*	2015	**LPL** ($n = 101$) **HP** ($n = 98$) (1:1 randomization)	III	90-day major morbidity	**Major morbidity** 31% versus 26% ($p = 0.53$) **Re-operation** 20% versus 6% ($p = 0.01$) **Mortality** 14% versus 12% ($p = 0.67$)	Among patients with likely perforated diverticulitis the use of LPL versus resection did not reduce severe post-operative complications and led to worse outcomes in secondary endpoints. LPL for treatment of perforated diverticulitis is not supported
Schultz et al. [149] *SCANDIV trial* *RCT*	2017	**LPL** ($n = 101$) **HP** ($n = 98$) (1:1 randomization)	III	90-day major morbidity(1 year results)	**Major morbidity** 34% versus 27% ($p = 0.32$) **Deep sepsis** 32% versus 13% ($p = 0.006$) **Unplanned re-operation rate** 27% versus 10% ($p = 0.01$) **Stoma rate** 14% versus 42% ($p < 0.001$)	The advantages of laparoscopic lavage should be weighed against the risk of secondary intervention (if sepsis is unresolved). Assessment to exclude malignancy (although uncommon) is advised

(continued)

Table 16.5 (continued)

Authors	Year	Groups	Hinchey grade	Primary endpoints	Results	Conclusions
Angenete et al. [147] *DILALA trial* *RCT*	2016	**LPL** ($n = 39$) **HP** ($n = 36$) (1:1 randomization)	III	1-year re-operation rate (short-term results)	**Short-term re-operation rate** LPL 13% versus 17% ($p = 0.63$) **Operative time** ($p < 0.0001$) **Morbidity** NS	LPL as treatment for patients with perforated diverticulitis Hinchey III was feasible and safe in the short term
Thornell et al. [150] *DILALA trial* *RCT*	2016	**LPL** ($n = 43$) **HP** ($n = 40$) (1:1 randomization)	III	1-year re-operation rate	**Re-operation rate** 28% versus 63% ($p = 0.004$) **Morbidity** NS **Mortality** NS	LPL reduced the need for re-operations, had a similar safety profile to the HP and may be an appropriate treatment of choice for acute perforated diverticulitis with purulent peritonitis
Gehrman et al. [142] *DILALA trial* *RCT*	2016	**LPL** ($n = 43$) **HP** ($n = 40$) (1:1 randomization)	III	1-year re-operation rate (1-year medical costs)	**Costs** 8983€ at 1 year–19,794€/expected life years	The significant cost reduction in this study support the routine use of laparoscopic lavage as treatment for complicated diverticulitis with purulent peritonitis

References

1. Shahedi K, et al. Long-term risk of acute diverticulitis among patients with incidental diverticulosis found during colonoscopy. Clin Gastroenterol Hepatol. 2013;11(12):1609–13.
2. Everhart JE, Ruhl CE. Burden of digestive diseases in the United States part II: lower gastrointestinal diseases. Gastroenterology. 2009;136:741–54.
3. Sandler RS, Everhart JE, Donowitz M, et al. The burden of selected digestive diseases in the United States. Gastroenterology. 2002;122:1500–11.
4. Beranbaum SL, Zausner J, Lane B. Diverticular disease of the right colon. Am J Roentgenol Radium Ther Nucl Med. 1972;115(2):334–48.
5. Imaeda H, Hibi T. The burden of diverticular disease and its complications: west versus east. Inflamm Intest Dis. 2018;3(2):61–8.
6. Weizman AV, Nguyen GC. Diverticular disease: epidemiology and management. Can J Gastroenterol. 2011 Jul;25(7):385–9.
7. Collins D, Winter DC. Modern concepts in diverticular disease. J Clin Gastroenterol. 2015;49(5): 358–69.
8. Makela J, Kiviniemi H, Laitinen S. Prevalence of perforated sigmoid diverticulitis is increasing. Dis Colon Rectum. 2002;45(7):955–61.
9. Bolers RS, Jordan SM. The clinical significance of diverticulosis. Gastroenterology. 1958;35(6): 579–82.
10. Rafferty J, Shellito P, Hyman NH, Buie WD. Standards Committee of American Society of Colon and Rectal Surgeons. Practice parameters for sigmoid diverticulitis. Dis Colon Rectum. 2006;49(7):939–44.
11. Parks TG. Natural history of diverticular disease of the colon. A review of 521 cases. BMJ. 1969;4(5684):639–42.
12. Stollman N, Raskin JB. Diverticular disease of the colon. Lancet. 2004;363(9409):631–9.
13. Aydin HN, Remzi FH. Diverticulitis: when and how to operate? Dig Liver Dis [Internet]. 2004;36(7):435–45.
14. Petruzziaello L, Iacopini L, Bulajic M, et al. Review article: uncomplicated diverticular disease of the colon. Aliment Pharmacol Ther. 2006;23(10):1379–91.
15. Etzioni DA, Mack TM, Beart RW Jr, et al. Diverticulitis in the United States: 1998–2005: changing patterns of disease and treatment. Ann Surg. 2009;249:210–7.
16. Parks TG. Natural history of diverticular disease of the colon. Clin Gastroenterol. 1975;4:53–69.
17. Stollman NH, Raskin JB. Diagnosis and management of diverticular disease of the colon in adults. Ad hoc practice parameters Committee of the American College of Gastroenterology. Am J Gastroenterol. 1999;94:3110–21.
18. Touzios JG, Dozois EJ. Diverticulosis and acute diverticulitis. Gastroenterol Clin North Am. 2009;38:513–25.
19. Klarenbeek BR, de Korte N, van der Peet DL, et al. Review of current classifications for diverticular disease and a translation into clinical practice. Int J Color Dis. 2012;27:207–14.
20. Annibale B, Lahner E, Maconi G, et al. Clinical features of symptomatic uncomplicated diverticular disease: a multicenter Italian survey. Int J Color Dis. 2012;27:1151–9.
21. Nguyen GC, Sam J, Anand N. Epidemiological trends and geographic variation in hospital admissions for diverticulitis in the United States. World J Gastroenterol. 2011 17:1600–5.
22. Martel J, Raskin JB. History, incidence, and epidemiology of diverticulosis. J Clin Gastroenterol. 2008;42:1125–7.
23. Kohler L, Sauerland S, Neugebauer E. Diagnosis and treatment of diverticular disease: results of a consensus development conference. The Scientific Committee of the European Association for Endoscopic Surgery. Surg Endosc. 1999;13: 430–6.
24. Pemberton J, De J, Black M, et al. Progress in surgical management of diverticulosis of the sigmoid colon. Surg Gynecol Obstet. 1947;85:523–34.
25. Hughes L. Postmortem survey of diverticular disease of the colon. I. Diverticulosis and diverticulitis. Gut. 1969;10:336–44.
26. Humes DJ, Solaymani-Dodaran M, Fleming KM, et al. A population based study of perforated diverticular disease incidence and associated mortality. Gastroenterology. 2009;136:1198–205.
27. Ambrosetti P, Jenny A, Becker C, et al. Acute left colonic diverticulitis—compared performance of computed tomography and water-soluble contrast enema: prospective evaluation of 420 patients. Dis Colon Rectum. 2000;43:1363–7.
28. Salem TA, Molloy RG, O'Dwyer PJ. Prospective, five-year follow-up study of patients with symptomatic uncomplicated diverticular disease. Dis Colon Rectum. 2007;50:1460–4.
29. Covino M, et al. Acute diverticulitis in elderly patients: does age really matter? Dig Dis. 2021;39(1): 33–41.
30. Covino M, Petruzziello C, Onder G, Migneco A, Simeoni B, Franceschi F, et al. A 12-year retrospective analysis of differences between elderly and oldest old patients referred to the emergency department of a large tertiary hospital. Maturitas. 2019;120:7–11.
31. You H, et al. The management of diverticulitis: a review of the guidelines. Med J Aust 2019;211(9):421–7.
32. Pietrzak A, Bartnik W, Szczepkowski M, Krokowicz P, Dziki A, Regula J, et al. Polish interdisciplinary consensus on diagnostics and treatment of colonic diverticulosis. Pol Przegl Chir. 2015;87(4):203–20. https://doi.org/10.1515/pjs-2015-0045.
33. Binda GA, Cuomo R, Laghi A, et al.; Italian Society of Colon and Rectal Surgery. Practice parameters for the treatment of colonic diverticular disease: Italian

Society of Colon and Rectal Surgery (SICCR) guidelines. Tech Coloproctol. 2015;19(10):615–626.
34. Feingold D, Steele S, Lee S, et al. Practice parameters for the treatment of sigmoid diverticulitis. Dis Colon Rectum. 2014;57:284–94.
35. Leifeld L, Germer CT, Bohm S, et al. S2k guidelines diverticular disease/diverticulitis. Z Gastroenterol. 2014;52(7):663–710.
36. Kruis W. Comment of the letter to the editor by Prof. M. Ebert. Z Gastroenterol. 2014;52(9):1110.
37. Andersen JC, Bundgaard L, Elbrond H, Laurberg S, Walker LR, Stovring J. Danish national guidelines for treatment of diverticular disease. Dan Med J. 2012;59(5):C4453.
38. Sartelli M, et al. 2020 update of the WSES guidelines for the management of acute colonic diverticulitis in the emergency setting. World J Emerg Surg. 2020;15(1):1–18.
39. Wilkins T, Embry K, George R. Diagnosis and management of acute diverticulitis. Am Fam Physician. 2013;87(9):612–20.
40. Agresta F, Ansaloni L, Baiocchi GL, et al. Laparoscopic approach to acute abdomen from the Consensus Development Conference of the Societa Italiana di Chirurgia Endoscopica e nuove tecnologie (SICE), Associazione Chirurghi Ospedalieri Italiani (ACOI), Societa Italiana di Chirurgia (SIC), Societa Italiana di Chirurgia d'Urgenza e del Trauma (SICUT), Societa Italiana di Chirurgia nell'Ospedalita Privata (SICOP), and the European Association for Endoscopic Surgery (EAES). Surg Endosc. 2012;6(8):2134–64.
41. Fozard J, Armitage N, Schofield J, Jones O. ACPGBI position statement on elective resection for diverticulitis. Color Dis. 2011;13:1–11.
42. Tursi A, Picchio M, Elisei W, et al. Management of patients with diverticulosis and diverticular disease: consensus statements from the 2nd international symposium on diverticular disease. J Clin Gastroenterol. 2016;50:S101–7.
43. Andeweg C, Mulder I, Felt-Bersma R, et al. Guidelines of diagnostics and treatment of acute left-sided colonic diverticulitis. Dig Surg. 2013;30:278–92.
44. Alonso S, Pera M, Parés D, et al. Outpatient treatment of patients with uncomplicated acute diverticulitis. Color Dis. 2010;12:278–82.
45. Tursi A. Efficacy, safety, and applicability of outpatient treatment for diverticulitis. Drug Healthc Patient Saf. 2014;6:29–36.
46. van Dijk S, Bos K, de Boer M, et al. A systematic review and meta-analysis of outpatient treatment for acute diverticulitis. Int J Color Dis. 2018;33:505–12.
47. Hinchey EJ, Schaal PG, Richards GK. Treatment of perforated diverticular disease of the colon. Adv Surg. 1978;12:85–109.
48. Sher ME, Agachan F, Bortul M, et al. Laparoscopic surgery for diverticulitis. Surg Endosc. 1997;11:264–7. https://doi.org/10.1007/s004649900340.
49. Wasvary H, Turfah F, Kadro O, et al. Same hospitalization resection for acute diverticulitis. Am Surg. 1999;65:632–5.
50. Kaiser AM, Jiang J-K, Lake JP, et al. The management of complicated diverticulitis and the role of computed tomography. Am J Gastroenterol. 2005;100:910–7.
51. Ambrosetti P, Beeker C, Terrier F. Colonic diverticulitis: impact of imaging on surgical management—a prospective study of 542 patients. Eur Radiol. 2002;12:1145–9.
52. Gentile V, et al. Perioperative and postoperative outcomes of perforated diverticulitis Hinchey II and III: Open Hartmann's procedure vs. laparoscopic lavage and drainage in the elderly. Int J Surg. 2014;12:S86–9.
53. Monson JRT. Management of acute diverticulitis: is less more? Dis Colon Rectum. 2011;54:126–8.
54. Wiegard N, Geltzeiler CB, Tsikitis VL. Trends in the surgical management of diverticulitis. Ann Gastroenterol. 2015;28(1):25.
55. Kreis ME, Jauch KW. Diverticular disease—Update 2006. In: Neugebauer EAM, Sauerland S, Fingerhut A, Millat B, Buess GF, editors. EAES guidelines for endoscopic surgery. New York: Springer; 2006. p. 157–60.
56. Farmakis N, Tudor RG, Keighley MR. The 5-year natural history of complicated diverticular disease. Br J Surg. 1994;81(5):733–5. [PubMed: 8044566].
57. Broderick-Villa G, Burchette RJ, Collins JC, Abbas MA, Haigh PI. Hospitalization for acute diverticulitis does not mandate routine elective colectomy. Arch Surg. 2005;140:576–81.
58. Hussain A, Mahmood H, Subhas G, EL-Hasani S. Complicated diverticular disease of the colon: do we need to change the classical approach? A retrospective study of 110 patients in Southeast England. World J Emerg Surg. 2008;3:5.
59. Anaya DA, Flum DR. Risk of emergency colectomy and colostomy in patients with diverticular disease. Arch Surg. 2005;140(7):681–5. [PubMed: 16027334]
60. Eglinton T, Nguyen T, Raniga S, Dixon L, Dobbs B, Frizelle FA. Patterns of recurrence in patients with acute diverticulitis. Br J Surg. 2010;97(6):952–7.
61. Binda GA, Karas JR, Serventi A, Sokmen S, Amato A, Hydo L, et al. Primary anastomosis vs nonrestorative resection for perforated diverticulitis with peritonitis: a prematurely terminated randomized controlled trial. Color Dis. 2012;14(11):1403–10. [PubMed: 22672447]
62. Lange VJ. Treatment of perforated diverticulitis with generalized peritonitis: past, present, and future. World J Surg. 2010;34:587–93.
63. Van De Wall BJM, et al. Diverticulitis in young versus elderly patients: a meta-analysis. Scand J Gastroenterol. 2013;48(6):643–51.
64. Abraha I, et al. Laparoscopic versus open resection for sigmoid diverticulitis. Cochrane Database Syst Rev. 2017;11:CD009277.

65. Li D, Baxter NN, McLeod RS, Moineddin R, Wilton AS, Nathens AB. Evolving practice patterns in the management of acute colonic diverticulitis: a population-based analysis. Dis Colon Rectum. 2014;57(12):1397–405.
66. Chapman J, Davies M, Wolff B, Dozois E, Tessier D, Harrington J, et al. Complicated diverticulitis: is it time to rethink the rules? Ann Surg. 2005;242(4):576–81; discussion 581–3. [PubMed: 16192818]
67. Pittet O, Kotzampassakis N, Schmidt S, Denys A, Demartines N, Calmes JM. Recurrent left colonic diverticulitis episodes: more severe than the initial diverticulitis? World J Surg. 2009;33(3):547–52. [PubMed: 19148697]
68. Salem L, Veenstra DL, Sullivan SD, Flum DR. The timing of elective colectomy in diverticulitis: a decision analysis. J Am Coll Surg. 2004;199(6):904–12. [PubMed: 15555974
69. Shaikh S, Krukowski ZH. Outcome of a conservative policy for managing acute sigmoid diverticulitis. Br J Surg. 2007;94(7):876–9. [PubMed: 17380481]
70. Hall JF, Roberts PL, Ricciardi R, et al. Long-term follow-up after an initial episode of diverticulitis: what are the predictors of recurrence? Dis Colon Rectum. 2011;54:283–8.
71. Salem L, Anaya DA, Flum DR. Temporal changes in the management of diverticulitis. J Surg Res. 2005;124:318–23.
72. Morris AM, Regenbogen SE, Hardiman KM, Hendren S. Sigmoid diverticulitis: a systematic review. JAMA Surg. 2014;311:287–97.
73. Ricciardi R, Baxter NN, Read TE, Marcello PW, Hall J, Roberts PL. Is the decline in surgical treatment for diverticulitis associated with an increase in complicated diverticulitis? Dis Colon Rectum. 2009;52:1558–63.
74. Köckerling F. Emergency surgery for acute complicated diverticulitis. Visc Med. 2015;31(2):107–10.
75. Stocchi L. Current indications and role of surgery in the management of sigmoid diverticulitis. World J Gastroenterol. 2010;16:804–17.
76. Eusebio EB, Eisenberg MM. Natural history of diverticular disease of the colon in young patients. Am J Surg. 1973;125:308–11.
77. Freischlag J, Bennion RS, Thompson JE. Complications of diverticular disease of the colon in young people. Dis Colon Rectum. 1986;29:639–43.
78. Köhler L, Sauerland S, Neugebauer E. Diagnosis and treatment of diverticular disease: results of a consensus development conference. The Scientific Committee of the European Association for Endoscopic Surgery. Surg Endosc. 1999;13:430–6.
79. Wong WD, Wexner SD, Lowry A, Vernava A 3rd, Burnstein M, Denstman F, et al. Practice parameters for the treatment of sigmoid diverticulitis–supporting documentation. The Standards Task Force. The American Society of Colon and Rectal Surgeons. Dis Colon Rectum. 2000;43:290–7.
80. Binda GA, Mataloni F, Bruzzone M, Carabotti M, Cirocchi R, Nascimbeni R, et al. Trends in hospital admission for acute diverticulitis in Italy from 2008 to 2015. Tech Coloproctol. 2018;22:597–604.
81. Vather R, Broad JB, Jaung R, Robertson J, Bissett IP. Demographics and trends in the acute presentation of diverticular disease: a nation study. ANZ J Surg. 2015;85:744–8.
82. Lidor AO, Segal JB Wu AW, et al. Older patients with diverticulitis have low recurrence rates and rarely need surgery. Surgery. 2011;150:146–53
83. Katz LH, Guy DD, Lahat A, Gafter-Gvili A, Bar-Meir S. Diverticulitis in the young is not more aggressive than in the elderly, but it tends to recur more often: systematic review and meta-analysis. J Gastroenterol Hepatol. 2013;28:1274–81.
84. Lidsky ME, Marosky Thacker JK, Lagoo-Deenadayalan SA, Scarborough JE. Advanced age is an independent predictor for increased morbidity and mortality after emergent surgery for diverticulitis. Surgery. 2012;152:465–72.
85. Ünlü C, van de Wall BJ, Gerhards MF, et al. Influence of age on clinical outcome of acute diverticulitis. J Gastrointest Surg. 2013;17:1651–6.
86. Beyer-Berjot L, et al. Emergency surgery in acute diverticulitis: a systematic review. Dis Colon Rectum. 2020;63(3):397–405.
87. Costa G, et al. The use of emergency laparoscopy for acute abdomen in the elderly: the FRAILESEL Italian multicenter prospective cohort study. Updates Surg. 2020:1–13.
88. Costa G, Tomassini F, Tierno SM, Venturini L, Frezza B, Cancrini G, Mero A, Lepre L. Emergency colonic surgery: analysis of risk factors predicting morbidity and mortality. Chir Ital. 2009;61:565–71.
89. Desserud KF, Veen T, Søreide K. Emergency general surgery in the geriatric patient. Br J Surg. 2016;103(2):e52–61. https://doi.org/10.1002/bjs.10044.
90. McLean RC, McCallum IJ, Dixon S, O'Loughlin P. A 15-year retrospective analysis of the epidemiology and outcomes for elderly emergency general surgical admissions in the north east of England: a case for multidisciplinary geriatric input Int J Surg. 2016;28:13–21.
91. Jacobs M, Verdeja JC, Goldstein HS. Minimally invasive colon resection (laparoscopic colectomy). Surg Laparosc Endosc Percutan Tech. 1991;1:144–50.
92. Bruce CJ, Coller JA, Murray JJ, Schoetz DJ Jr, Roberts PL, Rusin LC. Laparoscopic resection for diverticular disease. Dis Colon Rectum. 1996;39(10 Suppl):S1–6.
93. Dwivedi A, Chahin F, Agrawal S, Chau WY. Tootla A, Tootla F, et al. Laparoscopic colectomy vs open colectomy for sigmoid diverticular disease. Dis Colon Rectum. 2002;45:1309–14.
94. Lauro A, Alonso Poza A, Cirocchi R, Doria C, Gruttadauria S, Giustozzi G, et al. Laparoscopic surgery for colon diverticulitis. Minerva Chir. 2002;57:1–5.

95. De Chaisemartin C, Panis Y, Mognol P, Valleur P. Laparoscopic sigmoid resection for diverticulitis: is learning phase associated with increased morbidity? Ann Chir. 2003;128:81–7.
96. Lawrence DM, Pasquale MD, Wasser TE. Laparoscopic versus open sigmoid colectomy for diverticulitis. Am Surg. 2003;69:499–503.
97. Masoomi H, Buchberg B, Nguyen B, Tung V, Stamos MJ, Mills S. Outcomes of laparoscopic versus open colectomy in elective surgery for diverticulitis. World J Surg. 2011;39:2143–8.
98. Alves A, Panis Y, Slim K, Heyd B, Kwiatkowski F, Mantion G, et al. French multicentre prospective observational study of laparoscopic versus open colectomy for sigmoid diverticular disease. Br J Surg. 2005;92:1520–5.
99. Anania G, Vedana L, Santini M, Scagliarini L, Giaccari S, Resta G, et al. Complications of diverticular disease: surgical laparoscopic treatment. G Chir. 2014;35:126–8.
100. Enagore AJ, Duepree HJ, Delaney CP, Dissanaike S, Brady KM, Fazio VW. Cost structure of laparoscopic and open sigmoid colectomy for diverticular disease: similarities and differences. Dis Colon Rectum. 2002;45:485–90.
101. Yang CY, Chaudhry OO, Halabi WJ, et al. Outcomes of laparoscopic colorectal surgery: data from the Nationwide Inpatient Sample 2009. Am J Surg. 2012;204:952–7.
102. Senagore AJ, Duepree HJ, Delaney CP, Dissanaike S, Brady KM, Fazio VW. Cost structure of laparoscopic and open sigmoid colectomy for diverticular disease: similarities and differences. Dis Colon Rectum. 2002;45:485–90.
103. Klarenbeek BR, Bergamaschi R, Veenhof AA, et al. Laparoscopic versus open sigmoid resection for diverticular disease: follow-up assessment of the randomized control Sigma trial. Surg Endosc. 2001;25:1121–6.
104. Gervaz P, Inan I, Perneger T, Schiffer E, Morel P. A prospective randomized single-blind comparison of laparoscopic versus open sigmoid colectomy for diverticulitis. Ann Surg. 2010;252:3–8.
105. Young-Fadock TM, Solomon CG. Diverticulitis. N Engl J Med. 2018;379:1635–42.
106. Rogers AC, Collins D, O'Sullivan GC, Winter DC. Laparoscopic lavage for perforated diverticulitis: a population analysis. Dis Colon Rectum. 2012;55:932–8.
107. Francis NK, et al. EAES and SAGES 2018 consensus conference on acute diverticulitis management: evidence-based recommendations for clinical practice. Surg Endosc. 2019;33(9):2726–41.
108. Letarte F, Hallet J, Drolet S, et al. Laparoscopic emergency surgery for diverticular disease that failed medical treatment: a valuable option? Results of a retrospective comparative cohort study. Dis Colon Rectum. 2013;56:1395–402.
109. Turley RS, Barbas AS, Lidsky ME, Mantyh CR, Migaly J, Scarborough JE. Laparoscopic versus open Hartmann procedure for the emergency treatment of diverticulitis: a propensity-matched analysis. Dis Colon Rectum. 2013;56:72–82.
110. Letarte F, Hallet J, Drolet S, et al. Laparoscopic versus open colonic resection for complicated diverticular disease in the emergency setting: a safe choice? A retrospective comparative cohort study. Am J Surg. 2015;209:992–8.
111. Rea JD, Herzig DO, Diggs BS, Cone MM, Lu KC. Use and outcomes of emergent laparoscopic resection for acute diverticulitis. Am J Surg. 2012;203:639–43.
112. Titu LV, Zafar N, Phillips SM, Greenslade GL, Dixon AR. Emergency laparoscopic surgery for complicated diverticular disease. Color Dis. 2009;11:401–4.
113. Vennix S, Musters GD, Mulder IM, et al. LADIES Trial Collaborators. Laparoscopic peritoneal lavage or sigmoidectomy for perforated diverticulitis with purulent peritonitis: a multicentre, parallel-group, randomised, open-label trial. Lancet. 2015;386:1269–77.
114. Cirocchi R, et al. The role of emergency laparoscopic colectomy for complicated sigmoid diverticulitis: a systematic review and meta-analysis. Surgeon. 2019;17(6):360–9.
115. Jimenez Rodriguez RM, Segura-Sampedro JJ, Flores-Cortres ML, Fl-Bernal F, Marttres-Cortg VP, Ciuro FP, Ruiz JP. Laparoscopic approach in gastrointestinal emergencies. World J Gastroenterol. 2016;22:2701–10.
116. Agresta F, Campanile FC, Podda M, Cillara N, Pernazza G, Giaccaglia V, Ciccoritti L, Ioia G, Mandaln S, La Barbera C, Birindelli A, Sartelli M, Di Saverio S, Joined Italian Surgical Societies Working Group. Current status of laparoscopy for acute abdomen in Italy: a critical appraisal of 2012 clinical guidelines from two consecutive nationwide surveys with analysis of 271,323 cases over 5 years. Surg Endosc. 2017;31:1785–95.
117. Mandrioli M, Inaba K, Piccinini A, Biscardi A, Sartelli M, Agresta F, Catena F, Cirocchi R, Jovine E, Tugnoli G, Di Saverio S. Advances in laparoscopy for acute care surgery and trauma. World J Gastroenterol. 2016;22(2):668–80.
118. Pucher PH, Carter NC, Knight BC, Toh S, Tucker V, Mercer SJ. Impact of laparoscopic approach in emergency major abdominal surgery: single-centre analysis of 748 consecutive cases. Ann R Coll Surg Engl. 2018;100:279.
119. Tadlock MD, Karamanos E, Skiada D, et al. Emergency surgery for acute diverticulitis: which operation? A National Surgical Quality Improvement Program study. J Trauma Acute Care Surg. 2013;74:1385–91.
120. Saunders DI, Murray D, Pichel AC, Varley S, Peden CJ, Emergency Laparotomy Network UK. Variations in mortality after emergency laparotomy: the first report of the UK Emergency Laparotomy Network. Br J Anaesth. 2012;109:368–75.

121. Green G, Shaikh I, Fernandes R, Wegstapel H. Emergency laparotomy in octogenarians: a 5-year study of morbidity and mortality. World J Gastrointest Surg. 2013;5:216.
122. Al-Temimi MH, Griffee M, Enniss TM, Preston R, Vargo D, Overton S, Kimball E, Barton R, Nirula R. When is death inevitable after emergency laparotomy? Analysis of the American College of Surgeons National Surgical Quality Improvement Program database. J Am Coll Surg. 2012;215:503.
123. Morris CR, et al. Incidence of perforated diverticulitis and risk factors for death in a UK population. Br J Surg. 2008;95(7):876–81.
124. Zdichavsky M, Granderath FA, Blumenstock G, Kramer M, Kuper MA, Konigsrainer A. Acute laparoscopic intervention for diverticular disease (AIDD): a feasible approach. Langenbecks Arch Surg. 2010;395:41–8.
125. Cirocchi R, Trastulli S, Farinella E, Desiderio J, Listorti C, Parisi A, et al. Is inferior mesenteric artery ligation during sigmoid colectomy for diverticular disease associated with increased anastomotic leakage? A meta-analysis of randomized and non-randomized clinical trials. Color Dis. 2012;14:e521–9.
126. Cirocchi R, Trastulli S, Desiderio J, Listorti C, Boselli C, Parisi A, et al. Treatment of Hinchey stage III-IV diverticulitis: a systematic review and meta-analysis. Int J Color Dis. 2013;28(4):447–57. [PubMed: 23242271]
127. Abbas S. Resection and primary anastomosis in acute complicated diverticulitis: a systematic review of the literature. Int J Color Dis. 2007;22:351–7.
128. Morris A, Regenbogen S, Hardiman K, Hendren S. Sigmoid diverticulitis: a systematic review. J Am Med Assoc. 2014;311:287–97.
129. Agaba EA, Zaidi RM, Ramzy P, et al. Laparoscopic Hartmann's procedure: a viable option for treatment of acutely perforated diverticulitis. Surg Endosc. 2009;23(7):1483–6.
130. Lauro A, Alonso Poza A, Cirocchi R, Doria C, Gruttadauria S. Laparoscopic surgery for colon diverticulitis. Minerva Chir. 2002;57(1):1–5.
131. Fleming FJ, Gillen P. Reversal of Hartmann's procedure following acute diverticulitis: is timing everything? Int J Color Dis. 2009;24:1219–25.
132. Tadlock MD, Karamanos E, Skiada D, Inaba K, Talving P, Senagore A, et al. Emergency surgery for acute diverticulitis: which operation? A national surgical quality improvement program study. J Trauma Acute Care Surg. 2013;74(6):1385–91.
133. Regenbogen S, Hardman K, Hendren S, Morris A. Surgery for diverticulitis in the 21st century: a systematic review. J Am Med Assoc. 2014;149:292–302.
134. Stollman N, Smalley W, Hirano I, AGA Institute Clinical Guidelines Committee. American Gastroenterological Association Institute guideline on the management of acute diverticulitis. Gastroenterology. 2015;149:1944–9.
135. Floch M, Longo W. United States guidelines for diverticulitis treatment. J Clin Gastroenterol. 2016;50:53–6.
136. Zingg U, Pasternak I, Dietrich M, et al. Primary anastomosis vs Hartmann's procedure in patients undergoing emergency left colectomy for perforated diverticulitis. Color Dis. 2010;12:54–60.
137. Oberkofler CE, Rickenbacher A, Raptis DA, et al. A multicenter randomized clinical trial of primary anastomosis or Hartmann's procedure for perforated left colonic diverticulitis with purulent or fecal peritonitis. Ann Surg. 2012;256:819–26.
138. Biondo S, Lopez Borao J, Millan M, Kreisler E, Jaurrieta E. Current status of the treatment of acute colonic diverticulitis: a systematic review. Colorectal Dis. 2011;14:e1–e11.
139. Lee EC, Murray JJ, Coller JA, Roberts PL, Schoetz DL Jr. Intraoperative colonic lavage in nonelective surgery for diverticular disease. Dis Colon Rectum. 1997;40:669–74.
140. Afshar S, Kurer MA. Laparoscopic peritoneal lavage for perforated sigmoid diverticulitis. Color Dis. 2011;14:135–42.
141. Constantinides VA, Tekkis PP, Athanasiou T, et al. Primary resection with anastomosis vs. Hartmann's procedure in nonelective surgery for acute colonic diverticulitis: a systematic review. Dis Colon Rectum. 2006;49:966–81.
142. Myers E, Hurley M, O'Sullivan GC, Kavanagh D, Wilson I, Winter DC. Laparoscopic peritoneal lavage for generalized peritonitis due to perforated diverticulitis. Br J Surg. 2008;95:97–101.
143. Karoui M, Champault A, Pautrat K, Valleur P, Cherqui D, Champault G. Laparoscopic peritoneal lavage or primary anastomosis with defunctioning stoma for Hinchey 3 complicated diverticulitis: results of a comparative study. Dis Colon Rectum. 2009;52:609–15.
144. Afshar S, Kurer MA. Laparoscopic peritoneal lavage for perforated sigmoid diverticulitis. Color Dis. 2012;14:135–42.
145. McDermott FD, Heeney A, Kelly ME, Steele RJ, Carlson GL, Winter DC. Systematic review of preoperative, intraoperative and postoperative risk factors for colorectal anastomotic leaks. Br J Surg. 2015;102:462–79.
146. Angenete E, Thornell A, Burcharth J, et al. Laparoscopic lavage is feasible and safe for the treatment of perforated diverticulitis with purulent peritonitis: the first results from the randomized controlled trial DILALA. Ann Surg. 2016;263:117–22.
147. Schultz JK, Yaqub S, Wallon C, et al.; SCANDIV Study Group. Laparoscopic lavage vs primary resection for acute perforated diverticulitis: the SCANDIV randomized clinical trial. JAMA. 2015;314:1364–1375.
148. Schultz JK, Wallon C, Blecic L, et al.; SCANDIV Study Group. One-year results of the SCANDIV randomized clinical trial of laparoscopic lavage ver-

sus primary resection for acute perforated diverticulitis. Br J Surg. 2017;104:1382–1392.
149. Thornell A, Angenete E, Bisgaard T, et al. Laparoscopic lavage for perforated diverticulitis with purulent peritonitis: a randomized trial. Ann Intern Med. 2016;164:137–45.
150. Gehrman J, Angenete E, Björholt I, Bock D, Rosenberg J, Haglind E. Health economic analysis of laparoscopic lavage versus Hartmann's procedure for diverticulitis in the randomized DILALA trial. Br J Surg. 2016;103:1539–47.
151. Bretagnol F, Pautrat K, Mor C, Benchellal Z, Huten N, de Calan L. Emergency laparoscopic management of perforated sigmoid diverticulitis: a promising alternative to more radical procedures. J Am Coll Surg. 2008;206:654–7.
152. Alamili M, Gögenur I, Rosenberg J. Acute complicated diverticulitis managed by laparoscopic lavage. Dis Colon Rectum. 2009;52:1345–9.
153. Toorenvliet BR, Swank H, Schoones JW, Hamming JF, Bemelman WA. Laparoscopic peritoneal lavage for perforated colonic diverticulitis: a systematic review. Color Dis. 2010;12:862–7.
154. Cirocchi R, Trastulli S, Vettoretto N, et al. Laparoscopic peritoneal lavage: a definitive treatment for diverticular peritonitis or a "bridge" to elective laparoscopic sigmoidectomy?: a systematic review. Medicine (Baltimore). 2015;94:e334.
155. Gaertner WB, Kwaan MR, Madoff RD, et al. The evolving role of laparoscopy in colonic diverticular disease: a systematic review. World J Surg. 2013;37:629–38.
156. Nelson RS, Ewing BM, Wengert TJ, Thorson AG. Clinical outcomes of complicated diverticulitis managed nonoperatively. Am J Surg. 2008;196:969–74.
157. Liang S, Russek K, Franklin ME Jr. Damage control strategy for the management of perforated diverticulitis with generalized peritonitis: laparoscopic lavage and drainage vs. laparoscopic Hartmann's procedure. Surg Endosc. 2012;26:2835–42.
158. Radé F, Bretagnol F, Auguste M, Di Guisto C, Huten N, de Calan L. Determinants of outcome following laparoscopic peritoneal lavage for perforated diverticulitis. Br J Surg. 2014;101:1602–6.
159. Angenete E, Bock D, Rosenberg J, Haglind E. Laparoscopic lavage is superior to colon resection for perforated purulent diverticulitis—a meta-analysis. Int J Color Dis. 2017;32:163–9.
160. Shaikh FM, Stewart PM, Walsh SR, Davies RJ. Laparoscopic peritoneal lavage or surgical resection for acute perforated sigmoid diverticulitis: a systematic review and meta-analysis. Int J Surg. 2017;38:130–7.
161. Swank HA, Mulder IM, Hoofwijk AG, Nienhuijs SW, Lange JF, Bemelman WA, Dutch Diverticular Disease Collaborative Study Group. Early experience with laparoscopic lavage for perforated diverticulitis. Br J Surg. 2013;100:704–10.

Small Bowel Obstruction

17

Carlo Alberto Ammirati, Marco Ettore Allaix, and Mauro Zago

17.1 Introduction

Small bowel obstruction (SBO) accounts for about 15% of all hospital admissions for surgical gastrointestinal emergencies and 15% of admissions to the emergency room for abdominal pain.

It is an urgent condition that is associated with significant patient's morbidity and mortality, since it occurs more frequently in the elderly population than in young patients. Most frequent causes of SBO are adhesions (65%), hernias (10%), and tumors (5%) [1].

During the last 20 years, several advances in the diagnosis and treatment have been performed, aiming at improving the outcomes and reducing the treatment invasiveness. For instance, the implementation of the nonoperative management and the use of laparoscopy have reduced the number of unneeded laparotomies and lowered the postoperative complications [2].

The aim of this chapter is to revise pathophysiology, clinical presentation, diagnosis, and management of most common causes of SBO in the elderly.

C. A. Ammirati · M. E. Allaix (✉)
Department of Surgical Sciences, University of Torino, Torino, Italy
e-mail: marcoettore.allaix@unito.it

M. Zago
General and Emergency Surgery Division, A. Manzoni Hospital, Lecco, Italy
e-mail: m.zago@asst-lecco.it

17.2 Epidemiology

Intra-abdominal adhesions account for up to 70% of SBO in both young and elderly patient populations [1]. Formation of adhesions is related to the healing of the wounds after an operation, and it strictly depends on several factors, including the surgical technique, tissue inflammation, and use of foreign materials. The wide increase in the use of the laparoscopic approach has led to a significant reduction in both rate of adhesions formation after abdominal surgery and need for surgery for SBO, when compared to the open approach. This is mainly due to smaller incisions and overall, less tissue trauma, and lower intraoperative bleeding than open surgery [2].

Another factor that influences the adhesion formation is the surgical site, with the rate of SBO that increases from 0.05% after cesarean section to about 10% after colorectal resection [3].

SBO recurrence is quite common, ranging from 12% at 1 year to 20% at 5 years after an episode nonoperatively treated and varying from 8% after 1 year to 16% at 5 years in patients undergoing operative treatment [4].

17.3 Pathophysiology

In case of SBO, accumulation of intestinal contents leads to small bowel dilation proximal to the point of obstruction. The stasis of intestinal

F. Agresta et al. (eds.), *Emergency laparoscopic surgery in the elderly and frail patient*,
https://doi.org/10.1007/978-3-030-79990-8_17

fluids determines further gas production, mainly due to bacterial overgrowth and food fermentation. As a consequence, wall edema develops, and absorptive functions of the small bowel mucosa are lost. The sequestered fluids progressively transudate from the bowel lumen into the abdominal cavity. Fluids sequestration, along with vomit, leads to loss of fluids and subsequent hypovolemia. In addition, the decreased bowel perfusion due to mural edema, increased intraluminal pressure, and hypovolemia results in bowel ischemia with bacterial translocation and eventually in bowel necrosis. The risk of peritonitis significantly increases with the duration of failed medical treatment.

17.4 Clinical Presentation and Differential Diagnosis

Symptoms vary according to the severity, site, duration, and cause of SBO. Classic clinical manifestation of SBO includes abdominal (crampy, intermittent, or constant when ischemia occurs) pain and distention, nausea, vomiting, and progressive obstipation. Fever is a common sign of bowel ischemia and overwhelming sepsis [1].

Clinical examination usually reveals classical signs of dehydration, such as hypotension, tachycardia, and mucosal dryness. The evaluation of the abdomen shows moderate and localized to severe and diffuse distention according to the site of SBO (proximal vs. distal). During the first phase, bowel sounds appear hyperactive, aiming at overcoming the obstruction; then, they progressively disappear due to mural edema and muscular fatigue. Abdominal inspection reveals the presence of surgical scars from previous operations and allows to rule out the presence of incarcerated hernias of the abdominal wall [5]. Presence of rebound tenderness, guarding, and rigidity of the abdomen are clinical signs of bowel ischemia and possible perforation.

Blood tests are usually nonspecific, showing hemoconcentration, electrolyte derangement, and renal failure [6].Several conditions must be taken into consideration in the differential diagnosis of SBO: postoperative ileus, ileus secondary to excessive use of narcotics, and acute mesenteric ischemia.

17.5 Radiology

When SBO is suspected, *plain abdominal films* are commonly obtained in both dependent and nondependent positions. Sensitivity of abdominal x-rays for SBO widely ranges between 60 and 93%, according to the radiologist experience and patient's position used [7]. While abdominal x-rays could allow to detect abnormal small bowel dilation and the presence of air-fluid levels, they do not assess the location and the cause of SBO and the presence of bowel ischemia.

In case a laparoscopic approach is suggested, plain film is not enough for surgical planning in the vast majority of cases.

There are growing evidences that point-of-care ultrasound (US) in diagnosing SBO has sensitivity comparable to plain film [8–10]. Notwithstanding, the use of US is not widespread. The main US finding of SBO is the visualization of both dilated and empty small bowel loops, which is highly sensitive for the diagnosis of SBO. Additional findings are detection of free fluid, evaluation of peristalsis, measurement of dilated loops, pattern of the bowel wall, and assessment of bowel wall viability with color flow mapping and power Doppler. US is not as sensitive as CT in detecting the site and the nature of obstruction and can replace plain film as first-step imaging [10].

Abdominal CT scan is key in defining the exact site of SBO and the grade of dilatation of the small bowel loops, and in assessing signs of bowel ischemia (mural thickening and decreased enhancement, edema of the mesentery, pneumatosis), and/or perforation. The CT scan also distinguishes between partial and complete SBO, and low-grade versus high-grade SBO. A complete SBO occurs when the CT scan shows a severe discrepancy between the diameter of loops proximal to the transition point and distal small bowel, with no passage of gas or fluid. Incomplete high-grade SBO is similar to the complete SBO; however, it differs for minimal passage of intestinal contents beyond the point of obstruction. Low-grade SBO is characterized by mild discrepancy in the diameters of the loops, proximal and distal to the transition point; the CT scan shows the presence of gas and liquids in the distal small bowel and right colon.

17.6 Management

The management of patients with SBO can be operative or nonoperative. Among several classifications that have been proposed over years, there are two models predicting the need for surgery: the one proposed by Zielinski et al. [11] that is based on three radiological and clinical signs (mesenteric edema, absence of small bowel feces sign, and obstipation) and that by Baghdadi et al. [12], which includes radiologic findings, sepsis criteria, and comorbidities.

Nonoperative management should be always considered the first option in patients presenting with SBO without signs of peritonitis, small bowel strangulation, or intestinal ischemia. Even though the risk of SBO recurrence is slightly inferior after surgery than after conservative treatment, postoperative morbidity and mortality are high, especially in patients older than 80 years and postoperative quality of life is significantly impaired [13, 14].

Nonoperative management includes nil per os, insertion of nasogastric tube for gastric decompression, and liquid infusion. The success rate of this conservative strategy ranges between 70 and 90% [11]. Surgery should not be delayed more than 72 h if nonoperative management fails to solve the SBO episode, since complications rates are higher, the need for small bowel resection is more common, the hospital stay is longer, and mortality rates significantly increase.

The oral administration of Gastrografin®, a water-soluble radiopaque solution, is part of the conservative treatment in patients diagnosed with SBO. It has a therapeutic effect due to its osmolarity that is six times higher than that of extracellular fluids, it promotes the passage of fluids from the bowel wall into the intestinal lumen, thus reducing edema. In addition, it enhances small bowel peristalsis. It has been demonstrated that Gastrografin lowers the need for surgery, the length of hospital stay, and shortens the time to SBO resolution [15, 16]. However, the persistence of SBO-related symptoms, along with the lack of passage of Gastrografin in the ascending colon at plain films 6–8 h after oral administration, denotes failure of this treatment. The administration of Gastrografin® should be preferably included in a precise institutional algorithm [17]. There are some risk factors for failure: patient's age higher than 65 years, multiple previous open operations, and previous surgical treatment for SBO.

When a patient with SBO is selected for surgery, the choice is between an open and a laparoscopic approach. The last 15 years have witnessed a significant adoption of the minimally invasive approach in centers with extensive experience in laparoscopic surgery. However, main concerns remain the limited working space and the risk of iatrogenic injuries to the bowel.

Main contraindication to the laparoscopic approach to SBO is the patient's hemodynamic instability. Otherwise, it is recommended in stable patients and in those with suspected bowel ischemia too. Laparoscopy is associated with better short-term and long-term outcomes than open surgery. In particular, cardiorespiratory complication and deep venous thrombosis rates are lower, and resumption of gastrointestinal function occurs earlier [18, 19]. Predictors of success are less than two previous abdominal open surgeries, nonmedian incisions, single-band adhesion, treatment within 24 h from the onset of symptoms, and surgeon experience in laparoscopic surgery.

One of the most important factors that must be taken into consideration when planning the management strategy for SBO is the patient's age. For instance, elderly patients are more likely to have comorbidities that make the recovery after surgery prolonged with significant impairment of patient's functional status and quality of life. This might be due to the very limited use of the laparoscopic approach in elderly patients in Italy, as recently showed by the results of the FRAILESEL Italian Multicenter Prospective Cohort Study

[20]. On the other hand, delayed surgery more than 24 h after an attempt of nonoperative treatment in elderly patients might be associated with increased risk of acute renal failure and myocardial infarction secondary to stopping oral medications for the treatment of comorbidities. However, these statements are based on very limited amount of research, in the absence of high-quality evidence.

Most interesting, Springer et al., analyzing a series of SBO in an elder population, showed a higher rate of bowel resection (29%) among those who underwent delayed surgery (median 2 days). Surgery after failed nonoperative management was associated with a mortality of 14% versus 3% for those who underwent immediate surgery [21].

17.7 Laparoscopic Surgical Strategy and Technique: Tips and Tricks

Proper positioning of the patient is paramount for an effective laparoscopic adhesiolysis. Tilting of the table in every position during the operation for pulling away the dilated loops is frequently required, and sometimes a change of the side of the main operator. All the following issues should be meticulously checked before starting the operation: both arms should be along the patient's sides, shoulders keepers (and feet keepers in obese) must be in place, the table remote control should be efficient, and the nasogastric tube and the urinary catheter are in place.

Atraumatic graspers and cold scissors are the most important instruments. The use of a 30° telescope is strongly advisable. A preoperative individual planning based on CT-imaged evaluation is essential for deciding where the first trocar should be placed. In general, on the opposite quadrant of the presumed site of the obstructive band, and far from previous surgical scars.

No evidences are available for supporting the use of open laparoscopy versus Veress needle versus optic trocar for the induction of pneumoperitoneum. Gentle blunt dissection with a 30° telescope directly against parietal adhesions, when needed, is a clever maneuver for getting enough space for the second trocar. Additional ports are inserted as needed. Using a 5-mm angled scope allows to employ any port [22].

The first step is to pull away the dilated loops by gravity, gaining the workspace, focusing on the transition point. Dissection is done with cold scissors and blunt dissection. There is a high risk of immediate and/or delayed thermal injuries using energy devices.

Identification of the last ileal loop and a gentle handling of empty loops allow to get the occlusive point.

The technique is a mix of sharp and blunt dissection.

Handling dilated loops is forbidden, due to the risk of tearing. Grasping the mesentery could be an alternative, when required.

After fixing the occlusive band, there is no need for further explorations.

An inadvertent enterotomy can be laparoscopically repaired.

Unexpected findings need for resection, inadvertent enterotomy not manageable laparoscopically, and inability to find the transition point are reasons for conversion. Incision could be tailored in size and site according to the requirements.

A tailored laparotomy can be facilitated by an exploratory laparoscopy in particular cases: obstructing small bowel mass (endometriosis, neoplasia, carcinosis) or when facing with biliary ileus (laparoscopic identification of the impacted stone and a tailored laparotomy for enterotomy and stone extraction) [22].

Viability assessment could be safely done by laparoscopy, directly warming bowel loops with a jet of heated saline, waiting until 20 min for reassessment.

Five Things You Should Know About

- Intra-abdominal adhesions account for up to 70% of SBO in both young and elderly patient populations and it is burdened by considerable recurrence rate, ranging from 12% at 1 year to 20% at 5 years after an episode nonoperatively treated and varying from 8% after 1 year to 16% at 5 years in patients undergoing operative treatment.

- Symptoms are generally aspecific and vary according to the severity, site, duration, and cause of SBO, including abdominal pain, distention, nausea, vomiting, progressive obstipation, and fever which is a common sign of bowel ischemia and overwhelming sepsis.
- Abdominal X-rays and US may play a role during first steps of SBO diagnosis, with good sensitivity and specificity, as they can detect indirect signs of SBO, but they did not highlight the cause or the location of obstruction, as CT scan.
- Nonoperative management should be always considered the first option in patients presenting with SBO without signs of peritonitis, small bowel strangulation, or intestinal ischemia and it includes nil per os, insertion of nasogastric tube for gastric decompression, and liquid infusion; oral administration of water-soluble contrast agent may have a therapeutic as well as diagnostic role.
- Despite limited working space and the risk of iatrogenic bowel injuries, laparoscopic technique is associated with better short-term and long-term outcomes than open surgery; main contraindications are represented by hemodynamic instability.

References

1. Rami Reddy SR, Cappel MS. A systematic review of the clinical presentation, diagnosis, and treatment of small bowel obstruction. Curr Gastroenterol Rep. 2017;19:28.
2. Pey KZ, Asuzu D, Davis KA. Will laparoscopic lysis of adhesion become the new standard of care? Evaluating trends and outcomes in laparoscopic management of small-bowel obstruction using the American College of Surgeons National Surgical Quality Improvement Project Database. Surg Endosc. 2017;31:2180–6.
3. Ten Broek RP, Issa Y, van Santbrink EJ, et al. Burden of adhesions in abdominal and pelvic surgery: systematic review and met-analysis. BMJ. 2013;347:f5588.
4. Foster NM, McGory ML, Zingmode DS, et al. Small bowel obstruction: a population-based appraisal. J Am Coll Surg. 2006;203:170–6.
5. Azargury D, Liu RC, Morgan A. Small bowel obstruction. J Trauma Acute Care Surg. 2015;79:661–8.
6. Maung AA, Johnson DC, Piper GL, et al. Evaluation and management of small-bowel obstruction. J Trauma Acute Care Surg. 2012;73:S362–9.
7. Maglinte DD, Reyes BL, Harmon BH, et al. Reliability and role of plain film radiography and CT in the diagnosis of small-bowel obstruction. AJR Am J Roentgenol. 1996;167:1451–5.
8. Jang TB, Schindler D, Kaji AH. Bedside ultrasonography for the detection of small bowel obstruction in the emergency department. Emerg Med J. 2011;28:676–8.
9. Guttman J, Stone MB Kimberly HH, et al. Point-of-care ultrasonography for the diagnosis of small bowel obstruction in the emergency department. CJEM. 2015;17:206–9.
10. Zago M, Mariani D, Kurihara H, Baiocchi G, et al. In: Agresta F, Campanile FC, Anania G, Bergamini C, editors. Emergency laparoscopy. Switzerland: Springer International Publishing; 2016. p. 117–36.
11. Zielinski MD, Eiken PW, Bannon MP, et al. Small bowel obstruction-who needs an operation? A multivariate prediction model. World J Surg. 2010;34:910–9.
12. Baghdadi YMK, Morris DS, Choudhry AJ, et al. Validation of the anatomic severity score developed by the American Association for the Surgery of Trauma in small bowel obstruction. J Surg Res. 2016;204:428–34.
13. Clarke A, Murdoch H, Thomas MJ, et al. Mortality and postoperative care after emergency laparotomy. Eur J Anaesthesiol. 2011;28:16–9.
14. Saunders DI, Murray D, Pichel AC, et al. Variations in mortality after emergency laparotomy: the first report of the UK Emergency Laparotomy Network. Br J Anaesth. 2012;109:368–75.
15. Ceresoli M, Coccolini F, Catena F, et al. Water-soluble contrast agent in adhesive small bowel obstruction: a systematic review and meta-analysis of diagnostic and therapeutic value. Am J Surg. 2016;211:1114–25.
16. Branco BC, Barmparas G, Schnuriger B, et al. Systematic review and meta-analysis of the diagnostic and therapeutic role of water-soluble contrast agent in adhesive small bowel obstruction. Br J Surg. 2010;97:470–8.
17. Costa G, Ruscelli P, Balducci G, et al. Clinical strategies for the management of intestinal obstruction and pseudo-obstruction. Ann Ital Chir. 2016;87:105–17.
18. Krielen P, Di Saverio S, ten Broek R, et al. Laparoscopic versus open approach for adhesive small bowel obstruction, a systematic review and meta-analysis of short term outcomes. J Trauma Acute Care Surg. 2020;88:866–74.
19. Sallinen V, Di Saverio S, Haukijarvi E, et al. Laparoscopic versus open adhesiolysis for adhesive small bowel obstruction (LASSO): an international, multicentre, randomized, open-label trial. Lancet. 2019;4:278–86.

20. Costa G, Fransvea P, Podda M, et al.; ERASO (Elderly Risk Assessment and Surgical Outcome) Collaborative Study Group. The use of emergency laparoscopy for acute abdomen in the elderly: the FRAILESEL Italian Multicenter Prospective Cohort Study. Updates Surg. 2020;72:513–525.
21. Springer JE, Bailey JG, Davis PJB, et al. Management and outcomes of small bowel obstruction in older adult patients: a prospective cohort study. Can J Surg. 2014;57:379–84.
22. Zago M, Bozzo S, Centurelli A, et al. Laparoscopic and ultrasound assisted management of gallstone ileus after biliointestinal bypass: case report and review of literature. Ann Ital Chir. 2016;87:S2239253X16025676.

Incarcerated Inguinal and Crural Hernias

18

Alberto Sartori, Umberto Bracale, Andrea Bianchin, Emanuele Pontecorvi, Jacopo Andreuccetti, Vania Silvestri, and Francesco Corcione

18.1 Incarcerated Inguinal and Crural Hernias

The inguinal hernia is probably the surgical pathology that affects the majority of the population in the Western world; it has been calculated, for example, that about 1.65 million visits are made each year within the American healthcare system [1, 2]. In fact, the chance of developing an inguinal hernia during one's lifetime is relatively high and the rates are 27–43% for men and 3–6% for women [2–4]. While the groin hernia is more in the male, the femoral hernia is more frequently diagnosed in the female.

The risk factors associated with the onset of a hernia in the crural groin region are numerous and have been summarized in Table 18.1 [1]. Among the main risk factors, besides the sex of the patient, there is obesity, a pathology that is rapidly increasing in the world; this problem has assumed enormous proportions, almost pandemic in western regions so that the term "globesity" has been coined [5–8]. Obesity is also related to the onset of many other diseases such as diabetes mellitus, sleep apnea syndrome and asthma, non-alcoholic cirrhosis, and many others [8]. Obesity and associated diseases result in medically and surgically fragile patients.

Age is another risk factor involved in the formation of a hernia in the crural groin region, probably due to the progressive change of elastic fibers, with a progressive reduction of type I/III fibers in collagen metabolism [9, 10]. Some studies have shown that in elderly patients there is, on the one hand, a progressive reduction of oxytalan fibers, which are responsible for tissue resistance, and on the other hand, an increase in mature elastic fibers and elaunin, which are responsible for tissue elasticity. The degeneration of the elastic fibers and collagen fibers present in the transversalis fascia mainly favors the onset of a direct inguinal hernia, while the degeneration of the fibers and their replacement with less elastic fibers at the level of the inner groin ring promote the onset of an indirect hernia [9, 10].

The World Health Organization defines the elderly as those patients who are over 65 years of age [11]. It has been estimated that in the Western world in 2019 there were more than 700 million people considered elderly, and this number is expected to double by 2050, when this

A. Sartori (✉)
Department of General Surgery, San Valentino Hospital, Montebelluna, Italy

U. Bracale · E. Pontecorvi · V. Silvestri · F. Corcione
Department of General Surgery and Surgical Speciality, University Federico II of Naples, Naples, Italy

A. Bianchin
Department of Anaesthesia and Intensive Care, San Valentino Hospital, Montebelluna, Italy

J. Andreuccetti
Department of General Surgery II, Spedali Civili, Brescia, Italy

F. Agresta et al. (eds.), *Emergency laparoscopic surgery in the elderly and frail patient*,
https://doi.org/10.1007/978-3-030-79990-8_18

Table 18.1 Risk factors associated with IH formation

Evidence Level—high	Evidence Level—moderate	Evidence Level—low	Evidence Level—very low
Inheritance	Primary hernia type	Race (significantly less common in black patient)	Pulmonary disease (COPD and chronic cough) possibly increasing the risk of IH formation
Gender (8–10 times more common in males)	Increased systemic levels of matrix metalloproteinase	Chronic constipation	
Age	Rare connective tissue disorders	Tobacco use (inversely correlated)	
Collagen type I/III metabolism		Socio-occupational factors	
Obesity			
Prostatectomy history			

population will make up about 20% of the total [11, 12]. Therefore, the increase in life expectancy—associated with an increase in obesity and associated diseases and the high incidence of hernia pathologies of the crural groin region—makes us assume that, in the near future, clinicians and surgeons will have to treat more fragile and elderly patients with inguinal and femoral hernias.

Taking into consideration what is written in the proposed guidelines of the Hernia Surge Group, the strategy of "watch and wait" is safely applicable in patients with asymptomatic hernias, however, it must be kept in mind that in 70% of cases these patients will become symptomatic within 5 years of diagnosis and that the risk of incarcerated and strangled intestinal loop could be a problem when addressed in emergency [1]. A scheduled surgery, regardless of the technique, allows the clinician to minimize the operating risks, as opposed to what happens in emergency surgery, where the percentage of complications and mortality increases regardless of the age of the patient [13, 14]. By analyzing now the problem of the surgical treatment of inguinal hernias in elderly and frail patients, we must consider that these patients generally have a minor functional reserve and the associated comorbidities can negatively affect short-term outcomes and postoperative mortality. It is essential, as advocated by several authors, to stratify the risk of elderly patients according to age, comorbidities, and some exogenous factors. In literature, there are many studies that, by stratifying the surgical risk of the geriatric population, have shown that postoperative complications, mortality, and readmission at 30 days are higher in the population over 80 years of age [15–17]. In addition, Subramaniam et al., after analyzing a cohort of 117,997 geriatric patients undergoing surgery and through a multivariate analysis, have concluded that there are also many exogenous variables that can affect 30-day readmission [15]. These variables are not always related to the patient's comorbidities. Therefore, clinicians should carefully evaluate, if possible in a multidisciplinary analysis, which surgical approach is most appropriate and which anesthesia is most suitable in the elderly and frail patient presenting with a strangulated groin hernia.

The data regarding the possibility of incarcerated hernia in the groin-femoral region are quite heterogeneous and often, as reported by Gallegos et al., the first sign of the presence of a hernia is its imprisonment [18]. The risk of imprisonment for inguinal hernia is 11–24%, while for femoral hernia it varies from 16 to 62% [13, 14, 18]. The content of the herniated sac of an incarcerated hernia more frequently comprised omentum, peritoneal fat, and intestine and more rarely the appendix, bladder, and appendages [13, 14]. Mortality and postoperative complications after urgent crural groin hernioplasty are associated not only with the patient's preoperative clinical condition, but also with the fact that hernioplasty is associated with intestinal resection [19]. Incarceration and strangulation of the contents of the hernia sac cause a microvascular congestion which leads to a progressive ischemia of the tissue. The ischemia caused by incarceration of an intestinal loop and the risk of having to resect it are directly proportional to the time between diagnosis and treatment [20–23]. In fact, the time that elapses between the event and the surgical treatment is very important because not only will the intestinal ischemia be greater with the possibility of having to resect the loop and the presence of contaminated fluid due to bacterial translocation, but also the distension of the intestinal loops that could compromise the possibility of access to the abdominal cavity with laparoendoscopic technique [20]. As described by Koizumi et al., it is therefore evident that the timing for the treatment of a strangulated inguinal hernia is fundamental for the outcome of the surgery and for the choice of the surgical approach to be used [20].

The first case of incarcerated inguinal hernia treated laparoscopically in emergency was described in 1993 by Watson et al., however, to date there is little literature on the subject and the cases, are few, probably due to the low incidence rate of incarcerated hernia and the technical skills required by the surgeon to treat them laparoscopically [24]. The Italian Registry of emergency-treated hernias in the elderly patient has collected a case history with 259 patients operated on, of which only 10 with laparoscopic technique [19]; also the guidelines published by the Hernia Surge Group have not openly endorsed the use of the laparoscopic approach in emergency, they have concluded that the surgical indications of choice are bilateral inguinal hernias and recurrences, while unilateral hernias should be addressed only by experienced surgeons [1].

The problems in the choice of surgical technique for the treatment of an incarcerated femoral groin hernia in the elderly and frail patient can be divided into two main groups: anesthesiological problems and technical feasibility problems.

From the anesthesiological point of view, laparoscopy represents a safe technique and it has been shown that there is a reduction in blood loss, lung infections, and consequently postoperative hospitalization, making it the gold standard for some operations. Some challenging side effects from the past are now considered relatively minor and there is no way to predict the decompensation of chronic heart or lung disease during laparoscopic surgery [25–27]. Clinicians must consider that in the elderly patient the residual lung volume, that is, the portion of air that is not expelled and therefore does not participate effectively in gas exchange, increases by 10% every decade of age; the final effect is that the elderly patient is more prone to atelectasis, hypoxemia, and pulmonary shunting as they decrease vital capacity and lung reserve [27, 28]. Moreover, arterial hypertension, insufficiency, and cardiac ischemia are common in patients over 55 years of age and atrial fibrillation affects about 80% of elderly patients causing a decrease in cardiac output. Some of the advantages obtained by using the laparoscopic technique may be in vain in these patients, especially if the volume of intra-abdominal gas insufflation is greater than 15 mmHg, the positions on the operating bed are extreme, and even more if the operating time increases [28, 29]. The elderly patient with strangulated hernia and bowel loop involvement often reaches ER dehydrated and hypovolemic, which combined with the need to increase the Trendelenburg position to remove the loops and increased intra-abdominal pressure can have a negative effect on the patient. Clinicians should consider valvular and coronary heart conditions as the patient may not tolerate the preload and afterload values of laparoscopy, which may decrease splanchnic and especially renal perfusion [27–29]. The decision to submit a patient with a strangulated hernia to general anesthesia cannot be entrusted only to the ASA classification system, which does not consider the patient's age, type of surgery, and anesthesiological technique; even predictive morbidity and postoperative mortality are not well defined by the ASA classification [30–32]. In literature, there are few studies that report the use of spinal anesthesia to perform laparoscopic hernioplasty and concern only scheduled operations, therefore, for urgent operations, anesthesia should be general, possibly with laryngeal mask [33]. While there is evidence of increased postoperative pulmonary and cardiological complications associated with general anesthesia compared to local anesthesia, there is not the same evidence of increased neurocognitive disorders. General anesthesia plays an important role in postoperative neurocognitive disorders, the most frequent of which is postoperative delirium, which can persist even more than a month after surgery and therefore this factor should also be considered in the elderly and frail patient. In concluding the analysis of the anesthesiological problem in the treatment of emergency inguinal hernia in the elderly and frail patient, both surgeon and anesthesiologist will need to share clinical views [26–29].

With regard to the second problem of technical feasibility, the guidelines offered by the Hernia Surge Group have highlighted characteristics related to patients with hernias that justify the use of plastic surgery as first choice according to Lichtestein [1]. Some common conditions are inguinoscrotal hernias, previous abdominal surgery, pelvic or vascular surgery, recurrences after laparoendoscopic surgery, and lack of experience and appropriate equipment. As we have already seen, the literature regarding the use of emergency laparoscopic techniques is scarce and this is also determined by the fact that laparoendoscopic techniques are not widely used even in scheduled operations. Currently the laparoendoscopic approach to inguinal hernia is more widespread in wealthy countries with varying percentages in Australia (55%) and Switzerland (40%) [1]. In 1992, Arregui et al. first described a transabdominal preperitoneal plastic surgery (TAPP) to repair an inguinal hernia [34]. This technique, which exploits the principle of the preperitoneal approach of Stoppa, is completely "tension free" [35]. Shortly after, an alternative to the TAPP was introduced into clinical practice, the total extraperitoneal patch plasty (TEPP) that uses the same principles as the TAPP as a complete dissection of the pelvic floor with the implantation of a large mesh covering the entire inguinocrural area. Thus, in the late 1990s, laparoscopic inguinal hernia repair (LIHR) gained a stable role in the treatment of inguinal hernia repair (IHR). However, the spread of the techniques and the choice of one rather than the other by the surgical community were uneven worldwide [36]. The spread of TAPP and TEPP was slowed down by distrust of both techniques, linked to the need for a long learning curve, costs, and the need for general anesthesia in comparison to the open approach. In the world there is no preference for one approach in particular; in fact from the Swedish registry there is a tendency toward the preperitoneal approach as well as in Switzerland; on the other hand, from the German Herniamed registry the trans abdominal approach is preferred, in fact out of almost 180,000 groin hernias most of them have been operated using the TAPP technique and only 20% using the TEPP technique [37, 38]. Recently, with the improvement of scientific evidence, the International Guidelines of the Hernia Surge Group have reported many statements and recommendations regarding the use of laparoscopy for the treatment of inguinal hernias [1]. They have reported that TAPP and TEPP have similar operating times and risks of postoperative complications, equal incidence of acute and chronic pain, and recurrence rate. They showed a higher frequency of visceral lesions and hernias on trocar in TAPP and a higher incidence of vascular lesions and conversions in TEPP. Regarding the superiority of technique between TAPP and TEPP, in the last 10 years numerous studies have been published. Bracale et al. in their network meta-analysis have shown how TAPP and TEPP have improved clinical outcomes compared to the open technique, but TAPP and TEPP are equally effective [39]. However, the published recommendations are based on the results of some RCTs and meta-analyses in which the authors did not exclude female patients, or those with bilateral hernia or recurrence. This problem could affect the daily clinical approach to primary primitive unilateral hernia. In fact, even Kockerling suggested that a distinction should be made between different hernias (unilateral primary, bilateral, in women, recurrent hernia, etc.) and that in the future they should also be considered scientifically as separate groups [38]. He also reported that "this considerably reduces the total number of studies available to answer key scientific questions. But this would mean that the remaining studies would allow more precise statements to be made for a specific subgroup of inguinal hernias."

Currently six systematic reviews and meta-analyses of literature are available for comparison between TEPP and TAPP [39–42]. Some of these articles [39–41] did not include enough RCTs to allow direct comparison between TEPP and TAPP. Other [43] included seven RCTs, with different inclusion criteria (female patients, recurrences, or bilateral inguinal hernias). A recent meta-analysis for comparison of TEPP with Chen's TAPP with 1519 randomized patients also included other RCTs. Most of these studies included female patients, recurrences, or bilateral inguinal hernias [44]. Therefore, the body of previous meta-analyses does not allow definitive conclusions to be drawn on clinical decision making for TAPP or TEPP in primary unilateral hernias [40, 45].

In order to examine possible differences between TEPP and TAPP for unilateral primary inguinal hernia in men, we report the results of RCTs [46–48] that directly compared both procedures on this cluster. Butler et al. [47] reported minimally higher costs for TEPP than for TAPP. Similarly, there was no difference in recurrence rate. Hamza et al.'s RCT found no difference in operating time, postoperative complications, postoperative pain, time to return to normal activity, and recurrence rates between TEPP and TAPP [46]. Gong et al. also found no difference in surgery time, postoperative complication rate, hospitalization, postoperative pain, and time to return to normal activities [48].

Günal et al.'s RCT also found no difference between TEPP and TAPP in postoperative complications, postoperative pain, or recurrence rate [49]. Therefore, it is clear that few RCTs with a small sample size are available for comparison of TEPP and TAPP for selective primary unilateral inguinal hernia repair in men. However, these RCTs found no difference for most of the results examined.

These results have been recently confirmed through the Herniamed hernia registry [50]. Kockerling et al. compared the results of 14,426 TEPP with 14,426 TAPPs performed through scheduled operations for primitive unilateral inguinal hernias in male patients and found no difference in intraoperative complications, complication-related reoperation, recurrence rate, and pain [50]. They found only a significant disadvantage of TAPP for postoperative complications (3.0% vs. 1.7%) due to the higher seroma rate in TAPP. However, the bleeding rate was higher in TEPP at 0.8% versus 1.1%. The higher rate of postoperative complication for TAPP, to be handled very carefully, could be partly explained by larger defects, more scrotal hernias, and older age. They concluded that a large registry analysis found no significant difference between TAPP versus TEPP regarding the outcome of selective primary unilateral hernia repair in men.

Again from the Herniamed registry, other results are available as to the analysis between TEPP and TAPP for the treatment of recurrent hernia following previous open primary surgery [1]. There was no difference in other postoperative complications between TEPP and TAPP for recurrent hernia repair.

Another important topic about TAPP and TEPP is a theoretically higher risk of bleeding than OR due to the extensive dissection involved. This problem has always been analyzed on the basis of data collected in Herniamed's registry [51]. Of 82,911 patients in the Herniamed registry who had undergone inguinal hernia repair, 11% were operated on while receiving antithrombotic therapy or with existing coagulopathy [51]. The secondary postoperative bleeding rate (3.91%) was significantly higher (quadrupled) in patients with coagulopathy or antithrombotic therapy than in the group without that 1.12% risk profile. The multivariable analysis also showed that open surgery, older age, higher ASA score, recurrence, male, and a large hernia defect were factors associated with a higher risk of postoperative bleeding. Patients receiving antithrombotic therapy or with existing coagulopathy who undergo inguinal hernia surgery have a fourfold increased risk for postoperative secondary bleeding [51]. The authors concluded that, despite the extensive dissection required during TEPP and

TAPP, the risk of hemorrhagic complications and complication-related surgery appears to be lower than OR [51].

Other important factors recently investigated are sexual function and fertility rates after a different approach for IHR. Many patients with inguinal hernia complain of preoperative sexual dysfunction. IHR should relieve these preoperative symptoms. There have been few studies that have examined the impact of IHR on sexual function.

A study based on a questionnaire conducted by Schouten et al. with 500 male patients undergoing TEPP found that one third of patients had pain from sexual activity [52]. In contrast, in a Danish national questionnaire study, Bischoff et al. found that dysfunction and reduced sexual activity due to pain was a significant problem after LIHR [53].

In a study by Štula et al., 53% of patients undergoing TAPP had antisperm antibodies (ASA) which is the only marker for the measurement of nonfertility [54]. A recent RCT was designed to compare sexual function, effect on fertility indices, sperm quality, and the presence of ASA in patients undergoing inguinal hernia in the operating room, TEPP, and TAPP [55]. The study included 121 patients with 41 patients in the TAPP group (Group 1), 40 in the TEPP group (Group 2), and the remainder in the OR group (Group 3). They concluded that CSR, OR, TEPP, or TAPP lead to improved sexual function and fertility indices and can have a significant impact on the patient's preoperative counseling in terms of choice of repair, depending on the expertise available in a particular hospital center [55]. A previous RCT from Bansal et al. comparing testicular and sexual function and quality of life following TAPP and TEPP for IHR, found that LHR improves testicular function, sexual function, and quality of life, but TEPP and TAPP are comparable in terms of long-term results [56].

Regarding the problem of incarcerated hernia in the elderly and frail patient, there are no RCTs and meta-analyses comparing TAPP and TEPP, so the results are those referable to retrospective monocentric studies, also in case history patients are heterogeneous in sex, age, comorbidity, and types of hernia. Ceresoli et al. have shown through a multivariate analysis that some comorbidities are independently associated with major complications of hernioplasty [19]. In addition, postoperative hospitalization, regardless of whether associated with intestinal resection, is greater in patients operated laparoscopically than those operated with open technique, and also for this reason, some surgeons do not prefer the laparoscopic approach. In literature, the surgical technique is the same as the one used for scheduled operations, however, we believe that it is advisable to perform the surgery with a 30° optic and to place at least two 10 mm trocars to allow the insertion of gauze and stitches without having to repeatedly extract the optics losing time and concentration. The positioning of the bladder catheter is not carried out routinely in scheduled operations, but it is advisable to position it in emergency situations especially in the elderly patient, to monitor diuresis possibly also postoperatively. Antibiotic prophylaxis according to the International Guidelines may not be performed, but during operations for incarcerated hernias it is advisable for possible bacterial translocation especially when an intestinal loop is incarcerated [1]. Leibl et al. also recommended to wash the abdominal cavity and remove any liquid; according to our experience, it is advisable to perform a culture swab of the liquid in order to choose a targeted antibiotic therapy [57]. The reduction of the intestinal loop or the contents is not always possible so, as recommended by Leibl et al., it is useful to make an incision in the inner groin ring to facilitate the reduction of the contents of the herniated sac [57]. In case of intestinal necrosis, the positioning of the mesh is still a question of debate, however, we believe that if contamination is reduced, it is possible to perform it safely [13]. The first advantage of using the laparoscopic technique is to perform an exploration of the abdominal cavity to verify the vitality of the intestinal loop. In the past, a mixed technique was recommended that would allow the exploration of the abdominal cavity by inserting the optics through the inguinal ring, and despite various limitations, it can still be considered suitable, especially in the fragile patient [13, 14]. The second advantage of the laparoscopic technique is the possibility to treat the hernia once the sac is reduced and while waiting and observing the state of the intestine to decide whether to resect it [13, 14]. We do not believe that, in the presence of a contralateral hernia, should plastic surgery be performed also on a possible asymptomatic hernia. In conclusion, following our experience, the treatment of incarcerated inguinal hernia should not be considered the gold standard and should be performed by experienced surgeons. An incarcerated hernia in the elderly and frail patient can be treated laparoscopically, but both surgeon and anesthesiologist must carefully evaluate the patient's general and abdominal conditions to avoid canceling the positive effects of laparoscopic surgery.

Five Things You Should Know About Incarcerated Inguinal and Crural Hernias in the Elderly and Frail Patient

- There is no evidence supporting an optimal approach for strangulated or incarcerated groin hernia.
- The time from onset to surgery is the most important prognostic factor in patients with strangulated groin hernias.
- Abdominal contrast-enhanced computed tomography (CT) provides important information about wall hernias and their contents.
- Laparoscopy may be a useful tool with the target of assessing bowel viability after spontaneous or manual reduction of hernia.
- An incarcerated hernia in the elderly and frail patient can be treated laparoscopically, but both surgeon and anesthesiologist must carefully evaluate the patient's general and abdominal conditions.

References

1. The Hernia Surge Group International guidelines for groin hernia management. Hernia 2018;22(1):1–165.
2. Kingsnorth A, LeBlanc K. Hernias: inguinal and incisional. Lancet. 2003;362:1561–71.
3. Fitzgibbons RJ, Ramanan B, Arya S, et al. Long-term results of a randomized controlled trial of a nonoperative strategy (watchful waiting) for men with minimally symptomatic inguinal hernias. Ann Surg. 2013;258(3):508–15.
4. Amato B, Moja L, Panico G et al. Should ice technique versus other open techniques for inguinal hernia repair. Cochrane Database Syst Rev. 2012;(4):CD001543.
5. De Luca M, Angrisani L, Himpens J, Busetto L, Scopinaro N, Weiner R, Sartori A, Stier C, Lakdawala M, Bhasker AG, Buchwald H, Dixon J, Chiappetta S, Kolberg HC, Sarwer DB, Suter M, Soricelli E, Bluher M, Villalonga R, Sharma A, Shikora S. Obes Surg. 2016;26(8):1659–96.
6. Rosemar A, Angeras U, Rosengren A, Nordin P. Effect of body mass index on groin hernia surgery. Ann Surg. 2010;252(2):397–401.
7. Rosemar A, Angerås U, Rosengren A. Body mass index and groin hernia: a 34-year follow-up study in Swedish men. Ann Surg. 2008;247(6):1064–8.
8. Ichioka K, Kohei N, Yoshimura K, Arai Y, Terai A. Impact of retraction of vas deferens in post-radical prostatectomy inguinal hernia. Urology. 2007;70(3):511–4.
9. Rosch R, Junge K, Knops M, Lynen P, Klinge U, Schumpelick V. Analysis of collagen-interacting proteins in patients with incisional hernias. Langenbeck's Arch Surg. 2003;387(11–12):427–32.
10. Zheng H, Si Z, Kasperk R, Bhardwaj SR, Schumpelick V, Klinge U, Klosterhalfen B. Recurrent inguinal hernia: disease of the collagen matrix? World J Surg. 2002;26(4):401–8.
11. Ortman JM, Velkoff VA, Hogan H. An aging nation: the older population in the United States population estimates and projections. Curr Popul Rep. 2016;2014:24–1145.
12. Etzioni DA, Liu JH, Maggard MA, Ko CY. The aging population and its impact on the surgery workforce. Ann Surg. 2003;238(2):170.
13. Mancini R, Pattaro G, Spaziani E. Laparoscopic trans-abdominal pre-peritoneal (TAPP) surgery for incarcerated inguinal hernia repair. Hernia. 2019;23:261–6.
14. Legnani GL, Rasini M, Pastori S, Sarli D. Laparoscopic trans-peritoneal hernioplasty (TAPP) for the acute management of strangulated inguino-crural hernias: a report of nine cases. Hernia. 2008;12:185–8.
15. Subramaniam S, Aalberg JJ, Divino CM. Age stratified analysis of pre-operative factors impacting unplanned thirty day readmission in geriatric general surgery. Am J Surg. 2019;218:77–81.
16. Polanczyk CA, Marcantonio E, Goldman L, et al. Impact of age on perioperative complications and length of stay in patients undergoing noncardiac surgery. Ann Intern Med. 2001;134(8):637–43.
17. Hamel MB, Henderson WG, Khuri SF, Daley J. Surgical outcomes for patients aged 80 and older: morbidity and mortality from major noncardiac surgery. J Am Geriatr Soc. 2005;53(3):424–9.
18. Gallegos NC, Dawson J, Jarvis M, Hobsley M. Risk of strangulation in groin hernias. Br J Surg. 1991;78:1171–3.

19. Ceresoli M, Carissimi F, Nigro A, Lepre L, Braga M, Costa G. List of Elderly Risk Assessment and surgical Outcome (ERASO) Emergency hernia repair in the elderly: multivariate analysis of morbidity and mortality from an Italian registry. Hernia. 2020.
20. Koizumi M, Sata N, Kaneda Y, Endo K, Sasanuma H, Sakuma Y, Ota M, Lefor AT, Yasuda Y. Optimal timeline for emergency surgery in patients with strangulated groin hernias. Hernia. 2014;18:845–8.
21. Kulah B, Duzgun AP, Moran M, Kulacoglu IH, Ozmen MM, Coskun F. Emergency hernia repairs in elderly patients. Am J Surg. 2001;182:455–9.
22. Kulah B, Kulacoglu IH, Oruc MT, Duzgun AP, Moran M, Ozmen MM, Coskun F. Presentation and outcome of incarcerated external hernias in adults. Am J Surg. 2001;181:101–4.
23. Rai S, Chandra SS, Smile SR. A study of the risk of strangulation and obstruction in groin hernias. Aust N Z J Surg. 1998;68:650–4.
24. Watson SD, Saye W, Hollier PA. Combined laparoscopic incarcerated herniorrhaphy and small bowel resection. Surg Laparosc Endosc. 1993;3:106–8.
25. Berger M, Acker L, Deiner S. Chapter 65. Geriatric anesthesia. In: Miller's anesthesia. 9th ed. Elsevier; 2020. pp. 2102–2114.
26. O'Connor K, Parekh R. Chapter 60. Laparoscopic surgery. In: Anesthesia secrets. 6th ed. pp. 385–387.
27. Gerges FJ, Kanazi GE, Jabbour-khoury SI. Anesthesia for laparoscopy. J Clin Anesth. 2006;18:67–78.
28. Luba K. Chapter 46. Complications of laparoscopic surgery. In: Complications in anesthesia. Elsevier; 2018. pp. 185–188.
29. Irwin MG, Ip KY, Hui YM. Anesthetic considerations in nonagenarians and centenarians. Curr Opin Anesthesiol. 2019;32:776–82.
30. Mayhew D, Mendonca V, Murthy BVS. A review of ASA physical status—historical perspectives and modern developments. Anaesthesia. 2019;74(3):373–9.
31. Jin Z, Hu J, Ma D. Postoperative delirium: perioperative assessment, risk reduction, and management. Br J Anaesth. 2020;125(4):492–504.
32. Hughes CG, Boncyk CS, Culley DJ, et al.; Perioperative Quality Initiative (POQI) 6 Workgroup. American Society for Enhanced Recovery and Perioperative Quality Initiative joint consensus statement on postoperative delirium prevention. Anesth Analg. 2020;130(6):1572–1590.
33. Sarakatsianou C, Gerogopoulou S, Baloyiannis I, Chatzimichail M, Vretzakis G, Zacharoulis D, Tzorvaras G. Spinal versus general anesthesia for transabdominal preperitoneal (TAPP) repair of inguinal hernia: interim analysis of a controlled randomized trial. Am J Surg. 2017;214(2):239–45.
34. Arregui ME, Davis CJ, Yucel O. Laparoscopic mesh repair in inguinal hernia using a preperitoneal approach: a preliminary report. Surg Laparosc Endosc. 1992;2:53–8.
35. Stoppa RE, Petit J, Henry X. Unsutured Dacron prosthesis in groin hernias. Int Surg. 1975;60(8):411–2.
36. Bittner R, Schwarz J. Primary unilateral not complicated inguinal hernia: our choice of TAPP, why, results and review of literature. Hernia. 2019;23:417–28.
37. Gass M, Scheiwiller A, Sykora M, Metzger J. TAPP or TEP for recurrent inguinal hernia? Population-based analysis of prospective data on 1309 patients undergoing endoscopic repair for recurrent inguinal hernia. World J Surg. 2016;40(10):2348–52. https://doi.org/10.1007/s00268-016-3545-7.
38. Kockerling F. TEP for elective primary unilateral inguinal hernia repair in men: what do we know? Hernia. 2019;23:439–59.
39. Bracale U, Melillo P, Pignata G, Di Salvo E, Rovani M, Merola G, Pecchia L. Which is the best laparoscopic approach for inguinal hernia repair: TEP or TAPP? A systematic review of the literature with a network meta-analysis. Surg Endosc. 2012;26:3355–66.
40. McCormack K, Wake BL, Fraser C, Vale L, Perez J, Grant A. Transabdominal pre-peritoneal (TAPP) versus totally extraperitoneal (TEP) laparoscopic techniques for inguinal hernia repair: a systematic review. Hernia. 2005;9:109–14.
41. Wake BL, McCormack K, Fraser C, Vale L, Perez J, Grant A Transabdominal pre-peritoneal (TAPP) versus totally extraperitoneal (TEP) laparoscopic techniques for inguinal hernia repair: (review). Cochrane Database Syst Rev. 2005. https://doi.org/10.1002/14651858.CD004703.pub2.
42. Wei FX, Zhang YC, Wei H, Zhang YL, Shao Y, Ni R. Transabdominal pre-peritoneal (TAPP) versus totally extraperitoneal (TEP) for laparoscopic hernia repair: a meta-analysis. Surg Laparosc Endosc Percutan Tech. 2015;25:375–83. https://doi.org/10.1097/SLE.0000000000000123.
43. Antoniou SA, Antoniou GA, Bartsch DK, Fendrich V, Koch OO, Pointner R, Granderath FA. Transabdominal preperitoneal versus totally extraperitoneal repair of inguinal hernia: a meta-analysis of randomized studies. Am J Surg. 2013;206:245–52.
44. Chen LS, Chen WC, Kang YN, Wu CC, Tsai LW, Liu MZ. Effects of transabdominal preperitoneal and totally extraperitoneal inguinal hernia repair: an update systematic review and meta-analysis of randomized controlled trials. Surg Endosc. 2019;33:418–28.
45. Köckerling F, Stechemesser B, Hukauf M, Kuthe A, Schug-Pass C. TEP vs Lichtenstein: which technique is better for the repair of primary unilateral inguinal hernias in men? Surg Endosc. 2015;30:3304–13.
46. Hamza Y, Gabr E, Hammadi H, Khalil R. Four-arm randomized trial comparing laparoscopic and open hernia repairs. Int J Surg. 2010;8:25–8.
47. Butler RE, Burke R, Schneider JJ, Brar H, Lucha PA Jr. The economic impact of laparoscopic inguinal hernia repair: results of a double-blinded, prospective, randomized trial. Surg Endosc. 2007;21:387–90.
48. Gong K, Zhang N, Lu Y, Zhu B, Zhang Z, Du D, Zhao X, Jiang H. Comparison of the open tension-free mesh-plug, transabdominal preperitoneal (TAPP), and totally extraperitoneal (TEP) laparoscopic tech-

niques for primary unilateral inguinal hernia repair: a prospective randomized controlled trial. Surg Endosc. 2011;25:234–9.
49. Günal Ö, Özer S, Gürleyik E, Bahcebasi T. Does the approach to the groin make a difference in hernia repair? Hernia. 2007;11:429–34.
50. Köckerling F, Bittner R, Kofler M, Mayer F, Adolf D, Kuthe A, Weyhe D. Lichtenstein versus total extra-peritoneal patch plasty versus transabdominal patch plasty technique for primary unilateral inguinal hernia repair. Ann Surg. 2017;15:15–85.
51. Kockerling F, Bittner R, Jacob DA, Seidelmann L, Keller T, Adolf D, Kraft B, Kuthe A. TEP versus TAPP: comparison of the perioperative outcome in 17,587 patients with a primary unilateral inguinal hernia. Surg Endosc. 2015;29:3750–60.
52. Schouten N, van Dalen T, Smakman N, Clevers GJ, Davids PHP, Verleisdonk EJMM, Tekatli H, Burgmans JP. Impairment of sexual activity before and after endoscopic totally extraperitoneal (TEP) hernia repair. Surg Endosc. 2012;26(1):230–4.
53. Bischoff JM, Linderoth G, Aasvang EK, Werner MU, Kehlet H. Dysejaculation after laparoscopic inguinal herniorrhaphy a nationwide questionnaire study. Surg Endosc. 2012;26(4):979–83.
54. Štula I, Družijanić N, Sapunar A, Perko Z, Bošnjak N, Kraljević D. Antisperm antibodies and testicular blood flow after inguinal hernia mesh repair. Surg Endosc. 2014;28(12):3413–20.
55. Gupta S, Krishna A, Jain M, Goyal A, Kumar A, Chaturvedi P, Sagar R, Ramachandran R, Prakash O, Kumar S, Seenu V, Bansal V. A three-arm randomized study to compare sexual functions and fertility indices following open mesh hernioplasty (OMH), laparoscopic totally extra peritoneal (TEP) and transabdominal preperitoneal (TAPP) repair of groin hernia. Surg Endosc. 2021;35(6):3077–84.
56. Bansal VK, Krishna A, Manek P, Kumar S, Prajapati O, Subramaniam R, Kumar A, Kumar A, Sagar R, Misra MC. A prospective randomized comparison of testicular functions, sexual functions and quality of life following laparoscopic totally extra-peritoneal (TEP) and trans-abdominal pre-peritoneal (TAPP) inguinal hernia repairs. Surg Endosc. 2017;31(3):1478–86.
57. Leibl BJ, Schnedt CG, Kraft K, Kraft B, Bittner R. Laparoscopic transperitoneal hernia repair of incarcerated hernias: is it feasible? Results of a prospective study. Surg Endosc. 2001;15(10):1179–83.

Incarcerated Incisional and Ventral Hernias in the Elderly and Frail Patient

19

Diego Cuccurullo, Carlo Sagnelli, Ernesto Tartaglia, and Giovanni D'Alterio

19.1 Introduction

Many studies have focused on the "frail elderly," although the criteria used for this population's definition are still unstandardized [1]. Conventionally, "elderly" has been defined as a chronological age of 65 years old or older. This is the fastest-growing sector of society. Frailty is conceptually defined as a clinically recognizable state in which older people's ability to cope with everyday or acute stressors is compromised by an increased vulnerability brought by the age-associated decline in physiological reserve and function across multiple organ systems. The growing importance of elderly patients in national health care systems is well documented because it can raise medical costs and affect patient quality of life.

Laparoscopic surgery has been widely accepted as a minimally invasive treatment to reduce the morbidity after conventional surgery, and several studies have demonstrated the feasibility of laparoscopy in the elderly with advantages that include improved quality of life, a minimal degree of pain, shorter hospital stay, early rehabilitation, and early return to social activity. Despite underlying comorbidities, patients older than 65 years tolerate laparoscopic procedures exceptionally well. Abdominal hernia repair is one of the most common procedures performed by general surgeons, with more than 200,000 done each year in the United States [2]. Treatment for incarcerated hernia is often delayed in elderly and frail patients due to unresponsiveness and insensitiveness to local pain, but an early diagnosis is fundamental to avoid strangulation [3, 4]. Strangulation is a potentially fatal complication of a hernia and should always be considered a surgical emergency. The risk is maximal in small- to medium-sized defects. In large and extensive defects, the viscera are often permanently herniated and if this goes on over an extended period of time, the risk of 'loss of domain (LOD) within the proper abdominal cavity can emerge. This means that the remaining lateral abdominal wall tissues chronically retract and there may be insufficient room for all the viscera within the revised abdominal cavity when the tissues are re-approximated. In patients with LOD hernias, the abdominal cavity is unable to fully accommodate the abdominal contents within its fascial boundaries, and the closure of the fascia can lead to high intra-abdominal pressures or abdominal compartment syndrome. Despite the prevalence of abdominal wall reconstruction procedures, there is little consensus about the indications for repair, optimum technique, or appropriate position of the prosthetic mesh. Given the wide variety of patient and hernia factors, no single approach will likely fit all abdominal wall repair types. Most surgeons agree that all incisional hernias should be repaired with

D. Cuccurullo (✉) · C. Sagnelli · E. Tartaglia
G. D'Alterio
Department of General Surgery, Monaldi Hospital, Naples, Italy

F. Agresta et al. (eds.), *Emergency laparoscopic surgery in the elderly and frail patient*,
https://doi.org/10.1007/978-3-030-79990-8_19

a prosthetic (synthetic or biologic or biosynthetic) mesh because recurrence rates are 10% after indirect repair. Conversely, following prosthetic procedures, the rate is reduced to 2.7% [5].

A prosthetic mesh can be placed as an in-lay (sewn to the fascial edge), an on-lay (sewn above the fascia), or a sub-lay (underneath the fascia). Subway mesh can be placed in the intraperitoneal, preperitoneal, or retro-rectus space. The in-lay (bridge technique) approach has been largely abandoned because of high recurrence rates. The on-lay (Chevrel technique) approach is discouraged because when the prosthetic mesh is placed in the subcutaneous position, it is at high risk for mesh infection. Most hernia surgeons agree that the prosthetic mesh should be placed as a sub-lay. Surgical options include the laparoscopic technique, robotic transabdominal retromuscular umbilical prosthetic (TARUP) repair, or an open repair [6].

19.2 Pathophysiology

The higher incidence of incisional hernias in the elderly could be attributed to several factors, and is thought to be a multifactorial process. Systemic chronic diseases like obesity, renal failure, diabetes, malnutrition, smoking, or long-term systemic medications including immunosuppressants and steroids, increase the likelihood of developing an incisional hernia. It should also be considered that the prevalence of comorbidities could lead to increased intraabdominal pressure, including constipation, ascites, hypertrophy of the prostate, or connective tissue disorders [7]. The high recurrence rate has emphasized the importance of research in the development of high-quality mesh materials. It has prompted further studies on primary tissue healing mechanisms and scar formation. The exact pathophysiology of abdominal wall hernias is believed to be multifactorial. Collagen is the principal component of the extracellular matrix of both primary and scar tissue. Balanced collagen maturation and degradation are a requirement for normal scar formation. Studies showed a decreased collagen I/III ratio in direct skin and fascia biopsies of patients with recurrent incisional hernias. They strongly suggested that the abnormal collagen metabolism in these patients leads to an impaired wound healing through an impaired constitutive collagen expression and formation [8].

Chronically increased intraabdominal pressure predisposes the weakest abdominal wall areas to develop hernias. Several risk factors for the early development of incisional hernias, such as wound infection and wrong suture technique have been suggested. Elderly patients, especially those older than 80, have associated several comorbid diseases and high American Society of Anesthesiologists (ASA) scores, thus putting these patients at a greater risk of intra- and postoperative complications that can favor the formation of the incisional hernia [9].

Treatment for incarcerated hernia is often delayed in elderly and frail patients due to unresponsiveness and insensitiveness to local pain. As the incarceration persists, venous reflux disorders will first occur with partial arterial perfusion to hernia contents. When the bowel is involved in the incarcerated hernial content, intestinal obstruction can result, with a considerable risk of bowel ischemia and necrosis.

19.3 Diagnosis

Preoperative imaging of the abdominal wall can help delineate the hernia's location, size, and complexity. In all patients undergoing complex abdominal surgery, the gold standard is abdominal pelvic unenhanced computed tomography (CT) scan at rest and during the Valsalva maneuver. CT is helpful to identify the presence of and the size of the defect. In emergency settings, when during the physical examination the surgeon suspects concomitant bowel strangulation inside the hernia sac, a contrast-enhanced CT scan should be carried out.

19.4 Identification of the Presence of Incarceration

Full exposure of the abdomen is required during physical examination. An incarcerated hernia is associated with poor prognosis, and it should be thus suspected if any of the following clinical findings are detected: severe abdominal pain, sepsis or septic shock, peritonitis, fever, tachycardia and leukocytosis with neutrophilia, bloody fluid in vomit or stools, and palpable and tender intestinal loops with rebound tenderness.

19.5 Preoperative Preparation

The effects of the aging process do not usually affect organ functions in normal conditions. However, during periods of stress (such as surgical procedures or prolonged illness), elderly patients may not meet the increased metabolic demand. Specific considerations must be given to the proper management of fluid and electrolyte replacement [10].

A comprehensive assessment before surgery must be carried out in elective surgery to exclude contraindications for general anesthesia (such as cirrhosis, severe heart, and lung disease). Physical examination is done to determine whether there are predisposing conditions that require particular perioperative attention, such as respiratory function assessment to prevent atelectasis and pneumonia, monitoring for possible cardiac complications, obesity, diabetes, hormone therapy, skin infections, cirrhosis, use of immunosuppressive agents, and immune dysfunction. We perform one-shot intravenous administration of Cefazolin 2 g, 30 min before surgery, unless the operation involves dissecting the bowel or the infarcted omentum. In case of intestinal obstruction, the insertion of a nasogastric tube is mandatory before inducing anesthesia, to hold the intestinal loops and avoid "ab ingestis" events.

19.6 Laparoscopic Technique

Despite extensive experience and considerable reduction of complications in recent years, laparoscopic treatment of complex abdominal hernias is a challenge even for the experienced laparoscopic surgeon. Laparoscopic repair of ventral and incisional hernias was introduced by Karl LeBlanc in 1993 [11]. Today, a laparoscopic approach is recommended to treat recurrent ventral hernias and obese patients, while it is a potential option for compensated cirrhotic and childbearing-age female patients [12].

The patient is usually placed in the supine position and the surgeon chooses the location of the trocars at the moment of surgery. In most cases, we put the first 10-mm trocar on the transverse umbilical line in the right upper quadrant, the second 10-mm trocar on the right iliac fossa on the anterior axillary line in the right lower quadrant, and an additional 5-mm trocar is placed in the right hypochondrium for the left hand of the first operator.

The abdominal skin is prepared following the conventional laparoscopic practice. The umbilical area is washed, and the patient is instructed to empty the bladder. The surgery is usually performed without an indwelling catheter. However, one can be placed for better operative field exposure after anesthesia, and removed on completion of the surgery.

The first step is the induction of the pneumoperitoneum with an open-Verres-assisted technique and the cautious access to the abdominal cavity.

The 10-mm trocar for the videoscope is placed in the lateral abdominal position. This large port site is also needed for the passage of the rolled-up mesh through the abdominal wall.

Under the laparoscopic vision, reduction of hernia contents is first attempted with squeezing from outside following the same procedures as in manual reduction. The procedure should be gently done. Sometimes, the external palpation and pressure to aid hernia contents reduction and exposure for adhesiolysis are helpful. Working space to conduct the adhesiolysis and repair may be limited. In the case of failure, the contents can be returned with the help of noninvasive intestinal forceps. The preferred site for retraction is the greater omentum, followed by the bowel. If the procedure still fails to return the hernial contents, forced retraction should be avoided. In this case, we can use bipolar forceps to dehydrate the omentum, or we can make a 1–2 cm incision to the narrow hernial ring. The omentum that is difficult to return can be resected, if necessary, followed by high ligation of the hernia sac and suture closure by layer before continuing the laparoscopic surgery.

When incarcerated hernia contents are returned into the abdomen, they can be flipped in the abdominal cavity to assess the presence of any damage, intestinal peristalsis, leakage of intestinal contents, elasticity, color, mesenteric artery pulses, and so on, to establish a comprehensive assessment of the strangulation.

Reestablishing the linea alba is an essential concept in abdominal wall reconstruction. Suppose the linea alba is seen as the tendinous insertion of the rectus abdominis muscle and oblique muscles; in that case, it is critical to achieving appropriate physiologic loading of the abdominal wall. It will allow us to have more contact surface between the peritoneal surface and the mesh. Since the approximation of the linea alba is rigid and uneasy with laparoscopic techniques, we proceed to close the defect according to the Chelala technique [13].

The measurement of the size of the defect after reducing the pneumoperitoneum is crucial for the surgery's success, both for what concerns the success of the intervention and an adequate choice of the mesh (Fig. 19.1).

The hernial orifices are closed by an extracorporeal suture technique with nonabsorbable monofilament sutures. The needle is inserted near the left edge of the defect, and once introduced into the abdominal cavity, the stitch is passed with the U-reversal technique. It is subsequently knotted on the outside, disappearing into the subcutaneous layer (Fig. 19.2).

An appropriately sized prosthetic mesh is tailored to overlap all the defect margins in each direction by at least 5 cm. The overlap is always calculated based on the size of the original defect. The possible closure of the defect would not allow us to reduce the overlap or mesh size. Points of reference on the mesh and corresponding points on the abdominal wall are marked to help orient the mesh after its introduction into the abdomen. The mesh is rolled up and is pushed into the abdomen through the 10-mm trocar.

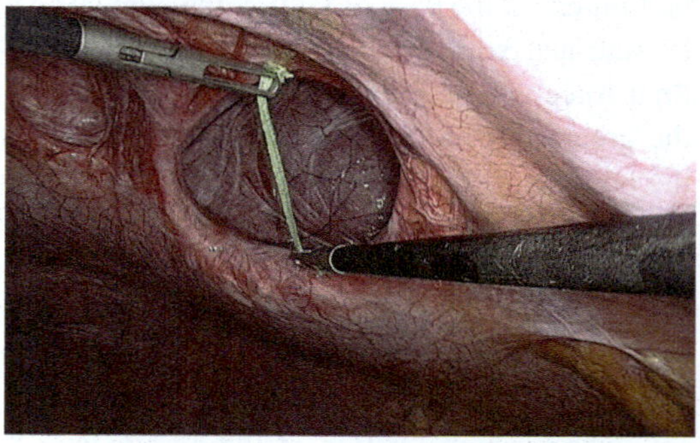

Fig. 19.1 Hernia defect was measured

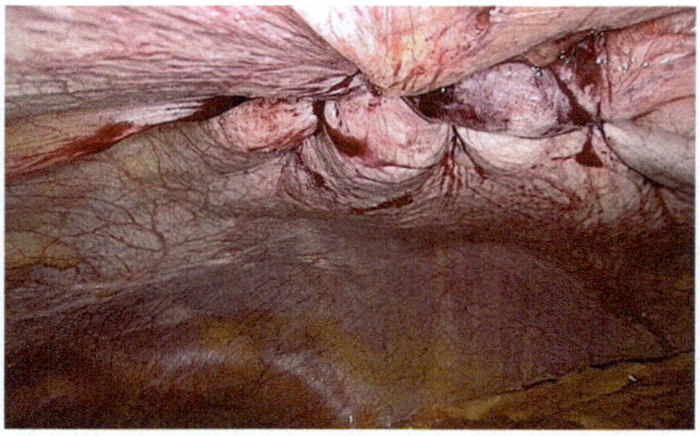

Fig. 19.2 Re-approximation of Linea Alba (laparoscopic image)

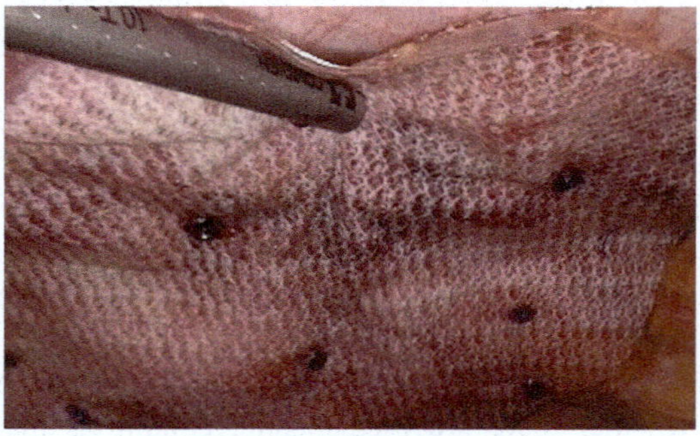

Fig. 19.3 "Chips chocolate cookie" (laparoscopic image)

After the mesh is positioned intracorporeally, the sutures are placed in the material before its insertion into the abdomen. The mesh is pulled through the abdominal wall with a Reverdin needle and tied with the knots buried subcutaneously. Additional full-thickness sutures are placed with a device for positioning totally absorbable takers, which are arranged according to an order defined as a "chips chocolate cookie" (Fig. 19.3), with particular attention not to leave spaces in which viscera could enter.

No drains are inserted. Fascial closure with sutures is performed at all 12–10 mm trocar sites.

To achieve early recovery after surgical procedures by maintaining preoperative organ function and reducing the stress response following surgery, the patient begins early feeding and spontaneous mobilization.

In specific situations, such as large defects or entero-atmospheric fistulas, we prefer an open technique [posterior component separation with transversus abdominis release (Rives, PCS + TAR)]. In these cases, particular attention must be given to avoid the onset of a compartment syndrome. Likewise, the laparoscopic approach is safe and effective for defects larger than 3 cm in diameter; old age, obesity, previous abdominal operations, recurrence, and strangulation are not absolute contraindications. Despite underlying comorbidities, individuals older than 65 years tolerate laparoscopic procedures exceptionally well. Complications and hospitalization are lower than in open procedures [14]. Ensuring an adequate overlap, careful adhesiolysis and correct prosthesis fixation are among the technical details recommended [15].

19.7 Conclusions

Laparoscopy for treatment of ventral and incisional abdominal wall hernias in elderly and frail patients is effective and advantageous in terms of improved postoperative outcomes, with reduction of short-term complications, including wound infection, deep vein thrombosis, metabolic, and electrolyte imbalances. Early mobilization, early resumption of the oral intake, and less postoperative hospital stay are among the most relevant advantages of minimally invasive surgery.

Five Things You Should Know About the Emergency Laparoscopic Approach in Incarcerated Incisional and Ventral Hernias in the Elderly and Frail Patient

- Treatment for incarcerated hernia is often delayed in elderly and frail patients due to unresponsiveness and insensitive to local pain. An early diagnosis is fundamental to avoid strangulation.
- Strangulation is a potentially fatal complication of a hernia and should always be considered a surgical emergency. The risk is maximal in small- to-medium-sized defects. In large defects, the viscera are often permanently herniated and if this goes on over an extended period of time, the risk of they 'loss of domain' (LOD) within the actual abdominal cavity, can emerge.
- Despite the prevalence of this procedure, there is little consensus about the indications for repair, optimum technique, or appropriate position of the prosthetic mesh in abdominal wall reconstruction. Given the wide variety of patient and hernia factors, no single approach will likely suffice to repair all abdominal wall defects.
- Most surgeons agree that all incisional hernias should be repaired with prosthetic (synthetic or biologic or biosynthetic) mesh because recurrence rates are almost 10% following direct repair. In contrast, in prosthetic procedures, the rate is reduced to 2.7%.
- Laparoscopy seems to be a good option also in elderly and frail patients with ventral or incisional hernia.

References

1. Preston SD, Southal AR, Nel M, Das SK. Geriatric surgery is about disease, not age. J R Soc Med. 2008;101(8):409–15. https://doi.org/10.1258/jrsm.2008.080035.
2. Rutkow IM. Demographic and socioeconomic aspects of hernia repair in the United States in 2003. Surg Clin N Am. 2003;83(5):1045–51, v–vi.
3. Lindmark M, Strigård K, Löwenmark T, Dahlstrand U, Gunnarsson U. Risk factors for surgical complications in ventral hernia repair. World J Surg. 2018;42(11):3528–36. https://doi.org/10.1007/s00268-018-4642-6).
4. Claes K, Beckers R, Heindryckx E, et al. Retrospective observational study on the incidence of incisional hernias after colorectal carcinoma resection with follow-up CT scan. Hernia. 2014;18:797–802.
5. Nguyen MT, Berger RL, Hicks SC, Davila JA, Li LT, Kao LS, Liang MK. Comparison of outcomes of synthetic mesh vs suture repair of elective primary ventral herniorrhaphy: a systematic review and meta-analysis. JAMA Surg. 2014;149(5):415–21. https://doi.org/10.1001/jamasurg.2013.5014. PMID: 24554114.

6. Museums F, Van Cleven S, Pletinckx P, et al. Robotic transabdominal retromuscular umbilical prosthetic hernia repair (TARUP): observational study on the operative time during the learning curve. Hernia. 2018;22:1101–11. https://doi.org/10.1007/s10029-018-1825-x.
7. Fischer JP, Wink JD, Nelson JA, Kovach SJ. Among 1,706 cases of abdominal wall reconstruction, what factors influence the occurrence of major operative complications? Surgery. 2014;155(2):311–9. issn:0039-6060. https://doi.org/10.1016/j.surg.2013.08.014.
8. White B, Osier C, Gletsu N, et al. Abnormal primary tissue collagen composition in the skin of recurrent incisional hernia patients. Am Surg. 2007;73(12):1254–8. https://doi.org/10.1177/000313480707301213.
9. Caglià P, Tracia A, Borzì L, Amodeo L, Tracia L, Leroux M, Amodeo C. Incisional hernia in the elderly: risk factors and clinical considerations. Int J Surg. 2014;12(Suppl 2):S164–9. https://doi.org/10.1016/j.ijsu.2014.08.357. Epub 2014 Aug 23. PMID: 25157994.
10. Evers BM, Townsend CM Jr, Thompson JC. Organ physiology of aging. Surg Clin N Am. 1994;74(1):23–39. https://doi.org/10.1016/s0039-6109(16)46226-2. PMID: 8108769.
11. LeBlanc KA, Booth WV. Laparoscopic repair of incisional abdominal hernias using expanded polytetrafluoroethylene: preliminary findings. Surg Laparosc Endosc. 1993;3(1):39–41. PMID: 8258069.
12. Silecchia G, Campanile FC, Sanchez L, Cuccurullo D, et al. Laparoscopic ventral/incisional hernia repair: updated consensus development conference based guidelines [corrected] [published correction appears in Surg Endosc. 2015 Sep;29(9):2485]. Surg Endosc. 2015;29(9):2463–84. https://doi.org/10.1007/s00464-015-4293-8.
13. Chelala E, Baraké H, Estievenart J, Dessily M, Charara F, Allé JL. Long-term outcomes of 1326 laparoscopic incisional and ventral hernia repair with the routine suturing concept: a single institution experience. Hernia. 2016;20(1):101–10. https://doi.org/10.1007/s10029-015-1397-y.
14. Weber DM. Laparoscopic surgery: an excellent approach in elderly patients. Arch Surg. 2003;138(10):1083–8. https://doi.org/10.1001/archsurg.138.10.1083. PMID: 14557124.
15. Cuccurullo D, Piccoli M, Agresta F, Magnone S, Corcione F, Stancanelli V, Melotti G. Laparoscopic ventral incisional hernia repair: evidence-based guidelines of the first Italian consensus conference. Hernia. 2013;17(5):557–66. https://doi.org/10.1007/s10029-013-1055-1. Epub 2013 Feb 12. PMID: 23400528.

20 Abdominal Trauma in the Elderly

Francesco Virdis, Matthew Martin, Mansoor Khan,
Isabella Reccia, Gaetano Gallo, Mauro Podda,
and Salomone Di Saverio

20.1 Introduction

The population over the age of 60 years continues to rapidly increase in size, particularly in high-income countries, due to increasing life expectancy, declining birth rates, advances in the care of chronic diseases, and a more active lifestyle. This major expansion of the elderly population naturally leads to an increased number of older adults presenting to emergency departments following trauma. Due to a greater number of comorbidities and a higher risk of severe disability and death, the impact of injuries in geriatric patients varies considerably from the younger patients; their response to even minor injuries is impaired by a weaker mechanism of compensation as well as the likelihood that ongoing chronic medical conditions and/or medications may dull their physiologic response to the stress of trauma and increase their risk for complications.

To reduce morbidity and mortality of the elderly in trauma, a higher index of suspicion for injuries, strict monitoring programs, and carefully tailored resuscitation practices are critical in order to optimize outcomes. Studies suggest that medical background and preexisting comorbidities may be more important than chronological age [1–4]. Overall, for trauma care involving the elderly, system-based modifications may improve geriatric patients outcomes, from the availability of a dedicated geriatric care team that may reduce rates of delirium, functional decline, and discharge to long-term care facilities, to a lower trauma activation threshold which may result in a mortality improvement up to 30% in this group of trauma patients [5, 6]. Multiple authors have reported a significantly higher risk of under-triage in patients ≥65 years old, and corresponding increased morbidity and mortality

F. Virdis
Department of Trauma Surgery, Barts Health, Royal London Hospital, London, UK

M. Martin
Department of General and Trauma Surgery, Scripps Mercy Hospital, San Diego, CA, USA

M. Khan
Department of General and Trauma Surgery, Brighton and Sussex University Hospital NHS Trust, Brighton, UK
e-mail: mansoorkhan@nhs.net

I. Reccia
Department of Hepato-biliary and Pancreatic Surgery, Imperial College, Hammersmith Hospital, London, UK

G. Gallo
Department of Medical and Surgical Sciences, Universita' degli Studi "Magna Græcia" di Catanzaro, Catanzaro, Italy

M. Podda
Policlinico Universitario Duilio Casula, AOU Cagliari, Department of Emergency Surgery, Monserrato, Italy

S. Di Saverio (✉)
Department of General Surgery, San Benedetto del Tronto General Hospital, San Benedetto del Tronto, Italy

F. Agresta et al. (eds.), *Emergency laparoscopic surgery in the elderly and frail patient*,
https://doi.org/10.1007/978-3-030-79990-8_20

among elderly patients who are under-triaged [7]. Geriatric patients with severe injuries may not express the physiologic criteria for trauma team activation, with up to 63% of them with severe injury [Injury Severity Score (ISS) > 15] who do not meet standard trauma team activation threshold based on heart rate or blood pressure [8, 9].

20.2 Changes in the Elderly

There are multiple physiological and anatomical changes that influence the epidemiology and the response to trauma in the elderly (Table 20.1). Along with postural changes, balance shifting due to peripheral proprioception, cerebellar function and oculovestibular integrity, reduced motor strength, and deterioration of visual acuity, older adults have reduced vital capacity, functional residual capacity, and forced expiratory volume (FEV1), which decreases respiratory reserve and restricts the ability to tolerate even minor-to-moderate trauma. The decreased pulmonary reserve in elderly trauma patients is particularly highlighted by the large body of literature showing significantly higher mortality and morbidity rates among elderly patients with rib fractures compared to younger cohorts [10–12].

The reduced cardiac output makes compensation less effective with the myocardium less sensitive to catecholamines, which can result in a less profound tachycardic response to bleeding, pain, or anxiety. In addition to the physiologic deficit, this can also result in error or under-triage by the managing clinician due to misinterpretation of the patient's physiological response to trauma. The blood pressure can be affected by the age-related increase in systemic vascular resistance, and therefore a "normal" blood pressure can be misleading in a situation of hypoperfusion [13].

Interpretation of vital signs critically varies among older patients; a large retrospective review of geriatric blunt trauma patients showed heart rates above 90 beats per minute and systolic blood pressure less than 110 mm Hg (rather than the usual cutoff of 90 mm Hg for younger patients) correlates with increased mortality in this population [13].

Additional commonly encountered comorbidities in the elderly include ischemic heart disease, arrhythmias, metabolic conditions (i.e., diabe-

Table 20.1 Physiological system changes in the elderly

System	Physiological changes	Consequences
Pulmonary	Decreased vital capacity Decreased gas exchange Decrease cough reflex Smaller alveolar surface area Decreased chest wall compliance	Reduced respiratory reserve Increased risk for respiratory failure Increased risk for pneumonia Reduced tolerance for rib fractures
Cardiac	Decreased cardiac output Decreased sensitivity to catecholamines Increased afterload Fixed cardiac output Fixed heart rate (Beta blockers)	Reduced cardiac reserve Vital signs may not reflect severity of injury Misleading response to hypovolemia Increased risk of dysrhythmias and schema
Renal	Decreased GFR Decreased renal mass Decreased sensitivity to ADH and aldosterone	Increased risk of traumatic injury Increased susceptibility to fluid overload Reduced clearance of certain medications
Musculoskeletal	Loss of muscle mass and subcutaneous fat Osteoporosis Degenerative changes	Increased risk of fracture Decreased mobility Difficult oral intubation Increased risk of hypothermia Difficult rehabilitation
Neurologic	Decreased autoregulatory capability Brain atrophy	Increased susceptibility to injury from Decreased cerebral perfusion Increased risk for occult injury
Immune	Impaired immune response	Increased risk of infection

tes, osteoporosis), liver disease, renal failure, malnutrition, and poor physical conditioning. Medications such as anticoagulants, antiplatelet agents, beta-blockers, or other vasoactive substances may interfere with physiological responses, worsening the effects of hypovolemia.

Although age has been found to be associated with the risk for adverse outcomes after traumatic injury, this relationship is not linear or perfectly correlated. Multiple methodologies have been proposed to attempt to better characterize a given patient's degree of physical and physiologic impairment that have may have an even stronger impact on risk than age alone. These have included various scoring systems utilizing physiologic and laboratory data (APACHE, SAPS), number and types of comorbidities (Charlson Comorbidity Index), and most recently "frailty" scores [1, 2, 14, 15]. There is a burgeoning body of literature demonstrating the critical role that frailty and assessment of frailty status plays in the elderly response to trauma. There are currently numerous methods and scoring systems for assessing frailty in elderly trauma patients that can be derived from clinical data, physical assessment, laboratory data, or even administrative variables. The Trauma-Specific Frailty Index (TSFI, see Fig. 20.1) is a well-validated and trauma-specific frailty assessment tool that can be easily calculated from 15 variables, and that has been shown to have powerful predictive ability for outcomes regardless of patient's chronologic age [16, 17].

Trauma Specific Frailty Index (TSFI)			
Fifteen Variable Trauma Specific Frailty Index			
Comorbidities			
Cancer history	YES (1)	No (0)	
Coronary Heart Disease	MI (1)	CABG (0.75)	PCI (0.5)
	Medication (0.25)	None (0)	
Dementia	Severe (1)	Moderate (0.5)	Mild (0.25)
	No (0)		
Daily Activities			
Help with grooming	Yes (1)	No (0)	
Help managing money	Yes (1)	No (0)	
Help doing housework	Yes (1)	No (0)	
Help toileting	Yes (1)	No (0)	
Help walking	Wheelchair (1)	Walker (0.75)	Cane (0.5)
	No (0)		
Health Attitude			
Feel less useful	Most time (1)	Sometimes (0.5)	Never (0)
Feel sad	Most time (1)	Sometimes (0.5)	Never (0)
Feel effort to do everything	Most time (1)	Sometimes (0.5)	Never (0)
Falls	Within last month (1)	Present not in last month (0.5)	None (0)
Feel lonely	Most time (1)	Sometimes (0.5)	Never (0)
Function			
Sexual active	Yes (0)	No (1)	
Nutrition			
Albumin	<3 (1)	>3 (0)	

Fig. 20.1 Trauma-Specific Frailty Index scoring system utilizing 15 variables (With permission from McCusker A, Khan M, Kulvatunyou N, Zeeshan M, Sakran JV, Hayek H, et al. Sarcopenia defined by a computed tomography estimate of the psoas muscle area does not predict frailty in geriatric trauma patients. Am J Surg. 2019;218(2):261–5)

20.3 Mechanisms of Injury

Falls and motor vehicle accidents are the most common mechanisms of injury in the elderly, and are associated with significantly higher mortality and morbidity compared to similarly injured younger patients. For patients with a severe injury or multiple injuries, up to one-third of all older adult patients presenting with an ISS greater than 15 can be expected to die during the index hospital admission [13].

About three-quarters of all trauma in old adults are due to falls, often occurring from a standing position and broadly classified as mechanical versus syncopal. In many trauma centers, these elderly falls have risen to epidemic proportions, and have overtaken motor vehicle collisions as the most common mechanism of injury [18, 19]. Road traffic accidents are the second most common mechanism of injury among the elderly (they often are victims of automobile-pedestrian accidents) and the most frequent cause of traumatic mortality. The over-75-year age group is second only to 16–25 years old in the frequency of these accidents.

Around 25% of the elderly victims of motor vehicle accident are diagnosed with a thoracic injury (frequently rib fractures), which can worsen preexisting cardiopulmonary disease and increase the risks of pneumonia and respiratory failure. Whereas isolated rib fractures are near uniformly survivable in younger patients, there is a well-documented stepwise increase in mortality based on the number of fractured ribs in the elderly population [10, 20, 21]. Many trauma centers have now adopted policies of automatic ICU admission for any elderly patient with rib fractures in order to provide closer monitoring and a higher level of initial care and pulmonary toilet [22–24].

Penetrating trauma and assaults are less frequent in patients over 65 years but still represent up to 14% of the total admissions in the elderly population of the USA. In these cases, similar to pediatric patients, the managing physicians should always maintain a high index of suspicion for elder abuse and also consider the possibility of self-harm and suicidal ideology (Fig. 20.2).

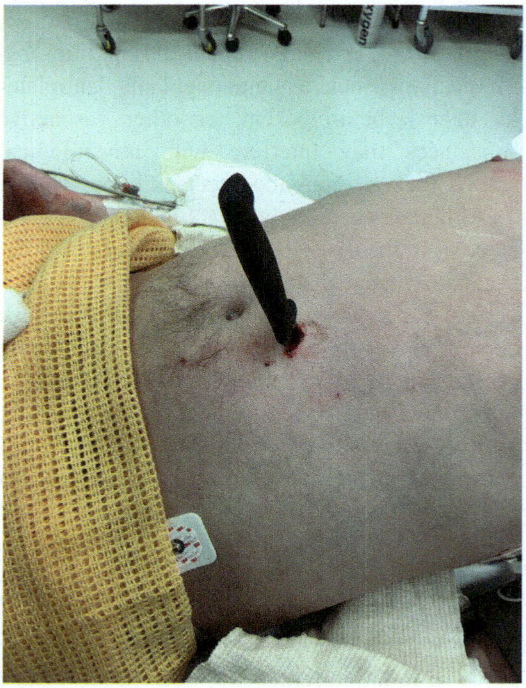

Fig. 20.2 Self-stab in an elderly patient

20.4 Abdominal Trauma in the Elderly

The management of abdominal trauma starts in the emergency department with fluid and blood resuscitation, strict hemodynamic monitoring, and early diagnosis of injuries. Abdominal injury patterns in the geriatric patients does not differ significantly from the younger patients, with the same mechanisms and grades of solid organ injury. However, in the elderly, reduced pain sensation and increased weakness of the abdominal wall, may make the abdominal examination more difficult and less reliable. The concomitant use of analgesic or psychoactive medications in the elderly may also result in a decreased pain response as well as more subtle abdominal exam findings even in the presence of major intraabdominal injury.

Diagnostic imaging tools should be liberally utilized to rule out intraperitoneal hemorrhage, hollow viscus perforation, or other operative abdominal injury. Focused assessment with sonography for trauma (FAST) should be performed in abdominal trauma patients as an adjunct to the primary survey and to assist with initial triage decisions. Although a clearly positive FAST exam is highly reliable, the well described weakness of the FAST exam is the high false-negative rate. It is also critical to appreciate that the FAST exam does not evaluate the retroperitoneum and is not reliable for identifying hollow viscus injuries. Computed tomography (CT) scan should be immediately obtained in most stable patients when an intraabdominal injury is suspected. Older patients at risk for significant injury and who have an unreliable exam (e.g., dementia, head injury), or who are intubated/sedated should be freely imaged when possible and consistent with the goals of care. CT scan in this population should be done with intravenous contrast whenever possible, although the association with contrast-induced nephropathy is a common concern. However, data from numerous studies suggest that contrast-induced nephropathy in elderly trauma patients is rare, regardless of the history of diabetes mellitus, age, creatinine, or high ISS [25, 26]. More recent data even suggest that there is no association between intravenous contrast and acute kidney injury with the use of modern contrast agents [25, 27, 28].

Early surgical consultation is mandatory for known or suspected intraabdominal injury in relation to a more difficult assessment in older patients and the considerations about type of management.

Nonoperative management (NOM) of abdominal solid organ injuries has been, in the past, documented as associated with increased failure rates in older patients compared to younger cohorts [29]. In fact, multiple authors have previously recommended age over 55 years as an absolute or relative contraindication to NOM [30–33].

However, more recent studies agreed that age should not represent an independent criteria to consider NOM since results showed that the majority of adults older than 55 years with splenic and hepatic trauma can be successfully managed without surgical intervention [33–35].

A multicenter study of the Eastern Association for the Surgery of Trauma confirmed that most patients >55 years of age with blunt splenic injuries can be treated with NOM, however, it demonstrates that failure of conservative management in this group of patients is associated with increased morbidity and mortality [13].

These authors concurred that age alone should no longer be considered a contraindication to nonoperative management of blunt liver and spleen injuries [13]. However, the managing trauma team must be particularly vigilant in the elderly patient undergoing NOM, with close serial clinical and laboratory evaluations coupled with a low threshold for converting to operative management if needed. Delay to definitive surgical intervention in the elderly patient with ongoing major hemorrhage or the development of peritonitis due to hollow viscus perforation carries a significantly higher morbidity and mortality rate versus younger cohorts with better physiologic reserve and tolerance.

The success rate of NOM in properly selected elderly blunt trauma patients has been reported around 62–85% in recent studies. Conservative management in liver trauma has been reported with a successful rate of 90% and a failure rate ranging from 5 to 15% across all age groups [33, 36–39].

Surgical indications in the geriatric abdominal trauma (both blunt and penetrating) follow the standard criteria, including hemorrhagic shock nonresponding to primary resuscitation, diffuse peritonism, radiological or high clinical suspicious of hollow viscus perforation, and diaphragmatic injury. The decision to manage patients conservatively following penetrating abdominal trauma should be made by experienced surgeons with the availability to provide vigilant follow-up and prompt intervention.

Hollow viscus injury in older patients is linked to high morbidity and mortality; physiological changes and declines in systems function, comorbidities, and long-standing metabolic disorders reduce survival in these patients.

There is no available evidence suggesting that different surgical techniques should be used in geriatric patients as opposed to younger ones. As predictable, compared to younger patients, the elderly have a generally poorer outcome when a surgical approach is required. Angioembolization (AE) has an increasingly important role in the NOM of solid organ injuries in the elderly and it can be used either as the primary therapeutic procedure when NOM is pursued or as an adjunct to the surgical intervention when hemostasis is not satisfactory.

20.5 Trauma Laparoscopy in the Elderly

Although all patient populations have been shown to benefit from the use of minimally invasive surgery, the older population derives particular benefit from the use of laparoscopic techniques. The benefits offered by laparoscopy with reduced postoperative pain, improved mobilization, shorter hospital stay, and fewer complications may be favorable in the prognosis of patients with significant comorbidity and impaired physiologic reserve [40]. Unless specifically contraindicated, the evidence supports the use of laparoscopic surgery in the elderly [13].

The risk of cardiovascular mortality compared with open surgery is lower in the minimally invasive approach but, still, laparoscopy may lead to distinctive hemodynamic and ventilatory effects that may increase the risk of cardiovascular complications in high-risk populations such as the older population.

Laparoscopy surgery may worsen conditions, including congestive heart failure, ischemic heart disease, valvular heart disease, congenital heart disease, and pulmonary hypertension.

Studies have shown that mechanical and neurohormonal responses are responsible for hemodynamic consequences related to increased intraabdominal pressure [13].

High intraabdominal pressure can lead to compression or reduced flow in major vessels such as the inferior vena cava and aorta, reduced splanchnic blood supply, and diaphragmatic displacement.

This is even more important to take into consideration in old frail trauma patients where a multi-systemic or isolated trauma can further compromise the physiology of the patient, therefore the decision to proceed with laparoscopic exploration must consider these factors.

Having said this, indications for laparoscopic approach in abdominal trauma of the elderly do not differ from the younger counterpart. In hemodynamically stable patients, laparoscopy reached a recognized role as a diagnostic tool in blunt and penetrating trauma of the abdomen [41]. In case of diagnostic doubts, with ambiguous CT scan findings or discordance between the clinical picture and the radiological report, studies have demonstrated good accuracy of laparoscopy in exposing abdominal injuries, when performed by surgeons with appropriate skills; this results in a lower rate of nontherapeutic laparotomy [42] as well as a shorter hospital stay, better respiratory management, and less postoperative pain when compared to the open approach [43].

The efficacy of laparoscopy may be particularly evident in cases of trauma patients with diagnostic imaging reporting free intraabdominal fluid not attributable to hepatic or splenic injury or in those with increasing abdominal pain, tenderness, and signs of ongoing sepsis compatible with hollow viscus injury. Preservation of the bowel within the abdominal cavity is considered an extra gain of the laparoscopic approach in frail patients such as the elderly, resulting in less fluid and temperature loss, coagulopathy, and postoperative paralytic ileus.

The laparoscopic approach may be indicated in the treatment of abdominal injuries [44], including primary repair of diaphragmatic, stomach, small and large bowel perforation, or in a delayed approach of complications related to hepatic trauma such biloma, abscess, or necrosis [13].

In high-grade splenic injuries [45] where nonoperative management has failed, and where interventional radiology is not available [46] or when dealing with complications of angioembolization, laparoscopic splenectomy can be an excellent alternative to open splenectomy [47].

When performing a therapeutic intervention, if the damage is diagnosed preoperatively, trocars can be inserted following the location of injury identified with the CT scan [44].

Contraindications for laparoscopic approach in trauma in the elderly are the same than the

Table 20.2 Contraindications for laparoscopy approach in trauma

Absolute	Relative
Hemodynamic instability	Generalized peritonitis
Transient or nonresponders with hemorrhagic or septic shock	Severe COPD with severe hypercapnia
Severe cardio-pulmonary dysfunction	Evisceration
Severe traumatic brain injury	Previous laparotomy
Inability to tolerate pneumoperitoneum	Multiple or complex intraabdominal injuries

younger counterpart and they include hemodynamic instability, hypovolemic or septic shock, serious cardio-respiratory impairment, severe brain injury, and inability to tolerate pneumoperitoneum [48] (Table 20.2).

20.6 Diagnostic Laparoscopy Technique

Intubation and general anesthesia is required to perform a complete trauma diagnostic laparoscopy.

The patient on the operative table should be positioned as per the standard rules of trauma surgery, supine, with the operative field extending from the chin to above the knees, between the posterior axillary lines and with both arms fully abducted, in case an emergency conversion to laparotomy or/and thoracotomy is required (i.e., abdominal injuries nonmanageable laparoscopically, hemodynamic instability, suspicion of thoracic injuries).

Initial trocar placement is done per the attending preference using Veress needle (consider possible risks related to distended bowel in trauma as well as loss of muscle mass and subcutaneous fat typical in the elderly), open Hasson technique, or direct optical trocar entry. Either a 5 or 10 mm trocar is first placed around the umbilical level and slow insufflation is utilized to achieve adequate pneumoperitoneum (12–14 mm Hg), strictly monitoring the patient's vitals and response.

If the first exploration of the abdominal cavity allows proceeding laparoscopically, two more trocars can be inserted under direct vision in the left-upper and lower quadrants to permit a methodical exploration of the abdomen and run the entire bowel. Two more trocars may be inserted in the right quadrants to better explore the left hemi-abdomen if required, or as needed to perform any therapeutic interventions such as suturing or stapling [48].

Exploration of the abdomen should be methodical; it does not matter where the surgeon begins as long as he/she utilizes a sensible and organized sequence that will cover all of the abdominal compartments. It can start from the right upper quadrant and advance clockwise.

Reverse Trendelenburg position allows better access and visualization of the supramesocolic region for the evaluation of spleen, liver and gallbladder, diaphragm, stomach, and duodenum, followed by exploration of transverse and descending colon and the mesocolon.

The Trendelenburg position will then facilitate the exploration of the rectum, Douglas pouch, and the pelvic organs the cecum, and right colon.

The small bowel can be explored from the ileo-cecal valve to the ligament of Treitz once the omentum has been moved upwards; grabbing the mesenteric fat to avoid iatrogenic injuries, the small bowel must be explored on both its mesenteric and antimesenteric side to rule out any damage, particularly in cases of penetrating trauma [48].

The lesser sac should usually be opened and explored; this can be done holding up the stomach and the transverse colon, pulling them apart to stretch the gastrocolic ligament and making a hole in its left side, which is usually less vascular. All zones (I–III) of the retroperitoneum can be readily visualized during a standard laparoscopic exploration, and if there are no visible abnormalities or clinical/imaging concerns for a retroperitoneal injury then no further evaluation is required. However, if there are signs of a major retroperitoneal injury that requires exploration (typically an expanding, pulsatile, or Zone 1 hematoma), then prompt conversion to standard laparotomy should be performed.

20.7 Anticoagulation

Emergency trauma surgery is associated with higher rates of morbidity and mortality as compared to routine surgery with bleeding representing one of the major contributors to poor outcomes; it concurs up to 40% of trauma-related deaths and it increases in-patient complications rates such as sepsis and multiorgan failure [49, 50].

Since anticoagulant therapy increasingly became more widespread, with the introduction of non-vitamin K oral anticoagulants such as rivaroxaban, apixaban, and edoxaban, bleeding control in trauma surgery became even more challenging. Acute coagulopathy and bleeding occur between 25 and 35% among trauma patients with up to 3% of whom are on anticoagulant therapy [51–53].

Despite that overall risk of bleeding linked to non-vitamin K oral anticoagulant is well known, there are not sufficient data on the risk of bleeding in the context of surgical intervention. To reduce the risk of bleeding in anticoagulated patients, reversal of the specific agent should usually be performed before the surgical intervention. Options available include pharmacologic interventions such as prothrombin complex concentrate (PCC), activated prothrombin complex concentrate (aPCC), recombinant activated factor VII, and fresh frozen plasma (FFP). More recent reversal agents have been also developed, including idarucizumab and andexanet alfa, and others are still under investigation [13]. However, the risk of bleeding from the initial injuries as well as operative bleeding complications must always be balanced with the competing risk of thrombotic or thromboembolic events that are also frequently present in the elderly patient cohort. In most cases where the traumatic injury has been managed definitely by surgery, resumption of anticoagulation can be performed as early as 24-h postsurgery. However, this risk/benefit analysis and decision on the exact timing for resumption of anticoagulation is a complex and multifactorial decision that must be individualized to each patient based on their clinical and injury factors.

Five Things You Should Know About Laparoscopy for Abdominal Trauma in the Elderly

- CT scan with intravenous contrast should be obtained in stable patients when an intraabdominal injury is suspected; contrast-induced nephropathy in elderly trauma patients is rare (or nonexistent), regardless of history of diabetes mellitus, age, creatinine, and high ISS.
- Older populations have major advantages from laparoscopic techniques, when indicated.
- Indications and techniques for a laparoscopic approach in abdominal trauma of the elderly does not differ significantly from their younger counterparts, but closer attention must be paid to their physiologic response and tolerance to general anesthesia and abdominal insufflation.
- Reduce the risk of bleeding in anticoagulated patients through reversal of the specific agent before the surgical intervention if warranted.
- Decreased sensitivity to catecholamines and impaired compensatory tachycardia, anticoagulants, antiplatelet agents, beta-blockers, and other cardioactive/vasoactive medications may interfere with physiological responses and worsen the effects of hypovolemia.

References

1. Joseph B, Pandit V, Rhee P, Aziz H, Sadoun M, Wynne J, et al. Predicting hospital discharge disposition in geriatric trauma patients: is frailty the answer? J Trauma Acute Care Surg. 2014;76(1):196–200.
2. Joseph B, Pandit V, Zangbar B, Kulvatunyou N, Hashmi A, Green DJ, et al. Superiority of frailty over age in predicting outcomes among geriatric trauma patients: a prospective analysis. JAMA Surg. 2014;149(8):766–72.
3. Maxwell CA, Mion LC, Mukherjee K, Dietrich MS, Minnick A, May A, et al. Preinjury physical frailty and cognitive impairment among geriatric trauma patients determine postinjury functional recovery and survival. J Trauma Acute Care Surg. 2016;80(2):195–203.
4. Zhao F, Tang B, Hu C, Wang B, Wang Y, Zhang L. The impact of frailty on posttraumatic outcomes in older trauma patients: a systematic review and meta-analysis. J Trauma Acute Care Surg. 2020;88(4):546–54.
5. Demetriades D, Karaiskakis M, Velmahos G, Alo K, Newton E, Murray J, et al. Effect on outcome of early

intensive management of geriatric trauma patients. Br J Surg. 2002;89(10):1319–22.

6. Demetriades D, Martin M, Salim A, Rhee P, Brown C, Chan L. The effect of trauma center designation and trauma volume on outcome in specific severe injuries. Ann Surg. 2005;242(4):512–7; discussion 7–9.
7. Lehmann R, Beekley A, Casey L, Salim A, Martin M. The impact of advanced age on trauma triage decisions and outcomes: a statewide analysis. Am J Surg. 2009;197(5):571–4; discussion 4–5.
8. Demetriades D, Sava J, Alo K, Newton E, Velmahos GC, Murray JA, et al. Old age as a criterion for trauma team activation. J Trauma. 2001;51(4):754–6; discussion 6–7.
9. Chang DC, Bass RR, Cornwell EE, Mackenzie EJ. Undertriage of elderly trauma patients to state-designated trauma centers. Arch Surg. 2008; 143(8):776–81; discussion 82.
10. Bulger EM, Arneson MA, Mock CN, Jurkovich GJ. Rib fractures in the elderly. J Trauma. 2000;48(6):1040–6; discussion 6–7.
11. Schmoekel N, Berguson J, Stassinopoulos J, Karamanos E, Patton J, Johnson JL. Rib fractures in the elderly: physiology trumps anatomy. Trauma Surg Acute Care Open. 2019;4(1):e000257.
12. Stawicki SP, Grossman MD, Hoey BA, Miller DL, Reed JF 3rd. Rib fractures in the elderly: a marker of injury severity. J Am Geriatr Soc. 2004;52(5): 805–8.
13. Martin JT, Alkhoury F, O'Connor JA, Kyriakides TC, Bonadies JA. 'Normal' vital signs belie occult hypoperfusion in geriatric trauma patients. Am Surg. 2010;76(1):65–9.
14. Gabbe BJ, Magtengaard K, Hannaford AP, Cameron PA. Is the Charlson comorbidity index useful for predicting trauma outcomes? Acad Emerg Med. 2005;12(4):318–21.
15. Korkmaz Toker M, Gulleroglu A, Karabay AG, Bicer IG, Demiraran Y. SAPS III or APACHE IV: which score to choose for acute trauma patients in intensive care unit? Ulus Travma Acil Cerrahi Derg. 2019;25(3):247–52.
16. McCusker A, Khan M, Kulvatunyou N, Zeeshan M, Sakran JV, Hayek H, et al. Sarcopenia defined by a computed tomography estimate of the psoas muscle area does not predict frailty in geriatric trauma patients. Am J Surg. 2019;218(2):261–5.
17. Joseph B, Pandit V, Zangbar B, Kulvatunyou N, Tang A, O'Keeffe T, et al. Validating trauma-specific frailty index for geriatric trauma patients: a prospective analysis. J Am Coll Surg. 2014;219(1):10–7.e1.
18. Cox S, Roggenkamp R, Bernard S, Smith K. The epidemiology of elderly falls attended by emergency medical services in Victoria, Australia. Injury. 2018;49(9):1712–9.
19. Sartini M, Cristina ML, Spagnolo AM, Cremonesi P, Costaguta C, Monacelli F, et al. The epidemiology of domestic injurious falls in a community dwelling elderly population: an outgrowing economic burden. Eur J Pub Health. 2010;20(5):604–6.
20. Van Vledder MG, Kwakernaak V, Hagenaars T, Van Lieshout EMM, Verhofstad MHJ, South West Netherlands Trauma Region Study Group. Patterns of injury and outcomes in the elderly patient with rib fractures: a multi-center observational study. Eur J Trauma Emerg Surg. 2019;45(4):575–83.
21. Bergeron E, Lavoie A, Clas D, Moore L, Ratte S, Tetreault S, et al. Elderly trauma patients with rib fractures are at greater risk of death and pneumonia. J Trauma. 2003;54(3):478–85.
22. Naar L, El Hechi MW, van Erp IA, Mashbari HNA, Fawley J, Parks JJ, et al. Isolated rib cage fractures in the elderly: do all patients belong to the intensive care unit? A retrospective nationwide analysis. J Trauma Acute Care Surg. 2020;89(6):1039–45.
23. Kelley KM, Burgess J, Weireter L, Novosel TJ, Parks K, Aseuga M, et al. Early use of a chest trauma protocol in elderly patients with rib fractures improves pulmonary outcomes. Am Surg. 2019;85(3):288–91.
24. Bakhos C, O'Connor J, Kyriakides T, Abou-Nukta F, Bonadies J. Vital capacity as a predictor of outcome in elderly patients with rib fractures. J Trauma. 2006;61(1):131–4.
25. McGillicuddy EA, Schuster KM, Kaplan LJ, Maung AA, Lui FY, Maerz LL, et al. Contrast-induced nephropathy in elderly trauma patients. J Trauma. 2010;68(2):294–7.
26. Finigan R, Pham J, Mendoza R, Lekawa M, Dolich M, Kong A, et al. Risk for contrast-induced nephropathy in elderly trauma patients. Am Surg. 2012;78(10):1114–7.
27. Colling KP, Irwin ED, Byrnes MC, Reicks P, Dellich WA, Reicks K, et al. Computed tomography scans with intravenous contrast: low incidence of contrast-induced nephropathy in blunt trauma patients. J Trauma Acute Care Surg. 2014;77(2):226–30.
28. Liu Y, Hong D, Wang AY, Guo R, Smyth B, Liu J, et al. Effects of intravenous hydration on risk of contrast induced nephropathy and in-hospital mortality in STEMI patients undergoing primary percutaneous coronary intervention: a systematic review and meta-analysis of randomized controlled trials. BMC Cardiovasc Disord. 2019;19(1):87.
29. Antonacci N, Di Saverio S, Ciaroni V, Biscardi A, Giugni A, Cancellieri F, et al. Prognosis and treatment of pancreaticoduodenal traumatic injuries: which factors are predictors of outcome?. Journal of Hepato-Biliary-Pancreatic Sciences. 2011;18(2):195–201.
30. Longo WE, Baker CC, McMillen MA, Modlin IM, Degutis LC, Zucker KA. Nonoperative management of adult blunt splenic trauma. Criteria for successful outcome. Ann Surg. 1989;210(5):626–9.
31. Smith JS Jr, Wengrovitz MA, DeLong BS. Prospective validation of criteria, including age, for safe, nonsurgical management of the ruptured spleen. J Trauma. 1992;33(3):363–8; discussion 8–9.
32. Godley CD, Warren RL, Sheridan RL, McCabe CJ. Nonoperative management of blunt splenic injury in adults: age over 55 years as a powerful indicator for failure. J Am Coll Surg. 1996;183(2):133–9.

33. Barone JE, Burns G, Svehlak SA, Tucker JB, Bell T, Korwin S, et al. Management of blunt splenic trauma in patients older than 55 years. Southern Connecticut Regional Trauma Quality Assurance Committee. J Trauma. 1999;46(1):87–90.
34. Cocanour CS, Moore FA, Ware DN, Marvin RG, Duke JH. Age should not be a consideration for nonoperative management of blunt splenic injury. J Trauma. 2000;48(4):606–10; discussion 10–2.
35. Myers JG, Dent DL, Stewart RM, Gray GA, Smith DS, Rhodes JE, et al. Blunt splenic injuries: dedicated trauma surgeons can achieve a high rate of nonoperative success in patients of all ages. J Trauma. 2000;48(5):801–5; discussion 5–6.
36. Falimirski ME, Provost D. Nonsurgical management of solid abdominal organ injury in patients over 55 years of age. Am Surg. 2000;66(7):631–5.
37. Albrecht RM, Schermer CR, Morris A. Nonoperative management of blunt splenic injuries: factors influencing success in age >55 years. Am Surg. 2002;68(3):227–30; discussion 30–1.
38. Richardson JD. Changes in the management of injuries to the liver and spleen. J Am Coll Surg. 2005;200(5):648–69.
39. Hurtuk M, Reed RL 2nd, Esposito TJ, Davis KA, Luchette FA. Trauma surgeons practice what they preach: the NTDB story on solid organ injury management. J Trauma. 2006;61(2):243–54; discussion 54–5.
40. Mandrioli M, Inaba K, Piccinini A, Biscardi A, Sartelli M, Agresta F, et al. Advances in laparoscopy for acute care surgery and trauma. World J Gastroenterol. 2016;14;22(2):668–80. https://doi.org/10.3748/wjg.v22.i2.668.
41. Cirocchi R, Birindelli A, Inaba K, Mandrioli M, Piccinini A,Tabola R, et al. Laparoscopy for Trauma and the Changes in its Use From 1990 to 2016: A Current Systematic Review and Meta-Analysis. Surg Laparosc Endosc Percutan Tech. 2018;28(1):1–12. https://doi.org/10.1097/SLE.0000000000000466.
42. Menegozzo CAM, Damous SHB, Alves PHF, Rocha MC, Collet E Silva FS, Baraviera T, et al. "Pop in a scope": attempt to decrease the rate of unnecessary nontherapeutic laparotomies in hemodynamically stable patients with thoracoabdominal penetrating injuries. Surg Endosc. 2020;34(1):261–7. https://doi.org/10.1007/s00464-019-06761-7. Epub 2019 Apr 8.
43. Di Saverio S. Emergency laparoscopy: a new emerging discipline for treating abdominal emergencies attempting to minimize costs and invasiveness and maximize outcomes and patients' comfort. J Trauma Acute Care Surg. 2014;77(2):338–50. https://doi.org/10.1097/TA.0000000000000288.
44. Birindelli A, Podda M, Segalini E, Cripps M, Tonini V, Tugnoli G, et al. Is the minimally invasive trauma surgeon the next (r)evolution of trauma surgery? Indications and outcomes of diagnostic and therapeutic trauma laparoscopy in a level 1 trauma centre. TraumaLap Study Group. Updates Surg. 2020;72(2):503–12. https://doi.org/10.1007/s13304-020-00739-0. Epub 2020 Mar 26.
45. Birindelli A, Segalini E, Affinita A, Tugnoli G, Di Saverio S. Laparoscopic splenectomy with selective intra-corporeal ligation of splenic hilar vessels for high grade splenic injury - video vignette. Colorectal Dis. 2017. https://doi.org/10.1111/codi.13988. Online ahead of print.
46. Segalini E, Gori A, Birindelli A, Gavriilidis P, Affinita A, Tartaglia D et al. Laparoscopic concomitant management of an incidental splenic artery aneurysm and splenectomy for trauma after unsuccessful endovascular treatment - a video vignette. Colorectal Dis. 2020;22(1):107–8. https://doi.org/10.1111/codi.14840. Epub 2019 Sep 17.
47. Birindelli A, Martin M, Khan M, Gallo G, Segalini E, Gori A, et al. Laparoscopic splenectomy as a definitive management option for high-grade traumatic splenic injury when non operative management is not feasible or failed: a 5-year experience from a level one trauma center with minimally invasive surgery expertise.Updates Surg. 2021. https://doi.org/10.1007/s13304-021-01045-z. Online ahead of print.
48. Di Saverio S, Birindelli A, Podda M, Segalini E, Piccinini A, Coniglio C, et al. Trauma laparoscopy and the six w's: Why, where, who, when, what, and how?. J Trauma Acute Care Surg. 2019;86(2):344–67. https://doi.org/10.1097/TA.0000000000002130.
49. Kauvar DS, Wade CE. The epidemiology and modern management of traumatic hemorrhage: US and international perspectives. Crit Care. 2005;9(Suppl 5):S1–9.
50. Spahn DR, Cerny V, Coats TJ, Duranteau J, Fernandez-Mondejar E, Gordini G, et al. Management of bleeding following major trauma: a European guideline. Crit Care. 2007;11(1):R17.
51. Brohi K, Singh J, Heron M, Coats T. Acute traumatic coagulopathy. J Trauma. 2003;54(6):1127–30.
52. Dossett LA, Riesel JN, Griffin MR, Cotton BA. Prevalence and implications of preinjury warfarin use: an analysis of the National Trauma Databank. Arch Surg. 2011;146(5):565–70.
53. Spahn DR, Bouillon B, Cerny V, Coats TJ, Duranteau J, Fernandez-Mondejar E, et al. Management of bleeding and coagulopathy following major trauma: an updated European guideline. Crit Care. 2013;17(2):R76.

Further Reading

Rodriguez A, Barraco RD, Ivatury RR. Geriatric trauma and acute care surgery. Springer International Publishing; 2018. https://doi.org/10.1007/978-3-319-57403-5.

Guidelines

American College of Surgeons. Geriatric trauma management guidelines. https://www.facs.org/-/media/files/quality-programs/trauma/tqip/geriatric_guidelines.ashx.

EAST Practice Management Guidelines Work Group. Eastern Association for the Surgery of Trauma, practice management guidelines for geriatric trauma. https://www.east.org/Content/documents/practicemanagementguidelines/geriatric.pdf.

NHS London Major Trauma System: management of elderly major trauma patients—Second Edition. https://www.c4ts.qmul.ac.uk/downloads/pan-london-major-trauma-system-elderly-trauma-guidancesecond-editiondecember-2018.pdf.

21 Laparoscopic Approach to Acute Mesenteric Ischemia in Elderly Patients

Marco Milone, Anna D'Amore, Michele Manigrasso, and Bruno Amato

21.1 Introduction

Acute mesenteric ischemia (AMI) is a rare but life-threatening disease that can cause mesenteric infarction, intestinal necrosis, and systemic inflammatory response.

The etiologies of AMI are classified into obstructive and nonobstructive visceral ischemia (NOMI, nonobstructive mesenteric ischemia). The obstructive origin includes an acute arterial occlusion due to vascular embolism (EAMI, acute embolic mesenteric ischemia) or to thrombosis (TAMI, acute thrombotic mesenteric ischemia) and an acute venous occlusion due to thrombosis (VAMI, acute venous mesenteric ischemia).

AMI is a life-threatening disease with a mortality rate of 50–69%. The diagnosis of AMI, in fact, represents a very difficult enigma because there are no specific signs or early routine clinical tests, significantly retarding, in this way, not only the detection of disease but also its treatment.

At present, the gold standard for diagnosis is the high-resolution computed tomography angiography (CTA), with high values of sensitivity and specificity (93.3% and 95.9%, respectively), but these values seem to change according to each etiological type. In fact, NOMI is diagnosed by excluding other etiologies; it represents the most important diagnostic problem because there are no specific radiological features on computed tomography angiography, which usually shows a normal bowel wall.

Early diagnosis and timely application treatment are the key determinants for improving prognosis. Some studies have demonstrated that early laparoscopic approach can be lifesaving with a 50% reduction in mortality compared with delayed intervention or conservative management. Diagnostic laparoscopy is also feasible as a bedside approach in the intensive care unit (ICU), avoiding time delay for awaiting operating room availability and preventing adverse events in patients with critical medical condition, including those on mechanical ventilation or unstable vital sign.

Moreover, laparoscopy may be a valid alternative to CTA in patients with kidney failure or other contraindications to iodate contrast injection. However, the laparoscopic approach to acute mesenteric ischemia has some limits because the laparoscopic diagnosis of AMI is influenced by the stage of bowel damage, the etiology of the ischemia, and the surgeon's experience and on the level of his learning curve, considering also that a low pressure of CO_2 pneumoperitoneum is advised.

M. Milone (✉) · A. D'Amore · M. Manigrasso
B. Amato
Department of Clinical Medicine and Surgery, University "Federico II" of Naples, Naples, Italy

F. Agresta et al. (eds.), *Emergency laparoscopic surgery in the elderly and frail patient*,
https://doi.org/10.1007/978-3-030-79990-8_21

21.2 Diagnostic Value of Laparoscopy in AMI

21.2.1 First-Look Exploration

First-look diagnostic laparoscopy (DL) can improve prognosis, allowing early recognition of AMI as shown by some studies.

Gonenc et al. [1] focused the attention on the positive impact of DL on the prognosis of the patients with suspected AMI. Fifty-three patients, undergoing DL for suspected AMI, were included in the study. In 20 cases (22.6%), DL was negative; in 43 cases (77.4%), DL detected AMI. In detail, subtotal or total necrosis of the bowel was present in 27 patients (62.8%), while in 16 patients (37.2%), there was subtotal or total ischemia. Revascularization with thrombectomy or embolectomy was performed. During second-look laparoscopy, eight patients were found to have necrosis, and thus six patients underwent successful revascularization while two patients received small bowel partial resection and anastomosis. These patients underwent a third-look laparoscopy to check the remaining small bowel and the anastomosis, which appeared healthy. Despite the encouraging results, this study has several flaws: first, it is retrospective, then the group of patients is heterogeneous and the time between the onset of symptoms and admission is not known exactly.

Some authors have described the use of indocyanine green (ICG) fluorescence imaging in early diagnosis of AMI.

ICG fluorescence imaging captures the fluorescence of indocyanine green injected into the body using a digital video camera. Indocyanine becomes excited by infrared light and emits infrared fluorescence that can easily transmit through about 10 mm of human soft tissue. Intravenously injected ICG is transported to peripheral vessels within a few seconds. In a tissue or an organ where blood flow is inhibited, the fluorescence emission of ICG weakens. The evaluation of blood flow using ICG fluorescence imaging is applied to breast reconstruction, coronary artery bypass grafting, and colorectal resection. This technique makes possible to objectively assess the quality of tissue perfusion, which is indispensable when deciding on the viability of the intestine after AMI.

The first application of fluorescein has been proposed in 1993 by Kam and Scheeres [2]. Paral et al. [3] confirmed on porcine model the feasibility of this procedure using the specific optical system in the follow-up of AMI patients. Alemanno et al. [4] decided to adopt this technique in order to early detect and treat an intestinal ischemia in a 68-year-old patient previously treated with a thoracic endovascular aortic repair (TEVAR) procedure for a type-B aortic dissection. The day after the TEVAR the patient developed abdominal pain with melena. A surgical evaluation and a CT scan were performed, but there were no signs of intestinal ischemia. However, after 2 h, the abdomen appeared distended, the diuresis stopped, and lactates increased; thus, a diagnostic laparoscopy with the support of intraoperative near-infrared indocyanine green fluorescence angiography was performed. The fluorescence system demonstrated a hypo-perfused area of the ascending colon allowing an ileocolic resection. Opening the operatory specimen, the mucosa of the colon appeared totally ischemic with a normal serosa. In fact, when ischemia occurs, the oxygen supply is interrupted and the necrosis of the enteral mucosa occurs within 3 h, while the necrosis of the full thickness of the bowel wall occurs within 6 h. A diagnosis during these "golden hours," like in this case report, is the most important factor for a successful treatment.

Karampinis et al. [5] demonstrated that ICG can also reduce extended bowel resection. Authors provided a retrospective analysis on 52 patients with acute mesenteric ischemia who received an operation using indocyanine green (ICG) fluorescence angiography. In 34 of 52 cases (65%), ICG angiography findings corresponded with the surgeon's clinical assessment. However, in 18 cases (35%), ICG angiography provided additional information concerning tissue perfusion. Twelve of those 18 patients did not survive the acute phase. In the other six cases, ICG fluorescence angiography resulted in a substantial change in operative strategy. Alexander et al. [6] described a case of AMI in which the patient successfully underwent percutaneous superior mesenteric artery (SMA) angioplasty with stenting followed by laparoscopy with indocyanine green (ICG) fluorescence imaging to confirm sufficient bowel and viability. On the 15th day after SMA stenting (18th in-hospital day), the patient was discharged in a good state of health with medical recommendations. Kim et al. [7] used early diagnostic laparoscopy for suspicious of AMI after cardiac surgery in two patients to show favorable outcomes. In the first case, the patient underwent off-pump coronary artery bypass grafting (CABG) for arteriosclerosis obliterans (ASO) and after 3 days developed abdominal pain with increasing levels of white blood cell (WBC) and C-reactive protein (CRP). On the fourth postoperative day, about 200 mL of blood appeared in the intraperitoneal drain. Computed tomographic angiography (CTA) showed pneumatosis intestinalis with maintained perfusion of the celiac axis and superior mesenteric artery, suggesting nonocclusive mesenteric ischemia (NOMI). Two hours after the CTA scan, a bedside laparoscopy in the ICU was performed, showing a few local ischemic spots without definite evidence of perfusion deficit. The patient was treated in a conservative way with fasting for 14 days and a combination of third-generation cephalosporin and metronidazole for 14 days. In the second case, the patient underwent mechanical aortic valve replacement for severe aortic stenosis, and on the third postoperative day, he developed abdominal pain, fever, and elevated levels of CRP and lactate. CTA showed, also in this case, several features suggesting of NOMI. The general surgery service recommended close observation. On the fifth postoperative day, a follow-up CTA was performed, and it showed features suggesting of microperforation. After performing DL, which demonstrated small bowel ischemia, the operation was converted to median laparotomy and resection of the ischemic segments of the small bowel, end-to-end anastomosis, and an ileostomy were performed. In the study, the patients underwent different postoperative cares, avoiding invasive surgical exploration in the first case and performing surgical resection in the second case. The authors demonstrated that the early application of DL in cardiac surgical patients with a suspicion of AMI might be a good strategy to avoid unnecessary laparotomy and to achieve better results.

Furthermore, diagnostic laparoscopy could be a less invasive alternative to laparotomy for the diagnosis of AMI in the critical setting, as shown by Tshomba et al. [8]. The authors retrospectively analyzed the results of a diagnostic protocol for the early detection of AMI in patients with aortic acute dissection (AoD). The protocol started in January 2004, and patients were selected for diagnostic laparoscopy if they had imaging suggesting impairment of flow to the visceral vessels, clinical signs and symptoms suggesting AMI, and lab tests suggesting AMI. In this way, laparoscopy can reduce the number of unnecessary laparotomies overall in elderly critically ill patients. If there were not these conditions, watchful waiting and CTA were the preferred management strategy. The authors observed 202 consecutive AoD treated in the same center (71 acute type A AoD; 131 acute and chronic type B AoD), and only in 17 patients AMI was suspected. Diagnostic laparoscopy (DL) was used in nine cases, in three cases during the medical treatment and in six cases after surgical or endovascular revascularization. In one case, AMI was diagnosed and the patient underwent emergency revascularization. The authors also implemented diagnostic laparoscopy in patients with kidney failure or other contraindications of iodate contrast injection.

Cocorullo et al. [9] have tried to give a contribution for the validation of laparoscopic approach in case of NOMI both for the first and the second looks to detect and remove necrotic bowel avoiding risks related with laparotomy. In a retrospective analysis of 32 consecutive patients admitted from January 1, 2006 to December 31, 2015, in the ICU of Paolo Giaccone University Hospital of Palermo, AMI was diagnosed by multislice CT, and if clinical conditions were permissive, selective angiography was done. Surgical approach was used if necrosis was already present or suspected. In their experience, laparoscopy was positively used in these patients, and no morbidity was recorded to laparoscopic procedure with a reduction of mortality probably due to the avoidance of a nontherapeutic laparotomy.

21.2.2 Second-Look Exploration

In the last years, laparoscopy has evolved as an alternative to laparotomy for the second look in the management of AMI to keep patients away from the effects of a progressive ischemia. AMI, either occlusive or nonocclusive, is frequently a progressive entity with repeated attacks of emboli or low-flow state which could cause ischemic challenge in the bowel even after surgical or medical management.

Second-look laparotomy, or relaparotomy, was introduced in 1965 by Shaw [10] to overcome the difficulty in assessing the adequacy of bowel resection during surgery. It included a routine re-exploration of the abdomen 24–48 h after the first operation, not just to distinguish between necrotic and healthy bowel but also to allow time for application of supportive measures.

The exact indication for second-look laparotomy is still controversial. Some surgeons choose an aggressive strategy with a second-look procedure in every patient undergoing bowel resection and primary anastomosis, while others suggest a more selective approach.

However, a second-look laparotomy is a calculated risk to AMI patients, who are at high risk of infection, malnutrition, hemodynamic instability, and multiple organ failure. Laparoscopy, as a minimally invasive approach, could allow the surgeon to avoid inflicting damage in an additional surgical procedure.

Anadol et al. [11] and Meng et al. [12] demonstrated that second-look laparoscopy not only gives the same information of a standard second-look laparotomy saving AMI patients from additional surgical trauma but also presents important advantages such as a shorter operative time and anesthesia, the chance of more explorations, and the possibility of avoiding unnecessary laparotomies.

Yanar et al. [13] investigated the role of second-look laparoscopy in patients with AMI and underwent the use of laparoscopy in the intensive care unit under sedation or analgesia. Authors provided a retrospective analysis on 71 patients who received an operation for the treatment of AMI. In 14 patients, a second-look laparoscopy exploration was performed. The indications for a second look were low-flow state, bowel resection, and anastomosis or mesenteric thromboembolectomy performed during the first operation. In 13 patients, the second-look laparoscopic examination revealed normal bowel viability, but in one patient, intestinal necrosis was detected. In two of the patients, a third operation was necessary to correct anastomotic leakage.

21.3 The Role of Laparoscopy in the Treatment of AMI

The first step in the treatment of AMI is bowel revascularization. The second step is the evaluation of bowel viability considering signs of adequate perfusion as mesenteric vessel pulsation, normal color of the bowel mucosa, peristalsis, and bleeding from cut surfaces.

The role of laparoscopy in treatment of AMI is not standardized but laparoscopic primary access could be an important therapeutic tool, as shown by Alemanno et al. [4]. The authors performed an ileocolic resection during a diagnostic laparoscopy with the support of intraoperative indocyanine green fluorescence angiography in a 68-year-old patient treated with a TEVAR procedure for a type-B aortic dissection.

Five Things You Should Know About Laparoscopic Approach to Acute Mesenteric Ischemia in Elderly Patients

- The gold standard for the diagnosis of AMI is CTA, which provides high rates of sensitivity and specificity.
- Early diagnostic laparoscopy in the suspicion of acute mesenteric ischemia is related with a 50% reduction of mortality compared with delayed intervention or conservative management. Diagnostic laparoscopy is also feasible as a bedside approach in the ICU. Furthermore, laparoscopy may be a valid alternative to CTA

in patients with kidney failure or other contra-indications to iodate contrast injection.

- First-look diagnostic laparoscopy with the use of indocyanine green fluorescence imaging can improve prognosis, allowing early recognition of AMI.
- Second-look laparoscopy not only gives the same information of a standard second-look laparotomy saving AMI patients from additional surgical trauma but also presents important advantages.
- The role of laparoscopy in the treatment of AMI is not standardized, but laparoscopic primary access could be an important therapeutic tool.

References

1. Gonenc M, Dural CA, Kocatas A, Buyukasik S, Karabulut M, Alis H. The impact of early diagnostic laparoscopy on the prognosis of patients with suspected acute mesenteric ischemia. Eur J Trauma Emerg Surg. 2013;39(2):185–9. https://doi.org/10.1007/s00068-013-0253-y.
2. Kam D, Scheeres D. Fluorescein-assisted laparoscopy in the identification of arterial mesenteric ischemia. Surg Endosc. 1993;7:75–8.
3. Paral J, Ferko A, Plodr M, et al. Laparoscopic diagnostics of acute bowel ischemia using ultraviolet light and fluorescein dye: an experimental study. Surg Laparosc Endosc Percutan Tech. 2007;17(4):291–5. https://doi.org/10.1097/SLE.0b013e3180dc9376.
4. Alemanno G, Somigli R, Prosperi P, et al. Combination of diagnostic laparoscopy and intraoperative indocyanine green fluorescence angiography for the early detection of intestinal ischemia not detectable at CT scan. Int J Surg Case Rep. 2016;26:77–80. https://doi.org/10.1016/j.ijscr.2016.07.016.
5. Karampinis I, Keese M, Jakob J, et al. Indocyanine green tissue angiography can reduce extended bowel resections in acute mesenteric ischemia. J Gastrointest Surg. 2018;22(12):2117–24. https://doi.org/10.1007/s11605-018-3855-1.
6. Alexander K, Ismail M, Alexander M, et al. Use of ICG imaging to confirm bowel viability after upper mesenteric stenting in patient with acute mesenteric ischemia: case report. Int J Surg Case Rep. 2019;61:322–6. https://doi.org/10.1016/j.ijscr.2019.07.077.
7. Kim SH, Hwang HY, Kim MJ, Park KJ, Kim KB. Early laparoscopic exploration for acute mesenteric ischemia after cardiac surgery [published online ahead of print, 2019 Apr 19]. Acute Crit Care. 2020;35(3):213–7. https://doi.org/10.4266/acc.2018.00423.
8. Tshomba Y, Coppi G, Marone EM, et al. Diagnostic laparoscopy for early detection of acute mesenteric ischaemia in patients with aortic dissection. Eur J Vasc Endovasc Surg. 2012;43(6):690–7. https://doi.org/10.1016/j.ejvs.2012.03.017
9. Cocorullo G, Mirabella A, Falco N, et al. An investigation of bedside laparoscopy in the ICU for cases of non-occlusive mesenteric ischemia. World J Emerg Surg. 2017;12:4. https://doi.org/10.1186/s13017-017-0118-5.
10. Shaw RS. The "second look" after superior mesenterial embolectomy or reconstruction for mesenteric infarction. In: Current surgical management. Philadelphia: W. B. Sounders Company; 1965. p. 509.
11. Anadol AZ, Ersoy E, Taneri F, Tekin EH. Laparoscopic "second-look" in the management of mesenteric ischemia. Surg Laparosc Endosc Percutan Tech. 2004;14(4):191–3. https://doi.org/10.1097/01.sle.0000136677.39377.62.
12. Meng X, Liu L, Jiang H. Indications and procedures for second-look surgery in acute mesenteric ischemia. Surg Today. 2010;40(8):700–5. https://doi.org/10.1007/s00595-009-4140-4.
13. Yanar H, Taviloglu K, Ertekin C, et al. Planned second-look laparoscopy in the management of acute mesenteric ischemia. World J Gastroenterol. 2007;13(24):3350–3. https://doi.org/10.3748/wjg.v13.i24.3350.

Open Abdomen in the Elderly

22

Giovanni Bellanova, Simone Frassini, Stefania Cimbanassi, Osvaldo Chiara, Sergio Ribaldi, and Gregorio Tugnoli

22.1 Introduction

Open abdomen (OA) treatment definition is when abdominal wall layers are purposefully left open (fascial edges and skin) after a laparotomy [1].

OA should not be compared to a laparostomy, because this approach has an important role treating a lot of abdominal affections, in particular septic condition: therefore, it has to be considered a crucial step in a clinical strategy, not only a simple surgical technique.

Comparing open abdomen to the surgical concept of laparostomy, OA is a sort of functional progress: clinical indications remain the same, but negative pressure wound therapy (NPWT) and injections in open abdomen treatment have an importance against abdominal sepsis and abdominal compartment syndrome (ACS). Although OA has well-known physiological origins, there are still not clear evidences supporting a more widespread application [2, 3].

OA is a surgical emergency option in case of patients with critical conditions—hemodynamical instability or septic shock—due to trauma or other abdominal acute disease.

Damage control surgery (DCS)—that includes specifically OA treatment—is a key step in the damage control resuscitation (DCR) approach to a severely injured patient. Traditionally, OA was indicated in trauma surgery to avoid intra-abdominal hypertension (IAH) and abdominal compartment syndrome (ACS), common causes of multiorgan failure (MOF) and mortality. Temporary abdominal closure in OA technique allows an easy way for surgical second-look when needed to check abdominal cavity condition, for example, in case of ischemic injury or when bowel anastomosis is performed.

OA, when performed for emergency and acute care surgery, has major morbidity and complications compared to trauma surgery application: enteroatmospheric fistula, intra-abdominal abscesses, frozen abdomen, and a more difficult definitive abdominal wall closure are typical [4].

Focusing on the OA application in the elderly population, there are really few evidences in scientific literature: however, is clear how this population could be more affected by surgical

G. Bellanova
Chirurgia Generale, PO Camberlingo, Francavilla Fontana, ASL Brindisi, Francavilla Fontana, Italy

S. Frassini · S. Cimbanassi
Chirurgia Generale, Trauma Team ASST Niguarda, Milan, Italy

O. Chiara
Università degli Studi di Milano, Dipartimento Fisiopatologia Trapianti—Chirurgia Generale, Trauma Team, ASST Niguarda, Milan, Italy

S. Ribaldi
Chirurgia d' Urgenza e del Trauma, Dipartimento di Emergenza, Policlinico Umberto I, Rome, Italy

G. Tugnoli (✉)
Chirurgia del Trauma, Dipartimento Emergenza, Ospedale Maggiore, Bologna, Italy
e-mail: gregorio.tugnoli@ausl.bologna.it

F. Agresta et al. (eds.), *Emergency laparoscopic surgery in the elderly and frail patient*
https://doi.org/10.1007/978-3-030-79990-8_22

complication in case of open abdomen. In a retrospective multicenter study, only age and important fascial retraction were associated to intraoperative mortality as independent prognostic factors [5].

Age is a negative prognostic factor not only for intraoperative mortality but also for the possibility of definitive fascia closure and in-hospital complications rate [6–8].

Open abdomen is the final step of emergency laparotomy when performed in DCS, avoiding loss of time for definitive surgical abdominal closure: the purpose is a fast admission of severe unstable patients to the intensive care unit in order to stabilize vital parameters after damage source control. In case of trauma, the control of bleeding is the intraoperative priority during DCS, while in case of emergency surgery laparotomy, the goal is the control of infectious source. After acute care management and resuscitation, patient is admitted to the operating room for a surgical second-look, definitive treatment—if necessary—and abdominal wall closure (last step of damage control treatment).

Acute care and septic control improvement decreased the open abdomen necessity, but it is still indicated in case of abdominal compartment syndrome. Septic resuscitation after surgery is typically treated with aggressive fluid supplement: bowel distension, edema, and cavity contamination can cause an increase in endocavitary volume and intra-abdominal pressure, not allowing an easy surgical closure of the abdominal wall.

Surgery for intestinal ischemia, pancreatic necrosectomy, bowel resection without direct anastomosis, or important abdominal sepsis can need an operative second-look: OA technique is useful also for these conditions.

The commonly accepted indications for open abdomen are as follows:

- IAH, intra-abdominal hypertension
- DCS in trauma
- Severe sepsis with abdominal origin
- Severe acute pancreatitis treatment

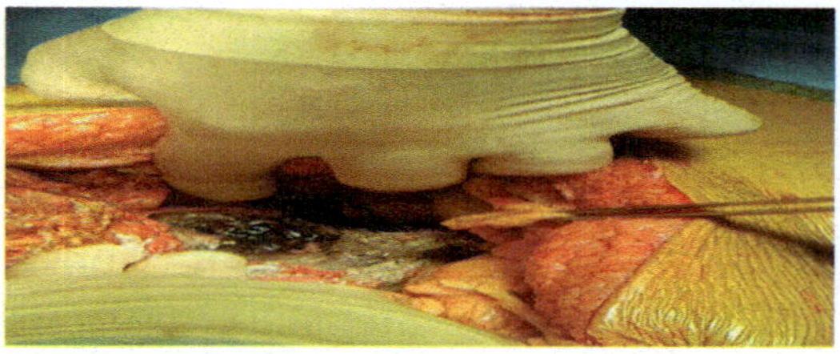

Acute necrotizing pancreatitis treatment

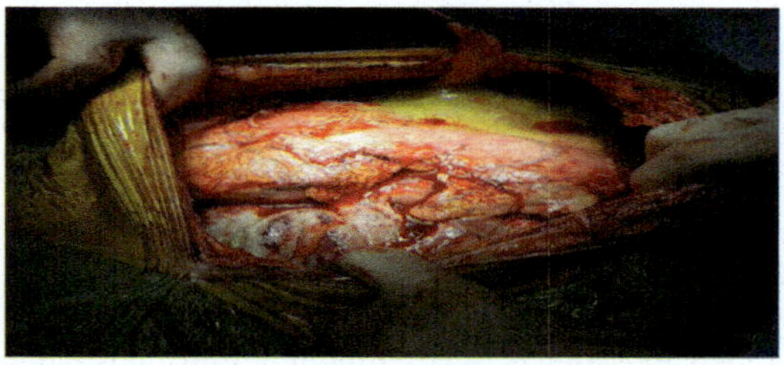

Severe peritonitis treatment

Normal intra-abdominal pressure (IAP) is from 5 to 7 mm Hg, while IAH is a clinical condition with IAP values of 12–20 mm Hg. Abdominal compartment syndrome is formally diagnosed in case of IAP > 25 mm Hg associated with hypotension, organs hypoperfusion, edema, bowel ischemia, kidney injury, and ongoing multiorgan failure (MOF).

IAH classification:

- Normal values: 5–7 mm Hg
- Grade 1 IAH: 12–15 mm Hg
- Grade 2 IAH: 16–20 mm Hg
- Grade 3 IAH: ACS: 21–25 mm Hg
- Grade 4 IAH: ACS: > 25 mm Hg

Although trauma surgery is the main OA application, new concept of damage control surgery and open abdomen—performed not only in trauma but also in septic and emergency surgery patients—needs a complete awareness of the technique by general surgeons. A proper management of OA is fundamental taking care of acute care surgery patients, in particular, in case of IAH or when abdominal wall is purposefully left open: targets are a correct fluid balance, protection from external agents, and finally to prevent loss of abdominal domain for an early definitive closure.

There are a lot of classification for open abdomen, one we are proposing appears as the most complete:

- Grade 1: OA without adherence between bowel and abdominal wall
  - 1A: Clean OA
  - 1B: Contaminated OA
  - 1C: Enteric leak
- Grade 2: OA with adherence or fixity
  - 2A: Clean OA
  - 2B: Contaminated OA
  - 2C: Enteric leak
- Grade 3: Frozen abdomen
  - 3A: Clean OA
  - 3B: Contaminated OA
- Grade 4: Frozen abdomen with enteroatmospheric fistula

22.2 Technique

Negative pressure wound therapy (NPWT), especially when combined with skin and fascial approximation, appears as the most appropriate method for OA management with and improved rate of early abdominal wall closure. NPWT needs commercial devices to be packed in the correct way, in order to drain peritoneal fluids, to facilitate nursing, and to prevent fascial retraction. OA and NPTW use are recommended with level of evidence (LoE) I and grade of recommendation (GoR) B.

After abbreviate laparotomy, there are some different surgical techniques to perform open abdomen, taking into account personnel skills, hospital facilities, and the availability of commercial devices.

In 2014, Italian Consensus Conference about OA after trauma surgery suggested commercial devices application with LoE I, limiting several inexpensive and homemade techniques for clear disadvantages like difficulty in nursing and abdominal lavage [9].

Key concepts in OA management are as follows:

- Peritoneal cavity lavage and damage source control
- Bowel protection
- Care and approximation of fascial layer
- Skin approximation
- Controlled suction of fluids
- 48-h check of OA and dressing renewal
- Definitive damage control
- Skin and fascial closure as soon as possible, at least at eighth postoperative day

In literature, there are a lot of OA techniques description:

1. Skin closure

   In this technique, only skin layer is closed with running suture or clips: after this treatment, only surgical second-look is possible.
2. Bogota bag

   This technique is based on antiadherent plastic bag placed over bowel loops and skin closure.

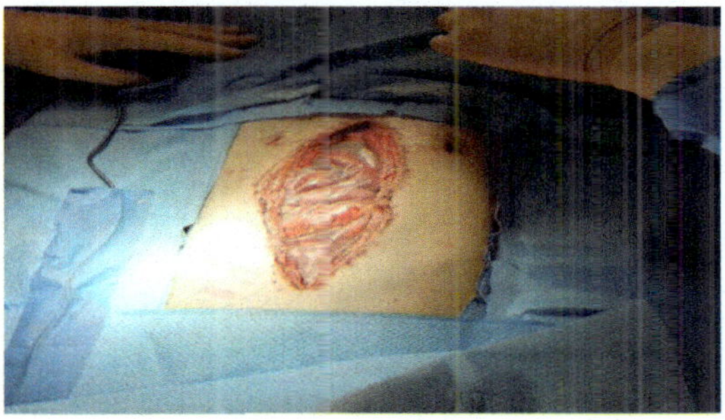

3. Opsite sandwich technique

   This OA technique consists in positioning a laparotomic gauze between two adhesive sterile drapes, above antiadherent plastic bag directly in contact with bowel loops. In the context that medication, it's necessary to place tubes for irrigation and suction.

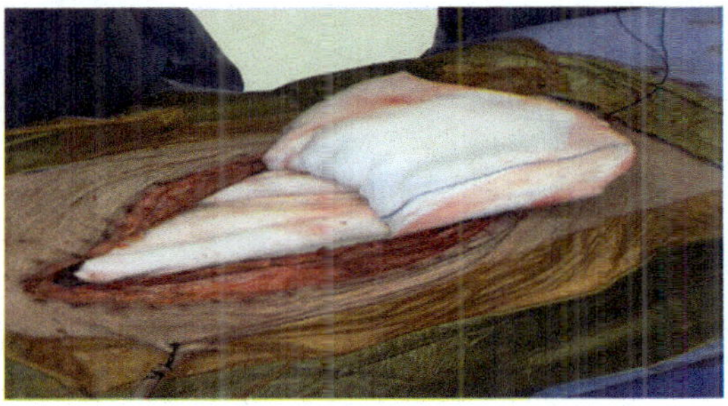

4. Zipper

   This technique is based on abdominal zip placement to make faster and easier surgical second-look.

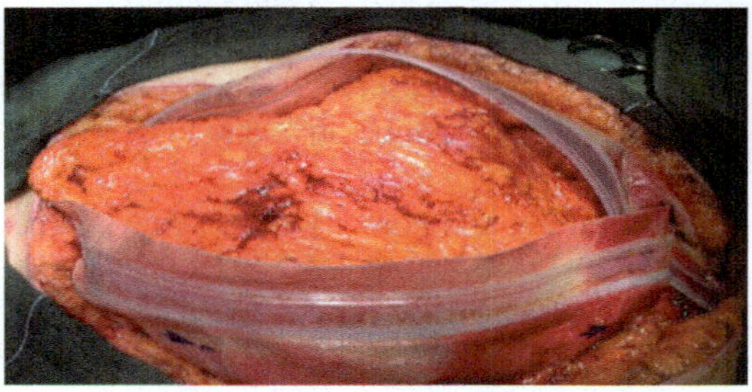

5. Adsorbable patch placement

   It's the case when some adsorbable patches are placed next to the fascial and skin suture to promote abdominal wall layers closure.

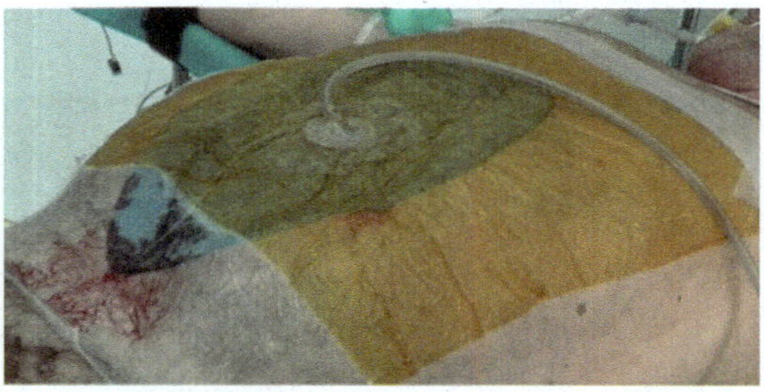

6. Negative pressure system

   With this technique, there is a negative pressure supported by commercial devices promoting peritoneal lavage and drainage: the most common system provides an equal negative pressure all over abdominal cavity. In case of negative pressure wound therapy during OA, it's possible to drain infected fluid and improving nursing care for fluid balance and dressing change.

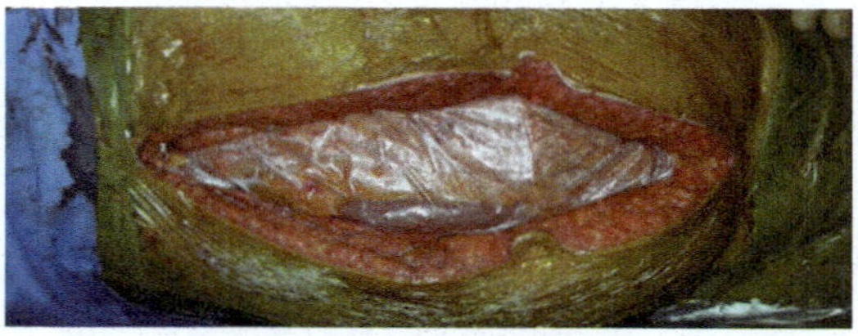

Similar, but homemade, the Barker Wound Management: above plastic layer over bowel loops, a laparotomic gauze with aspiration is placed for a NPWT effect.

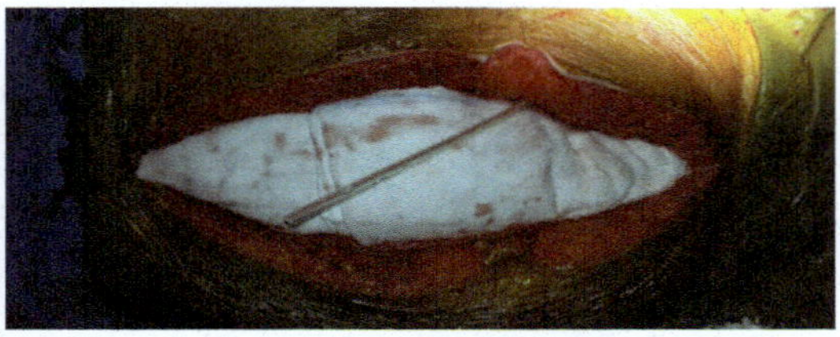

About fluid for peritoneal lavage, there are not evidences regarding quality and quantity. Currently, there are studies matched computer-controlled irrigation system and continue instillation techniques.

22.3 Results

Open abdomen is effective but there are complications about this technique: in particular, when skin and fascia closure is delayed, complications are possible [10].

Enteroatmospheric fistula are typical complications after OA, with a complex management, high rate of mortality, and morbidity over 40%. Due to the difficult management of this patients, associated with high complication rate and risk of acute fluid imbalance, a multidisciplinary point of view is necessary; early fascial closure—if possible, within eight postoperative days—should be gold standard to avoid tissue retractions and all the complications listed above.

Open abdomen closure is a major surgery, because fascial and muscular layers are defined surgically as "difficult to manage" [11]. Techniques differ from patient to patient, and some of them are typically treated with "planned hernia" approach: when primary skin and fascial closure is not possible, for example, for severe septic condition, could be ideal to program surgery on a second time. In literature, there are some different techniques described for fascial reconstruction: with LoE, biological meshes are gold standard for definitive surgery. Resuming, primary fascial closure is related with risk of hernia after some months, on the other hand could be an idea to plan more complex approach with bridges techniques before component-separation surgery. Tissue contamination and surgical difficulties often require instillations and NPWT, but in case of biological mesh, negative pressure is contraindicated.

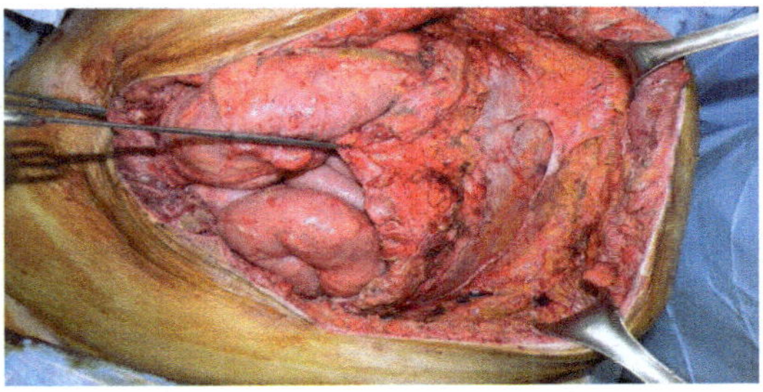

In conclusion, OA is a possible surgical technique also in elderly population, but it's clear the association with high mortality and morbidity: cautions and attention are required for worst clinical cases and OA indications should be proper.

Five Things You Should Know About Open Abdomen

- OA should be considered as a part of a damage control strategy.
- The use of industrial dressings should be preferred because they guarantee a safer control of the suction pressure.
- Dressing changes should be done no later than every 48 h. On that occasion, it is necessary to provide for a complete mitigation of the intestinal loops in order to open any collections.
- The duration of OA directly affects the possibility of a direct closure of the abdomen.
- In case of need for a prolonged period of OA, a planned ventral hernia is an acceptable outcome.

References

1. Sarani B, Martin N. Management of the open abdomen in adults. UpToDate. Wolters Kluwer Health; 2012.
2. Kirkpatrick AW, Coccolini F, Ansaloni L, et al. Closed or open after source control laparotomy for severe complicated intra-abdominal sepsis (the COOL trial): study protocol for a randomized controlled trial. World J Emerg Surg. 2018;13:26. https://doi.org/10.1186/s13017-018-0183-4.
3. Coccolini F, Catena F, Montori G, et al. IROA: the international register of open abdomen. An international effort to better understand the open abdomen: call for participants. World J Emerg Surg. 2015;10:37. https://doi.org/10.1186/s13017-015-0029-2.
4. Coccolini F, Biffl W, Catena F, et al. The open abdomen, indications, management and definitive closure. World J Emerg Surg. 2015;10:32.
5. Sartelli M, Catena F, Ansaloni L, Coccolini F, et al. Complicated intra-abdominal infections worldwide: the definitive data of the CIAOW study. World J Emerg Surg. 2014;9:37.
6. Acosta S, Bjarnason T, Petersson U, et al. Multicentre prospective study of fascial closure rate after open abdomen with vacuum and mesh-mediated fascial traction. Br J Surg. 2011;98:735–43.
7. Morais M, Gonçalves D, Bessa-Melo R, et al. The open abdomen: analysis of risk factors for mortality and delayed fascial closure in 101 patients. Porto Biomed J. 2018;3(2):e14.
8. Coccolini F, et al. Open abdomen and age; results from IROA (international register of open abdomen). Am J Surg. 2020;220(1):229–36. https://doi.org/10.1016/j.amjsurg.2019.11.022.
9. Chiara O, et al. International consensus conference on open abdomen in trauma. J Trauma Acute Care Surg. 2016;80:173–83.
10. Coccolini F, et al. The open abdomen in trauma and non trauma patients: WSES guideline. WJES. 2018;13:7.
11. Piccoli M, et al. Complex abdominal wall management: evidence-based guidelines of Italian consensus conference. Updates Surg. 2019;71:255–72.

Gynaecologic Emergencies

23

Emanuele Botteri, Giulia Montori, Luca Ansaloni, and Federico Coccolini

23.1 Introduction

Even though gynaecological emergencies occur most commonly in young women, geriatric gynaecological disorders are now increasing in number due to the ageing of the general population. Nowadays, we assume that certain elderly specific conditions are more important than chronological age alone in predicting surgical outcome [1–4]. Among the clinical manifestations of frailty, we record cognitive impairment, poor exercise capacity and diminished functional status. Each of these factors may prejudice the ability of the body to cope with acute stressors such as surgery.

Diagnostic laparoscopy is effective and safe for discerning the cause of abdominal pain. It allows a definitive diagnosis in 98% of cases [3–5].

The 1970s laparoscopy has become the gold standard for several gynaecological diseases, however, its diffusion in emergency cases is not so wide [6–9]. In particular, there is a lack in specific guidelines and evidence-based literature. The most frequent exclusion criteria for the enrolment in clinical trials are extreme age and a high ASA score, so elderly patients are often underrepresented in surgical trials. Several patients who have undergone diagnostic laparoscopy have avoided laparotomy because they were successfully treated with a laparoscopic procedure. A mini-invasive approach in emergency situations carries with it well-known advantages such as elective procedure, in particular, swifter mobilization and the resumption of oral intake, less pain and blood loss.

Emergency physicians should take care to adapt to women's challenges and to consider age-specific disorders. However, few statistics and few literature data are available concerning these patients.

Common gynaecological disorders occurring in postmenopausal age women that require urgent treatment are: intra-abdominal haemorrhage, adnexal torsion, traumatic injuries and rupture of pyometra.

23.2 Intra-abdominal Haemorrhage in the Elderly

In young and childbearing age females, intra-abdominal haemorrhage can occur due to different conditions: ectopic pregnancy, ruptured

E. Botteri (✉)
Montichiari Surgery, ASST Spedali Civili Brescia, Brescia, Italy

G. Montori
Surgical Oncology, IRCCS CRO National Cancer Institute, Aviano, Italy

L. Ansaloni
Unit of General Surgery, IRCCS San Matteo Hospital, University of Pavia, Pavia, Italy

F. Coccolini
Emergency Surgery Unit and Trauma Center, Pisa University Hospital, Pisa, Italy

F. Agresta et al. (eds.), *Emergency laparoscopic surgery in the elderly and frail patient*,
https://doi.org/10.1007/978-3-030-79990-8_23

haemorrhagic cysts and less frequently by ruptured endometrioma, uterine rupture and ruptured hydrosalpinx.

Clinical symptoms present more frequently with abdominal pain and tenderness, and only rarely with hypovolaemia and haemodynamic instability.

In the elderly, intra-abdominal haemorrhage can occur extremely rarely. Principal causes can be uterine leiomyomas, and less frequently leiomyosarcoma. This disease can occur with tumour rupture and intra-abdominal haemorrhage [10, 11].

Intraperitoneal haemorrhage is rare and can be caused due to torsion or avulsion of a pedunculated leiomyoma [11]. More severe haemorrhages from leiomyomas are exceptional and may result from different causes: spontaneous or traumatic leiomyoma rupture, rupture of a subserosal vein or superficial dilated vein, or from a ruptured arterial aneurysm or arterial vessel arising from the uterine arteries [11]. Venous bleeding is more frequent than arterial bleeding [11]. A leiomyoma's size greater than 10 cm is also considered to be a risk factor for vein rupture and bleeding [12].

Moreover, other causes of intraperitoneal bleeding reported in the literature are: laceration, avulsion, torsion, or rupture of a degenerative fibroid or fibroid capsule [13, 14].

Trauma is another cause of pelvic intraperitoneal bleeding.

Diagnosis can be performed looking at the conditional status and laboratory tests, as well as imaging modalities, such as ultrasound (US), computed tomography (CT) scan and magnetic resonance imaging (MRI) [11]. MRI and CT scans should always be performed in stable patients [11]. FAST (Focused Assessment with Sonography for Trauma) ultrasound should be performed, instead, in unstable patients to identify intra-abdominal fluid [11–15]. Despite the rarity of this condition, no data about the preferential surgical technique approach are published in the literature.

However, as recommended by the World Society of Emergency Surgery (WSES) as well as other scientific societies dealing with emergency surgery, the decision to perform laparoscopy or open surgery is dependent upon the haemodynamic status. Moreover, in the case of suspected leiomyosarcomas, during abdominal exploration, open approach is mandatory and total abdominal hysterectomy with bilateral salpingo-oophorectomy should be performed [11]. In unstable patients, open surgery is mandatory to stop bleeding rapidly and to encourage fast resuscitation; whilst in stable patients, especially in expert hand, laparoscopic surgery can be more performing to detect the bleeding origin, to treat them and to give faster recovery with less length of stay [11–17].

In elderly patients, the choice of different approaches should also consider the presence of other co-morbidities, the clinical status and the drug history [18, 19].

23.3 Adnexal Torsion in Elderly

The risk of adnexal torsion is increased in reproductive age females and in pregnant women with a rate of 2.7–60% of cases and lower in the postmenopausal age range [20, 21]. Moreover, it is almost always associated with an enlarged ovarian mass and the risk is increased when there is a size mass greater than 8 cm [20]. In addition to these physiological clinical conditions, ovarian tumours can cause ovarian torsion (50–60%), as well as mature cystic teratomas (dermoid tumours) (25% rate of benign tumours) [20–22]. Research into postmenopausal women is mainly reported in descriptive studies and retrospective chart reviews, so the data are very limited [23].

Clinically, women present an acute, intermittent, unilateral pelvic pain that can change with different positional shifts [21, 22]. Frequently, they also present gastrointestinal symptoms, such as nausea and vomiting. For this reason, differential diagnosis like appendicitis, bowel obstruction and mesenteric ischaemia should be excluded [20]. Upon physical examination, a tender mass can be appreciated.

Pelvic ultrasound with a Colour Doppler (US-CD) can be useful to detect an increased flow can be highly predictive of an adnexal torsion [20–

24]. However, in the case of a normal CD flow, adnexal torsion cannot be excluded and an intraoperative diagnosis can often be made [20–22].

Moreover, a contrast-enhanced CT scan can be a useful tool to evaluate also other causes of abdominal pain. However, no clear and well-defined CT criteria are found in the literature to suggest ovarian torsion. Frequently, asymmetric ovarian enlargement can be a suspicious finding in ovarian torsion. In contrast, enhanced CT peripheral follicles surrounding an enlarged ovary, ovarian haemorrhage, free pelvic fluid, inflammatory fat stranding adjacent to the ovary, a thickened uterine tube, uterine deviation towards the side of torsion or a twisted vascular pedicle can suggest this disorder. CT can also suggest the risk of ovarian malignancy. However, in the case of a completely normal CT scan, the risk of torsion is low [23].

To avoid the risk of ovarian loss, diagnosis should be made as soon as possible [22–24].

Treatment of adnexal torsion still consists of surgical reduction [20]. The treatment can be more conservative especially in younger patients and in the case of a benign suspect disease (only adnexal reduction and possibly oophoropexy, stitching ovarian stroma to the pelvic sidewall) or more aggressive, especially in the case of severe vascular impairment (a salpingo-oophorectomy) [20, 25, 26]. With the conservative approach, the laparoscopic success rate is near to 88% with high satisfaction rates for women. These treatments can be performed with the laparoscopic approach [27]. Risk of injuring the ureter (runs inferiorly and laterally to the infundibulopelvic ligament) should always be kept in mind.

In postmenopausal age, considering the risk of malignancies (3–25% vs. 1% in premenopausal age), extensive surgery can be necessary [22, 28–31]. Some authors reported an increased rate of conversion to laparotomy in elderly patients and in the case of ovarian necrosis [22]. An increased risk of laparotomic total abdominal hysterectomy and bilateral salpingo-oophorectomy and staging surgery (including pelvic wash for cytology, hysterectomy and adnexectomy, omentectomy and lymph node sampling) is required [22]. However, the possibility to perform a frozen pathological section study can help minimize the risk of conversion, only in the case of malignancy [22, 32].

In the case of desmoid tumours, the laparoscopic approach can be safe but it is mandatory to avoid the risk of cyst rupture and intraoperative spillage of sebaceous fluid, placing the patient at risk of chemical peritonitis [31]. Different types of dissections are reported in the literature, including blunt dissection, use of an endobag and the creation of a posterior colpotomy, or aqua dissection [31]. Some authors found that intraoperative spillage was more common with sharp dissection; others found less spillage in patients treated by enucleation and removal via a colpotomy or with hysterectomy than endobag removal [31]. However, no serious complications are reported in any of the cases with a risk of chemical peritonitis lower than 0.2% [31]. Moreover, copious and immediate peritoneal washing can minimize the risk of peritonitis [31].

23.4 Traumatic Injuries and Cuff Dehiscence Post-hysterectomy

Traumatic gynaecological emergencies are rare and in the majority of cases are treated in the Emergency Department or treated conservatively with analgesics, ice packs or sitz baths [33]. However, in some cases, (extended lacerations more than 3 cm, or lacerations involving hymen, urethra, anus, vaginal bleeding with unclear source, very large hematomas, involvement of adjacent structures, necroses, rapid expansion hematoma) an operative exploration and possibly repair is mandatory [33]. These traumatic conditions can occur in women of any age and the risk of potential sexual abuse should be always investigated.

Although rare, vaginal cuff dehiscence is a serious event that can develop after hysterectomy. It is defined as 'a full thickness separation, partial or total of the anterior and posterior edges of the vaginal cuff' [34, 35]. It occurs typically 5–7 weeks after surgery and is often caused by sexual intercourse or other traumatic aetiology, when vaginal cuff fusion is insufficient. The lowest incidence of the disease is after total vaginal hysterectomy (0.08–0.15%) and it grows after abdominal and laparoscopic total hysterectomy (0.15–0.25% and 0.64–1.35% respectively) [36, 37].

Atrophic vaginitis, tobacco use, poorly controlled diabetes mellitus, irradiation and long-term steroid treatment are well-known risk factors for vaginal cuff dehiscence [37]. Indeed, it is not clear whether a hysterectomy performed for malignant conditions represents a risk factor for dehiscence. Women may manifest increased vaginal discharge and bleeding, lower abdominal pain and discomfort. History of hysterectomy and any of these complaints should mean that the patient is referred for a pelvic and speculum examination. Vaginal cuff dehiscence is a surgical emergency because prolapse of pelvic content may happen with life-threatening consequences such as bowel occlusion or necrosis. Not only is the ileum involved, prolapse of the omental sheet, appendix and fallopian tube have also been reported.

Vaginal cuff dehiscence can be managed both with the transvaginal or transabdominal approach. For the latter, literature describes laparoscopy and laparotomy according to the initial clinical condition.

In the presence of an unstable patient with diffuse peritonitis, immediate laparotomy is mandatory with peritoneal drainage, vaginal cuff closure and possibly bowel resection.

In medically stable patients without signs of bowel necrosis or diffuse peritonitis, vaginal surgery could be considered. This has the advantage of being minimally invasive, but it does not allow an accurate observation of the abdominal cavity [38]. Laparoscopy allows a good visualization of the intraperitoneal side of the vaginal cuff and the abdomen as a whole. The first successful repair performed with laparoscopy was reported in 2002 by Lledo. In a recent paper, Thomopoulos et al. [39] reported the results of 116 vaginal cuff dehiscence repair collected between 1864 and 2016 and they found that laparoscopy was used in only 2% of the cases but a satisfactory outcome was achieved in all cases. Several other case reports share the same results [40, 41].

Regarding technical features, the cuff can be repaired in one or two layers. In literature, there are some randomized trials and retrospective analysis comparing these two methods [42–45]. The reports indicate that a two-layer continuous suture using absorbable barbed threads is more effective and safer for vaginal cuff repair.

A systemic review performed by Bogoglio et al. [46] found that the use of absorbable barbed suture significantly reduces operative time.

23.5 Pyometra Perforation

The collection of pus in the uterine cavity is known as pyometra [47]. It is a rare disease in the general population with an incidence of 0.1–0.5% but it is found more frequently in postmenopausal women representing 13.6% of gynaecological admission [48, 49]. Genital tract malignancies and the consequences of radiotherapy are the main cause of pyometra. Several other benign conditions, such as senile cervicitis, uterine fibrosis, endometrial lesions (leiomyoma or polyps) and congenital cervical anomaly can induce pyometra.

The classical symptoms are lower abdominal pain, vaginal discharge and bleeding even if more than 50% of unperforated pyometra are asymptomatic [50–52]. Spontaneous perforation of pyometra is a life-threatening yet rare condition with an incidence of 0.01–0.05% [5]. Uterine perforation is usually located in the fundus (77%), alternatively, it can involve the anterior wall (4%) [53]. Ultrasonography has high sensitivity in assessing pyometra, so it is the first investigation required. It has a limited role in the diagnosis of perforation due to the inability to demonstrate the uterine breach and the limited sonographic window available.

The gold standard radiological evaluation used for acute abdomen is the total abdomen CT scan. It can show pneumoperitoneum and intra-abdominal fluid, which frequently leads to the misdiagnosis of gastrointestinal perforation. Sagittal and coronal reformats reconstructions in multi-detector computerized tomography are very helpful in depicting the site and size of uterine breach. Septic shock and multiple organ failure are the most significant factors in high mortality linked to pyometra perforation (close to 40%) [54]. Prompt medical therapy based on fluid resuscitation and wide-broad spectrum antibiotics is required. Urgent surgical management relies on hysterectomy and salpingo-oophorectomy. Once more, the initial clinical conditions of patients drive us in the choice of the approach. Immediate laparotomy is mandatory in severely ill or unstable patients.

Laparoscopy is rarely used although it could be performed by experienced surgeons in stable patients. Searching in the literature we found fewer than 90 cases of ruptured pyometra from 1949 to 2020 and in only one patient laparoscopy was used with good results [55].

Five Things You Should Know About Gynaecologic Emergencies in the Elderly and Frail Patient

- Laparoscopy in gynaecological emergency is nowadays underemployed. There are few evidence-based level 1 recommendations, so the choice of laparoscopic approach is left to surgeon's experience.
- Laparoscopy for gynaecological disorders in elderly patients seems to share the same advantages found in younger women. Probably, a minimally invasive approach plays a key role in a good recovery and in the lowering of complication after surgery also in aging.
- Principal cause of intra-abdominal bleeding is rupture of leiomyomas and less frequently leyomyosarcomas. In stable patients, benign disease, and experienced hands, laparoscopy can be safe.
- Adnexal torsion is rare in elderly, however, the surgical approach of adnexal reduction should take into account the risk of malignancy.
- Laparoscopic sutures are safe and effective for the closure of vaginal cuff dehiscence. Experienced surgeon should face this condition because there are some risks of visceral injuries during the reduction of herniated organs.

Conflict of Interest The authors declare no source of funding or conflict of interest.

References

1. Unger CA, Hickman LC, Mitchell-Handley B, Barber MD, Ridgeway B. The incidence of perioperative adverse events in the very elderly undergoing urogynecologic surgery. Female Pelvic Med Reconstr Surg. 2016;22:425–9.
2. Greer JA, Northington GM, Harvie HS, Segal S, Johnson JC, Arya LA. Functional status and postoperative morbidity in older women with prolapse. J Urol. 2013;190:948–52.
3. Sozuer EM, Bedirli A, Ulusal M, et al. Laparoscopy for diagnosis and treatment of acute abdominal pain. J Laparoendosc Adv Surg Tech. 2000;10:203–7.
4. Salky BA, Edye MB. The role of laparoscopy in the diagnosis and treatment of abdominal pain syndromes. Surg Endosc. 1998;12:911–4.
5. Navez B, d'Udekem Y, Cambier E, et al. Laparoscopy for management of nontraumatic acute abdomen. World J Surg. 1995;19:382–6.
6. Ou CS, Rowbotham R. Laparoscopic diagnosis and treatment of nontraumatic acute abdominal pain in women. J Laparoecdo Adv Surg Tech. 2000;10 41–5.
7. Cohen SB, Weisz B, Seidman DS, et al. Accuracy of the preoperative diagnosis in 100 emergency laparoscopies performed due to acute abdomen in nonpregnant women. J Am Assoc Gynecol Laparosc. 2001;8:92–4.
8. Magos AL, Baumann R, Turnbull AC. Managing gynaecological emergencies with laparoscopy. BMJ. 1989;299:371–4.
9. Taylor EW, Kennedy CA, Dunham RH, et al. Diagnostic laparoscopy in women with acute abdominal pain. Surg Laparosc Endosc. 1995;5:125–8.
10. Juhasz-Böss I, Gabriel L, Bohle RM, Horn LC, Solomayer EF, Breitbach GP. Uterine leiomyosarcoma. Oncol Res Treat. 2018;41(11):680–6.
11. Elkbuli A, Shaikh S, McKenney M, Boneva D. Life-threatening hemoperitoneum secondary to rupture of a uterine leiomyoma: a case report and review of the literature. Int J Surg Case Rep. 2019;61:51–5.
12. Horowitz E, Dekel A, Feldberg D. Massive hemoperitoneum due to rupture of an artery overlying a uterine leiomyoma: a case report. Acta Obstet Gynecol Scand. 2005;84:408–9.
13. Nigam A, Raghunandan C, Yadav R. Twisted subserosal leiomyoma in a non-gravid uterus: a rare cause of acute abdomen. J Obstet Gynaecol. 2014;34:657–8.
14. Schwitkis A, Shen S, Vos E, Torbati S. Spontaneous hemoperitoneum from rupture of massive leiomyoma. Clin Pract Cases Emerg Med. 2017;1(2):148–9.
15. American College of Surgeons, Committee on Trauma. Advanced trauma life support: student course manual. 10th ed. 2018.

16. Agresta F, Campanile FC, Podda M, Cillara N, Pernazza G, Giaccaglia V, et al. Current status of laparoscopy for acute abdomen in Italy: a critical appraisal of 2012 clinical guidelines from two consecutive nationwide surveys with analysis of 271,323 cases over 5 years. Surg Endosc. 2017;31(4):1785–95.
17. Beuran M, Negoi I, Hostiuc S, Catena F, et al. Laparoscopic approach has benefits in gynecological emergencies—even for massive hemoperitoneum. Chirurgia (Bucur). 2016;111(1):48–53.
18. Kanasaki H, Oride A, Miyazaki K. Laparoscopic surgery in elderly patients aged 65 years and older with gynecologic disease. ISRN Obstet Gynecol. 2012;2012:678201.
19. McWilliams GD, Hill MJ, Dietrich CS 3rd. Gynecologic emergencies. Surg Clin N Am. 2008;88(2):265–83.
20. Lawrence LL. Unusual presentations in obstetrics and gynecology. Emerg Med Clin North Am. 2003;21(3):649–65.
21. Balci O, Energin H, Görkemli H, Acar A. Management of adnexal torsion: a 13-year experience in single tertiary center. J Laparoendosc Adv Surg Tech A. 2019;29(3):293–7.
22. Robertson JJ, Long B, Koyfman A. Myths in the evaluation and management of ovarian torsion. J Emerg Med. 2017;52(4):449–56.
23. Hiller N, Appel Baum L, Simanovsky N, et al. CT features of adnexal torsion. AJR Am J Roentgenol. 2007;189(1):124–9, 19g, 21g.
24. Nagel TC, Sebastian J, Malo JW. Oophoropexy to prevent sequential or recurrent torsion. J Am Assoc Gynecol Laparosc. 1997;4(4):495–8.
25. Zweizig S, Perron J, Grubb D, et al. Conservative management of adnexal torsion. Am J Obstet Gynecol. 1993;168(6 Pt 1):1791–5.
26. Cohen SB, Wattiez A, Seidman DS, et al. Laparoscopy versus laparotomy for detorsion and sparing of twisted ischemic adnexa. JSLS. 2003;7(4):295–9.
27. Herman GH, Shalev A, Ginath S, Kerner R, Keidar R, Bar J, Sagiv R. Clinical characteristics and the risk for malignancy in postmenopausal women with adnexal torsion. Maturitas. 2015;81:57–61.
28. Ozcan A, Mumusoglu S, Gokcu M, et al. Differentiated therapy in pre- and postmenopausal adnexal torsion based on malignancy rates: a retrospective multicentre study over five years. Int J Surg. 2016;29:95–100.
29. Lee RA, Welch JS. Torsion of the uterine adnexa. Am J Obstet Gynecol. 1967;97:974–7.
30. Promecene PA. Laparoscopy in gynecologic emergencies. Semin Laparosc Surg. 2002;9(1):64–75.
31. Aulestia SN, Cantele H, Leyba JL, Navarrete M, Llopla SN. Laparoscopic diagnosis and treatment in gynecologic emergencies. JSLS. 2003;7(3):239–42.
32. Manning S. Genital complaints at the extremes of age. Emerg Med Clin North Am. 2019;37(2):193–205.
33. Nichols D. Late postoperative complications. 4th ed. Baltimore: Lippincott Williams & Wilkins Company; 1996.
34. Falcone T. Vaginal cuff dehiscence after hysterectomy. Obstet Gynecol. 2012;120:511–2.
35. Ceccaroni M, Berretta R, Malzoni M, Scioscia M, Roviglione G, Spagnolo E, Rolla M, Farina A, Malzoni C, De Iaco P, Minelli L, Bovicelli L. Vaginal cuff dehiscence after hysterectomy: a multicenter retrospective study. Eur J Obstet Gynecol Reprod Biol. 2011;158:308–13.
36. Uccella S, Ceccaroni M, Cromi A, Malzoni M, Berretta R, De Iaco P, Roviglione G, Bogani G, Minelli L, Ghezzi F. Vaginal cuff dehiscence in a series of 12,398 hysterectomies: effect of different types of colpotomy and vaginal closure. Obstet Gynecol. 2012;120:516–23.
37. Matthews CA, Kenton K. Treatment of vaginal cuff evisceration. Obstet Gynecol. 2014;124:705–8.
38. Lledó JB, Roig MP, Serra AS, Astaburuaga CR, Giménez FD. Laparoscopic repair of vaginal evisceration: a case report. Surg Laparosc Endosc Percutan Tech. 2002;12:446–8.
39. Thomopoulos T, Zufferey G. Totally laparoscopic treatment of vaginal cuff dehiscence: a case report and systematic literature review. Int J Surg Case Rep. 2016;25:79–82.
40. Matsuhashi T, Nakanishi K, Hamano E. Laparoscopic repair of vaginal evisceration after abdominal hysterectomy for uterine corpus cancer: a case report and literature review. J Nippon Med Sch. 2017;84:90–5.
41. Agrawal A, Huang K-G, Mendoza MCV. Emergency laparoscopic repair of coitus induced vaginal cuff dehiscence: a case report Agrawal et al. J Med Case Rep. 2020;14:40.
42. Shen CC, Hsu TY, Huang FJ, Roan CJ, Weng HH, Chang HW, Chang SY. Comparison of one- and two-layer vaginal cuff closure and open vaginal cuff during laparoscopic-assisted vaginal hysterectomy. J Am Assoc Gynecol Laparosc. 2002;9:474–80.
43. Jeung IC, Baek JM, Park EK, Lee HN, Kim CJ, Park TC, Lee YS. A prospective comparison of vaginal stump suturing techniques during total laparoscopic hysterectomy. Arch Gynecol Obstet. 2010;282:631–8.
44. Cronin B, Sung VW, Matteson KA. Vaginal cuff dehiscence: risk factors and management. Am J Obstet Gynecol. 2012;206:284–8.
45. Bogliolo S, Musacchi V, Dominoni M, Cassani C, Gaggero CR, De Silvestri A, Gardella B, Spinillo A. Barbed suture in minimally invasive hysterectomy: a systematic review and meta-analysis. Arch Gynecol Obstet. 2015;292:489–97.
46. Kutuk MS, Ozgun MT, Tas M, Uludag S. Spontaneous uterine perforation due to pyometra. J Obstet Gynaecol. 2013;33(3):322–3.
47. Sawabe M, Takubo K, Esaki Y, Hatano N, Noro T, Nokubi M. Spontaneous uterine perforation as a serious complication of pyometra in elderly females. Aust N Z J Obstet Gynaecol. 1995;35(1):87–91.
48. Inui A, Nitta A, Yamamoto A, Kang SM, Kanehara I, Tanaka H, et al. Generalized peritonitis with pneumoperitoneum caused by the spontaneous perforation of

pyometra without malignancy: report of a case. Surg Today. 1999;29(9):935–8.
49. Nuamah NM, Hamaloglu E, Konan A. Spontaneous uterine perforation due to pyometra presenting as acute abdomen. Int J Gynecol Obstet. 2005;92:145–6.
50. Chen PH, Hsien L, Lee SL, Chang CY, Chang CC. Pneumoperitoneum caused by perforation of pyometra associated with a lost intrauterine device and perforated malignancy of the sigmoid colon. Taiwan J Obstet Gynecol. 2011;50(1):124–5.
51. Imachi M, Tanaka S, Ishikawa S, Matsuo K. Spontaneous perforation of pyometra presenting as generalized peritonitis in a patient with cervical cancer. Gynecol Oncol. 1993;50(3):384–8.
52. Kitai T, Okuno K, Ugaki H, et al. Spontaneous uterine perforation of pyometra presenting as acute abdomen. Case Rep Obstet Gynecol. 2014;2014:738568.
53. Yildizhan B, Uyar E, Şişmanoğlu A, et al. Spontaneous perforation of pyometra. Infect Dis Obstet Gynecol. 2006;2006:26786.
54. Huseyin K, Lale TS, Burak Y. A case of obstructed hemivagina and ipsilateral renal anomaly syndrome complicated with pyometra: tips and tricks for laparoscopic hemi-hysterectomy. Fertil Steril. 2019;112(1):177–9.
55. Hur HC, Donnellan N, Mansuria S, Barber RE, Guido R, Lee T. Vaginal cuff dehiscence after different modes of hysterectomy. Obstet Gynecol. 2011;118:794–801.

Bedside Laparoscopy in the Elderly and Frail Patient

24

Carlo Bergamini, Giovanni Alemanno, Alessio Giordano, Alessandro Bruscino, Gherardo Maltinti, Desiré Pantalone, Jacopo Martellucci, and Paolo Prosperi

24.1 Definition and Rationale for Use

Laparoscopy performed at bedside is a valuable diagnostic tool that can be used safely and efficiently in the evaluation of intra-abdominal pathologies, especially in the frail patients admitted to the Intensive Care Unit, when conventional methods are equivoques or difficult to be performed.

Progress in critical care management, especially timely, aggressive resuscitation, has resulted in a subset of intensive care patients, dependent on a multitude of technical devices ranging from monitors, to ventilators, to medication dosimeters. These patients' courses can be complicated by unexpected new disease processes at any given moment, resulting in acute deterioration unless recognized and managed promptly and accurately. The abdomen is a notorious "black hole" for such unforeseen adverse events, such as septic foci, secondary perforations, hemorrhages, or missed injuries [1, 2].

The conventional diagnostic evaluation usually includes history/physical examination/serum investigations, plain film X-rays, ultrasonography (US), and computed tomography (CT), the latter requiring transport to the radiology suite. However, their application is sometimes frustrating for the following reasons:

1. History may bring suboptimal information in ICU patients from their impaired mental status due to metabolic encephalopathy, brain injury or pharmacologic sedation. Moreover, abdominal examination is often impaired because of different reasons, such as a possible spinal cord injury, a postoperative abdomen, and immunocompromised state which underlies a condition of frailty and hyporeactivity. Therefore, the physical exam is often unhelpful, aiding in diagnosis of only 43–69% of the time with intra-abdominal abscesses [3]. On the other hand, serum investigations can often be nonspecific in the critically ill subjects, with leukocytosis, renal impairment, and a lactic acidosis, all being relatively frequent but nonspecific findings.
2. In the absence of pneumo-peritoneum, plain film X-rays have limited utility and rarely drive the decision to operate.
3. While US of the abdomen has the advantage of portability, it is mostly utilized for the evaluation of the biliary tree, pleural space, cardiac dysfunction, free fluid in the abdomen, and hypovolemia, but is less useful in the frequent case of the presence of bowel gaseous

C. Bergamini (✉) · G. Alemanno · A. Giordano
A. Bruscino · G. Maltinti · D. Pantalone
J. Martellucci · P. Prosperi
Emergency Surgery Department, University Hospital of Careggi, Florence, Italy
e-mail: desire.pantalone@unifi.it; prosperip@aou-careggi.toscana.it

F. Agresta et al. (eds.), *Emergency laparoscopic surgery in the elderly and frail patient*,
https://doi.org/10.1007/978-3-030-79990-8_24

distension and therefore it is limited as a diagnostic tool. It is also not likely to be diagnostic in cases of mesenteric ischemia. Diagnostic yield from US examination of the abdomen is also operator-dependent. For instant, in the traumatically injured patient, the sensitivity of US for detection of acalculous cholecystitis is only 30% [4].

4. Additionally, unlike plain film X-rays and US, CT requires transport that presents a risk for the hemodynamically unstable patient. Actually, most of these patients are hemodynamically labile requiring multiple vasopressors and escalating ventilatory support thereby imposing significant risks during patient transport for imaging or even to the operating room. Life-threatening complications during patient transport, including hypotension, respiratory distress, central line disconnections, and dysrhythmias are not uncommon and have been reported to occur in up to 45% of ICU patient transports [5]. Furthermore, though CT is an excellent diagnostic modality for intra-abdominal pathology, studies have shown limited utility in the critically ill patient: the accuracy of CT in critically ill patients varies between 78 and 89% and can be nonspecific in subtle cases of mesenteric ischemia of recent onset [6]. Its sensitivities is as low as 33–48% for detection of acalculous cholecystitis in the ICU population [7]. Moreover, in some studies, the average time to perform a bedside laparoscopy was less than that needed to obtain a CT scan [8].
5. Diagnostic peritoneal lavage (DPL) is used often to investigate suspected intra-abdominal pathology in patients too unstable for transport; however, DPL has a similar risk profile to diagnostic laparoscopy and does not provide definitive information [9].
6. Finally, the association between occult intra-abdominal infection and organ dysfunction has been deemed sufficiently strong enough to justify empiric laparotomy for the patient with progressive organ dysfunction but no defined focus of infection. However, exploratory laparotomy has not demonstrated an overall decrease in mortality given the large percentage of negative or nontherapeutic results. Of note, laparotomies under these circumstances are associated with reported morbidity rates ranging from 5 to 22%. These data may further encourage diagnostic laparoscopy, which seems to avoid useless laparotomies in up to 25–50% of these patients, particularly in the setting of acalculous cholecystitis, with much less morbidity than a "blinded" laparotomy [10].

24.2 History of Application

The oldest documentation of attempts at minimally invasive surgery comes from the beginning of this century. The technique of insufflation with carbon dioxide and the use of the Verres needle were described in the 1930. Though this concept of diagnostic, or even therapeutic, access to the abdomen without formal laparotomy appeared exciting, several decades passed before it received widespread acceptance. The introduction of the safer open technique for insufflation and trocar insertion and the advent of video laparoscopy with its superior view of the abdominal cavity resulted in an enthusiastic, explosive expansion of applications for diagnosis and surgical procedures by laparoscopic techniques in the 1990. The simplicity of laparoscopy itself, the limited requirement of instruments and personnel, have made this modality attractive for applications outside the operating room setting, such as the ICU or the emergency room. In 1989, Iberti et al. reported the use of bedside laparoscopy in the ICU to diagnose gangrenous bowel after aortic reconstruction surgery [11]. In 1991, Berci reported the use of emergency mini-laparoscopy with the use of a 4-mm laparoscope in the emergency department and in the ICU with local anesthesia and intravenous sedation in both trauma patients and critically ill patients [12]. Since 1992, there have been increasing number of reports of diagnostic laparoscopy in the ICU with a total of several hundred patients.

24.3 Advantages and Indications

Most reports consider the use of laparoscopy in the critically ill patient as a diagnostic tool of high accuracy, which is well tolerated by these high risk frail patients and it avoids nontherapeutic laparotomies and their associated morbidity, cost, or risky transport to the radiology department or operating room. On the contrary, bedside diagnostic laparoscopy (BDL) in the ICU may offer the potential for an accurate assessment in the suspected intra-abdominal pathologies, thanks to a direct intra-abdominal visualization.

Percentages of patients who may avoid an open laparotomy range from 30 to 65%, and 50% of the septic patients with a bedside laparoscopy diagnosis are followed by a causal therapeutic intervention [13].

Complications related to the transportation of critically ill patients include hemodynamic instability, respiratory distress, and airway occlusion due to intra-orotracheal tube dislocation [14].

However, BDL must be applied with sticks indications in order to avoid dangerous side effects. The Agency for Healthcare Research and Quality lists such pathophysiological indications for BDL in ICU patients [15, 16]:

1. *Unexplained sepsis, with or without abdominal pain, systemic inflammatory response syndrome (SIRS), or multiorgan failure with no obvious indication for laparotomy.* Common intra-abdominal conditions causing septic shock in the critically ill patients consist of acalculous cholecystitis, acute mesenteric ischemia, pancreatitis, visceral perforation, and intra-abdominal collections. Acalculous cholecystitis is common in these patients due to a combination of prolonged fasting, opioid analgesics, and low cardiac output states [17]. Any delay in the recognition or management of these conditions can lead to multiple organ dysfunction syndrome and mortality rates that approach 100%. In this subset of patients, it is therefore critical that a rapid diagnosis is achieved, and definitive intervention performed. Intra-abdominal pathology may be also the primary cause of sepsis and hence admission to a critical care unit. Speaking about acute mesenteric ischemia (AMI), nowadays the gold standard for diagnosis is CT, which offers a good accuracy in AMI detection with high values of sensitivity and specificity, but it is well-known that these values are not similar in each etiological type [18]. Nonocclusive mesenteric ischemia mechanism is an exclusion diagnosis. It presents the most important diagnostic problems due to lack of specific radiological features on CT, which usually shows a normal bowel wall and a high variability of its contrast enhancement ranging from absent or diminished to increased. In this setting, laparoscopy could be a feasible and safe surgical approach for diagnosis of ischemic tract of bowel and to removing it [19].
2. *Increase in abdominal distension in the absence of bowel obstruction.* Such condition may arise from ischemic colitis, colic paralysis due to functional (Ogilvie syndrome) or infective (pseudo-membranous colitis) etiology, which may degenerate to the life-threatening condition of toxic megacolon or abdominal compartment syndrome if not rapidly diagnosed and healed.
3. *Unexplained metabolic (lactic) acidosis.* Lactic acidosis (LA), defined as a serum lactate of ≥4 mmol/L, is a common finding in critically ill patients since some conditions, such as hypovolemia and septic shock (e.g., intra-abdominal pathology), cause impaired oxygen delivery to tissues [20]. Moreover, there is a reduced hepatic and renal clearance. It is an indicator of higher morbidity and mortality especially in patients who are relatively unstable. Diagnosing the intra-abdominal cause of LA in critically ill patients remains challenging. Patients are usually too unwell to undergo radiological investigations like CT scan. In such cases, suspicion of an intra-abdominal catastrophe often results in an emergency laparotomy which carries its own morbidity and mortality. In these patients, BDL is thought to be a useful diagnostic tool for the investigation of intra-abdominal cause

of LA in critically ill patients when medical causes of LA have been excluded, like cardiorespiratory, renal, alcohol, or drug-related. An intra-abdominal source of pathology is found in 43% of patients undergoing BDL for these indications.

Patients who have undergone open-heart surgery or major vascular surgery utilizing extracorporal circulation have rather frequently complications with the above-mentioned pathophysiological patterns, and especially with ischemic origin [21]. Morbidity ranges from 0.3 to 13%; ischemic mesenterial, complications, cholecystitis, and hyperamylasemia or acute pancreatitis are the most important morbidities. Several risk factors for the development of abdominal pathology have been defined, including patient age (>70 years), preoperative New York Heart Association (NYHA) classification (NYHA 4), duration of cardiopulmonary bypass, and need for blood transfusion [22]. The diagnosis of abdominal abnormalities is often extremely difficult in critically ill patients, because these patients often do not show typical symptoms due to sedation or activity. Moreover, they often have numerous other conditions that may be responsible for changes in physical status or laboratory parameters. Therefore, the early diagnosis of abdominal complications is a clinical challenge, but it is of utmost importance because early diagnosis and especially early treatment are the key determinants of clinical outcome.

The use of bedside diagnostic laparoscopy has also been proposed in post-traumatic intra-abdominal injuries for both blunt and penetrating mechanisms, to facilitate a faster diagnosis in the emergency room [23]. Its use in this setting has been extensively analyzed by Stefanidis and colleagues in a review [24]. Most of the anectodical reports on trauma patients concern trauma-diagnostic of penetrating mechanisms, in particular, peritoneal penetration that leads to thoraco-abdominal or tangential diaphragmatic injury, trans-diaphragmatic pericardial window, evaluation of presence and extent of hemoperitoneum, evaluation for seat-belt injuries, acute abdomen after blunt mechanism with a negative CT. However, a more extensive discussion of this indication is beyond the scope of this book as there is no direct correlation between trauma and the frailty or elderly condition of the patient.

24.4 Contraindications and Potential Adverse Effects

The physician should be aware of patient selection and understand the absolute and relative contraindications for DL, which can be summarized as follows:

Absolute contraindications for DL:

1. Prior abdominal surgeries, that can make laparoscopy difficult and increase potential risk due to intra-abdominal adhesions, that is enterotomy.
2. Uncorrected coagulopathy.
3. Known or obvious indication for therapeutic intervention such as perforation or peritonitis.
4. Suspected intra-abdominal compartment syndrome.
5. Intestinal obstruction with associated massive bowel dilation.
6. Wound dehiscence.
7. Clear indications of bowel injuries such as the presence of bile or evisceration.

Should any of these circumstances be present, an exploratory laparotomy is mandated.

Are instead relative contraindications:

1. Morbid obesity.
2. Pregnancy.
3. Presence of anterior abdominal wall infection.
4. Recent laparotomy (4–6 weeks).
5. Extensive adhesions from previous surgery.
6. Aorto-iliac aneurysmal disease.
7. Decreased distensibility of the abdomen, such as that due to diffuse carcinomatosis or tuberculous peritonitis or in patients with augmented volume in the abdominal cavity such as bowel nonobstructive distention that interferes with visual access.

These conditions are to be evaluated very carefully when considering diagnostic laparoscopy.

The potential negative impact of the physiologic consequences of peritoneal insufflation is increased in an already critically ill patient, including the chemical effect of carbon dioxide and the inherent increased intra-peritoneal pressure associated with pneumo-peritoneum and adequate insufflation, and this is to be considered when planning the procedure [25].

Moreover, the increased intra-abdominal pressure elevates the diaphragm and subsequently results in the collapse of basal lung tissue. Potential deleterious respiratory effects include decreased functional residual capacity, ventilation perfusion mismatch, increased intra-pulmonary shunting of blood leading to hypoxemia and increased alveolar arterial oxygen gradient. Increasing the frequency of mechanical ventilation with positive end-expiatory pressure (PEEP) and increasing the fraction of inspired oxygen during the procedure will decrease the intra-operative atelectasis and improve the gas exchange and oxygenation.

Compression of the vena cava may occur during insufflation yielding decreased pre-load (thus cardiac output) and increased vascular resistance in the arterial circulation. This effect can be minimized with adequate fluid resuscitation. Furthermore, limiting insufflation pressures (<10 mm Hg) leads to less hemodynamic compromise. Cardiac arrhythmias including bradycardia from vagal stimulation, premature ventricular contractions, or ventricular tachycardia can also occur and should be closely monitored.

Hypercarbia can also result due to the reabsorption of the carbon dioxide into the circulation. If coupled with hypo-ventilation, it can yield acidosis and further depression of the cardio-pulmonary system. The use of continuous end-tidal carbon dioxide monitoring may help to prevent worsening acidosis in these circumstances.

If the procedure is kept short and is performed at low insufflation pressures, the physiologic alterations that do occur are of little or no consequence. Bedsides laparoscopy should therefore be used primarily as a diagnostic tool or only for basic straightforward, short interventions, such as coagulating a minor bleeder or placing a drain. These recommendations also keep the necessary equipment simple and the required sedation less complex and not necessarily dependent on an anesthesiologist.

24.5 Results and Complications

When proposing the use of a novel surgical approach, three aspects should be critically evaluated: feasibility, safety, and efficacy. After an advantage is shown over the current approach, recommendations can be made to adopt the newer modality.

The feasibility of diagnostic laparoscopy in the critically ill patient, both in the ICU at the patient's bedside and in the operating room was shown by several small series and case reports. The equipment (camera, monitor, and insufflator) is readily available on a mobile cart, and the number of instruments required for diagnostic laparoscopy is small. The procedure is therefore simple to accomplish outside the operating room environment [26, 27].

Because only small incisions are involved, with no exposure of the abdominal contents, diagnostic laparoscopy can be performed in the ICU using standard sterile equipment, with a low infection rate. The procedure is feasible even in the "difficult" abdomen, as in patients after open laparotomy. Extra care is needed when gaining access to the reoperated abdomen, and the use of open approach is recommended.

The safety of laparoscopy in critically ill patients was questioned because of two common conditions observed in these patients: hemodynamic instability and abdominal sepsis. As above reported, the use of CO_2 pneumo-peritoneum was shown to be associated with adverse hemodynamic effects, of which the cardiovascular and respiratory are the most prominent. These effects may be even more pronounced in the high-risk patient, causing temporary myocardial failure. Experimental studies demonstrated hemodynamic compromise in septic animals undergoing laparoscopy, mostly related to hypercarbia and acidosis [28].

Despite these concerns, conflicting data may be found in the literature regarding the occurrence and significance of these adverse effects. Specifically, there is a discrepancy between the experimental studies and the actual results in high-risk patients subjected to laparoscopy, and even when hemodynamic parameters are affected, the overall clinical significance of these measured changes is not clear. In many series, no significant hemodynamic changes were observed, even in patients who were dependent on high-dose amine support [8].

It should be remembered that ICU laparoscopy is performed under optimal monitoring conditions, and that the cardiovascular effects of laparoscopy are readily reversible by disinflation. The combination of slow insufflation and low abdominal pressure minimizes the adverse hemodynamic effects of laparoscopy. By its nature, diagnostic laparoscopy is a short procedure, so the effects of CO_2 pneumo-peritoneum are minimized. The use of alternative gases, such as N_2O, to reduce the chemical effects of CO_2, is also possible. Nitrous oxide may also be associated with less discomfort in patients who are not under general anesthesia.

The use of laparoscopy in a critically ill patient with abdominal sepsis is also a source of concern. Some experimental studies showed increased bacterial growth in the CO_2 peritoneal environment, but other models showed conflicting results, with similar or better outcome compared with laparotomy. An augmenting effect of pneumo-peritoneum on bacterial translocation was suspected but disproved. Despite theoretical concerns that pneumo-peritoneum may increase bacterial spread, results of many studies showed a decrease in infectious complications, so laparoscopy was considered a safe option for the diagnosis and treatment of peritonitis [29].

As laparoscopy is associated with less stress and a reduced acute-phase response, it appears that there is better preservation of immune function. As there are also fewer parietal complications such as wound infection and dehiscence, laparoscopy may be a safer option in the diagnosis of abdominal sepsis.

The efficacy of ICU laparoscopy was repeatedly demonstrated. The diagnostic accuracy is greater than 90% and was always better than ultrasound, CT scan, or diagnostic peritoneal lavage. Retroperitoneal pathology, which is less evident by laparoscopy, might be misdiagnosed. However, with careful exploration, the retroperitoneum organs, like the pancreas, are still accessible. A routine inspection of the lesser sac could help to obviate this problem [19].

The efficacy of ICU laparoscopy is also measured by the effect on further management. Avoiding an unnecessary laparotomy is important in these patients, and a change in management occurred in 33% of the patients [19].

In some cases, the diagnosed pathology can be treated laparoscopically, either in the ICU or after transfer to the operating room.

The overall prognosis in this group of patients is poor. However, when considering patient outcome, ICU diagnostic laparoscopy may affect treatment decisions even in the unsalvageable patient. Arriving at a correct diagnosis is important to the patient's family, as well as to the physician, before deciding to withdraw or implement further costly efforts [29].

In patients with findings that require laparotomy, such as mesenteric ischemia or necrotizing pancreatitis, initial laparoscopy does not significantly increase the operative risk. The slightly increased operating times are marginal, since experienced surgeons can perform the procedure in 10–15 min.

Complication rates of diagnostic laparoscopy range from 1 to 9%. Thus, even in critically ill patients, the procedure can be performed without increasing the standard risk [30].

The Society of American Gastrointestinal and Endoscopic Surgeons (SAGES) recommends that BDL is technically feasible and can be applied safely in appropriately selected ICU patients (grade B). According to this Society, it is generally well-tolerated in the ICU population with overall morbidity rates reported from 0 to 8% with no mortality directly associated with the procedure being described [31–33].

The positive outcome of bedside diagnostic laparoscopy can be guaranteed with three major factors: cooperation among anesthesiologists and the surgeon in the decision-making of whether to perform a bedside laparoscopy; single-bed isolated room setting, that guarantee an optimal operating room-like environment; and daily emergency surgery technical skills of surgeon. As the level of intraperitoneum pressure is the most critical intra-procedure parameter, the range of 8–15 mm Hg is suggested, because this is usually well-tolerated and does not compromise mechanical ventilation or the hemodynamic parameters in critically ill patients.

The most severe procedures-related complications is visceral perforation, pneum-operitoneum-induced bradycardia, intra-peritoneal hemorrhage and post-procedure ascitic leak from trocar site. Level II and III data demonstrate diagnostic accuracy ranging between 90 and 100% with the main limitation being the evaluation of retroperitoneal structures. Therefore, despite the technical challenges associated with bedside laparoscopy, it offers a viable alternative to exploratory laparotomy which has traditionally yielded higher mortality rates, particularly in ICU patients with multisystem organ failure [16].

24.6 Technique: Rules and Pitfalls

BDL procedures are performed in an isolated single bedroom of the ICU ward. Standard laparoscopy equipment required to perform a BDL in the ICU includes an insufflator, image processor, light source, cautery, camera head, lens, light cord, trocars, instruments, suture, and monitor (Fig. 24.1 and Table 24.1).

We recommend an experienced surgical team, nurse, and technician; an individual to serve as assistant for unexpected needs; an anesthesiologist (Fig. 24.1).

Excellent communication between the surgeon and anesthesiologist is required as the patient is mechanically ventilated and invasive arterial blood pressure, electrocardiogram, pulse oximetry, and end-tidal carbon dioxide are constantly monitored. When required, hemodynamic support is established by noradrenaline infusion. This monitoring is typical for a critically ill patient. While inhaled anesthetic may be used in the ICU, we recommend total intravenous anesthesia (TIVA) to minimize the equipment that must be transferred from the operative room.

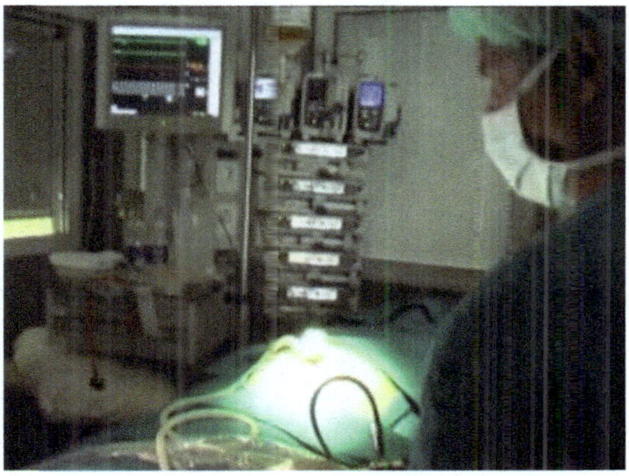

Fig. 24.1 Scenario of BDL in ICU

Table 24.1 List of equipment needed to perform a BDL

Laparoscopic mobile tower	Operative materials	Backup equipment
Insufflator	Laparoscopic instruments	Open set
Image processor	Needle drivers	Lap sponges
Light source	Clip appliers	Suture
Cautery	Various sutures	Open suction
Monitor	Ports	Retraction instruments
Second monitor	Coagulating substrates	Lighting (overhead and headlamp)
–	Bipolar vessel sealing system or harmonic scalpel of choice	–

All the staff present in the room wear protective clothing, a surgical cap, gloves, and a surgical mask. Sterility is warranted by adherence to routine operating-room protocols and sterilization of the operating site with povidone-iodine. The anesthesiologist on duty directs the administration of total intravenous anesthesia, ventilation, and hemodynamic support

The patient is in a supine position and Trendelenburg or anti-Trendelenburg movements are assured to obtain the most appropriate laparoscopic view (e.g., diaphragmatic exploration).

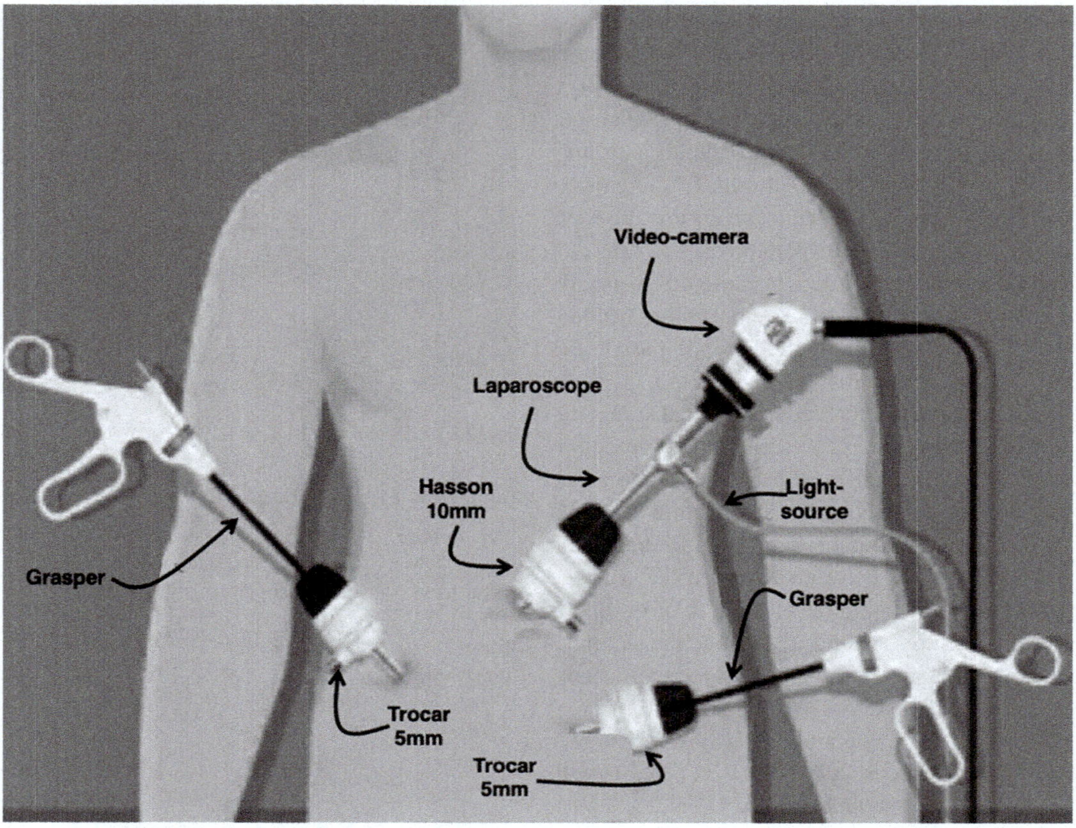

Fig. 24.2 Trocars placement for a BDL procedure

Trocars are placed into the paraumbilical region, as shown in Fig. 24.2.

The surgeon should utilize 5-mm ports and instruments to minimize equipment needs. We prefer the open Hasson technique to access the peritoneal space; however, the method most comfortable for the operating surgeon should be used. Pneumo-peritoneum should be limited to 8–10 mm Hg pressure, rather than the standard 15 mm Hg pressure, to decrease CO_2 absorption, minimize effect on preload, and reduce blood pressure. It is technically feasible to avoid chemical paralytics and perform BDL under local anesthetic and low insufflation pressure.

The use of alternative gases such as N_2O, helium and air has been described with the potential benefit of decreased hypercarbia/acidosis; however, both air and N_2O pose a significant risk of nitrogen or air embolus. However, usually low pressure (8–10 mm Hg) CO_2 is familiar to the OR team, readily available, safe, and does not compromise the ability to successfully visualize the peritoneal cavity.

The surgeon is careful to avoid injury to the bowel or cause bleeding. When the procedure is complete, the patient is monitored for any signs of bleeding at additional port sites following removal, and the umbilical port site is carefully sutured starting from the fascia.

Five Things You Should Know About Bedside Laparoscopy (BDL) in the Elderly

- The BDL finds its ideal application in ICU patients, and, to a lesser extent, in the emergency room.
- The indications to BDL in ICU are actually very strict: sepsis, abdominal distension and lactic acidosis of unknown origin, after a full diagnosis attempt has been made, including CT scan.

- Among the various diseases for which BDL represents an efficient and useful tool for a better management, the acute mesenteric ischemia is surely the most relevant since its time-dependent prognosis may be significantly affected by an early laparoscopic approach sometimes also avoiding moving the patients to the Radiology Unit.
- In critically ill patients, the procedure can be performed without increasing the standard risk.
- Given the advantages offered by this method, especially in patients hospitalized in ICU, it would be advisable for a laparoscopic equipment to always be kept in close proximity to the ICU, in case an urgent BDL is needed.

References

1. Rehm CG. Bedside laparoscopy. Crit Care Clin. 2000;16:101–12.
2. Crandall M, West MA. Evaluation of the abdomen in the critically ill patient: opening the black box. Curr Opin Crit Care. 2006;12(4):333–9.
3. Calandra T, Cohen J. The international sepsis forum consensus conference on definitions of infection in the intensive care unit. Crit Care Med. 2005;33:1538–48.
4. Brandt CP, Priebe PP, Eckhauser ML. Diagnostic laparoscopy in the intensive care patient: avoiding the nontherapeutic laparotomy. Surg Endosc. 1993;7:168–72.
5. Beckmann U, Gillies DM, Berenholtz SM, et al. Incidents relating to the intrahospital transfer of critically ill patients. An analysis of the reports submitted to the Australian incident monitoring study in intensive care. Intensive Care Med. 2004;30:1579–85.
6. Norwood S, Civetta J. Abdominal CT scanning in critically ill surgical patients. Ann Surg. 1985;202:166–75.
7. Mirvis SE, Vainright JR, Nelson AW. The diagnosis of acalculous cholecystitis: a comparison of sonography, scintigraphy, and CT. Am J Radiol. 1986;147:1171–5.
8. Peris A, Matano S, Manca G, et al. Bedside diagnostic laparoscopy to diagnose intraabdominal pathology in the intensive care unit. Crit Care. 2009;13:R25.
9. Lee MJ, Sperry JL, Rosengart MR. Evaluating for acute mesenteric ischemia in critically ill patients: diagnostic peritoneal lavage is associated with reduced operative intervention and mortality. J Trauma Acute Care Surg. 2014;77:441–7.
10. Martin ND, Patel SP, Chreiman K, et al. Emergency laparotomy in the critically ill: futility at the bedside. Crit Care Res Pract. 2018;2018:6398917.
11. Iberti TJ, Salky BA, Onofrey D. Use of bedside laparoscopy to identify intestinal ischemia in postoperative cases of aortic reconstruction. Surgery. 1989;105:686–9.
12. Berci G, Sackier JM, Paz-Partlow M. Emergency laparoscopy. Am J Surg. 1991;161:332–5.
13. Koganti D, Hazen BJ, Dente CJ, Nguyen J, et al. The role of diagnostic laparoscopy for trauma at a high-volume level one center. Surg Endosc. 2021;35(6):2667–70. https://doi.org/10.1007/s00464-020-07687-1.
14. Kleffmann J, Pahl R, Deinsberger W, et al. Intracranial pressure changes during intrahospital transports of neurocritically ill patients. Neurocrit Care. 2016;25:440–5.
15. Zemlyak A, Heniford BT, Sing RF. Diagnostic laparoscopy in the intensive care unit. J Intensive Care Med. 2015;30:297–302.
16. Marrero JJ, Christmas AB. Bedside laparoscopy in the ICU. In: Taylor D, Sherry S, Sing R, editors. Interventional critical care. Cham: Springer; 2016. https://doi.org/10.1007/978-3-319-25286-5_34.
17. Laurila J, Syrjälä H, Laurila PA, et al. Acute acalculous cholecystitis in critically ill patients. Acta Anaesthesiol Scand. 2004;48:986–91.
18. Bourcier S, Oudjit A, Goudard G, et al. Diagnosis of non-occlusive acute mesenteric ischemia in the intensive care unit. Ann Intensive Care. 2016;6:112. https://doi.org/10.1186/s13613-016-0213-x.
19. Cocorullo G, Mirabella A, Falco N, et al. An investigation of bedside laparoscopy in the ICU for cases of non-occlusive mesenteric ischemia. World J Emerg Surg. 2017;12:4. https://doi.org/10.1186/s13017-017-0118-5.
20. Sajid MA, Khan KS, Hanif Z. Diagnostic laparoscopy to investigate unexplained lactic acidosis in critically ill patients—a descriptive single centre cohort study. Ann Med Surg (Lond). 2018;36:231–4
21. Nilsson J, Hansson E, Andersson B. Intestinal ischemia after cardiac surgery: analysis of a large registry. J Cardiothorac Surg. 2013;8:156. https://doi.org/10.1186/1749-8090-8-156.
22. Dong G, Liu C, Xu B, et al. Postoperative abdominal complications after cardiopulmonary bypass. J Cardiothorac Surg. 2012;7:108. https://doi.org/10.1186/1749-8090-7-108.
23. Wood D, Berci G, Morgenstern L. Mini-laparoscopy in blunt abdominal trauma. Surg Endosc. 1988;2:184–9.
24. Stefanidis D, Richardson WS, Chang L, et al. The role of diagnostic laparoscopy for acute abdominal conditions: an evidence-based review. Surg Endosc. 2009;23:16–23.
25. Grabowski JE, Talamini MA. Physiological effects of pneumoperitoneum. J Gastrointest Surg. 2009;13:1009–16.
26. Kelly JJ, Puyana JC, Callery MP, et al. The feasibility and accuracy of diagnostic laparoscopy in the septic ICU patient. Surg Endosc. 2000;14:617–21.
27. Alemanno G, Prosperi P, Di Bella A, et al. Bedside diagnostic laparoscopy for critically ill patients in the

intensive care unit: retrospective study and review of literature. J Minim Access Surg. 2019;15:56–62.
28. Hatipoglu S, Akbulut S, Hatipoglu F, et al. Effect of laparoscopic abdominal surgery on splanchnic circulation: historical developments. World J Gastroenterol. 2014;20:18165–76.
29. Rosin D, Haviv Y, Kuriansky J, et al. Bedside laparoscopy in the ICU: report of four cases. J Laparoendosc Adv Surg Tech A. 2001;11:305–9.
30. Hackert T, Kienle P, Weitz J, et al. Accuracy of diagnostic laparoscopy for early diagnosis of abdominal complications after cardiac surgery. Surg Endosc. 2003;17:1671–4.
31. https://www.sages.org/publications/guidelines/guidelines-for-diagnostic-laparoscopy/.
32. Jaramillo EJ, Trevino JM, Berghoff KR, et al. Bedside diagnostic laparoscopy in the intensive care unit: a 13-year experience. JSLS. 2006;10:155–9.
33. Bergamini C, Alemanno G, Giordano A, et al. The role of bed-side laparoscopy in the management of acute mesenteric ischemia of recent onset in post-cardiac surgery patients admitted to ICU. Eur J Trauma Emerg Surg. 2020. https://doi.org/10.1007/s00068-020-01500-3.

Emergency Video-Assisted Thoracoscopy in the Elderly

25

Nicola Tamburini, Francesco D'Urbano, Pio Maniscalco, Francesco Quarantotto, Francesco Bagolini, Alessandro Bertani, and Giorgio Cavallesco

25.1 Introduction

Video-assisted thoracoscopic surgery (VATS), like any other minimal access surgery, offers considerable benefits to patients compared to traditional thoracic procedures: it positively influences postoperative pain, morbidity, and mortality. Furthermore, it has been largely demonstrated that VATS can reduce hospital stay when compared to thoracotomy [1]. For these reasons, in the last decade, VATS has become a popular surgical approach, and nowadays, it is used to diagnose and treat a variety of conditions within the chest cavity [2]. The application of VATS in acute settings was originally reported in a series evaluating diaphragmatic injuries [3]. Over the last years, in addition to detecting diaphragmatic injuries, numerous other indications have evolved as a result of increasing familiarity and acceptance of the VATS technique worldwide [4–6]. Indications for subacute thoracoscopy following trauma include empyema, treatment of thoracic duct injury, and removal of symptomatic foreign bodies. Furthermore, VATS has been used for chest trauma in hemodynamically stable patients who have an indication for urgent thoracic exploration within 24 h following presentation [7, 8]. The surgical treatment of elderly patients with chest injuries is a great challenge: elderly patients have up to four-fold greater morbidity and mortality rate compared with younger patients [9–11]. Because of increased underlying comorbidities and decreased physiologic reserve in the geriatric population, the severely injured elderly patient requires intensive monitoring, aggressive management, and comprehensive care [12]. For these reasons, VATS is increasingly used in the treatment of thoracic injuries in elderly patients too [13, 14].

25.2 Indications for Thoracoscopy

Although the majority of hemodynamically stable patients with thoracic injuries can initially be managed with tube thoracostomy and close observation, some patients may progress to develop acute and chronic complications requiring operative therapy. Thoracoscopy has a role in both diagnosis and treatment of chest injuries. Hemodynamic stability is an important prerequisite, since thoracoscopy is not an approach to be used in the initial assessment of hemodynamically unstable injured patients. In patients

N. Tamburini · F. D'Urbano · P. Maniscalco
F. Quarantotto · F. Bagolini · G. Cavallesco (✉)
Department of Morphology, Experimental Medicine and Surgery, Section of Chirurgia 1, Sant'Anna Hospital, University of Ferrara, Ferrara, Italy
e-mail: cgg@unife.it

A. Bertani
Division of Thoracic Surgery and Lung Transplantation, Department for the Treatment and Study of Cardiothoracic Diseases and Cardiothoracic Transplantation, IRCCS ISMETT, Palermo, Italy

F. Agresta et al. (eds.), *Emergency laparoscopic surgery in the elderly and frail patient*,
https://doi.org/10.1007/978-3-030-79990-8_25

experiencing thoracic injury with hypovolemic shock, emergency thoracotomy remains the most appropriate option. Further, thoracoscopy is contraindicated in patients unable to tolerate lung deflation with single-lung ventilation [14].

25.3 Hemothorax

The most common causes of hemothorax can be divided into traumatic, iatrogenic, and nontraumatic causes as shown in Table 25.1.

The majority (85%) of patients with hemothorax are managed by tube thoracostomy. Guidelines recommend referral for surgery for acute blood loss over 1500 mL or recorded ongoing drainage of more than 200–400 mL over 2–4 h [15]. Hemothorax typically progresses in three manners: complete spontaneous reabsorption of blood within several weeks, progression to fibrothorax, or infection with empyema formation. In the initial management of hemothorax, CT scan is an important tool to detect the bleeding site and to identify other sources of hemorrhage than the intercostal arteries (ICAs). In case of active bleeding from ICAs transcatheter arterial embolization (TAE) is a safe and effective measure to arrest bleeding in hemodynamically stable patients [16].

The majority of hemothoraces following blunt trauma are easily treated by drainage and re-expansion of the lung. If bleeding continues, underlying factors, such as coagulopathy, acidosis, and hypothermia should all be sought and addressed. Particular attention should be paid to the elderly on various forms of anticoagulation. Normally, bloody effusions are entirely resorbed after 4–6 weeks without causing infection. However, some patients may experience retained hemothorax because of malposition or poor drainage of chest tubes. Retained hemothorax is defined as residual clots at least 500 mL large, or in which at least one-third of the blood in the pleural space cannot be drained by a chest tube after 72 h of initial treatment revealed by a computed tomography (CT) scan [17, 18]. In the past, the primary method for treating retained hemothorax was to perform an additional tube thoracostomy or exploratory thoracotomy.

Jones et al. in 1981 first described the role of VATS in the initial management of patients with hemothorax. They found that thoracotomy could be avoided in the majority of stable patients with high chest tube output and bleeding was stopped in most cases with electrocautery [19].

For patients undergoing VATS surgery, single-lung ventilation is ideal, allowing adequate visualization. If the patient is unable to tolerate this for underlying lung pathology or significant contusion, double-lung ventilation with intermittent apnea is an option. Patients should be placed in the lateral decubitus position with flexing of the table to allow widening of the intercostal spaces.

The initial incision for the camera placement is in the sixth or seventh space or at the site of the tube thoracostomy. The thoracic cavity is entered under vision. The placement of additional ports may be determined after the initial inspection with the thoracoscope, with current evidence, single or multiport approaches are equally acceptable. After insertion of the thoracoscope, the adhesions should be released by blunt digital dissection or sharp endoscopic

Table 25.1 Most frequent causes of hemothorax

Traumatic	Iatrogenic	Non-traumatic
Penetrating or lacerating chest trauma (lung blood vessels, chest wall, diaphragm, pleural adhesions, mediastinum, large vessels, abdomen)	Cardiac or lung surgery Pleural techniques (thoracentesis, pleural biopsy, drains) Insertion of catheter in the subclavian vein Percutaneous lung biopsy	Neoplasias (primary or metastatic) Pulmonary embolism Catamenial hemothorax Anticoagulant treatment Hematological diseases (hemophilia, thrombocytopenia) Intrapleural fibrinolytics Aorta dissection or rupture

electrocoagulated dissection. Full-lung collapse is crucial for inspecting the entire pleural cavity. Blood and clots are removed by using a standard suction instrument or a suction–irrigator system. A sample of fluid is routinely collected for microbiological assessment. In patients with organized thoracic collections, carefully dissecting and peeling away the outer layer with sponge sticks and ring forceps typically enables the outer layer to be removed from the visceral and parietal pleura, thus completely releasing the trapped lung. Following adequate drainage and washout of the hemithorax, a chest drain should be placed prior to closure. It is crucial to ensure that the lung fully expands to occupy the space. If there is residual space, blood can recollect and lead to postoperative complications.

There is evidence in the literature that VATS, in well-selected patients, is superior to tube thoracostomy and leads to decreased post-traumatic infection length of ventilatory dependency and overall hospital stay [20]. Increased age is associated with a decreased respiratory function. As chest wall compliance decreases secondary to structural changes, such as vertebral collapse and kyphosis, inspiratory capacity decreases. Furthermore, it needs to be remembered that injured lungs have a compromised compliance and the presence of low suction might be advisable to promote drainage of pleural fluid.

25.4 Diaphragmatic Injury

Diaphragmatic injuries account for 3% of all trauma cases and up to 8% of trauma surgical explorations. It may be due to both a severe blunt trauma, from motor vehicle accidents, and penetrating trauma, from knife or gunshot wounds. Diaphragmatic hernias are more common in the elderly population and they have higher associated mortality than younger age groups [21]. The mechanism of diaphragmatic injury is often high impact injuries which lead to a sudden increase in intra-abdominal pressure causing rupture. The right diaphragm is protected by the liver; hence, 80% of ruptures occur on the left.

Diagnosing a diaphragmatic rupture after trauma is a challenge for both emergency radiologists and surgeons. The initial radiograph can be diagnostic, however, in one series of elderly patients with traumatic hernias, 50% of initial radiographs were normal. A normal admission radiograph can result in delays in diagnosis and delay to operative repair which increases rates of surgical complications such as time of ventilatory support and death [22]. Even CT scanning can be non-definitive, it has a low sensitivity (53–74%) [23]. Atelectasis, pulmonary contusions, hemothorax, and intra-abdominal pathology can mask diaphragmatic injury.

Two principles must be observed when repairing acute traumatic diaphragmatic hernias: complete reduction of the herniated organs back into the abdomen and watertight closure of the diaphragm to avoid recurrence. The role of VATS in this situation is invaluable as it has a 100% sensitivity and allows for repair at the same time [24]. Thoracoscopy provides excellent visualization of the posterior recesses of the thoracic cavity, areas not often seen well with the laparoscope. The patient should be placed into the Trendelenburg position to facilitate adequate visualization of the diaphragm. Nasogastric tube placement is important to deflate the stomach and can facilitate reduction of any herniation. Simple interrupted sutures should be enough to repair most of the acute defects [25] and mesh repairs should be reserved for chronic or large defects.

25.5 Esophageal Perforation

Esophageal perforation is a rare condition occurring in 3 out of 100,000 people in the United States. The advances in diagnostic and therapeutic endoscopic interventions have led to iatrogenic perforation as the most common etiology (Table 25.2) [26].

Iatrogenic perforation is common in the hypopharynx or the distal esophagus while spontaneous rupture may occur in the posterolateral wall of the esophagus just above its diaphragmatic hiatus. Esophageal perforations can present in different ways depending on several factors including the etiology of the perforation, the location of

Table 25.2 Causes of esophageal perforation

Etiology	Incidence (%)
Iatrogenic	59
Spontaneous	15
Foreign body ingestion	12
Trauma	9
Operative injury	2
Tumor	1
Other causes	2

the perforation (cervical, intrathoracic, or intra-abdominal), the severity of contamination, injury of nearby mediastinal structures (i.e., trachea or pericardium), and the time elapsed from the perforation until treatment. Common symptoms include chest pain, dysphagia, dyspnea, subcutaneous emphysema, epigastric pain, fever, tachycardia, and tachypnea. Early diagnosis is very important because it significantly decreases morbidity and mortality [27]. Computed tomography (CT scan) of the chest and abdomen should be performed when esophageal perforation is suspected. It has the advantage of showing intrathoracic or intra-abdominal collections that require percutaneous or surgical drainage. The principles of management in esophageal perforation are to eliminate the focus of infection and inflammation, prevent further contamination of the mediastinum with adequate drainage and antibiotics, restore alimentary tract continuity and establish nutritional support [28]. For those who receive surgical intervention, within the first 24 h, the published mortality is 13% [29]. Traditionally, upper and middle third perforations are approached via thoracotomy with primary closure, esophagectomy, use of esophageal T-tube, exclusion-diversion, and mediastinal drainage. However, few studies have demonstrated the efficacy of VATS approach in esophageal perforations but further studies are needed to clarify its role in primary repair [30]. In selected cases of esophageal perforation, thoracoscopy can be applied by using the same surgical principles as in the open thoracotomy approach. Advantages of the video-thoracoscopic approach are the excellent view of the whole thoracic cavity and adequate debridement and proper drainage of all pleural cavity areas. Either primary closure or an esophageal T-tube can be used to close the esophageal leak. By avoiding a major thoracotomy, the patient benefits from less postoperative pain, a decrease in wound-related complications, and a faster postoperative recovery. Over the last decade, stent grafting of esophageal perforations has been increasingly adopted with promising results. VATS debridement and drainage can be used in combination with stent positioning allowing for control of the septic focus [31]. VATS in association with endoscopic techniques may be particularly suited for the elderly patient population, as the significant morbidity of a thoracotomy or laparotomy may be avoided [32].

25.6 Descending Necrotizing Mediastinitis

Descending necrotizing mediastinitis (DNM) is a severe complication of infection originating from the neck, most commonly an oropharyngeal or odontogenic focus, which spreads in the cervical fascial spaces and descends into the mediastinum. Early diagnosis is essential because DNM can rapidly progress to septic shock and organ failure. At present, the cervicothoracic CT scan is the gold standard for diagnosis. Odontogenic sources, tonsillar and pharyngeal abscesses, sialadenitis, injury by a foreign body, or catheterization are common origins of DNM. Elderly patients are immunocompromised with comorbidities, such as diabetes mellitus, malnutrition, renal failure, liver cirrhosis, and underlying malignancy. This alone may significantly compromise patient outcomes and be a predicting factor for mediastinal spreading.

Early aggressive intervention and medical optimization can stop the progression of descending mediastinitis and to septic shock, drastically improving survival. Transcervical drainage alone may be effective for localized DNM in the upper mediastinum, whereas combined cervical drainage and mediastinum drainage may provide adequate drainage for DNM extending to the lower anterior mediastinum. In case of DNM extent into the anterior and lower posterior mediastinum, the optimal treatment should include radical surgical debridement of affected tissue through an open thoracic approach [33, 34]. However, these invasive methods are high-risk approaches for elderly and critically ill patients with overwhelming sepsis and may lead to unfavorable outcomes with complications. In 2004, Isowa et al. first reported the successful management of descending necrotizing mediastinitis patients with VATS [35]. At around that time, more and more authors advocated VATS as one of the treatments for DNM and emphasized the excellent visualization of the entire thoracic cavity, the lower degree of invasiveness, and favorable outcome [36, 37]. Patients are positioned with full lateral decubitus and under direct vision of thoracoscope, the mediastinal pleura around all abscess pockets is opened and the pus drained through it. In all patients, chest tubes are positioned in the mediastinum through the opening of mediastinal pleura for drainage of mediastinal pus.

Five Things You Should Know About Emergency Video-Assisted Thoracoscopy in the Elderly

- VATS have a role in both diagnosis and treatment of chest injuries in hemodynamically stable patients.
- Chest trauma is the most common cause of hemothorax, the majority of hemothoraces are managed by tube thoracostomy.
- VATS, in well-selected patients, is superior to tube thoracostomy in decreased post-traumatic infection, length of ventilatory dependency, and overall hospital stay.
- The role of VATS in diaphragmatic injuries is invaluable as it has a high sensitivity for diagnosis and allows for repair at the same time.
- VATS may be particularly suited for the elderly patient population, as the significant morbidity of a thoracotomy or laparotomy may be avoided.

References

1. McKenna RJ, Houck W, Fuller CB. Video-assisted thoracic surgery lobectomy: experience with 1,100 cases. Ann Thorac Surg. 2006;81:421–6.
2. Swanson SJ, Herndon JE, D'Amico TA, et al. Video-assisted thoracic surgery lobectomy: report of CALGB 39802—a prospective, multi-institution feasibility study. J Clin Oncol. 2007;25:4993–7.
3. Ochsner MG, Rozycki GS, Lucente F. Prospective evaluation of thoracoscopy for diagnosing diaphragmatic injury and thoraco-abdominal trauma: a preliminary report. J Trauma. 1993;34:704–10.
4. Cetindag IB, Neideen T, Hazelrigg SR. Video-assisted thoracic surgical applications in thoracic trauma. Thorac Surg Clin. 2007;17:73–9.
5. Ahmed N, Jones D. Video-assisted thoracic surgery: state of the art in trauma care. Injury. 2004;35:479–849.
6. Smith JW, Franklin GA, Harbrecht BG, et al. Early VATS for blunt chest trauma: a management technique underutilized by acute care surgeons. J Trauma. 2011;71:102–7.
7. Goodman M, Lewis J, Guitron J, Reed M, et al. Video-assisted thoracoscopic surgery for acute thoracic trauma. J Emerg Trauma Shock. 2013;6:106–9
8. Manlulu AV, Lee TW, Thung KH, Wong R, et al. Current indications and results of VATS in the evaluation and management of hemodynamically stable thoracic injuries. Eur J Cardiothorac Surg. 2004;25:1048–53.
9. Holcomb JB, McMullin NR, Kozar RA, et al. Morbidity from rib fractures increases after age 45. J Am Coll Surg. 2003;196:549–55.
10. Evans L. Age and fatality risk from similar severity impacts. J Traffic Med. 2001;29:10–9.
11. Victorino GP, Chong TJ, Pal JD. Trauma in the elderly patient. Arch Surg Chicago. 2003;138:1093–8.
12. Demetriades D, Karaiskakis M, Velmahos G, et al. Effect on outcome of early intensive management of geriatric trauma patients. Br J Surg. 2002;89:1319–22
13. Carrillo EH, Heniford BT, Etoch SW, et al. Video-assisted thoracic surgery in trauma patients. J Am Coll Surg. 1997;184:316–24.
14. Huang WY, Lu IY, Yang C, et al. Efficiency analysis of direct video-assisted thoracoscopic surgery in elderly patients with blunt traumatic hemothorax without an initial thoracostomy. Biomed Res Int. 2016;2016:3741426.
15. ATLS Subcommittee; American College of Surgeons' Committee on Trauma; International ATLS Working Group. Advanced trauma life support (ATLS®): the ninth edition. J Trauma Acute Care Surg. 2013;74:1363–6.
16. Tamburini N, Carriel N, Cavallesco G, et al. Technical results, clinical efficacy and predictors of outcome of intercostal arteries embolization for hemothorax: a two-institutions' experience. J Thorac Dis. 2019;11(11):4693–9.
17. Carrillo EH, Richardson JD. Thoracoscopy in the management of hemothorax and retained blood after trauma. Curr Opin Pulm Med. 1998;4:243–6.
18. Casos SR, Richardson JD. Role of thoracoscopy in acute management of chest injury. Curr Opin Crit Care. 2006;12:584–9.

19. Jones JW, Kitahama A, Webb WR, McSwain N. Emergency thoracoscopy: a logical approach to chest trauma management. J Trauma. 1981;21(4): 280–4.
20. Chou YP, Kuo LC, Soo KM, et al. The role of repairing lung lacerations during video-assisted thoracoscopic surgery evacuations for retained haemothorax caused by blunt chest trauma. Eur J Cardiothorac Surg. 2014;46:107–11.
21. Lewis JD, Starnes SL, Pandalai PK, et al. Traumatic diaphragmatic injury: experience from a level I trauma center. Surgery. 2009;146(4):578–83; discussion 583–4.
22. Hsu YP, Chen RJ, Fang JF, et al. Blunt diaphragmatic rupture in elderly patients. Hepatogastroenterology. 2005;52(66):1752–8.
23. Jaroslaw K. ESTS textbook of thoracic surgery. Cracow: Medycyna Praktyczna; 2015.
24. Paci M, Ferrari G, Annessi V, et al. The role of diagnostic VATS in penetrating thoracic injuries. World J Emerg Surg. 2006;1:30.
25. Parelkar SV, Oak SN, Patel JL, et al. Traumatic diaphragmatic hernia: management by video assisted thoracoscopic repair. J Indian Assoc Pediatr Surg. 2012;17:180–3.
26. Brinster CJ, Singhal S, Lee L, et al. Evolving options in the management of esophageal perforations. Ann Thorac Surg. 2004;77:1475–83.
27. White RK, Morris DM. Diagnosis and management of esophageal perforations. Am Surg. 1992;58: 112–9.
28. Bufkin BL, Miller JI Jr, Mansour KA. Esophageal perforation: emphasis on management. Ann Thorac Surg. 1996;61:1447–52.
29. Fell SC. Esophageal perforation. In: Patterson G, Cooper JD, Deslauriers J, et al., editors. Pearson's thoracic & esophageal surgery. 3rd ed. Philadelphia, PA: Churchill Livingston; 2008. p. 792–808.
30. Haveman JW, Nieuwenhujis VB, Kobold JPM, et al. Adequate debridement and drainage of the mediastinum using open thoracotomy or video-assisted thoracoscopic surgery for Boerhaave's syndrome. Surg Endosc. 2011;25:2492–7.
31. Mavroudis CD, Kucharczuk JC. Acute management of esophageal perforation. Curr Surg Rep. 2014;2:34.
32. Benns M, Richardson JD. Thoracic diseases in the elderly for geriatric trauma and emergency care. In: Luchette F, Yelon J, editors. Geriatric trauma and critical care. Cham: Springer; 2017.
33. Kocher GJ, Hoksch B, Caversaccio M, et al. Diffuse descending necrotizing mediastinitis: surgical therapy and outcome in a single-centre series. Eur J Cardiothorac Surg. 2012;42:e66–72.
34. Freeman RK, Vallieres E, Verrier ED, et al. Descending necrotizing mediastinitis: an analysis of the effects of serial surgical debridement on patient mortality. J Thorac Cardiovasc Surg. 2000;119:260–7.
35. Isowa N, Yamada T, Kijima T, et al. Successful thoracoscopic debridement of descending necrotizing mediastinitis. Ann Thorac Surg. 2004;77:1834–7.
36. Min HK, Choi YS, Shim YM, et al. Descending necrotizing mediastinitis: a minimally invasive approach using video-assisted thoracoscopic surgery. Ann Thorac Surg. 2004;77:306–10.
37. Chen KC, Chen JS, Kuo SW, et al. Descending necrotizing mediastinitis: a 10-year surgical experience in a single institution. J Thorac Cardiovasc Surg. 2008;136:191–8.

Palliative Surgery for Oncologic Elderly Patients in Emergency

26

Nereo Vettoretto, Emanuele Botteri, Dhimiter Cuka, Alessandra Marengoni, and Giuseppe Romanelli

26.1 Introduction

The purpose for the treatment of cancer in elderly is often different from that of younger patients. Several times palliative surgery is performed in order to treat or reduce the risk of complication of advanced cancer. Hence, radical oncological surgery can develop a higher risk of postoperative complications, thus reducing the life expectancy and, most of all, its residual quality. Other reasons for a higher prevalence of palliative surgery rely on the impossibility for old patients to face aggressive perioperative chemotherapy and radiotherapy due to their reduced functional reserves.

Surgical care in the elderly always becomes a tailored treatment which must focus on patient's quality of life rather than on disease-free survival, and it is also embedded in a cost-effectiveness scenario.

N. Vettoretto (✉) · E. Botteri
Montichiari Surgery, ASST Spedali Civili Brescia, Brescia, Italy

D. Cuka
Surgical Clinic, University of Brescia, Brescia, Italy

A. Marengoni · G. Romanelli
Department of Clinical and Experimental Sciences, University of Brescia, Brescia, Italy
e-mail: alessandra.marengoni@unibs.it; giuseppe.romanelli@unibs.it

26.2 Epidemiology

Cancer occurs tenfold more frequently in elderly in comparison to younger patients [1]; thus, due to the growing life expectancy, neoplasm is an increasingly common lifetime event. Epidemiological data show a higher risk of developing any invasive cancer in men compared to women [2]. In the two decades starting from 2010 to 2030, the cancer incidence will increase by approximately 45%. This is mainly driven by cancer diagnosis in elderly patients, with an expected 67% increase in this population. As in 2030 patients aged more than 65 years are predicted to comprise 20% of the total world population, this group is anticipated to account for 70% of all cancer diagnoses [3].

Cancer survival usually decreases with age, but different degrees of variability are reported, depending on anatomical region and cancer type [4].

26.3 Multidimensional Geriatric Evaluation in the Emergency Surgical Patient

Older patients with cancer are a very heterogeneous group including both fit and frail individuals. A great discrepancy between chronological and biological age may be present due to the different speeds of the aging process across

F. Agresta et al. (eds.), *Emergency laparoscopic surgery in the elderly and frail patient*,
https://doi.org/10.1007/978-3-030-79990-8_26

individuals; in particular, cognitive and functional status, prevalence of co-morbidities, and polypharmacy may have huge variations. The Comprehensive Geriatric Assessment (CGA) is a specific tool for the assessment of the old person; it evaluates several health domains, such as the cognitive-behavioral, functional-dependency, socio-environmental, and relational status of the patient, including the identification of any latent deficits, such as pre-frailty. Several tools have been employed to evaluate the different domains of the CGA; one of the most widely used and with the largest evidence in oncology and surgery is the multidimensional prognostic index (MPI) [5, 6]. The MPI is an algorithm including information from eight domains of the CGA: activities of daily living, instrumental activities of daily living, short portable mental status questionnaire, cumulative illness rating scale, mini-nutritional assessment, Exton-Smith scale for bed scores, medication use, and cohabitation.

26.4 An Overview of Palliative Cancer Surgery

Despite age and functional status, some clinical scenarios can only be managed with surgery, for example, complications of locally advanced cancers. However, it seems difficult to propose a standard of care because very little level 1 evidences are reported. In fact, patients over 70 years old are often excluded from clinical randomized trials [7], so elderly people are still managed on the basis of assumptions proposed for younger patients. This attitude appears completely unjustified considering that nowadays almost half of the patients requiring emergent surgery are over 70 years old and have a sixfold greater mortality compared to those aged 50 or under as reported in NELA project [8]. Furthermore, several small studies show a mortality rate ranging from 32 to 42% in the over 80s age group undergoing emergent abdominal surgery [9].

The National Confidential Enquiry into Perioperative Death (NCEPOD) published in 2010 [10] highlighted the reasons leading to these poor outcomes, including the delay in admission or to theatre, the inappropriate admission under medical specialties, and the poor operative assessment.

The aim of a good palliation surgery is to alleviate symptoms effectively, carrying the shortest possible hospitalization, thereby improving the quality of life in this age group. Laparoscopy could represent a useful tool to reach these goals; in fact, it is worldwide related to improvement in enhanced discharge, intraoperative blood loss, early return in normal bowel function, less wound infections, and post-operative morbidity. The advantages of minimally invasive surgery have been observed in both elective and emergency settings, although a specific experience and skill are recommended for the latter condition.

26.5 Palliation for Colorectal Obstructions

Malignant bowel obstruction (MBO) is a condition which is often seen in the pre-terminal stages of abdominal cancers, which make a patient unable to eat and, if not treated, brings intermittent abdominal pain, nausea, and vomiting. MBO occurs in several gastrointestinal, gynecological, pancreatic, and urologic cancers, and the incidence reaches 30% [11] of hospital admissions. As age increases, also the rate of emergency admissions for colorectal cancer increases (from 28% between 75 and 84 years to 29% in over 85 years old patients) [12]. At the very beginning, a conservative approach can be attempted with the use of intravenous hydration and gastric decompression with a nasogastric tube. Medical therapies include the administration of analgesics, high-dose steroids, and octreotide with some rate of clinical relief. Palliative surgery enables the patients to resume oral food intake and to achieve a discharge from the hospital. Unfortunately, palliative surgery for MBO is associated with high mortality and morbidity rate and often worsens the quality of life of patients with limited life span [13]. There are several factors affecting the outcomes of the surgery: some technical factors are related to poor prognosis such as the location of obstruction in the small bowel rather than large bowel, an extended peritoneal carcinosis, multiple sites of obstruction, and the finding of a palpable mass [14]. Among patient-related variables, we consider both physiological and chronological ages, performance and nutritional status, the presence of ascites, the comorbidity, the presence of a perioperative chemotherapy or radiotherapy treatment as well as psychological status and social support [15]. Nevertheless, some score systems have been proposed in order to predict the outcomes after palliative surgery but none of them reached a strong validation. Another debated item is whether to resect a stage IV colorectal cancer with unresectable liver metastases in order to prevent obstructive or hemorrhagic complications, but this goes beyond our present aim of discussion [16].

Probably palliative surgery is the first option in the treatment of MBO when technically feasible in a patient with a good performance status.

Whenever facing an MBO, three kinds of procedures can be proposed: resection, internal bypass, and ostomy (colostomy or ileostomy) formation.

When possible, resection carries the best outcomes if compared to other palliative procedures in terms of symptom relief and survival [17]. There is general agreement in considering resection surgery as the procedure with the lower incidence of re-obstruction due to malignant progression [18]. Moreover, resection is mandatory, when feasible, in the presence of perforation with active spread of enteric fluid in abdominal cavity or abscesses, while proximal ostomy and drainage carry poorer outcome but is recommended whenever the cancer is unresectable. Internal bypass is a faster procedure, feasible in the majority of cases without unintentional vascular or visceral injuries. Both in bypass and in resections, an anastomosis has to be performed, and this obviously exposes patients to the risk of anastomotic leakage. Internal visceral bypasses can be ileocolic anastomoses for obstructive right colon cancers or transverse-sigmoid colo-colic anastomoses or ileo-sigmoid anastomoses for distal transverse, splenic flexure, and descending colon obstruction [19]. There are no significant data in the literature, apart from case series or case reports, which can state other than the feasibility of these procedures.

Ostomy formation is a simple and fast option to treat MBO. It does not require any anastomosis, so it is feasible also in very ill patients of those with hemodynamic instability. Both ileostomy and colostomy are effective in the management of MBO. Colostomy has a lower output of liquid stool and carries a minor rate of skin inflammation compared to ileostomy. Data from literature support the use of colostomy when the obstacle is located in pelvis [20]. The choice between colostomy or endoscopic stent in obstruction of the left colon and rectum depends on the possibility of adjuvant cure with chemotherapy: in case of extremely frail patients who can obtain only palliative care, the stent is preferable for faster discharge and better quality of life, whether colostomy is less prone to complications with anti-angiogenics or other chemotherapies when indicated [21].

Finally, for extremely ill patients with MBO, especially in segments of the colon in which an endoscopic stent is difficult to position (transverse colon, splenic flexure), a cecostomy can be performed: it is feasible in local anesthesia and carries good results also when used as a "bridge" to resective surgery [22].

Laparoscopy appears to be a good tool, in experienced hands and for selected patients, to pursue the objective of minimizing the invasiveness and reduce the morbidity rate. Despite a good amount of literature analyzing the role of laparoscopy in urgent setting and in particular for colorectal disease (demonstrating faster functional recovery, lower risk of infections, less blood loss, shorter length of stay, and reduced ileus and pneumonia), very few works are published regarding its use in MBO [23].

Moreover, a recent systematic review regarding the management of bowel obstruction in the elderly does not describe any role for laparoscopy [24], and the recent guidelines by WSES recommend "*The use of laparoscopy in the emergency treatment of MBO … should be reserved to selected favourable cases and in specialized centers.*" Our experience in the palliative treatment of MBO with emergency laparoscopy is satisfactory, especially in the elderly, and the advantages of having less pain and ileus, without a significant rise in complications, are convincing us toward a wider use in these situations.

Evidence-based advantages of laparoscopic surgery for MBO, though, have thus not been confirmed.

26.6 Palliation for Gastric Cancer

Gastric neoplasms represent a leading cause of cancer death worldwide, being responsible of malignant bowel obstruction (MBO), upper gastrointestinal (GI) obstruction, perforation, or nutritional impairment. Survival for elective surgery is improving due to the progress of research and the standardization of lymphectomy. Unfortunately, there is a paucity of data regarding outcomes for the main complications.

Approximately, 5% of the upper GI bleeding is caused by cancer [25], and often it is the first presentation of the disease. Although in half of the cases the bleeding is chronic or occult, active bleeding is far from being a rare condition, ranging from 21 to 40% [26]. Clinical presentation mainly relies on melena, hematemesis, and coffee ground vomiting. Abdominal pain, when present, is mild without a clear peritonism. The symptoms are also determined by the speed of blood loss, in particular, low bleeding over time makes the patients pale and asthenic but, on the other hand, a rapid anemization can bring hemodynamic alterations up to hemorrhagic shock. The cornerstones for the diagnosis are CT scan with contrast and esophagogastroduodenoscopy. The patients' risk stratification can be done on the basis of validated scores (such as Rockall and Glasgow-Blatchford) as recommended by guidelines [27]. The treatment of gastric cancer bleeding is based on the clinical status and the effectiveness of the implemented treatment. Supportive medical therapy relies on proton pump inhibitors, intravenous fluids, and red blood cell transfusions. The first line of operative treatment is endoscopic with its several hemostatic procedures that can be used individually or in combination. The endoscopist deals with hemorrhage using electrocoagulation, clip, injecting, or spraying hemostatic agent. If the endoscopic treatment fails or an active cancer bleeding cannot be controlled, the patients might undergo trans-arterial embolization or surgery.

Palliative surgery for gastric cancer should be considered an option for the management of major bleeding and obstruction in the emergency setting. In fact, recently, an experts' panel concluded that surgical resection for incurable disease is considered inappropriate for those patients without major symptoms [28]. However, palliative surgery can be performed according to the clinical condition of the patients in both urgent and elective settings. Laparoscopic surgery for the elderly patients with gastric cancer seems to be a safe approach that shares the advantages of minimal invasiveness such as faster post-operative recovery, less blood loss, and reduced post-operative morbidity if performed by experienced surgeons. These results are corroborated by good quality literature data. For example, a meta-analysis retrieving 7 papers and collecting 845 patients showed perioperative good results with the disadvantage of a longer operative time [29]. In urgent setting, the outcomes probably are influenced by several factors: patients related, surgery related, and disease related. The largest casuistry regarding urgent surgery for gastric cancer is extrapolated from the US National Cancer Database [30]; it found that being elderly was a factor in all-cause mortality and morbidity; moreover, the likelihood of urgent surgery increased in older patients compared to patients aged 50–59 years. The work concluded that urgent surgery for gastric cancer is associated with significantly worse surgical and oncologic outcomes; in particular, it is related to an increased 90-day mortality, a worse lymph node retrieving, and a higher risk of positive margins. Unfortunately, this work does not mention laparoscopy at all.

Less invasive laparoscopic procedures related to obstructive palliation in the elderly with advanced gastric cancer comprehend gastroenterostomy [31]. The results for gastric outlet obstruction are still debated in comparison with endoscopic metallic stents [32] and endoscopic ultrasound (EUS)-guided gastroenterostomy (still experimental) [33]. Surgery can be performed by means of laparoscopy, and it is mostly to prefer in patients with a longer life expectancy [34]. Recently, a technical variation with a partition of the stomach has configured a lower rate of delayed gastric emptying [35].

Another emergency palliation for gastric outlet syndrome in advanced gastric cancer, whenever a neoadjuvant chemotherapy might be proposed, is laparoscopic nutritional jejunostomy which can offer an adequate nutritional support to these patients and is generally made in association with staging laparoscopy, peritoneal washing in search for malignant cytology, and port-a-cath positioning [36]. The surgery can also be performed in a single-port fashion [37], as we do in our institution.

26.7 Palliation for Pancreatic Cancer

Palliation for pancreatic neoplasm is often required, due to the fact that only 20% of patients have a resectable disease at the time of diagnosis [38]. The most common complications are jaundice, duodenal obstruction, and tumor-associated pain. Undoubtedly, percutaneous and endoscopic procedures are the gold standard for palliation, especially for the treatment of jaundice. Indeed, duodenal obstruction or strict contraindications to nonsurgical procedures (such as previous gastric surgery, especially with Roux-en-Y reconstruction, chronic skin infections, failure of percutaneous drainage or complication in biliary stenting, and recurrence of jaundice) might require surgery. Post-operative outcomes in terms of mortality and morbidity remain high, despite improvement throughout the decades. Jaundice, poor performance and nutritional status, comorbidity, and age over 70 years old are known risk factors for worse outcomes after palliative surgery. Patients with unresectable pancreatic cancer have to be referred to a multidisciplinary team in order to individualize the treatment. In the emergency setting, the mortality rate indeed approaches 25%. The recent introduction of minimally invasive surgery in the palliation of pancreatic unresectable and complicated cancer has been evaluated in few works in literature without any evidence-based advantages for the laparoscopic approach, even if some benefits (earlier discharge and lower use of morphine) are demonstrated. In the laparoscopic palliation of duodenal obstruction, morbidity, mortality, analgesic consumption, time to solid oral food intake, and operative time were not different from traditional open approach [39] even if the length of stay and blood loss were significantly reduced in the laparoscopic group.

The first palliative minimally invasive surgical procedure described for the jaundice was the laparoscopic cholecystojejunostomy [40] and, more recently, side-to-side hepatico-jejunostomy [41], although it is a technically demanding procedure, requiring advanced skills and expertise. In association, laparoscopic antecolic side-to-side gastrojejunostomy has been performed for the palliation of duodenal obstruction [42]. The use of antecolic way is preferred because it lessens the possibility of another obstruction due to tumor infiltration. In case of combined complication of obstruction and jaundice, a simple jejunal loop can be used for both anastomoses. A review of the literature analyzes the results of long-term patency of biliary bypass and the effectiveness of gastrojejunal anastomosis. For the jaundice treatment, hepatico-jejunostomy seems to be associated with a higher success rate and a lower risk of recurrent jaundice compared to cholecystojejunostomy [43]. An evidence-based advantage of laparoscopic palliation has to be demonstrated with further clinical trials.

Take-Home Messages

- Emergency surgery for cancer in the elderly is fast growing.
- Primary outcomes to be pursued in the frail and vulnerable patient must rely on different criteria from those traditionally considered.
- Multidimensional/multidisciplinary approach is the key to personalize the cure.
- Emergency complications of cancer have different approaches, and minimally invasive surgery is an option to be considered but requires advanced skills and expertise.
- Laparoscopic procedures for emergency care of cancer still need evidence-based studies.

References

1. Yancik R. Cancer burden in the aged: an epidemiologic and demographic overview. Cancer. 1997;80(7):1273–83.
2. Jemal A, Siegel R, Xu J, Ward E. Cancer statistics, 2010. CA Cancer J Clin. 2010;60(5):277–300. https://doi.org/10.3322/caac.20073.
3. McKoy JM, Samaras AT, Bennett CL. Providing cancer care to a graying and diverse cancer population in the 21st century: are we prepared? J Clin Oncol. 2009;27(17):2745–6. https://doi.org/10.1200/JCO.2009.22.4352.
4. De Angelis R, Sant M, Coleman MP, Francisci S, Baili P, Pierannunzio D, Trama A, Visser O, Brenner H, Ardanaz E, Bielska-Lasota M, Engholm G, Nennecke A, Siesling S, Berrino F, Capocaccia R, EUROCARE-5 Working Group. Cancer survival in Europe 1999-2007 by country and age: results of EUROCARE—5-a population-based study. Lancet Oncol. 2014;15(1):23–34. https://doi.org/10.1016/S1470-2045(13)70546-1.
5. Liuu E, Hu C, Valero S, Brunet T, Jamet A, Bureau ML, Pilotto A, Saulnier PJ, Paccalin M. Comprehensive geriatric assessment in older patients with cancer: an external validation of the multidimensional prognostic index in a French prospective cohort study. BMC Geriatr. 2020;20(1):295. https://doi.org/10.1186/s12877-020-01692-8.
6. Bureau ML, Liuu E, Christiaens L, Pilotto A, Mergy J, Bellarbre F, Ingrand P, Paccalin M, MPI_AGE Project Investigators. Using a multidimensional prognostic index (MPI) based on comprehensive geriatric assessment (CGA) to predict mortality in elderly undergoing transcatheter aortic valve implantation. Int J Cardiol. 2017;236:381–6. https://doi.org/10.1016/j.ijcard.2017.02.048.
7. Zulman DM, Sussman JB, Chen X, Cigolle CT, Blaum CS, Hayward RA. Examining the evidence: a systematic review of the inclusion and analysis of older adults in randomized controlled trials. J Gen Intern Med. 2011;26(7):783–90. https://doi.org/10.1007/s11606-010-1629-x.
8. NELA Project Team. First patient report of the National Emergency Laparotomy Audit, R Coll Anaesth. London; 2015.
9. Louis DJ, Hsu A, Brand MI, Saclarides TJ. Morbidity and mortality in octogenarians and older undergoing major intestinal surgery. Dis Colon Rectum. 2009;52(1):59–63. https://doi.org/10.1007/DCR.0b013e31819754d4.
10. Wilkinson K, Martin IC, Gough MJ, Stewart JAD, Lucas SB, Freeth H, Bull B. An age old problem: a review of the care received by elderly patients undergoing surgery 2010. In: A report by the national confidential enquiry into patient outcome and death. London; 2010. www.ncepod.org.
11. Feuer DJ, Broadley KE, Shepherd JH, Barton DP. Systematic review of surgery in malignant bowel obstruction in advanced gynecological and gastrointestinal cancer. The Systematic Review Steering Committee. Gynecol Oncol. 1999;75(3):313–22. https://doi.org/10.1006/gyno.1999.5594.
12. Surgery for colorectal cancer in elderly patients: a systematic review. Colorectal Cancer Collaborative Group. Lancet. 2000;356(9234):968–974.
13. Ferguson HJ, Ferguson CI, Speakman J, Ismail T. Management of intestinal obstruction in advanced malignancy. Ann Med Surg (Lond). 2015;4(3):264–70. https://doi.org/10.1016/j.amsu.2015.07.018.
14. Medina-Franco H, García-Alvarez MN, Ortiz-López LJ, Cuairán JZ. Predictors of adverse surgical outcome in the management of malignant bowel obstruction. Rev Invest Clin. 2008;60(3):212–6.
15. Henry JC, Pouly S, Sullivan R, Sharif S, Klemanski D, Abdel-Misih S, Arradaza N, Jarjoura D, Schmidt C, Bloomston M. A scoring system for the prognosis and treatment of malignant bowel obstruction. Surgery. 2012;152(4):747–56; discussion 756–7. https://doi.org/10.1016/j.surg.2012.07.009.
16. Cirocchi R, Trastulli S, Abraha I, Vettoretto N, Boselli C, Montedori A, Parisi A, Noya G, Platell C. Non-resection versus resection for an asymptomatic primary tumour in patients with unresectable stage IV colorectal cancer. Cochrane Database Syst Rev. 2012;(8):CD008997. https://doi.org/10.1002/14651858.CD008997.
17. Khan MR, Bari H, Zafar SN, Raza SA. Impact of age on outcome after colorectal cancer surgery in the elderly—a developing country perspective. BMC Surg. 2011;11:17. https://doi.org/10.1186/1471-2482-11-17.
18. Shariat-Madar B, Jayakrishnan TT, Gamblin TC, Turaga KK. Surgical management of bowel obstruction in patients with peritoneal carcinomatosis. J Surg Oncol. 2014;110(6):666–9. https://doi.org/10.1002/jso.23707.
19. Pisano M, Zorcolo L, Merli C, Cimbanassi S, Poiasina E, Ceresoli M, Agresta F, Allievi N, Bellanova G, Coccolini F, Coy C, Fugazzola P, Martinez CA, Montori G, Paolillo C, Penachim TJ, Pereira B, Reis T, Restivo A, Rezende-Neto J, Sartelli M, Valentino M, Abu-Zidan FM, Ashkenazi I, Bala M, Chiara O, De' Angelis N, Deidda S, De Simone B, Di Saverio S, Finotti E, Kenji I, Moore E, Wexner S, Biffl W, Coimbra R, Guttadauro A, Leppäniemi A, Maier R, Magnone S, Mefire AC, Peitzmann A, Sakakushev B, Sugrue M, Viale P, Weber D, Kashuk J, Fraga GP, Kluger I, Catena F, Ansaloni L. 2017 WSES guidelines on colon and rectal cancer emergencies: obstruction and perforation. World J Emerg Surg. 2018;13:36. https://doi.org/10.1186/s13017-018-0192-3.
20. Kucukmetin A, Naik R, Galaal K, Bryant A, Dickinson HO. Palliative surgery versus medical management for bowel obstruction in ovarian cancer. Cochrane Database Syst Rev. 2010;2010(7):CD007792. https://doi.org/10.1002/14651858.
21. Trigui A, Rejab H, Akrout A, Harbi H, Kachaou A, Fendri S, Frikha MF, Mzali R. Comparaison entre

stent endoscopique et colostomie pour les cancers coliques gauches en occlusion : revue de la littérature [Comparison between endoscopic stenting and colostomy in the management of obstructing cancer of the left colon: Literature review]. Presse Med. 2019;48(2):173–180. French. https://doi.org/10.1016/j.lpm.2019.01.007.
22. Perrier G, Peillon C, Liberge N, Steinmetz L, Boyet L, Testart J. Cecostomy is a useful surgical procedure: study of 113 colonic obstructions caused by cancer. Dis Colon Rectum. 2000;43(1):50–4. https://doi.org/10.1007/BF02237243.
23. Maeda Y, Shinohara T, Katayama T, Minagawa N, Sunahara M, Futakawa N, Hamada T. A laparoscopic approach is associated with a decreased incidence of SSI in patients undergoing palliative surgery for malignant bowel obstruction. Int J Surg. 2017;42:90–4. https://doi.org/10.1016/j.ijsu.2017.04.052
24. Santangelo ML, Grifasi C, Criscitiello C, Giuliano M, Calogero A, Dodaro C, Incollingo P, Rupealta N, Candida M, Chiacchio G, Riccio E, Pisani A, Tammaro V, Carlomagno N. Bowel obstruction and peritoneal carcinomatosis in the elderly. A systematic review. Aging Clin Exp Res. 2017;29(Suppl 1):73–8. https://doi.org/10.1007/s40520-016-0656-9.
25. Sheibani S, Kim JJ, Chen B, Park S, Saberi B, Keyashian K, Buxbaum J, Laine L. Natural history of acute upper GI bleeding due to tumours: short-term success and long-term recurrence with or without endoscopic therapy. Aliment Pharmacol Ther. 2013;38(2):144–50. https://doi.org/10.1111/apt.12347.
26. Schatz RA, Rockey DC. Gastrointestinal bleeding due to gastrointestinal tract malignancy: natural history, management, and outcomes. Dig Dis Sci. 2017;62(2):491–501. https://doi.org/10.1007/s10620-016-4368-y.
27. Gralnek IM, Dumonceau JM, Kuipers EJ, Lanas A, Sanders DS, Kurien M, Rotondano G, Hucl T, Dinis-Ribeiro M, Marmo R, Racz I, Arezzo A, Hoffmann RT, Lesur G, de Franchis R, Aabakken L, Veitch A, Radaelli F, Salgueiro P, Cardoso R, Maia L, Zullo A, Cipolletta L, Hassan C. Diagnosis and management of nonvariceal upper gastrointestinal hemorrhage: European Society of Gastrointestinal Endoscopy (ESGE) guideline. Endoscopy. 2015;47(10):a1–a46. https://doi.org/10.1055/s-0034-1393172.
28. Brar SS, Mahar AL, Helyer LK, Swallow C, Law C, Paszat L, Seevaratnam R, Cardoso R, McLeod R, Dixon M, Yohanathan L, Lourenco LG, Bocicariu A, Bekaii-Saab T, Chau I, Church N, Coit D, Crane CH, Earle C, Mansfield P, Marcon N, Miner T, Noh SH, Porter G, Posner MC, Prachand V, Sano T, van de Velde C, Wong S, Coburn NG. Processes of care in the multidisciplinary treatment of gastric cancer: results of a RAND/UCLA expert panel. JAMA Surg. 2014;149(1):18–25. https://doi.org/10.1001/jamasurg.2013.3959.
29. Wang JF, Zhang SZ, Zhang NY, Wu ZY, Feng JY, Ying LP, Zhang JJ. Laparoscopic gastrectomy versus open gastrectomy for elderly patients with gastric cancer: a systematic review and meta-analysis. World J Surg Oncol. 2016;14:90. https://doi.org/10.1186/s12957-016-0859-8.
30. Fisher BW, Fluck M, Young K, Shabahang M, Blansfield J, Arora TK. Urgent surgery for gastric adenocarcinoma: a study of the National Cancer Database. J Surg Res. 2020;245:619–28. https://doi.org/10.1016/j.jss.2019.07.073.
31. Kocic M, Inic M, Marjanovic B, Juskic M, Nikolic S. Gastroenteroanastomosis (GEA): method of choice in the advanced stomach cancer in older age. Arch Oncol. 2002;10(3):139.
32. Tsukada K. Metallic stent placement or gastroenterostomy for gastric outlet obstruction caused by gastric cancer? J Gastroenterol. 2005;40(10):1007–8. https://doi.org/10.1007/s00535-005-1700-2.
33. Ge PS, Young JY, Dong W, Thompson CC. EUS-guided gastroenterostomy versus enteral stent placement for palliation of malignant gastric outlet obstruction. Surg Endosc. 2019;33(10):3404–11. https://doi.org/10.1007/s00464-018-06636-3.
34. Manuel-Vázquez A, Latorre-Fragua R, Ramiro-Pérez C, López-Marcano A, la Plaza-Llamas R, Ramia JM. Laparoscopic gastrojejunostomy for gastric outlet obstruction in patients with unresectable hepatopancreatobiliary cancers: a personal series and systematic review of the literature. World J Gastroenterol. 2018;24(18):1978–88. https://doi.org/10.3748/wjg.v24.i18.1978.
35. Kumagai K, Rouvelas I, Ernberg A, Persson S, Analatos A, Mariosa D, Lindblad M, Nilsson M, Ye W, Lundell L, Tsai JA. A systematic review and meta-analysis comparing partial stomach partitioning gastrojejunostomy versus conventional gastrojejunostomy for malignant gastroduodenal obstruction. Langenbecks Arch Surg. 2016;401(6):777–85. https://doi.org/10.1007/s00423-016-1470-8.
36. Siow SL, Mahendran HA, Wong CM, Milaksh NK, Nyunt M. Laparoscopic T-tube feeding jejunostomy as an adjunct to staging laparoscopy for upper gastrointestinal malignancies: the technique and review of outcomes. BMC Surg. 2017;17(1):25. https://doi.org/10.1186/s12893-017-0221-2.
37. Mohiuddin SS, Anderson CE. A novel application for single-incision laparoscopic surgery (SILS): SIL jejunostomy feeding tube placement. Surg Endosc. 2011;25(1):323–7. https://doi.org/10.1007/s00464-010-1168-x.
38. Warshaw AL. Progress in pancreatic cancer. World J Surg. 1984;8:801–2. https://doi.org/10.1007/BF01656018.
39. Bergamaschi R, Mårvik R, Thoresen JE, Ystgaard B, Johnsen G, Myrvold HE. Open versus laparoscopic gastrojejunostomy for palliation in advanced pancreatic cancer. Surg Laparosc Endosc. 1998;8(2):92–6.
40. Raj PK, Mahoney P, Linderman C. Laparoscopic cholecystojejunostomy: a technical application in unresectable biliary obstruction. J Laparoendosc Adv Surg

Tech A. 1997;7(1):47–52. https://doi.org/10.1089/lap.1997.7.47.
41. Scott-Conner CE. Laparoscopic biliary bypass for inoperable pancreatic cancer. Semin Laparosc Surg. 1998;5(3):185–8. https://doi.org/10.1177/155335069800500305.
42. Röthlin MA, Schöb O, Weber M. Laparoscopic gastro- and hepaticojejunostomy for palliation of pancreatic cancer: a case controlled study. Surg Endosc. 1999;13(11):1065–9. https://doi.org/10.1007/s004649901174.
43. Gentileschi P, Kini S, Gagner M. Palliative laparoscopic hepatico- and gastrojejunostomy for advanced pancreatic cancer. JSLS. 2002;6(4):331–8.

Emergency Robotic Surgery for Acute Abdomen in the Elderly

27

Wanda Petz, Paolo Pietro Bianchi,
Graziano Pernazza, and Graziano Ceccarelli

27.1 Introduction

Robotic surgical systems have been introduced to overcome technical challenges of laparoscopy, therefore expanding applications of minimally invasive surgery.

The high-degree three-dimensional vision of the stable camera platform, the increased dexterity of endo-wristed instruments, tremor abolition, motion scaling and the possibility of simultaneously utilising two energetic devices are characteristics of robotic platforms that can ameliorate surgical performance [1, 2].

In recent years, robotic surgery has markedly increased its applications in all the fields of surgery [3], from upper gastrointestinal benign [4, 5] and malignant conditions [6, 7] to hepatobiliary [8] and pancreatic surgery [9], from colorectal [10] to bariatric and to hernia repair [11].

Actual evidence, even if not robust and definitive, suggests good clinical results, comparable oncologic outcomes and less conversion rate across multiple specialties in comparison to laparoscopic surgery, and less surgical trauma and therefore early recovery in comparison to open surgery [12–18].

Robotic surgery needs an appropriate training both for the surgeon and for the assistant, as well as for the operative room staff [19]: nurses have to manage the use of instrumentation, the docking and undocking of the system, and anaesthesiologists are required to deal with fixed patient position during the surgical procedure, and limited access to patient's thorax and arms due to the space of the robotic cart.

Robotic operations are generally longer than open and laparoscopic ones, and the "rigidity" of the system makes it mostly utilised in procedures with a restricted surgical field, although last generation platforms have been conceived to be more flexible and suitable in particular for multiquadrant surgery.

The high cost of the platform and instruments is one of the major concerns making the availability for surgery 24 h a day and 7 days a week extremely rare.

Therefore, emergency surgical procedures are rarely performed robotically [20], and literature about the employment of robotics in the

W. Petz (✉)
Department of Digestive Surgery, IEO European Institute of Oncology IRCCS, Milan, Italy
e-mail: wanda.petz@ieo.it

P. P. Bianchi
Division of General Surgery, University of Milano, Ospedale San Paolo, Milan, Italy

G. Pernazza
General Surgery Robotic Unit, Department of Surgery, San Giovanni Addolorata Hospital, Rome, Italy

G. Ceccarelli
Department of General Surgery, "San Giovanni Battista" Hospital, USL Umbria 2, Foligno, Perugia, Italy

F. Agresta et al. (eds.), *Emergency laparoscopic surgery in the elderly and frail patient*,
https://doi.org/10.1007/978-3-030-79990-8_27

emergency setting in general, and in the elderly patient in particular, is scarce.

However, some suggestions can be listed from published case reports and case series: in this chapter, we summarise actual evidence on emergency robotic surgery and the use of robotics in the elderly population, and finally try to provide some personal indications about this particular topic.

27.2 Robotic Surgery in the Emergency Setting

To our knowledge, the first report on emergency robotic abdominal procedures was the paper from Sudan in 2012 [21]. He presented two cases of complicated bariatric surgery in 40- and 59-year-old patients. In the first patient, who was readmitted after discharge and diagnosed with a stricture of the stomach tube, the choice of performing the second surgery robotically was dictated by the limited access of the surgeon to robotic platform during weekdays owing to hospital constraints and multidisciplinary usage of the system. To provide the patient with a second robotic operation, the surgeons chose to perform it during the weekend.

The second case was a proper emergency, with a patient presenting with acute abdomen and biliary peritonitis.

The initial laparoscopic exploration of the abdomen did not allow evidencing the site of perforation, and the conversion to a robotic procedure permitted the accurate diagnosis of a dehiscence of the duodenal stump and its treatment by a manual suture.

In 2014, Felli [22] reported about an 86-year-old patient admitted in emergency for massive intestinal bleeding and severe anaemia owing to a bleeding right colon cancer; the patient was haemodynamically stable, and after stabilisation with blood transfusion in the intensive care unit, she was successfully submitted to robotic right colectomy.

A series of 106 patients operated for uncomplicated, complicated or recurrent diverticulitis has been published in 2019 by Beltzer [23]; in that series, robotic and laparoscopic approaches were compared. Early postoperative results did not differ between the two groups, but in the robotic group there were more cases of complicated diverticulitis (diverticulitis with macroabscesses or relapsing diverticulitis with complications), suggesting a role of robotics in the emergency surgical treatment of complicated diverticular disease.

In 2020, Anderson [24] reported that robotic urgent subtotal colectomy for ulcerative colitis has the same perioperative outcomes as the same laparoscopic urgent procedure; in that series, sample size was small (6 patients in the robotic group and 13 in the laparoscopic group) and mean age was 41 years in the robotic and 34 years in the robotic group; however, efficacy and safety of robotic subtotal colectomy in the urgent setting were affirmed.

In 2020, Ceccarelli [25] published a personal series of five patients (among 31 operated during a 10-year period for uncomplicated giant hiatal hernia) admitted to the Emergency Department for severe abdominal and thoracic pain, nausea and vomiting owing to a complicated giant hiatal hernia; patients received a minimally invasive (laparoscopic and robotic) surgery with hernia reduction, hiatoplasty and fundoplication (Fig. 27.1). The robotic approach was perceived to guarantee more comfort and precision, and was judged as an interesting option to facilitate complex surgical tasks as management of complications of giant hiatal hernia.

Milone [26] reported the feasibility of robotic cholecystectomy in three patients (58, 75 and 53 years old) presenting with acute cholecystitis, but the most numerous series on this topic was published by Gangemi in 2017 [27]: in that experience, 686 patients receiving a robotic cholecystectomy were compared with 284 receiving a laparoscopic procedure. A significantly lower conversion rate to open surgery was shown in the robotic group, even in the presence of acute or gangrenous cholecystitis.

Robotic approach has been employed also for the treatment of Mirizzi syndrome, one of the most serious complications of cholelitiasis: some series have described robotic cholecystectomy

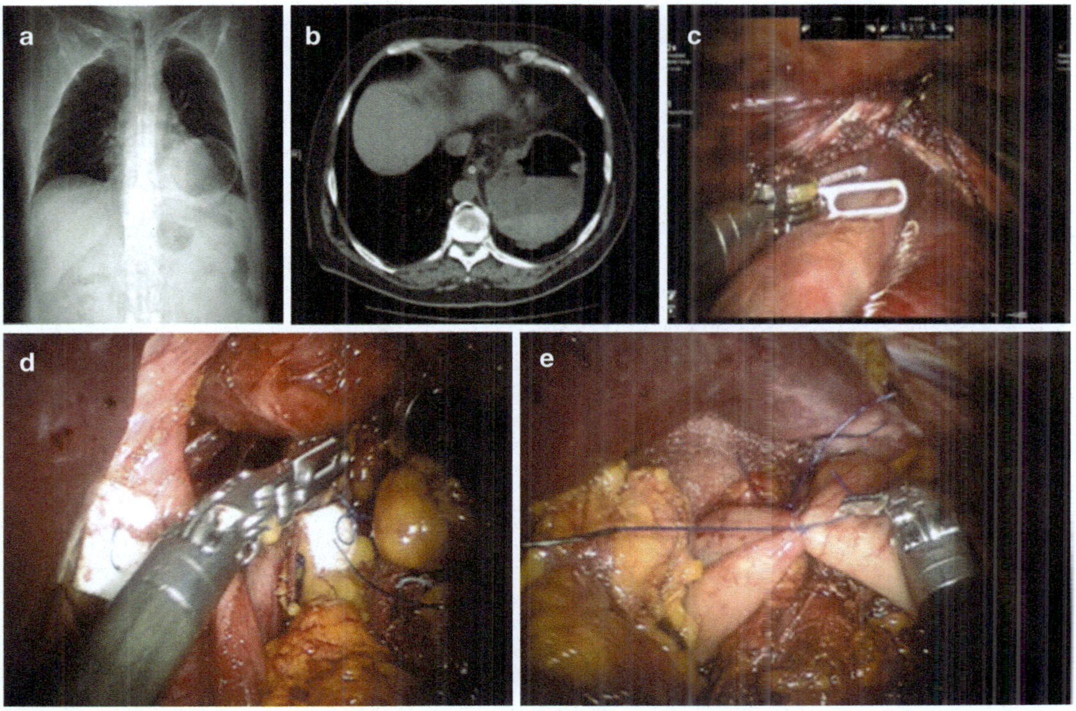

Fig. 27.1 Robotic repair of incarcerated paraesophageal hiatal hernia. (**a**) Chest X-ray showing giant paraesophageal hernia. (**b**) Thoracic CT scan showing giant paraesophageal hernia. (**c**) Hernia reduction in the abdominal cavity. (**d**) Robotic hiatoplasty. (**e**) Robotic anterior fundoplication

after endoscopic placement of a biliary stent to acutely decompress the common bile duct (Fig. 27.2).

In those series, robotic cholecystectomy was performed out from the true acute presentation with jaundice and fever; Lee [28] described five patients treated by endoscopic biliary stent placement and subsequent robotic partial cholecystectomy. There was no conversion to open surgery, and postoperative course was uneventful for all five patients; hospital stay was shorter in comparison with a historical series of 17 patients treated with the open approach.

Magge [29] reported about six patients who received a similar combined endoscopic and robotic approach; in that series, however, surgery was a complete cholecystectomy, associated with three cases to a Roux-en-Y hepatico-jejunostomy.

Authors conclude that the robotic approach is preferable to laparoscopy for the treatment of Mirizzi syndrome, facilitating complex dissection in an inflammatory and fibrotic milieu, reducing the very high conversion rate traditionally associated with laparoscopy and allowing for a minimally invasive treatment even in difficult cases.

27.3 Robotic Surgery in Elderly Patients

Concerns regarding the employment of robotic surgery in elderly patients derive mainly from the longer operative time and the fixed patient position during surgery, which may be difficult to tolerate for frail patients with cardiovascular or pulmonary comorbidities.

On the other hand, the proven advantages of laparoscopic over open surgery in elderly patients (reduced surgical trauma, early postoperative recovery and shorter hospital stay) [30–34] could be transferred to robotic surgery, which shares with laparoscopy the same minimally invasive approach.

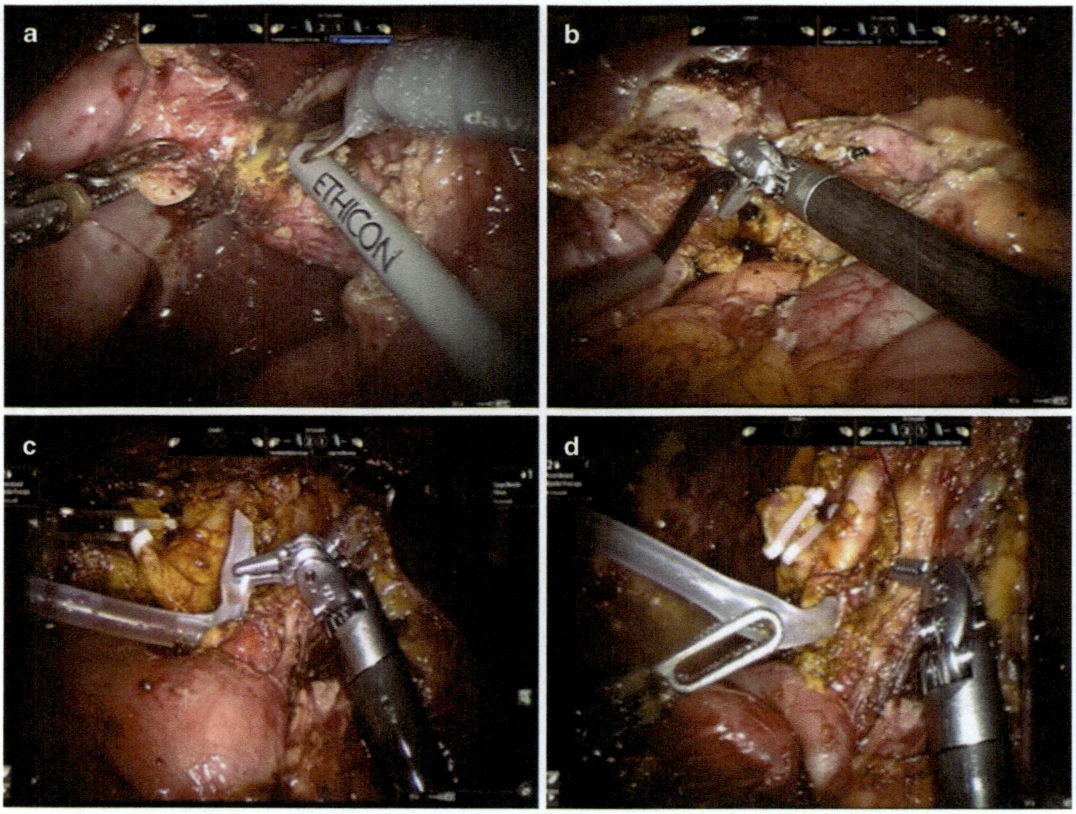

Fig. 27.2 (**a**) Opening of common bile duct. (**b**) Common bile duct exploration with a choedocoscope. (**c**) Insertion of a Kehr T-tube. (**d**) Procedure completed with T-tube in place

Actually, the minimally invasive approach to surgery for colon cancer in elderly patients has been considered, together with a multidisciplinary protocol of enhanced recovery policy, with early feeding and ambulation, one of the elements that can contribute to decrease the length of stay [33, 35, 36] and complications rate [37].

Furthermore, the reduced conversion rate that has been described in many surgical settings for the robotic in comparison to the laparoscopic approach [12, 13, 17] can represent a veritable benefit in the specific population of elderly and frail patients.

In the field of gynaecology and urology, some series have reported about the safe use of robotics in the elderly and even very elderly population [38–40].

Focusing on General Surgery, in 2010, Buchs [41] reported a series of 73 patients older than 70 years, receiving various robotic procedures with low, intermediate and high complexity levels.

In that paper, early clinical results were comparable to those of open and laparoscopic corresponding procedures, and no statistically significant differences in terms of conversion rate, transfusions, morbidity, mortality and readmission rate between the three groups of patients were observed.

In 2017, Ceccarelli [42] published a four-year robotic experience in general surgery focusing on results in elderly patients; the three more frequent major surgical procedures were right colectomy, gastric resection and liver resection, accounting for 171 patients.

Comparing patients younger than 65 years, between 65 and 79 years and older than 80 years, the authors found an increased incidence of overall complications and conversion rate in the 65–79 and the >80 group, reflecting higher comorbidities and ASA score and higher incidence of end-stage disease in these two groups.

However, the majority of complications were Clavien-Dindo I and II, while major complications and mortality rates did not differ among the three groups.

Same comparable results between patients younger ($n = 28$) and older ($n = 22$) than 70 years receiving a robotic colon or rectal resection were reported by Oldani in 2017 [43].

The largest series of minimally invasive colorectal surgery for cancer in elderly patients has been published in 2018 by De'Angelis [44]: in that paper, outcomes of 102 patients who received a laparoscopic resection were compared with those of 58 patients who received a robotic resection.

No statistically significant differences were found in postoperative complications, conversion rate, oncologic outcomes, overall and disease-free survival between the laparoscopic and the robotic groups.

27.4 Conclusions

All reported case series about the employment of robotics in emergency procedures and elderly patients come from very experienced robotic surgeons from high volume centres; so far, available literature data suggest that robotic surgery can be safely employed even in the emergency setting, provided that important key points are respected: patient must be haemodynamically stable, the choice of surgical approach must be agreed between surgeons, nurses and anaesthesiologists, and all the staff must have a wide experience in robotic elective surgery.

Interesting application of robotic surgery is the management of postponable complex emergencies after stabilisation of the acute clinical presentation, for example, cholecystectomy for Mirizzi syndrome after resolution of hyperbilirubinaemia with endoscopic biliary decompression, and the treatment of other common surgical complications as anastomotic leaks after colorectal surgery.

Some studies have affirmed the feasibility, safety and good clinical outcomes of repeated laparoscopy in the early management of colorectal anastomotic leaks [45, 46], and superiority of the laparoscopic over the open approach in terms of 30-day morbidity and length of hospital stay [47, 48].

The robotic approach in this setting, even still not described in the literature, could potentially provide the same benefits of laparoscopy and increase the precision of surgical dissection.

An issue deserving a special consideration is the appropriate training of the entire staff in executing a rapid robot undocking in case of extreme intraoperative emergency: a delayed undocking in the need of reanimation or rapid conversion to open surgery may result in fatality [49], and appropriate curricula for emergent undocking have proven their efficacy [50, 51], but have to be acquired by all the staff.

With the prerequisites of adequate surgical staff training and patient hemodynamic stability, the robotic assistance can allow for adequate surgical field exposure and precise intraoperative diagnosis and treatment of surgical complications.

In the specific population of elderly patients, the robotic technique should be considered as a part of the multidisciplinary pre-, intra- and post-operative approach which, combined with dietary optimisation, anaesthesiology management and rehabilitation, aims to provide these patients the best tolerated care.

The elevated cost of the robotic platform and of its maintenance limits at the moment its utilisation in urgent surgical procedures, even if expanding indications to robotic surgery may contribute to the amortisation of the purchase expenses.

Five Things You Should Know About Emergency Robotic Surgery for Acute Abdomen in the Elderly and Frail Patient

Robotic surgery is feasible even in the elderly patient and in the emergency setting.

- If patient is haemodynamically stable.
- If the choice of the robotic approach has been agreed upon with the anaesthesiologist.

- If the entire surgical team (included nurses, fellows and residents) has a solid experience in elective robotic surgery.
- If local organisation allows the use of the robotic platform even during night hours or weekends.
- For the treatment of postponable complex emergencies after stabilisation of the acute clinical presentation (e.g. cholecystectomy after biliary decompression in Mirizzi syndrome and treatment of anastomotic leaks in colorectal surgery).

References

1. Kim VB, Chapman WH, Albrecht RJ, et al. Early experience with telemanipulative robot-assisted laparoscopic cholecystectomy using Da Vinci. Surg Laparosc Endosc Percutan Tech. 2002;12:34–40.
2. Lanfranco AR, Castellano AE, Desai JP, et al. Robotic surgery. A current perspective. Ann Surg. 2004;239:14–21.
3. Stewart CL, Ituarte PHG, Melstrom KA, et al. Robotic surgery trends in general surgical oncology from the National Inpatient Sample. Surg Endosc. 2019;33:2591–601.
4. Pallabazzer G, Peluso C, de Bortoli N, et al. Clinical and pathophysiological outcomes of the robotic-assisted Heller–Dor myotomy for achalasia: a single-center experience. J Robot Surg. 2020;14(2):331–5. https://doi.org/10.1007/s11701-019-00988-1.
5. Damani T, Ballantyne G. Robotic foregut surgery. Surg Clin N Am. 2020:249–64.
6. Song J, Kang WK, Sung JO, et al. Role of robotic gastrectomy using da Vinci system compared with laparoscopic gastrectomy: initial experience of 20 consecutive cases. Surg Endosc. 2009;23:1204–11.
7. Ruurda JP, Van Der Sluis PC, Van Der Horst S, et al. Robot-assisted minimally invasive esophagectomy for esophageal cancer: a systematic review. J Surg Oncol. 2015;112:257–65.
8. Rong L, Wakabayashi G, Kim H-J, et al. International consensus statement on robotic hepatectomy surgery in 2018. World J Gastroenterol. 2019;25:1432–44.
9. Zureikat AH, Moser JA, Boone BA. 250 robotic pancreatic resections: safety and feasibility. Ann Surg. 2013;258:554–62.
10. Antoniou SA, Antoniou GA, Koch OO. Robot-assisted laparoscopic surgery of the colon and rectum. Surg Endosc. 2012;26:1–11.
11. Muysoms F, Cleven S, Pletinckx P, et al. Robotic transabdominal retromuscular umbilical prosthetic hernia repair (TARUP): observational study on the operative time during the learning curve. Hernia. 2018;22:1101–11.
12. Rouanet P, Bertrand MM, Jarlier M, et al. Robotic versus laparoscopic total mesorectal excision for sphincter-saving surgery: results of a single-center series of 400 consecutive patients and perspectives. Ann Surg Oncol. 2018;25:3572–9.
13. Jayne D, Pigazzi A, Marshall H, et al. Effect of robotic-assisted vs conventional laparoscopic surgery on risk of conversion to open laparotomy among patients undergoing resection for rectal cancer: the ROLARR Randomized Clinical Trial. JAMA. 2017;318(16):1569–80.
14. Sheng S, Zhao T, Wang X. Comparison of robot-assisted surgery, laparoscopic-assisted surgery, and open surgery for the treatment of colorectal cancer. A network meta-analysis. Medicine. 2018;97(34):e11817.
15. Bobo Z, Xin W, Jiang L, et al. Robotic gastrectomy versus laparoscopic gastrectomy for gastric cancer: meta-analysis and trial sequential analysis of prospective observational studies. Surg Endosc. 2019;33:1033–48.
16. Hu L, Yao L, Li X, et al. Effectiveness and safety of robotic-assisted versus laparoscopic hepatectomy for liver neoplasms: a meta-analysis of retrospective studies. Asian J Surg. 2018;41:401–16.
17. Guerrini GP, Lauretta A, Belluco C, et al. Robotic versus laparoscopic distal pancreatectomy: an up-to-date meta-analysis. BMC Surg. 2017;17:105.
18. Gavriilidis P, Roberts KJ, Sutcliffe RP. Comparison of robotic vs laparoscopic vs open distal pancreatectomy. A systematic review and network meta- analysis. HPB. 2019;21:1268–76.
19. Petz W, Spinoglio G, Choi GS, et al. Structured training and competence assessment in colorectal robotic surgery. results of a consensus experts round table. Int J Med Robot. 2016;12:634–41.
20. Bilgin EA, Bas M, Benlice C, et al. Totally laparoscopic and totally robotic surgery in patients with left-sided colonic diverticulitis. Int J Med Robot. 2020;16(1):e2068.
21. Sudan R, Desai SS. Emergency and weekend robotic surgery are feasible. J Robot Surg. 2012;6:263–6.
22. Felli E, Brunetti F, Disabato M. Robotic right colectomy for hemorrhagic right colon cancer: a case report and review of the literature of minimally invasive urgent colectomy. World J Emerg Surg. 2014;9:32.
23. Christian Beltzer C, Knoerzer L, Bachmann R, et al. Robotic versus laparoscopic sigmoid resection for diverticular disease: a single-center experience of 106 cases. J Laparoendosc Adv Surg Tech. 2019:1451–5.
24. Anderson M, Lynn P, Aydinli HH, et al. Early experience with urgent robotic subtotal colectomy for severe acute ulcerative colitis has comparable perioperative outcomes to laparoscopic surgery. J Robot Surg. 2020;14:249–53.
25. Ceccarelli G, Pasculli A, Bugiantella W. Minimally invasive laparoscopic and robot- assisted emergency treatment of strangulated giant hiatal hernias: report of five cases and literature review. World J Emerg Surg. 2020;15:37.

26. Milone M, Vertaldi S, Bracale U, et al. Robotic cholecystectomy for acute cholecystitis. Three case reports. Medicine. 2019;98:1–4.
27. Gangemi A, Danilkowicz R, Bianco F, et al. Risk factors for open conversion in minimally invasive cholecystectomy. JSLS. 2017;21:1–6.
28. Lee K, Chong C, Ma K, et al. A minimally invasive strategy for Mirizzi syndrome: the combined endoscopic and robotic approach. Surg Endosc. 2014;28:2690–4.
29. Magge D, Steve J, Novak S, et al. Performing the difficult cholecystectomy using combined endoscopic and robotic techniques: how I do it. J Gastrointest Surg. 2017;21:583–9.
30. Akiyoshi T, Kuroyanagi H, Oya M, et al. Short-term outcomes of laparoscopic rectal surgery for primary rectal cancer in elderly patients: is it safe and beneficial? Gastrointest Surg. 2009;13:1614–8.
31. Vignali A, Di Palo S, Tamburini A, et al. Laparoscopic vs. open colectomies in octogenarians: a case-matched control study. Dis Colon Rectum. 2005;48:2070–5.
32. Chautard J, Alves A, Zalinski S, et al. Laparoscopic colorectal surgery in elderly patients: a matched case-control study in 178 patients. J Am Coll Surg. 2008;206:255–60.
33. Senagore AJ, Madbouly KM, Fazio VW, et al. Advantages of laparoscopic colectomy in older patients. Arch Surg. 2003;138:252–6.
34. Cheung HY, Chung CC, Fung JT, Wong JC, Yau KK, Li MK. Laparoscopic resection for colorectal cancer in octoge- narians: results in a decade. Dis Colon Rectum. 2007;50:1905–10.
35. Ostermann S, Bucher P, Gervaz P, et al. Really so far from fast-track colorectal surgery in senior patients? Rev Med Suisse. 2009;5:1676–9.
36. Bardram L, Funch-Jensen P, Kehlet H. Rapid rehabilitation in elderly patients after laparoscopic colonic resection. Br J Surg. 2000;87:1540–5.
37. Allardyce RA, Bagshaw PF, Frampton CM, Frizelle FA, Hewett PJ, Rieger NA, et al. Australasian laparoscopic colon cancer study shows that elderly patients may benefit from lower postoperative complication rates following laparo- scopic versus open resection. Br J Surg. 2010;97:86–91.
38. Gallotta V, Conte C, D'Indinosante M, et al. Robotic surgery in elderly and very elderly gynecologic cancer patients. J Minim Invasive Gynecol. 2018;25:872–7.
39. Lee DJ, Rothberg MB, McKiernan JM, Benson MC, Badani KK. Robot-assisted radical cystoprostatectomy in complex surgical patients: single institution report. Can J Urol. 2009;16:4664–9.
40. Woods M, Thomas R, Davis R, Andrews PE, Ferrigni RG, Cheng J, Castle EP. Robot-assisted extended pelvic lymphade- nectomy. J Endourol. 2008;22:1297–302.
41. Buchs NC, Pietro Addeo P, Bianco FM, et al. Safety of robotic general surgery in elderly patients. J Robot Surg. 2010;4:91–8.
42. Ceccarelli G, Andolfi E, Biancafarina A, et al. Robot-assisted surgery in elderly and very elderly population: our experience in oncologic and general surgery with literature review. Aging Clin Exp Res. 2017;29(Suppl 1):S55–63.
43. Oldani A, Bellora P, Monni M, et al. Colorectal surgery in elderly patients: our experience with DaVinci Xi System. Aging Clin Exp Res. 2017;29(Suppl 1):S91–9.
44. de Angelis N, Abdalla S, Bianchi G, et al. Robotic versus laparoscopic colorectal cancer surgery in elderly patients: a propensity score match analysis. J Laparoendosc Adv Surg Tech. 2018;11:1334–45.
45. Chen W, Bansal S, Ke T, et al. Combined repeat laparoscopy and transanal endoluminal repair (hybrid approach) in the early management of postoperative colorectal anastomotic leaks: technique and outcomes. Surg Endosc. 2018;32:4472–80.
46. Marano A, Giuffrida MC, Giraudo C, et al. Management of peritonitis after minimally invasive colorectal surgery: can we stick to laparoscopy? J Laparoendosc Adv Surg Tech. 2017;27:342–7.
47. Wind J, Koopman AG, van Berge Henegouwen MI, et al. Laparoscopic reintervention for anastomotic leakage after primary laparoscopic colorectal surgery. BJS. 2007;94:1562–6.
48. Lee CM, Huh JW, Yun SH, et al. Laparoscopic versus open reintervention for anastomotic leakage following minimally invasive colorectal surgery. Surg Endosc. 2015;29:931–6.
49. Thompson J. Myocardial infarction and subsequent death in a patient undergoing robotic prostatectomy. AANA J. 2009;77:365–71.
50. Huser AS, Müller D, Brunkhorst V, et al. Simulated life- threatening emergency during robot-assisted surgery. J Endourol. 2014;28:717–21. https://doi.org/10.1089/end.2013.0762.
51. Ballas A, Cesta M, Gothard D. Emergency undocking curriculum in robotic surgery. Cureus. 11(3):e4321.

Part III

Perioperative Care

28 Enhanced Recovery After Emergency Surgery in the Elderly

Ugo Elmore, Andrea Vignali, Giulia Maggi, Roberto Delpini, and Riccardo Rosati

28.1 Introduction

The aging of the general population is increasing worldwide. As a consequence of this irreversible process, a higher number of elderly patients is currently requiring and will require surgery in the next years, in both elective and emergency settings. This latter circumstance deserves some considerations, since it has been well described that older patients undergoing emergency surgery have poorer outcome in terms of increased postoperative complications, increased functional dependence, and an increased risk of mortality [1, 2]. In daily routine practice, these complex frail patient candidates to elective major abdominal surgery are subjected to meticulous preoperative assessment to minimize modifiable risk factors. This process is limited or impossible in emergency situations. Under this view, one current hot topic of international literature is how to manage available resources to improve outcomes in this group of patients.

There is no "typical" older patient. A great heterogeneity exists between biological and chronological ages. Moreover, there is controversy about the cut-off value used to define a patient old, which has been called into dispute by several authors [3]. A preoperative comprehensive geriatric assessment (CGA), a multidisciplinary diagnostic and treatment approach, has been recently introduced. This process involves a careful observation of several parameters including also emotional, socio-economic, and cognitive status, which are crucial in the elderly daily life [4]. A preferable definition of this kind of patient is frail patients, defying frailty as a syndrome associated with vulnerability resulting from the age-related accumulation of deficiencies in different physiological systems [5]. This assessment will influence the decision-making process concerning invasive treatments and could help the caregiver team to adjust one or more perioperative aspects to the single patient. In fact, several nonsurgical options are already available and may represent valid alternatives for older or more fragile patients, not fit for surgery (antibiotics, percutaneous drainages such as cholecystectomy).

Once an operation is planned in both elective and emergency settings, the main goal will be to return patients to their preoperative status, through a reduction of surgical stress and an improvement of postoperative functional recovery.

Enhanced recovery after surgery (ERAS), a multidisciplinary approach initially developed for colon surgery [6] and now applied to the majority of surgical disciplines [7–10], should be considered. The main intuition of this protocol,

U. Elmore (✉) · A. Vignali · G. Maggi · R. Delpini
R. Rosati
Department of Surgery, San Raffaele Scientific Institute, University Vita-Salute, Milan, Italy
e-mail: elmore.ugo@hsr.it

F. Agresta et al. (eds.), *Emergency laparoscopic surgery in the elderly and frail patient*,
https://doi.org/10.1007/978-3-030-79990-8_28

in fact, relies on the application of pre-, intra-, and postoperative evidence-based measures to limit intraoperative fluid administration, reduces preoperative fasting, favors early mobilization, and promotes early postoperative feeding. Evidence is accumulating in the literature that protocol-driven care and consistent application of evidence-based standards of care in the perioperative period can substantially improve outcomes for high-risk and frail patients. Encouraging data have been recently published showing a lower incidence of grade III/IV Clavien–Dindo postoperative complications, shorter length of stay, lower postoperative mortality, and earlier intake and mobilization in elderly patients treated with ERAS protocol when compared to patients treated with traditional care [11–13].

The favorable results should be ascribed to the well-known properties of ERAS protocol of reducing insulin resistance, protein catabolism, as well as endocrine and inflammatory response following elective surgery [14–16]. Surgical stress response, however, is more intense when an emergency procedure is taken into account, and clinical consequences are dramatic when a frail patient is involved, with mortality rate of over 50% being reported [17]. The aim of the present narrative review is to analyze the potential benefit of the application of ERAS protocol on elderly and frail patients undergoing emergency operations. The first obstacle in reaching this target is represented by the lack of robust evidence in the international literature with only few papers dealing with the subject ERAS pathway, elderly, and emergency settings [18].

28.2 Eras in Emergency and Frail Patients

In an emergency setting scenario, when the adherence issue is considered, there are several preoperative items which could not be objectively been applied such as full preoperative counseling, complete optimization of medical conditions, preoperative pre-habilitation, nutritional supplementation, and carbohydrate loading. In addition, there is some evidence in the literature that also the adherence to postoperative items could be lower [19], in particular, in patients who develop postoperative complications, which are more common in emergency conditions. Moreover, patients undergoing emergency procedures might require an intensive care unit support that hampers an early mobilization, early feeding, and early removal of urinary catheter. Prolonged postoperative ileus, which is more common in the elderly, could also nullify benefits of early enteral nutrition. Skinner has recently reviewed the possible ERAS elements applicable in an emergency setting in the pre-, intra-, and postoperative periods and the inherent limitations [20] (Table 28.1).

The time-critical nature of emergency abdominal surgery requires tailored ERAS programs that suit the needs of these patients. Optimized perioperative cares, termed "modified ERAS pathways," have been applied to patients with obstructive colon cancer who underwent emergency surgery with associated clinical benefits in terms of fast recovery of bowel function, reduced

Table 28.1 Applicability of ERAS items in the emergency setting

Preoperative items	**Applicable**
Precounseling	No
Optimizing fluid hydration	Yes
Carbohydrate loading	No
Reduced starvation	No
No bowel preparation	Yes
Intraoperative items	**Applicable**
Laparoscopic surgery	Yes
Use of transverse incisions	Yes
No nasogastric tube	Possible
Use of regional anesthesia	Yes
Goal-directed fluid therapy	Yes
Prevention of hypothermia	Yes
Limited use of drainage	Possible
Postoperative items	**Applicable**
Early mobilization	Yes
Early hydration and nourishment	Possible
Adequate intravenous therapy	Yes
No wound drains	Possible
No nasogastric tube	Possible
Early removal catheter	Possible
Oral analgesia	Yes
Avoidance of systemic opiates	Possible

Adapted from Skinner et al. [20]

postoperative complications, and shorter hospital stay [19–22]. Similar results have been reported by a recently published meta-analysis, including 1334 elderly patients who underwent different abdominal emergency operations [23]. A significant reduction of postoperative major complications was reported when ERAS pathway was applied. In particular, a lower risk of pulmonary complications, paralytic ileus, and surgical site infection was found. Of relevance is the reported lower incidence of paralytic ileus, since gastrointestinal motility may take up to several days to recover, in particular, in the presence of peritonitis. Moreover, re-operation and re-admission rates were not affected by the application of ERAS pathway. The re-admission rate issue is another point of relevance in elderly and frail patients; during home recovery, they might be more vulnerable, due to socio-economic factor or lack of relative's support. Another possible benefit of the ERAS application in the elderly relies on the shorter length of stay, with a mean difference of 3 days when compared to conventional care, even after emergency surgery [23].

Their efficacy of ERAS in emergency, however, remains inconclusive given the pending challenges for modified ERAS protocol in the care of such patients. The heterogeneity of the emergency geriatric surgical population included in the aforementioned papers represents another possible bias. Moreover, preoperative ERAS as previously mentioned is arguably more difficult to adhere, and the target should be moved to identify intra- and postoperative elements that produce better outcomes. Gonec identified no naso-gastric tube (NGT) tube usage, early oral feeding, and use of NSAIDs medications as predictors of better outcome in ERAS patients who undergone emergency surgery, while intraoperative fluid management was indicated as predictive factor in a large series by the ERAS group society [24]. Of interest, Paduraru in a systematic review on ERAS, emergency surgery, and geriatric patients concluded that, despite a high application of ERAS items was feasible in emergency surgery as well in elderly patients, studies with fewer elements did not achieve poorer outcomes [18]. These data, however, need caution in their interpretation, due to the limitations related to the paucity of data available and the quality of the reports, and further studies are needed to reach definitive conclusions.

The great vulnerability of elderly patients requires additional efforts that should be focused on intraoperative phases. Among intraoperative ERAS items, the adoption of a mini-invasive approach has been probably represented one of the first steps toward the patient pathway optimization. Laparoscopy was initially contraindicated in the elderly, because of the hemodynamic and respiratory effects of carbon dioxide insufflation. In particular, CO_2 absorption across the peritoneal membrane can cause hypercapnia and significant acidosis in patients with severe cardiopulmonary disease. Moreover, diaphragmatic splinting, reduced venous return, and cardiac output related to CO insufflation could predispose the patient to myocardial infarction and basal atelectasis [25].

28.3 Eras and Laparoscopy

The wide experience on laparoscopy acquired by surgeons and anesthesiologists in the last three decades has reduced fears of pneumoperitoneum-related complications even in the elderly, as emerged by several studies which showed that mini-invasive approach was safe and effective, maintaining some of the short-term benefits observed in the younger population [25–27]. The combination of laparoscopy and ERAS hypothetically should represent the best perioperative strategy since both are aimed to reduce surgical stress response and organ dysfunction, thereby promoting a faster recovery after surgery [28]. A correct assessment of the impact of ERAS pathway over laparoscopy is extremely difficult and complex since they influence each other in reducing morbidity and length of stay (LOS), confounding the interpretation as recently stressed by Meillat in a paper on this issue [29].

A meta-analysis on this subject concludes that laparoscopic colorectal resection significantly reduced total LOS and number of complications when compared with open surgery even in the settings of suboptimal ERAS programs [30].

However, the benefits of laparoscopic colorectal resection remain to be proved within optimal ERAS programs.

The application of mini-invasive surgery in the emergency settings is another object of controversy, due to increased risk of dissemination and augmented contamination. Recent surgical guidelines, however, recognize laparoscopy as an effective procedure, in the hands of experienced surgeons, to treat various surgical emergencies [31]. The increased adoption of laparoscopy in emergency settings is confirmed by a recent Italian nationwide survey which documented an increase from 24.7% in 2010 to 30.3% in 2014, in particular, for acute appendicitis (44–64.7%) and Hinchey III acute diverticulitis (14–29.7%) [32]. However, the path is still debated as emerged by another Italian study including almost 2000 elderly patients undergoing abdominal emergency surgery [33]. In this study, about 1300 patients underwent open surgery, whereas 624 underwent laparoscopic surgery. Laparoscopy was implemented for the vast majority of cholecystectomies, half of appendectomies, and the minority of perforated gastroduodenal ulcer repair, adhesiolysis with/without small bowel resection, large bowel resection, and hernia repair. Despite encouraging results that have been reported favoring minimally invasive approach in terms of overall morbidity and mortality rates, in the elderly, emergency operations for acute abdomen are mainly performed through an open approach [32]. The author hypothesized that patient's poor preoperative clinical conditions and the lack of expertise during nighttime or weekend may influence the choice of surgical approach.

In conclusion, a high proportion of ERAS items for elective surgery could be applicable also in emergency surgery [34]; however, its application in elderly who undergo emergency surgery is quite difficult. Active participation and collaboration are required, which might be perceived as quite aggressive by this kind of frail patient. The paramount aspect that needs to be remembered is that the ERAS program is tailored to the patient, and adherence has not to be considered an end point if it is not useful for him. Thus, few studies have attempted to analyze whether a modified ERAS protocol could be useful for this category of patients even in emergency situations, and the interest in the scientific literature concerning this aspect has grown over the years. The lower trials of number of trials and studies available, however, indicate that this is a new area to expand and explore and, despite promising results have been published in terms of safety and efficacy, further studies are required to reach robust evidence.

Five Things You Should Know About Enhanced Recovery After Emergency Surgery in the Elderly

- Protocol-driven care and consistent application of evidence-based standards of care in the perioperative period can substantially improve outcomes for high-risk and frail patients including elderly patients.
- A high proportion of ERAS items for elective surgery could be applicable also in emergency surgery, with favorable outcomes in terms of postoperative complications, accelerated recovery of bowel function, and shorter postoperative hospital stay, without increasing for re-admission. A tailored ERAS pathway including frailty assessment and specific discharge strategy should be considered.
- The combination of laparoscopy and ERAS represents an optimal perioperative strategy since both promote a faster recovery after surgery and reduce perioperative surgical stress, which is of pivotal importance in frail and elderly patients.
- The simultaneous application of ERAS and laparoscopy in the elderly and emergency settings has resulted in safe and efficacy, with no adverse effect on postoperative outcome; however, no robust conclusion could be reached at the moment, due to the paucity and the retrospective nature of data currently available.
- More evidence is clearly required. The path is still long. The heterogeneity of care among different centers, the objective difficulty in obtaining an appropriate preoperative patient selection able to identify patients who can benefit most from the application of laparos-

copy and ERAS are the main obstacles. An active participation and collaboration and the creation of a dedicated multidisciplinary network are mandatory to better understand the feasibility and safety and the real impact of ERAS and laparoscopy on postoperative outcomes in frail and elderly patients in the context of an emergency setting.

References

1. Sheetz KH, Waits SA, Krell RW, et al. Improving mortality following emergent surgery in older patients requires focus on complication rescue. Ann Surg. 2013;258:614–7.
2. Svenningsen P, Manharan T, Fodd NB, et al. Increased mortality in the elderly after emergency abdominal surgery. Dan Med J. 2014;61:A4876.
3. Etzioni D, Liu J, Maggard M. The aging population and its impact on the surgery workforce. Ann Surg. 2003;238:170–7.
4. Pereira J, Paduraru M. Multimodal rehabilitation in geriatric emergency surgery. Chirurgia (Bucur). 2017;112:558–65.
5. Joseph B, Zangbar B, Pandit V. Emergency general surgery in the elderly: too old or too frail? J Am Coll Surg. 2016;222:805–13.
6. Kehlet H. Fast-track colorectal surgery. Lancet. 2008;371:791–3.
7. Kagedan D, Ahmed M, Devitt K. Enhanced recovery after pancreatic surgery: a systematic review of the evidence. HPB. 2015;17:11–6.
8. Pisarska M, Malczak P, Major P. Enhanced recovery after surgery protocol in oesophageal cancer surgery: systematic review and meta-analysis. PLoS One. 2017;12:3.
9. Małczak P, Pisarska M, Piotr M. Enhanced recovery after bariatric surgery: systematic review and meta-analysis. Obes Surg. 2017;27:226–35.
10. Hughes M, McNally S, Wigmore S. Enhanced recovery following liver surgery: a systematic review and meta-analysis. HPB. 2014;16:699–706.
11. Tejedor P, Pastor C, Gonzalez-Ayora S. Short-term outcomes and benefits of ERAS program in elderly patients undergoing colorectal surgery: a case-matched study compared to conventional care. Int J Color Dis. 2018;33:1251–8.
12. Millan M, Beatriz E, Aleidis C. ERAS programs in elderly patients: is there a limit? Int J Color Dis. 2018;33:1313.
13. Gonzalez-Ayora S, Pastor C, Guadalajara H. Enhanced recovery care after colorectal surgery in elderly patients. Compliance and outcomes of a multicenter study from the Spanish Working Group on ERAS. Int J Colorectal Dis. 2016;31:1625–31.
14. Ljungqvist O. Jonathan E. Rhoads lecture 2011: insulin resistance and enhanced recovery after surgery. JPEN J Parenter Enteral Nutr. 2012;36(4):389–98.
15. Ljungqvist O, Scott M, Fearon K. Enhanced recovery after surgery: a review. JAMA Surg. 2017;152:292–8.
16. Nisanevich V, Felsenstein I, Almogy G. Effect of intraoperative fluid management on outcome after intraabdominal surgery. Anesthesiology. 2005;103:25–32.
17. Al-Temimi M, Griffee M, Enniss T. When is death inevitable after emergency laparotomy? Analysis of the American College of Surgeons National Surgical Quality Improvement Program Database. J Am Coll Surg. 2012;215:503–11.
18. Paduraru M, Ponchietti L, Casas I. Enhanced recovery after surgery (ERAS)—the evidence in geriatric emergency surgery: a systematic review. Chirurgia (Bucur). 2017;112:546–57.
19. Roulin D, Blanc C, Muradbegovic M. Enhanced recovery pathway for urgent colectomy. World J Surg. 2014;38:2153–9.
20. Skinner A, Huddart S. The application of enhanced recovery after surgery in emergency abdominal surgery. Department of Anaesthesia, Royal Surrey County Hospital, Guildford.
21. Lohsiriwat V. Enhanced recovery after surgery vs conventional care in emergency colorectal surgery. World J Gastroenterol. 2014;20:13950–5.
22. Shang Y, Guo C, Zhang D. Modified enhanced recovery after surgery protocols are beneficial for postoperative recovery for patients undergoing emergency surgery for obstructive colorectal cancer: a propensity score matching analysis. Medicine. 2018;97:12348.
23. Hajibandeh S, Hajibandeh S, Bill V. Meta-analysis of enhanced recovery after surgery (ERAS) protocols in emergency abdominal surgery. World J Surg. 2020;44:1336–48.
24. ERAS Compliance Group. The impact of enhanced recovery protocol compliance on elective colorectal cancer resection: results from an international registry. Ann Surg. 2015;261:1153–9.
25. Brunt L, Quasebarth M, Dunnegan D. Outcomes analysis of laparoscopic cholecystectomy in the extremely elderly. Surg Endosc. 2001;15:700–5.
26. Adachi Y, Shiraishi N, Shiromizu A. Laparoscopy-assisted Billroth I gastrectomy compared with conventional open gastrectomy. Arch Surg. 2000;135:806–10.
27. Vignali A, Di Palo S, Tamburini A. Laparoscopic vs. open colectomies in octogenarians: a case-matched control study. Dis Colon Rectum. 2005;48:2070–5.
28. Vlug M, Wind J, Hollmann M. Laparoscopy in combination with fast track multimodal management is the best perioperative strategy in patients undergoing colonic surgery: a randomized clinical trial (LAFA-study). Ann Surg. 2011;254:868–75.
29. Meillat H, Brun C, Zemmour C. Laparoscopy is not enough: full ERAS compliance is the key to improvement of short-term outcomes after colectomy for cancer. Surg Endosc. 2020;34:2067–75.

30. Zhuang C, Ye X, Zhang X. Enhanced recovery after surgery programs versus traditional care for colorectal surgery: a meta-analysis of randomized controlled trials. Dis Colon Rectum. 2013;56:667–78.
31. Agresta F, Ansaloni L, Baiocchi G. Laparoscopic approach to acute abdomen from the consensus development conference of the SICE, ACOI, SIC, SICUT, SICOP, EASES. Surg Endosc. 2012;26:2134–64.
32. Agresta F, Campanile F, Podda M. Current status of laparoscopy for acute abdomen in Italy: a critical appraisal of 2012 clinical guidelines from two consecutive nationwide surveys with analysis of 271,323 cases over 5 years. Surg Endosc. 2017;31:1785–95.
33. Costa G, Fransvea P, Podda M. The use of emergency laparoscopy for acute abdomen in the elderly: the FRAILESEL Italian multicenter prospective cohort study. Updates Surg. 2020;72:513–25.
34. Lohsiriwat V, Jitmungngan R. Enhanced recovery after surgery in emergency colorectal surgery: review of literature and current practices. World J Gastrointest Surg. 2019;11:41–52.

29 Antibiotics in Emergency Abdominal Surgery in the Elderly

Massimo Sartelli

29.1 Introduction

Intra-abdominal infections (IAIs), although affect all age groups, take a greater toll on the elderly population than it does on younger populations. Given the increased mortality and morbidity associated with IAIs in the elderly population, and given the varied means of disease presentation, practitioners must have heightened indices of suspicion when treating these patients [1].

IAIs encompass a variety of pathological conditions, ranging from uncomplicated appendicitis to fecal peritonitis.

The treatment of patients with intra-abdominal infections involves both source control and antibiotic therapies [2].

Source control encompasses all measures undertaken to eliminate the source of infection, reduce the bacterial inoculum, and correct or control anatomic derangements to restore normal physiologic function. The procedure used to treat the infection depends on the anatomical site of infection, the degree of peritoneal inflammation, the generalized septic response, the patient's underlying condition, and the available resources of the treatment center.

M. Sartelli (✉)
Department of Surgery, Macerata Hospital,
Macerata, Italy

Antibiotic therapy is nevertheless important in the overall management of IAIs. Inappropriate antibiotic therapy may result in poor patient outcomes and the appearance of bacterial resistance. Initial antibiotic therapy is typically empirical in nature because they need immediate treatment (especially in critically ill patients), and microbiological data (culture and susceptibility results) usually require ≥24 h for the identification of pathogens and antibiotic susceptibility patterns.

Isolation and identification of bacterial strains take more time, and results of antibiotic susceptibility are usually only available after 48 h and later.

The decision tree for the empiric antibiotic regimen should depend mainly on three factors: presumed pathogens involved and risk factors for major resistance patterns, clinical patient's severity, and presumed/identified source of infection.

IAIs that affect elderly patients are challenging to manage, because the etiology, presentation, severity, and outcome differ from those of younger populations.

29.2 The Management of Infections in Elderly People

Infectious diseases pose a major challenge in the elderly persons for two main reasons: (1) the susceptibility to infection increases with age and

F. Agresta et al. (eds.), *Emergency laparoscopic surgery in the elderly and frail patient*,
https://doi.org/10.1007/978-3-030-79990-8_29

when infections occur they often present atypically; and (2) the diagnostic uncertainty is much more pronounced in the geriatric population [3].

Age is a well-established risk factor for infection but furthermore is a risk factor for prolonged length of hospital stay, increased incidence of complications, and significant and sustained decline in baseline functional status. Age-dependent changes in the immune system may affect the organism's ability to overcome external stressors. However, impaired immunity is much more associated with disease burden than the chronological age, and older adults with chronic diseases (e.g., diabetes mellitus, chronic obstructive pulmonary disease, or heart failure) are more susceptible to common infections [3].

Classical symptoms and signs such as fever are not common in the elderly. Although fever may be absent or blunted in many elderly patients, its detection in a geriatric patient should be taken seriously for the evaluation of infection, especially when compared to a younger patient [4]. Instead, infections are usually presented with changes in mental status including confusion, obtundation, agitation, delirium, poor oral intake, malaise, falls hypothermia, etc. The presence of hypothermia has been found to be a predictor of mortality in septic elderly patients [5]. In addition, due to dementia or altered mental status, a detailed history may not usually be obtained, and physical examination and diagnostic tests are difficult to perform. High blood cell count with left shift, acute phase biomarkers, such as procalcitonin and C-reactive protein, have similar diagnostic efficacy in the elderly and the younger patients [6, 7]. Thus, they can be considered as adjunctive diagnostic tools for infection, however, with limitations.

29.3 Antibiotic Therapy in Elderly Patients

Effective and safe antibiotic therapy is essential to keeping this vulnerable population healthy and preventing morbidity and mortality due to infection. To be able to provide effective antibiotic therapy to this population, all clinicians should understand the altered pharmacokinetics of antibiotics used in elderly patients due to comorbid conditions and the normal physiological changes associated with aging.

The antibiotic dosing regimen should be always established depending on host factors and properties of antibiotics agents. Antibiotic pharmacodynamics integrates the complex relationship between organism susceptibility and patient pharmacokinetics. Pharmacokinetics describes the fundamental processes of absorption, distribution, metabolism, and elimination and the resulting concentration-versus-time profile of an agent administered in vivo. The achievement of appropriate target site concentrations of antimicrobials is essential to eradicate the relevant pathogen. Suboptimal target site concentrations may have important clinical implications and may explain therapeutic failures, in particular, for bacteria for which in vitro MICs are high [8].

Rational and effective dosage and administration strategies based on pharmacodynamic breakpoints and detailed understanding of the pharmacokinetics of antibiotics in the elderly patients can increase the chances of achieving complete eradication of an infection in a timely manner. Importantly, this strategy helps prevent selection of drug-resistant bacteria and minimizes the toxic effects of antibacterial therapy in the elderly patient [9].

As persons age, the gastrointestinal tract undergoes a variety of morphological and functional changes leading to delayed gastric emptying, reduced splanchnic blood flow, and alterations in pH.

Key pharmacokinetic parameters such as the bioavailability of orally administered antibiotics are affected by these changes in the intraluminal environment. Therefore, when treating elderly patients with oral antibiotics, it is important to consider the impact, even if small, that these gastrointestinal changes may have on drug absorption [9].

Elderly patients tend to have an increased proportion of adipose tissue to lean mass compared to younger patients. With this increased fat content, lipophilic antibiotics are more readily soluble in tissue compartments, leading to increased half-lives of lipid-soluble drugs, including rifampin, fluoroquinolones, macrolides, oxazolidinones, and tetracyclines [10]. A concomitant decrease in total body water and lean mass contributes to decreased solubility of water-soluble drugs in tissue compartments, leading to increased plasma concentrations of hydrophilic antibiotics, including aminoglycosides, beta-lactams, and glycopeptides [10]. Due to this decreased total body water, elderly patients with severe infections should be administered full loading doses of beta-lactams, aminoglycosides, and glycopeptides when indicated.

As patients age, there is an increased risk for decreased clearance of drug from the body due to declining function of the lung, kidney, bladder, gastrointestinal, and circulatory system, which leads to drug accumulation [10].

Renal function declines as part of the normal aging process, even without concomitant renal disease. Therefore, it is paramount to assess renal function when considering the pharmacokinetics of antibiotics in elderly patients. The kidneys are essential for drug elimination of many antimicrobial agents, including but not limited to beta-lactams, glycopeptides, aminoglycosides, daptomycin, ciprofloxacin, levofloxacin, and trimethoprim/sulfamethoxazole. With decreased renal function leading to impaired drug clearance, renally eliminated drugs can accumulate in the body resulting in prolonged half-lives, high serum concentrations, and increased risk of toxicity. When renal replacement therapy is utilized in advanced kidney failure, drugs may be eliminated to a greater extent than with normal renal elimination, requiring patient- and agent-specific dosage adjustments.

In Table 29.1, recommended dosing regimens (according to renal function) of the most commonly used renally excreted antibiotics are illustrated [11].

29.4 Elderly Patients and Antimicrobial Resistance

Antimicrobial resistance (AMR) is one of the greatest threats to public health, sustainable development, and security worldwide. Its prevalence has increased alarmingly over the past decades. In 2008, the "ESKAPE" pathogen which refers to *Enterococcus faecium, Staphylococcus aureus,*

Table 29.1 Recommended dosing regimens (according to renal function) of the most commonly used renally excreted antibiotics

Renal function				
Antibiotic	Increased	Normal	Moderately impaired	Severely impaired
Piperacillin/ tazobactam	16/2 g q24 h CI or 3.375 q6 h EI over 4 h	4/0.5 g q6 h	3/0.375 g q6 h	2/0.25 g q6 h
Imipenem	500 mg q4 h or 250 mg q3 h over 3 h CI	500 mg q6 h	250 mg q6 h	250 mg q12 h
Meropenem	1 g q6 h over 6 h CI	500 mg q6 h	250 mg q6 h	250 mg q12 h
Ertapenem	ND	1 g q24 h	1 g q24 h	500 mg q24 h
Gentamycin	9–10 mg/kg q24 h[b]	7 mg/kg q24 h	7 mg/kg q36–48 h	7 mg/kg q48–96 h
Amikacin	20 mg/kg q24 h	15 mg/kg q24 h	15 mg/kg q36–48 h[b]	15 mg/kg q48–96 h
Ciprofloxacin	600 mg q12 h or 400 mg q8 h	400 mg q12 h	400 mg q12 h	400 mg q24 h
Levofloxacin	500 mg q12 h	750 mg q24 h	500 mg q24 h	500 mg q48 h
Vancomycin	30 mg/kg q24 h CI	500 mg q6 h	500 mg q12 h	500 mg q24–72 h
Teicoplanin	LD 12 mg/kg q12 h for 3–4 doses; MD 6 mg/kg q12 h	LD 12 mg/kg q12 h for 3–4 doses; MD 4–6 mg/kg q12 h	LD 12 mg/kg q12 h for 3–4 doses; MD 2–4 mg/kg q12 h	LD 12 mg/kg q12 h for 3–4 doses; MD 2–4 mg/kg q24 h
Tigecycline	LD 100 mg; MD 50 mg q12 h	LD 100 mg; MD 50 mg q12 h	LD 100 mg; MD 50 mg q12 h	LD 100 mg; MD 50 mg q12 h

Klebsiella pneumoniae, Acinetobacter baumannii, Pseudomonas aeruginosa, and *Enterobacter species* was proposed to highlight those pathogens where AMR is of particular concern and to emphasize which bacteria increasingly "escape" the effects of antibiotics [12]. These organisms are increasingly multi-drug, extensive-drug, and pan-drug resistant, and this process is accelerating globally.

The global nature of AMR calls for a global response, both in the geographic sense and across the whole range of sectors involved. Nobody is exempt from the problem, nor from playing a role in the solution. The impact of AMR worldwide is significant, because it may

- Lead to some infections becoming untreatable
- Lead to inappropriate empirical treatment in critically ill patients where an appropriate and prompt treatment is mandatory
- Increase length of hospital stay, morbidity, mortality, and cost; and
- Make necessary alternative antimicrobials which are more toxic, less effective, or more expensive

New mechanisms of resistance continue to emerge and spread globally, threatening our ability to treat common infections. An effective and cost-effective strategy to reduce AMR should involve a multi-faceted approach aimed at optimizing antibiotic use, strengthening surveillance and infection prevention and control, and improving patient and clinician education and awareness regarding the appropriate use of antibiotics.

Although most clinicians are aware of the problem of antimicrobial resistance, most underestimate this problem in their own hospital. Incorrect and inappropriate use of antibiotics and other antimicrobials, as well as poor prevention and control of infections, contributes to the development of such resistance.

Elderly patients are at increased risk of acquiring drug-resistant bacterial infections due to multiple factors including more frequent and prolonged contact with the health-care system, chronic disease states that impair immune function, immunosenescence that comes with normal aging, and use of medical devices prone to bacterial colonization including indwelling catheters. Patients and residents in long-term care facilities are more likely to be colonized with at least one multi drug resistant organisms (MDRO), including extended-spectrum beta-lactamase producers, methicillin-resistant Staphylococcus aureus, and vancomycin-resistant Enterococcus [13].

Compared to infections with antimicrobial-susceptible organisms, infection with an MDRO is associated with significantly increased mortality [14].

29.5 Conclusions

Given the increased mortality and morbidity associated with intra-abdominal infections in the elderly population, and given the varied means of disease presentation, clinicians must have heightened indices of suspicion when treating these patients. The decrease in the acuity of symptoms and delay in the presentation can make diagnosis difficult.

Older age is a well-established risk factor for infection and furthermore is a risk factor for prolonged length of hospital stay, increased incidence of complications, and significant and sustained decline in baseline functional status. Moreover, with an increasing elderly population and increasing antimicrobial resistance, it is important that health-care providers understand how to utilize antibiotics effectively and safely in this patient population.

Rational and effective dosage and administration strategies based on pharmacodynamic breakpoints and detailed understanding of the pharmacokinetics of antibiotics in the elderly patients can increase the chances of achieving complete eradication of an infection in a timely manner. Importantly, this strategy helps prevent the selection of drug-resistant bacteria and minimizes the toxic effects of antibacterial therapy in the elderly patient.

Five Things You Should Know About Antibiotics in Emergency Abdominal Surgery in the Elderly

- Older age is a well-established risk factor for infection which is a risk factor for prolonged length of hospital stay, increased incidence of complications, and significant and sustained decline in baseline functional status.
- Because of a variety of physiologic changes that occur as people age, infections may present with vague symptoms and longer histories.
- High blood cell count with left shift and acute phase biomarkers, such as procalcitonin and C-reactive protein, have similar diagnostic efficacy in the elderly and the younger patients. Thus, they can be considered as adjunctive diagnostic tools for infection, however, with limitations.
- With the increase of antibiotic use and the current growth in the number and proportion of elderly patients, it is essential that clinicians understand appropriate antibiotic pharmacotherapy in the elderly patient finding the right balance between maximizing clinical outcome and minimizing emergence of the development of resistance and the selection of resistant pathogens such as *Clostridium difficile*.
- Rational and effective dosage and administration strategies based on pharmacodynamic breakpoints and detailed understanding of the pharmacokinetics of antibiotics in the elderly patients can increase the chances of achieving complete eradication of an infection in a timely manner.

References

1. Podnos YD, Jimenez JC, Wilson SE. Intra-abdominal sepsis in elderly persons. Clin Infect Dis. 2002;35(1):62–8.
2. Sartelli M, Catena F, Abu-Zidan FM, Ansaloni L, Biffl WL, Boermeester MA, Ceresoli M, Chiara O, Coccolini F, De Waele JJ, Di Saverio S, Eckmann C, Fraga GP, Giannella M, Girardis M, Griffiths EA, Kashuk J, Kirkpatrick AW, Khokha V, Kluger Y, Labricciosa FM, Leppaniemi A, Maier RV, May AK, Malangoni M, Martin-Loeches I, Mazuski J, Montravers P, Peitzman A, Pereira BM, Reis T, Sakakushev B, Sganga G, Soreide K, Sugrue M, Ulrych J, Vincent JL, Viale P, Moore EE. Management of intra-abdominal infections: recommendations by the WSES 2016 consensus conference. World J Emerg Surg. 2017;12:22.
3. Beckett CL, Harbarth S, Huttner B. Special considerations of antibiotic prescription in the geriatric population. Clin Microbiol Infect. 2015;21(1):3–9.
4. Norman DC. Fever in the elderly. Clin Infect Dis. 2000;31:148–51.
5. Tiruvoipati R, Ong K, Gangopadhyay H, Arora S, Carney I, Botha J. Hypothermia predicts mortality in critically ill elderly patients with sepsis. BMC Geriatr. 2010;10:70.
6. Steichen O, Bouvard E, Grateau G, Bailleul S, Capeau J, Lefèvre G. Diagnostic value of procalcitonin in acutely hospitalized elderly patients. Eur J Clin Microbiol Infect Dis. 2009;28:1471–6.
7. Ticinesi A, Lauretani F, Nouvenne A, Porro E, Fanelli G, Maggio M, et al. C-reactive protein (CRP) measurement in geriatric patients hospitalized for acute infection. Eur J Intern Med. 2017;37:7–12. https://doi.org/10.1016/j.ejim.2016.08.026.
8. Sartelli M, Weber DG, Ruppé E, Bassetti M, Wright BJ, Ansaloni L, et al. Antimicrobials: a global alliance for optimizing their rational use in intra-abdominal infections (AGORA). World J Emerg Surg. 2016;11:33.
9. Noreddin AM, Haynes V. Use of pharmacodynamic principles to optimise dosage regimens for antibacterial agents in the elderly. Drugs Aging. 2007;24(4):275–92.
10. Giarratano A, Green SE, Nicolau DP. Review of antimicrobial use and considerations in the elderly population. Clin Interv Aging. 2018;13:657–67.
11. Pea F, Viale P. Bench-to-bedside review: appropriate antibiotic therapy in severe sepsis and septic shock–does the dose matter? Crit Care. 2009;13(3):214.
12. A global declaration on appropriate use of antimicrobial agents across the surgical pathway. Surg Infect (Larchmt). 2017;18(8):846–853.
13. March A, Aschbacher R, Dhanji H, et al. Colonization of residents and staff of a long-term-care facility and adjacent acute-care hospital geriatric unit by multiresistant bacteria. Clin Microbiol Infect. 2010;16(7):934–44.
14. Schwaber MJ, Carmeli Y. Mortality and delay in effective therapy associated with extended-spectrum beta-lactamase production in Enterobacteriaceae bacteraemia: a systematic review and meta-analysis. J Antimicrob Chemother. 2007;60(5):913–20.

30 Imaging and Interventional Radiology in Emergency Abdominal Surgery in the Elderly

Francesca Iacobellis, Gianluca Rasetto, Antonio Brillantino, Marco Di Serafino, Roberto Rizzati, and Luigia Romano

30.1 Imaging Approach to the Elderly Patients with Acute Abdominal Pain/Acute Abdomen

Acute abdominal pain is a common complaint in the emergency department, it can originate from many underlying conditions, and it should be of particular concern for elderly patients.

With the advent of modern-day imaging techniques, faster and more accurate diagnosis have been available to the emergency, and thus many patients with a clinical condition of acute abdomen—candidates to surgery—are instead treated with conservative measures, while others, clinically affected by a condition of acute abdominal pain that does not meet the criteria of acute abdomen, will undergo surgery, for example, patients suffering from acute appendicitis [1].

To this day, the most useful imaging techniques in the emergency study of acute abdominal pain are three: plain radiograph, ultrasonographic studies, and computed tomography (CT). Magnetic resonance imaging (MRI), with some exceptions, is not yet widely used in the diagnostic work-up of acute abdominal pain in elderly patients.

F. Iacobellis (✉) · M. Di Serafino · L. Romano
Department of General and Emergency Radiology, "Antonio Cardarelli" Hospital, Naples, Italy

G. Rasetto · R. Rizzati
Department of Clinical Diagnostic and Interventional Radiology, Ausl Ferrara, "SS. Annunziata" Hospital, Ferrara, Italy

A. Brillantino
Department of Emergency Surgery, "Antonio Cardarelli" Hospital, Naples, Italy

30.1.1 Abdominal Radiographs

Abdominal radiographs can be still considered the first-level imaging study in suspected diseases like gastrointestinal perforation and obstruction [2].

30.1.1.1 Main Findings

The most important pathological variations of the normal air pattern are those relative to the presence of free air and the small and large intestine pattern alteration. Free air is better seen on erect antero-posterior (AP) view, because air rises and it is found in the upper abdominal quadrants. Typically, free air is seen as a semilunar radiolucent bubble placed directly under the diaphragm or may also collect in the spaces between the bowel loops and form triangles or particular shapes in gas-filled bowel [3, 4]. Bowel dilatation is another important pathological finding. The underlying conditions of bowel dilatation are either mechanical obstruction or functional ileus, but the underlying causes of bowel obstruction cannot be diagnosed with an abdominal radiograph [5–10].

F. Agresta et al. (eds.), *Emergency laparoscopic surgery in the elderly and frail patient*,
https://doi.org/10.1007/978-3-030-79990-8_30

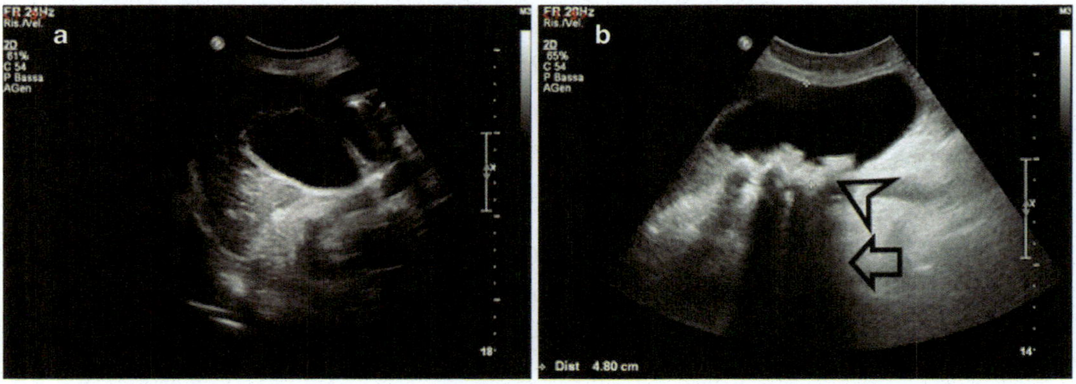

Fig. 30.1 Abdominal US study, transverse plane: (**a**) normal gallbladder with thin walls and homogeneous, anechoic content, (**b**) enlarged gallbladder (transverse length exceeding 4 cm) containing multiple gallstones, notice the highly reflective echogenic focus (arrowhead) and the posterior acoustic shadowing (arrow)

Foreign bodies are another important pathological finding, especially when they are metallic or glass, but not all the foreign bodies are radiopaque and in this case they may be harder to visualize [11–13].

30.1.1.2 Pros and Cons

Abdominal radiograph is a low-cost examination, easy to perform, and readily available; it can be performed on uncooperative patients with good results and, even though other imaging techniques are more sensitive and specific, it can still give much informations [14].

In emergency setting, abdominal radiograph is most useful to identify free air and to assess a possible bowel dilatation.

30.1.2 Ultrasound

Ultrasound (US) is an extremely useful tool in the emergency department, for both screening and diagnostic purposes. Thanks to its portability, accessibility, non-invasiveness and simple learning curve, it has become one of the most frequently adopted diagnostic techniques in the emergency department by non-radiologists. US has been proven useful in various emergencies, and it carries out a specific role in acute abdomen [15].

30.1.2.1 Main Findings

US allows the morphological and dynamic study of the abdominal wall, permitting the evaluation of abdominal wall hernias [16, 17].

Furthermore, US allows to detect some intra abdominal important findings. Free fluid in the abdomen can be easily detected at ultrasound imaging; it can be related to several urgent and emergency conditions as inflammatory, bleeding, infective, and neoplastic [18]. US can be used as screening, bedside tool for the fast detection of abdominal aortic aneurysm, eventually ruptured, during the initial patient assessment [15], and can evaluate the echostructure of the parenchymatous organs. US has high sensitivity and specificity in detecting gallstones (Fig. 30.1), and it can elicit the "Murphy's sign" using the ultrasound transducer, suspecting for gallbladder and biliary diseases [19].

30.1.2.2 Pros and Cons

US may suffer from some disadvantages: it is disturbed by gas and bones, is less effective in obese and uncooperative patients, and is an "operator-dependent" imaging technique; furtermore, it has lower panoramicity when compared to CT and does not allow an exaustive study of the abdominal vessels, frequently involved in the physiopathology of acute abdominal pain in elderly patients. On the other hand, it has several perks over other techniques: it is a bedside tool, does not adopt iodinated intravenous contrast medium and ionizing radiations; when the target organ can be closely approached, the contrast and spatial resolution of a high-frequency US may be higher than those of CT, and the dynamic, real-time properties of US are unique: it can directly assess bowel peristalsis and vessel blood flow, changes during Valsalva's maneuver, gravity, or compression. Moreover, US allows a detailed correlation of the area of maximum tenderness or palpable mass with the findings. In the case of intraperitoneal fluid, US-guided puncture is a safe and rapid way to determine its nature [20]. Lastly, according to ACR appropriateness criteria, US is the most appropriate imaging modality for patients suspected of having acute calculous cholecystitis [1].

30.1.3 CT Scan

In many cases of acute abdominal pain, CT with intravenous contrast medium of the abdomen and pelvis is the first-line imaging investigation, due to the high sensitivity and specificity and allowing a fast and accurate differential diagnosis among different causes of abdominal pain, both surgical and non-surgical [21, 22]. Compared to other imaging techniques, it can provide a more complete view of all the abdominal structures, without any limits related to the presence of bowel gas and abdominal fat [23].

30.1.3.1 Pathological Findings

CT scan may detect and localize many pathological findings, some of them less specific and common to different pathologies, others more specific. One of the most common, but non-specific, is the presence of abdominal free fluid and the fat stranding that can be recognized in infectious, inflammatory, malignant, or traumatic conditions [24]. Another non-specific finding is bowel wall thinning or thickening that may be the result of ischemic, infectious, or inflammatory etiologies [1, 25–28].

CT scan can accurately examine all the abdominal parenchymatous organs and the bowel, recognizing all signs of bowel obstruction and perforation [1]. Using intravenous contrast medium, it is possible to obtain an accurate and detailed study of the parenchymatous organs, looking for several different pathologies, and of the bowel wall vascularization, being able to recognize and characterize signs related to arterial, venous, or non-occlusive mesenteric ischemia and their stages [25–34].

CT allows to precisely localize the bowel loops, making detailed diagnosis of hernias and volvulus; this possibility, together with the signs of inflammation and ischemia can give an accurate identification of the causes and the state of the pathologic bowel orienting the treatment [23, 35, 36].

CT can clearly recognize free air for which it is specific and sensitive, and it can also frequently identify the exact site of gastrointestinal perforation when present [37–40].

30.1.3.2 Pros and Cons

CT is overall more sensitive and accurate than plain radiograph; it requires short time and minimal cooperation from the patient, and it can detect and localize many different pathologies. Furthermore, it can suggest alternative diagnoses if the suspected clinical diagnosis is unconfirmed, a major advantage considering the wide spectrum of diseases that can be responsible for acute abdominal pain [41]. On the other hand, it exposes the patient to a large dose of ionizing radiation [42]; however, in elderly patients, radiation has a lower chance to cause cancer than in younger and the literature promotes an early, liberal use of CT imaging due to its high panoramicity and accuracy [43].

30.2 Role of Radiology in Patient Management

Especially in an elderly population, it is crucial to discriminate between non-surgical and surgical patients and, among them, to establish the best therapeutic approach Enhanced CT represents the best choice to address these crucial points. The main points that have to be considered for candidating patients to laparoscopic approach are the presence of cardiovascular diseases such as pulmonary embolism, extensive pulmonary emphysema, or the presence of significant pleural effusion impairing respiration.

Furthermore, specific conditions regarding the surgical access need to be examined as the presence of abdominal wall hernias or abdominal wall adhesions from previous surgery.

Typical causes of abdominal pain/acute abdomen in the elderly include acute cholecystitis, incarcerated hernias, bowel obstruction, and appendicitis [44].

30.2.1 Acute Cholecystitis

US may constitute the first diagnostic step in suspected acute cholecystitis allowing to make the diagnosis and staging the grade of inflammation; however, CT in emergency setting gives more complete and detailed information to appropriately manage patients, especially in case of coexistent complications (Fig. 30.2) [45]. MRI may be considered as a second-level examination in cooperative patient when US does not provide a definitive diagnosis, or integrative to CT to better understand biliary anatomy or to better depict gallstones.

In acute cholecystitis, CT particularly helps in determining gallbladder wall perfusion or the presence of wall perforation with contiguous abscesses, coexistent signs of peritonitis, the relationships with adjacent organs, and exploring the whole biliary tree looking for migrated hyperdense gallstones that may change the therapeutic approach. In this last case, MRI may offer a further help in detecting and precisely localize migrated gallstones sending patients to endoscopic retrograde cholangiopancreatography or a combined endoscopic and surgical treatment, and to precisely assess the anatomy of the biliary system. CT can also make differential diagnosis with other conditions as cancer diseases.

In case of mild cholecystitis, early laparoscopic cholecystectomy may be indicated [45];

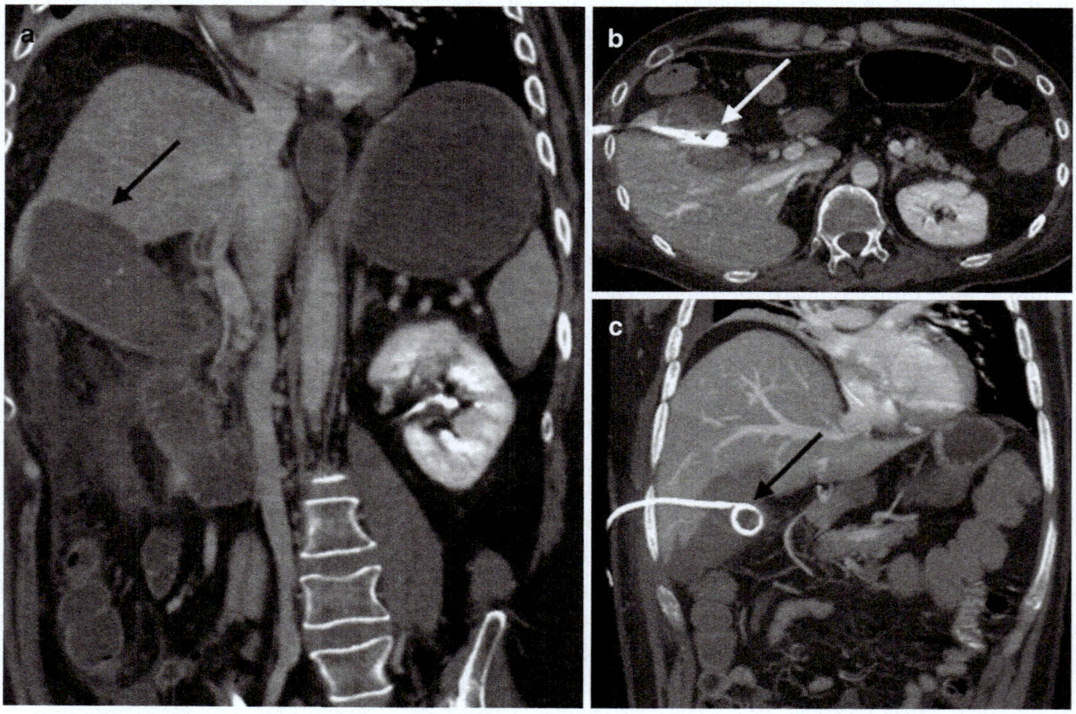

Fig. 30.2 Emergency CT examination of 74 patients with acute cholecystitis in coronal view (**a**). Note the distended gallbladder with irregular and inhomogeneous wall enhancement (**a**, arrow). As the patients could not undergo immediate surgery for the conditions, cholecystostomy was performed (**b**, axial plane; **c**, coronal plane, arrows)

otherwise, in case of complicated cholecystitis in high-risk patients, imaging may guide interventional approach consisting in cholecystostomy (Fig. 30.2) or in draining biliary or purulent collections. These procedures, usually performed US-guided, may help in stabilizing patients deferring the surgical approach.

30.2.2 Intestinal Diseases

30.2.2.1 Acute Appendicitis

In elderly patients, CT is preferred to US due to the fast execution time and panoramicity allowing detailed diagnosis. CT stages the appendix inflammation and allows the detection and characterization of related complications. Furthermore, several conditions may mimic acute appendicitis or can be associated with, so they need to be defined to properly assess patient and to ensure an appropriate treatment. The laparoscopic approach in elderly patients is still debated but seems to be safer than conventional open surgical approach due to its low invasiveness and faster recovery [46]. In this sense, CT helps precisely identifying appendix course, if there are adhesions, comorbidity, or specific complications requiring an open surgical approach as fistulization in adjacent anatomical structures. Furthermore, in case of abscess related to perforated appendicitis or to consequent surgical complications, CT is helpful in guiding percutaneous drainage of collections.

30.2.3 Diverticulitis

CT is the diagnostic method of choice for the diagnosis and staging of acute diverticulitis and its complications [47]. All different guidelines distinguish between simple and complicated diverticulitis; different stages imply a different management taking into consideration new imaging-guided therapeutic strategies, such as the positioning of percutaneous drainages.

In the early phase, imaging findings are represented by bowel wall thickening eventually associated with inflammatory involvement of the perivisceral fat; this stage can be followed by the appearance of bubbles of extraluminal air, perivisceral or distant abscesses, pneumoperitoneum, and free intraperitoneal fluid. Furthermore, septic and fistulizing complications can also manifest. CT may also detect, characterize, and quantify the active bleeding eventually present, sending the patient to the interventional radiology, endoscopist, surgeon, or to conservative therapy when indicated.

The treatment may be conservative up to the presence of abscesses of a maximum diameter of 4 cm, and if larger, a US- or CT-guided percutaneous drainage can be considered. Interventional radiology approach is also indicated in case of arterial active bleeding; indeed, a prompt endovascular embolization stabilizes the patient and allows to plan further treatment. If there are free air and fluid in the abdomen, the patient needs surgery; in these cases, the most appropriate surgical approach depends on the presence of comorbidity and on the technical surgical difficulties evaluable at CT.

The main imaging differential diagnosis of diverticulitis, especially in elderly patients, is with colon cancer (Fig. 30.3), and there are several imaging features that may help in this sense [48, 49]. Nevertheless, sometimes it is not possible to obtain a definite differential diagnosis; in these cases, endoscopic examination is needed to further characterize the abnormal findings.

30.2.4 Bowel Obstruction

Suspected bowel obstruction is a frequent diagnostic suspicion in elderly patients; it may occur due to functional or organic etiology [50]. This is the first differential diagnosis to make in case of bowel obstruction as the patient management is completely different. At abdominal radiograph, there are signs that can distinguish between these two different conditions (Fig. 30.4); US can give further elements as caliper of the bowel loops, bowel wall appearance, peristalsis, and if free fluid is present. However, CT helps in precisely identifying the etiology of bowel obstruction, orienting the following treatment. Indeed, in case of mechanical obstruction, it is important to define the level, the cause, and the severity, if the

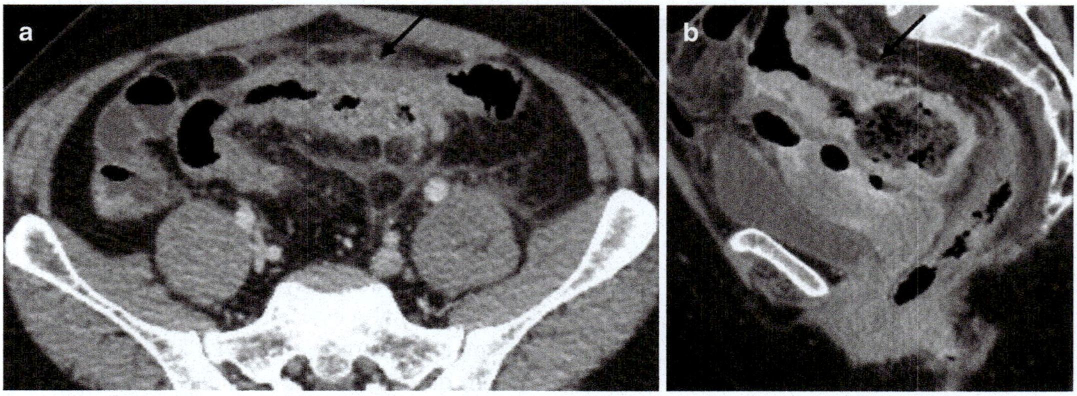

Fig. 30.3 CT in axial (**a**) and in sagittal views (**b**) of two different elderly patients presenting with acute pelvic pain, in the first case (**a**) related to acute diverticulitis (**a**, arrow) and in the second one (**b**) related to sigmoid cancer (**b**, arrow). Note the morphological differences between the different bowel wall thickenings and the fat stranding due to the peridiverticular inflammatory reaction (**a**), absent in the second case (**b**)

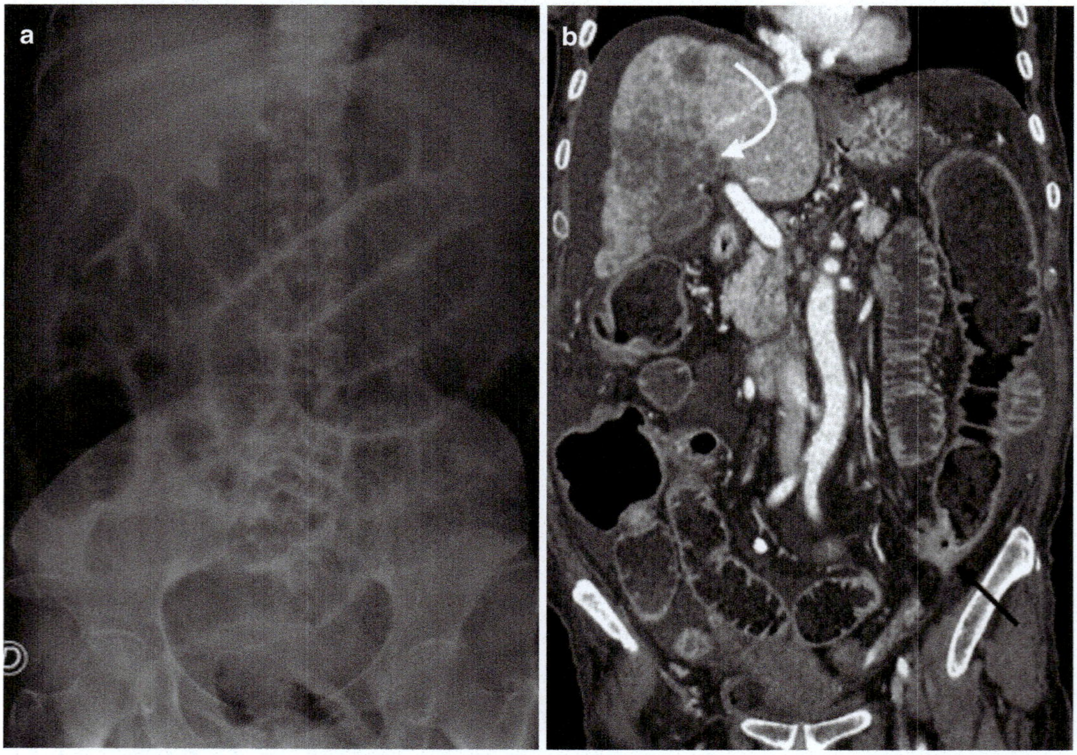

Fig. 30.4 Abdominal radiograph in AP projection (**a**) and CT in coronal view (**b**) of an 86-year-old male with intestinal obstruction. Note the small and large bowel overdistension due to mechanical ileus. CT (**b**) clarifies the etiology of obstruction due to colon cancer obstructing the lumen (**b**, straight arrow). Liver metastases are also present (**b**, curved arrow)

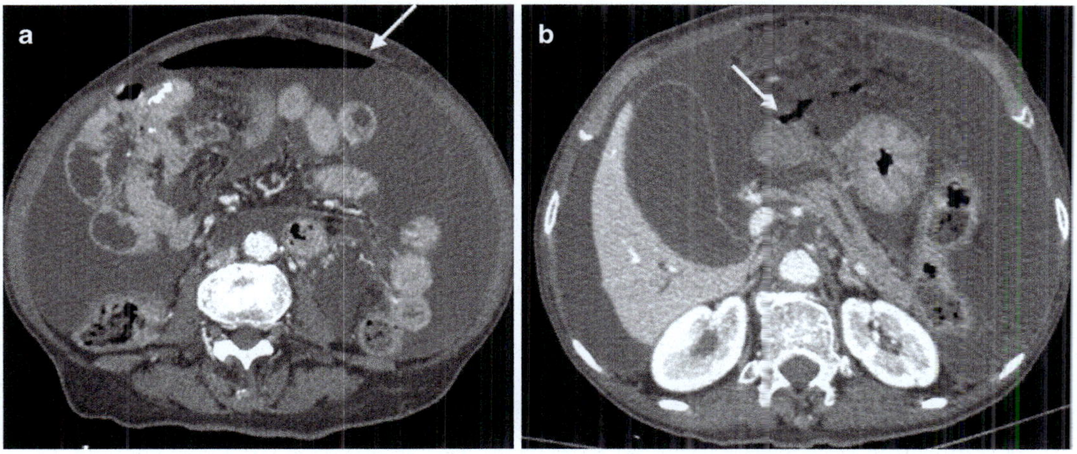

Fig. 30.5 CT of a 75-year-old male with acute abdomen. Note the pneumoperitoneum (**a**, arrow), due to gastric wall perforation (**b**, arrow)

obstruction is simple or with "closed loop" and if signs of ischemia or perforation are present. The detailed description of the patient status achieved by CT establishes the surgical emergency and approach deciding between a laparoscopic approach and open surgery (Figs. 30.4 and 30.5); in some cases, a temporary conservative approach can be also attempted [50].

30.2.5 Alimentary Tract Perforations

CT represents the best choice to make the diagnosis of alimentary tract perforations, excluding different diagnoses [50]. CT diagnosis can be so detailed that allows to make also prognostic evaluation [50]. The diagnosis of gastrointestinal perforation is based on direct CT findings as the presence of extraluminal air and discontinuity of the bowel wall (Fig. 30.4), and on indirect CT findings as bowel wall thickening, abnormal bowel wall enhancement, abscesses, and inflammatory mass or free fluid collection in the surrounding soft tissues adjacent to the bowel [50]. CT is highly sensitive for the detection of extraluminal free air such as small free air bubbles, pneumoperitoneum, and/or retropneumoperitoneum, in contrast to the low sensitivity of plain radiograph. Furthermore, the distribution of extraluminal free air suggests perforation location, planning a more specific surgical treatment. Sometimes, the administration of oral contrast medium can help to precisely detect the site of perforation; however, its adoption in emergency setting is controversial due to abdominal conditions that can impair its progression [50].

Five Things You Should Know About Imaging and Interventional Radiology in Emergency Abdominal Surgery in the Elderly

- CT with intravenous contrast medium is the primary imaging technique for elderly patients with acute abdomen.
- In acute abdominal pain, especially located in the right upper quadrant, US may be adopted as first imaging examination.
- Abdominal radiograph may be used as first-line imaging evaluation, usually associated with abdominal US, in patients with abdominal pain suspected for bowel obstruction or perforation, mainly to establish the priority to send patients to CT.
- CT allows a wide and complete depiction and differential diagnosis among the different causes of acute abdominal pain/acute abdomen orienting the following surgical, interventional, or conservative treatment.
- MRI may have a role in cooperative elderly patients with suspected biliary causes of acute abdominal pain.

References

1. Stoker J, van Randen A, Laméris W, et al. Imaging patients with acute abdominal pain. Radiology. 2009;253(1):31–46. https://doi.org/10.1148/radiol.2531090302.
2. Gupta H, Dupuy DE. Advances in imaging of the acute abdomen. Surg Clin North Am. 1997;77(6):1245–63. https://doi.org/10.1016/s0039-6109(05)70616-2.
3. Romano L, Pinto A, editors. Imaging of alimentary tract perforation. Springer; 2015.
4. Pinto A, Miele V, Schillirò ML, et al. Spectrum of signs of pneumoperitoneum. Semin Ultrasound CT MR. 2016;37(1):3–9. https://doi.org/10.1053/j.sult.2015.10.008.
5. James B, Kelly B. The abdominal radiograph. Ulster Med J. 2013;82(3):179–87.
6. Somma F, Faggian A, Serra N, et al. Bowel intussusceptions in adults: the role of imaging. Radiol Med. 2015;120(1):105–17.
7. Di Mizio R, Di Mizio V, Della Marra R, et al. Chapter 5. Radiological correlations. In: Di Mizio R, Scaglione, editors. Small-bowel obstruction CT features with plain film and US correlations. Springer; 2007. pp. 75–111.
8. Gangadhar K, Kielar A, Dighe MK, et al. Multimodality approach for imaging of non-traumatic acute abdominal emergencies. Abdom Radiol (NY). 2016;41(1):136–48. https://doi.org/10.1007/s00261-015-0586-6.
9. Grassi R, Di Mizio R, Pinto A, et al. Serial plain abdominal film findings in the assessment of acute abdomen: spastic ileus, hypotonic ileus, mechanical ileus and paralytic ileus. Radiol Med. 2004;108(1–2):56–70.
10. Iacobellis F, Laccetti E, Romano F, et al.: Imaging of bowel obstruction and bowel perforation. In: Cova A, editor. Pain imaging—a clinical-radiological approach to pain diagnosis. Springer; 2017.
11. Aras MH, Miloglu O, Barutcugil C, et al. Comparison of the sensitivity for detecting foreign bodies among conventional plain radiography, computed tomography and ultrasonography. Dentomaxillofac Radiol. 2010;39(2):72–8.
12. Grassi R, Faggian A, Somma F, et al. Application of imaging guidelines in patients with foreign body ingestion or inhalation: literature review. Semin Ultrasound CT MR. 2015;36(1):48–56. https://doi.org/10.1053/j.sult.2014.10.004.
13. Pinto A, Muzj C, Stavolo C, et al. Pictorial essay: foreign body of the gastrointestinal tract in emergency radiology. Radiol Med. 2004;107(3):145–52.
14. Nguyen LK, Wong DD, Fatovich DM, et al. Low-dose computed tomography versus plain abdominal radiography in the investigation of an acute abdomen. ANZ J Surg. 2012;82(1–2):36–41. https://doi.org/10.1111/j.1445-2197.2010.05632.x.
15. Nicola R, Dogra V. Ultrasound: the triage tool in the emergency department: using ultrasound first. Br J Radiol. 2016;89(1061):20150790. https://doi.org/10.1259/bjr.20150790.
16. Mazzei MA, Guerrini S, Cioffi Squitieri N, et al. The role of US examination in the management of acute abdomen. Crit Ultrasound J. 2013;5 Suppl 1(Suppl 1):S6. https://doi.org/10.1186/2036-7902-5-S1-S6.
17. Amadar DA, Jacobson JA, Morag Y, et al. Characteristic locations of inguinal region and anterior abdominal wall hernias: sonographic appearances and identification of clinical pitfalls. AJR Am J Roentgenol. 2007;188(5):1356–64. https://doi.org/10.2214/AJR.06.0638.
18. Erkek A, Yılmaz Aydın Y, Çiftçi H, et al. Significance of intra-abdominal free fluid detected in ultrasonography in the clinical assessment and outcomes of adult patients presenting to the emergency department due to abdominal pain. Cureus. 2019;11(10):e5948. https://doi.org/10.7759/cureus.5948.
19. Chawla A, Bosco JI, Lim TC, et al. Imaging of acute cholecystitis and cholecystitis-associated complications in the emergency setting. Singapore Med J. 2015;56(8):438–43; quiz 444. https://doi.org/10.11622/smedj.2015120.
20. Puylaert JB. Ultrasonography of the acute abdomen: gastrointestinal conditions. Radiol Clin N Am. 2003;41(6):1227–42, vii. https://doi.org/10.1016/s0033-8389(03)00120-9.
21. Wildman-Tobriner B, Ehieli WL, Dixon AX, et al. Computed tomography of the acute abdomen. Appl Radiol. 2019;48(6):32–9.
22. Romano S, Romano L. Utilization patterns of multidetector computed tomography in elective and emergency conditions: indications, exposure risk, and diagnostic gain. Semin Ultrasound CT MR. 2010;31(1):53–6. https://doi.org/10.1053/j.sult.2009.10.002. PMID: 20102696.
23. Gore RM, Miller FH, Pereles FS, et al. Helical CT in the evaluation of the acute abdomen. AJR Am J Roentgenol. 2000;174(4):901–13. https://doi.org/10.2214/ajr.174.4.1740901.
24. Thornton E, Mendiratta-Lala M, Siewert B, et al. Patterns of fat stranding. AJR Am J Roentgenol. 2011;197(1):W1–14. https://doi.org/10.2214/AJR.10.4375.
25. Reginelli A, Genovese E, Cappabianca S, et al. Intestinal ischemia: US-CT findings correlations. Crit Ultrasound J. 2013;5 Suppl 1(Suppl 1):S7. https://doi.org/10.1186/2036-7902-5-S1-S7.
26. Reginelli A, Iacobellis F, Berritto D, et al. Mesenteric ischemia: the importance of differential diagnosis for the surgeon. BMC Surg. 2013;13 Suppl 2(Suppl 2):S51. https://doi.org/10.1186/1471-2482-13-S2-S51.
27. Iacobellis F, Berritto D, Fleischmann D, et al. CT findings in acute, subacute, and chronic ischemic colitis: suggestions for diagnosis. Biomed Res Int. 2014;2014:895248. https://doi.

org/10.1155/2014/895248. Epub 2014 Aug 27. PMID: 25247191; PMCID: PMC4163450.
28. Berritto D, Iacobellis F, Mazzei MA, et al. MDCT in ischaemic colitis: how to define the aetiology and acute, subacute and chronic phase of damage in the emergency setting. Br J Radiol. 2016;89(1061):20150821. https://doi.org/10.1259/bjr.20150821.
29. Wiesner W, Khurana B, Ji H, et al. CT of acute bowel ischemia. Radiology. 2003;226(3):635–50. https://doi.org/10.1148/radiol.2263011540.
30. Scaglione M, Grassi R, Pinto A, et al. Positive predictive value and negative predictive value of spiral CT in the diagnosis of closed loop obstruction complicated by intestinal ischemia. Radiol Med. 2004;107(1–2):69–77. English, Italian. PMID: 15031698.
31. Romano S, Romano L, Grassi R, et al. Multidetector row computed tomography findings from ischemia to infarction of the large bowel. Eur J Radiol. 2007;61(3):433–41. https://doi.org/10.1016/j.ejrad.2006.11.002.
32. Woodhams R, Nishimaki H, Fujii K, et al. Usefulness of multidetector-row CT (MDCT) for the diagnosis of non-occlusive mesenteric ischemia (NOMI): assessment of morphology and diameter of the superior mesenteric artery (SMA) on multi-planar reconstructed (MPR) images. Eur J Radiol. 2010;76(1):96–102. https://doi.org/10.1016/j.ejrad.2009.05.012.
33. Bradbury MS, Kavanagh PV, Bechtold RE, et al. Mesenteric venous thrombosis: diagnosis and noninvasive imaging. Radiographics. 2002;22(3):527–41. https://doi.org/10.1148/radiographics.22.3.g02ma10527.
34. Lassandro F, Scaglione M, Rossi G, et al. Portomesenteric vein gas: diagnostic and prognostic value. Emerg Radiol. 2002;9(2):96–9. https://doi.org/10.1007/s10140-002-0206-y.
35. Vandendries C, Jullès MC, Boulay-Coletta I, et al. Diagnosis of colonic volvulus: findings on multidetector CT with three-dimensional reconstructions. Br J Radiol. 2010;83(995):983–90. https://doi.org/10.1259/bjr/35714052.
36. Reginelli A, Pezzullo MG, Scaglione M, et al. Gastrointestinal disorders in elderly patients. Radiol Clin N Am. 2008;46(4):755–71, vi. https://doi.org/10.1016/j.rcl.2008.04.013.
37. Solis CV, Chang Y, De Moya MA, et al. Free air on plain film: do we need a computed tomography too? J Emerg Trauma Shock. 2014;7(1):3–8. https://doi.org/10.4103/0974-2700.125631.
38. Saturnino PP, Pinto A, Liguori C, et al. Role of multidetector computed tomography in the diagnosis of colorectal perforations. Semin Ultrasound CT MR. 2016;37(1):49–53. https://doi.org/10.1053/j.sult.2015.10.007.
39. Pinto A, Scaglione M, Giovine S, et al. Comparison between the site of multislice CT signs of gastrointestinal perforation and the site of perforation detected at surgery in forty perforated patients. Radiol Med. 2004;108(3):208–17.
40. Grassi R, Romano S, Pinto A, et al. Gastro-duodenal perforations: conventional plain film, US and CT findings in 166 consecutive patients. Eur J Radiol. 2004;50(1):30–6. https://doi.org/10.1016/j.ejrad.2003.11.012.
41. Leschka S, Alkadhi H, Wildermuth S, et al. Multi-detector computed tomography of acute abdomen. Eur Radiol. 2005;15(12):2435–47. https://doi.org/10.1007/s00330-005-2897-4.
42. Cartwright SL, Knudson MP. Diagnostic imaging of acute abdominal pain in adults. Am Fam Physician. 2015;91(7):452–9.
43. Gardner CS, Jaffe TA, Nelson RC. Impact of CT in elderly patients presenting to the emergency department with acute abdominal pain. Abdom Imaging. 2015;40(7):2877–82. https://doi.org/10.1007/s00261-015-0419-7
44. Costa G, Massa G, ERASO (Elderly Risk Assessment for Surgical Outcome) Collaborative Study Group. Frailty and emergency surgery in the elderly protocol of a prospective, multicenter study in Italy for evaluating perioperative outcome (The FRAILESEL Study). Updates Surg. 2018;70(1):97–104 https://doi.org/10.1007/s13304-018-0511-y. Epub 2018 Jan 30. PMID: 29383680.
45. Yokoe M, Hata J, Takada T, et al. Tokyo guidelines 2018: diagnostic criteria and severity grading of acute cholecystitis (with videos). J Hepatobiliary Pancreat Sci. 2018;25(1):41–54. https://doi.org/10.1002/jhbp.515.
46. Wang D, Dong T, Shao Y, et al. Laparoscopy versus open appendectomy for elderly patients, a meta-analysis and systematic review. BMC Surg. 2019;19(1):54. https://doi.org/10.1186/s12893-019-0515-7
47. Sessa B, Galluzzo M, Ianniello S, et al. Acute perforated diverticulitis: assessment with multidetector computed tomography. Semin Ultrasound CT MR. 2016;37(1):37–48. https://doi.org/10.1053/j.sult.2015.10.003.
48. Ripollés T, Martínez-Pérez MJ, Gómez Valencia DP, et al. Sigmoid stenosis caused by diverticulitis vs. carcinoma: usefulness of sonographic features for their differentiation in the emergency setting. Abdom Imaging. 2015;40(7):2219–31.
49. Lips LM, Cremers PT, Pickhardt PJ, et al. Sigmoid cancer versus chronic diverticular disease: differentiating features at CT colonography. Radiology. 2015;275(1):127–35.
50. Iacobellis F, Laccetti E, Romano F, et al. Imaging of bowel obstruction and bowel perforation. In: Cova M, Stacul F, editors. Pain imaging. Cham: Springer; 2019. https://doi.org/10.1007/978-3-319-99822-0_17.

31 Anesthesia and Emergency Laparoscopy in the Elderly Patient

Concezione Tommasino

The care of elderly patients, undergoing emergency laparoscopy, requires good team-working with the purpose to improve all perioperative period qualities (Fig. 31.1). Implementing a multimodal and multidisciplinary pathway decreases hospital length of stay (LOS), loss of independence, and 30-day readmission rates for frail geriatric patients undergoing emergency surgery [1].

31.1 Physiology Considerations in the Elderly Patient

The physiological changes occurring with aging, especially when combined with coexisting diseases, create a very complex condition and have anesthetic implications [2] (Table 31.1).

31.2 Laparoscopy and Organ and System Modification

Laparoscopy in the geriatric population is feasible and safe [3]; however, positioning and pneumoperitoneum effects are cumulative, can induce pathophysiological changes (Tables 31.2 and 31.3), and increase perioperative complications.

C. Tommasino (✉)
Anesthesia and Intensive Care, San Paolo Hospital, University of Milan, Milan, Italy
e-mail: concezione.tommasino@unimi.it

In elderly patients undergoing laparoscopy surgery, the recent Italian intersociety consensus recommends the following [4]:

- Avoiding exaggerated or prolonged Trendelenburg or anti-Trendelenburg positions
- Avoiding unjustified prolongation of surgical times
- Using the lowest possible intraabdominal pressure (IAP), to minimize cardiovascular and respiratory effects
- Administering deep neuromuscular blockade, to allow low working pressures

31.3 Preoperative Care

Preoperative evaluation should include patient/caregiver interview and review of the available medical records (medical history, allergies, medication, and habitual level of function (METs)); direct physical examination (airway, lungs, and heart); ordering/reviewing pertinent tests and consultations, as necessary for anesthesia care (Table 31.4); together with the surgeon, goals of care discussion (quality of life, unnecessary/non-beneficial treatment) with both patient's next-of-kin and caregivers. Frailty assessment indicates when anesthesia tailoring becomes mandatory [2, 4], and in emergency cases the deficit accumulation frailty index can be appropriate, as it is calculated on the number of deficits the patient

F. Agresta et al. (eds.), *Emergency laparoscopic surgery in the elderly and frail patient*,
https://doi.org/10.1007/978-3-030-79990-8_31

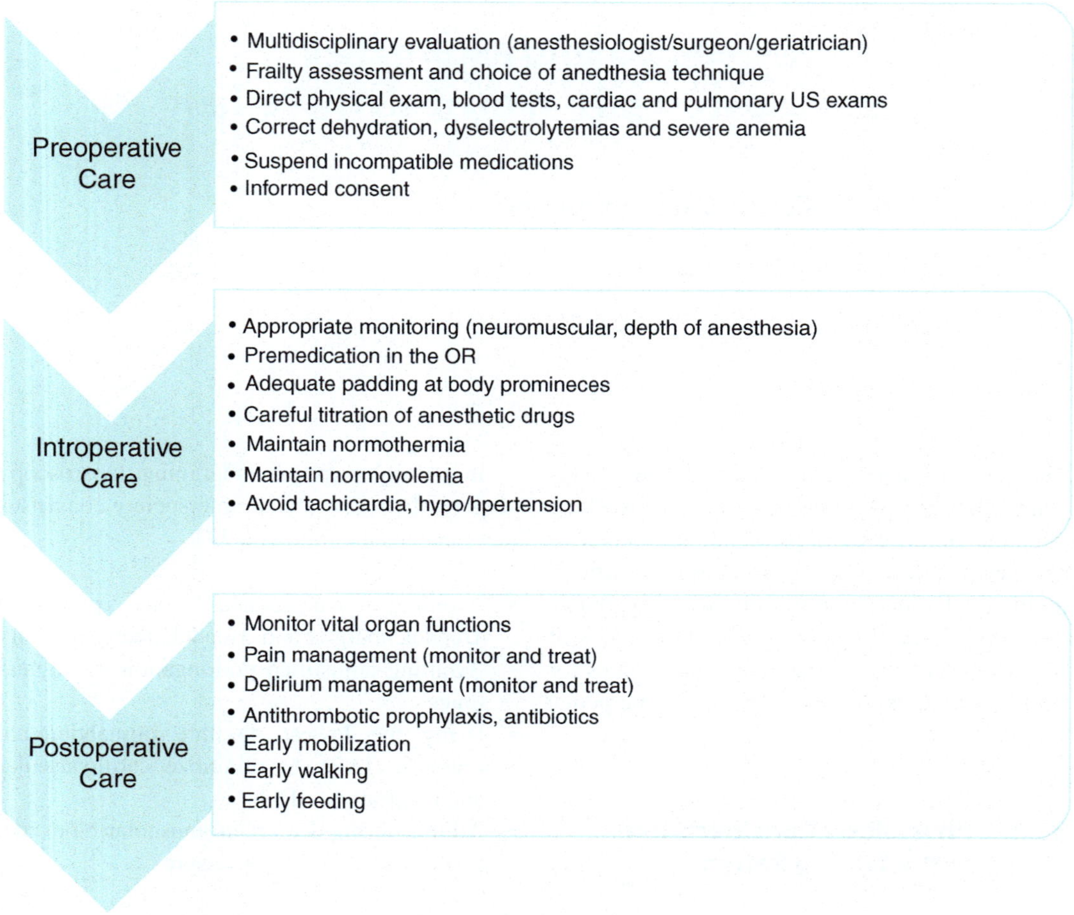

Fig. 31.1 Perioperative care for laparoscopic surgery in elderly patients. This is not an exhaustive list and highlights the most important targets for perioperative anesthesia care of the elderly patient undergoing laparoscopic emergency procedures. *OR* operating room, *US* ultrasound

presents and can be based on clinical notes, without physical performance-based measures [4, 5]. Frailty assessment improves the information anesthesiologists and surgeons will provide to the patient and/or caregivers, avoids futile treatments, and enhances the informed consent [6]. Polypharmacy is a major issue in the elderly, and medications are omitted/optimized which may be harmful [4]. In emergency, there is limited time for preoperative consultations or rehabilitation; however, correction of anemia, water and electrolyte disturbances, glycemic control, and thromboprophylaxis are possible even in emergency cases [7, 8]. Although cardiac evaluation may not change the course of the intervention, preoperative-focused echocardiography by the anesthesiologist does not delay surgery and affects diagnosis and management [9].

31.4 Intraoperative Care

Whether anesthetic technique has a significant impact on outcome in elderly is unclear, the choice between regional (RA) or general anesthesia (GA) is debated. Anesthesia technique will depend on both surgical requirements and patient comorbidities, and the major efforts should be to avoid perioperative tachycardia, hypo/hypertension, anemia, and volume derangement.

Table 31.1 Geriatric physiology and anesthetic implications

	Change with normal aging	Anesthetic implications
Cardiovascular system	• Decreased sympathetic tone • Decreased venous compliance and preload • Impaired baroreceptor response • Cardiac diastolic dysfunction	• Labile blood pressure • Sensitivity to hypotension and volume overload • Cardiac function decline with inadequate cardiac filling
Pulmonary system	• Increased pulmonary arterial pressure • Decreased response to hypoxia and hypercarbia • Decreased muscle mass and lung elasticity • Decreased cough reflex and esophageal motility	• Raised PAO_2–PaO_2 gradient • Sensitivity to hypoxia and hypercarbia • Increased dead space ventilation and work of breathing • Sensitivity to residual anesthetic effects • Aspiration risk
Gastrointestinal tract	• Reduced blood flow	• Risk of opioid-related gut mobility disturbance
Nervous system	• Decreased neurotransmitters • Decreased receptor density and increased receptor affinity	• Increased risk of postoperative cognitive dysfunction • Increased sensitivity to drugs' effect
Endocrine system	• Impaired glucose tolerance	• Increased intraoperative hyperglycemia
Hepatic/renal system	• Altered drug metabolism	• Decreased drug clearance
Hepatic metabolism	• Decreased hepatic blood flow • Reduced liver mass and functioning cells • Decreased cytochrome P450 system activity	• Reduced first-pass metabolism • Oxidative reaction (phase 1 metabolism) may be reduced with prolonged drug half-life • Conjugation (phase 2 metabolism) usually preserved • Difficult to predict precise individual effects
Renal excretion	• Reduced renal blood flow • Reduced glomerular filtration • Reduced tubular secretion	• Reduced excretion of drugs and metabolites → accumulation and prolonged effects
Body composition	• Decreased muscle mass • Increased body fat • Reduced total body water • Reduced plasma proteins	• Increased free fraction of drugs that bind plasmatic proteins • Lipophilic drugs → larger volume of distribution and longer duration of action • Hydrophilic drugs → increased serum concentration • Increased potential of drug–drug interaction
Thermoregulation	• Decreased muscle mass and vascular reactivity	• Increased risk of hypothermia

Table 31.2 Systemic effects of operative positioning

Positioning	Systemic effects
Trendelenburg, head-down position	• Increased venous return • Congestive heart failure • Cyanosis and edema of the face and the neck • Increased intracranial pressure (extreme head-down position) • Increased ocular pressure (extreme head-down position)
Reverse Trendelenburg, head-up position	• Reduced venous return • Reduced cardiac output • Hypotension
Lithotomy, legs up position	• Blood from legs to central body compartment • Increased preload
Lateral decubitus	• Inferior vena cava compression • Decreased venous return • Hypotension

Table 31.3 Physiologic effects due to pneumoperitoneum and positioning: What to do

			To do or not to do
CO_2 pneumoperitoneum	Hypercarbia	– Acidosis (>with pre-existing lung disease) – Cardiac arrhythmias	Progressive increase of minute ventilation
	Hypothermia	Core temperature can drop 0.3 °C for every 50 liters of instilled CO2	Normothermia • room T 22–24 °C • forced-air warming devices set to 38 °C • reduce operation time
Cardiocirculatory effects	Increased mean arterial pressure Increased systemic vascular resistance Increased central venous pressure Decreased cardiac output Decreased stroke volume	Decreased cardiac output may persist in older patients with pre-existing cardiac disease	Lowest possible inflation pressure • IAP: 8–10 mm Hg • adequate muscle relaxation
Pulmonary effects	Increased peak airway pressure Increased pulmonary vascular resistance Decreased functional residual capacity Decreased lung compliance		Appropriate PEEP to corresponding IAP • low tidal volume (6–8 mL/kg/bw) • PEEP (5–10 cm H_2O)
Neurologic effects	Hypercapnia Head-down position Elevated IAP	Increased intracranial pressure	No laparoscopy in patients with brain lesion or shunt
Splanchnic vasculature	Reduced splanchnic blood flow	Transient hepatocellular injury	Reduce IAP
Gastroesophageal reflux	Increased risk of reflux	Aspiration during surgery (>Trendelenburg position)	Maintenance of adequate endotracheal tube cuff pressure
Renal	Decreased blood flow Decreased glomerular filtration rate	Decreased urine output	Maintain adequate hydration Avoid hypovolemia and/or hypotension

IAP intraabdominal pressure, *PEEP* positive end-expiratory pressure

31.5 Anesthetic Technique

GA is thought to be the best choice for emergency laparoscopy: GA provides a secure airway, enables control of minute ventilation and proper handling of the CO_2 absorption, and facilitates muscle relaxation to optimize the surgical view, reducing the need for high IAP [10]. RA has been applied successfully in elective laparoscopy; however, operative positions are uncomfortable for the awake elderly patients, and when RA is combined with sedation, respiratory depression, and hypercapnia can be expected. GA may avoid the discomfort of intraoperative shoulder pain and is preferred for extensive procedures.

31.5.1 Premedication

Drug effect can be unpredictable, and elderly should be premedicated when monitored and supervised. Benzodiazepines may be questionable regarding risk–benefit ratio; however, midazolam in age-adjusted dosage (0.01–0.02 mg/kg iv) alleviates anxiety and nervousness and does not compromise cardiorespiratory function [11]. This represents the personal author approach, and

Table 31.4 Clinical examination and preoperative tests in emergency cases

System	Features of interest	Preoperative test
General	Nutritional state; skin and mucous membranes condition (anemia, hydration, perfusion); body temperature	Hemoglobin/hematocrit Type and Screen (blood loss) Na, K Glucose
Cardiovascular	Blood pressure, peripheral pulse (rate, rhythm, volume); jugular vein (volume, pulsation); heart sounds; carotid bruits; dependent edema Implantable defibrillators or pacemakers (indication, model, and location of the device)	ECG Coagulation studies (>patients on anticoagulant) Cardiac ultrasound exam
Respiratory	Pulmonary auscultation; cyanosis; dyspnea	Chest X-ray; pulmonary ultrasound exam (COPD, respiratory infection)
Airway and ventilation	Mouth opening; neck size and movement; dentition; beard; OSAS	Tracheal intubation screening tests (El-Ganzouri Risk Index)
Renal	Diuresis, dialysis	Creatinine, BUN, calculated GFR
Nervous	Peripheral and central dysfunction	GCS

COPD Chronic Obstructive Pulmonary Disease, *BUN* Blood Urea Nitrogen, *GRF* Glomerular Filtration Rate, *GCS* Glasgow Coma Scale, *OSAS* Obstructive Sleep Apnea Syndrome

the ongoing study [12] will give the final answer on the effects of midazolam on functional and cognitive recovery, postoperative delirium (POD), health-related quality of life, and mortality.

31.5.2 Positioning on the Operating Table

Positioning should be adjusted according to the patient's problems, considering skin (atrophy, injury) and musculoskeletal system (bone deformities, joint stiffness, presence of prostheses), taking care to place adequate padding at bony prominences [4].

31.5.3 Intraoperative Monitoring

Electrocardiogram (ECG), heart rate (HR), blood pressure (BP), airway pressures, O_2 saturation (SpO_2), end-tidal carbon dioxide (CO_2), neuromuscular blockade (NMB), and body temperature (T, patient's core T can drop 0.3 °C for every 50 L of instilled CO_2) need always to be monitored. During laparoscopy, central venous pressure does not reflect the patients' filling status; non-invasive cardiac monitoring systems are useful, and invasive monitoring should be considered in very high-risk patients. Depth of anesthesia monitoring (e.g., bispectral index monitoring (BIS)) is recommended to tailor hypnotic dose and avoid deep level of anesthesia, an independent risk factor for POD [13]. Furthermore, combination of low BP and low BIS (deep anesthesia) increases 90-day mortality [14].

31.6 General Anesthesia

Aging affects pharmacokinetics and pharmacodynamics. Old patients are routinely given anesthetic drugs greater-than-recommended doses for their age, and titration is mandatory [2] (Table 31.5), to avoid excessive cerebral nervous system (CNS) depression and cardiovascular side effects, especially hypotension which is independently associated with adverse outcome.

31.6.1 Hypnotic Drugs and Anesthesia Induction

Propofol is a good choice because of its rapid recovery time and few side effects (Table 31.5) [2, 15]. Age-adjusted induction dose with 1.0–1.5 mg/kg produces rapid hypnosis (<1 min), lasting 5–10 min; dose is reduced to 0.5–1.0 mg/kg if administered with any other agent,

Table 31.5 Dose adjustments for anesthetic drugs in elderly patients

Drug	Adjusted dosage for elderly patients
Midazolam	0.01–0.02 mg/kg premedication dose 0.05–0.15 mg/kg induction dose in premedicated patient 20% reduction in patients >55 years 75% reduction in patients >90 years
Propofol	Bolus: 1.0–1.5 mg/kg Infusion: 70–175 mcg/kg/min
Sevoflurane	MAC is reduced by 6.7% per decade of increasing age MAC 60 years ≅ 1.6% MAC 70 years ≅ 1.5% MAC 80 years ≅ 1.4% MAC 90 years ≅ 1.3%
Desflurane	MAC is reduced by 6.7% per decade of increasing age MAC 60 years ≅ 5.8% MAC 70 years ≅ 5.5% MAC 80 years ≅ 5.1% MAC 90 years ≅ 4.8%
Morphine	Intraoperative: 0.05–0.1 mg/kg Acute postoperative analgesia: 1–2 mg boluses titrated to effect
Fentanyl	0.5–1 mcg/kg for short-term analgesia
Remifentanil	Bolus: 0.25–0.5 mcg/kg Infusion: 0.01–0.06 mcg/kg/min
Dexmedetomidine	Infusion: 0.5 mcg/kg/h

MAC Minimum Alveolar Concentration

narcotics or benzodiazepines, as anesthetic depth is synergistically increased, and further reduced for patients of >70 years. Patients of >80 years exhibit less cognitive impairment with propofol as compared to other hypnotics. GA induction with midazolam is feasible, and the dose should be 0.1–0.15 mg/kg, with reduction to <0.1 mg/kg if synergistic drugs, such as opioids, are used.

31.6.2 Opioid Analgesics

Opioids provide the analgesic component of anesthesia, especially during TIVA. The old brain is sensitive to opioids, and frail patients are more sensitive to their respiratory depressant effects, and fentanyl, sufentanil, and alfentanil doses need to be decreased by 50% [15] (Table 31.5). Remifentanil has a very short context-sensitive half-time, is not influenced by hepatic or renal failure, and is independent of infusion duration. In the elderly, because of age-dependent reduction of both central compartment volume and clearance, a smaller remifentanil dose infusion is required (Table 31.5). Morphine is metabolized mainly in the liver (>90%); old patients, especially with renal insufficiency, have reduced the elimination of its metabolites, which explains the enhanced analgesia and the risk of adverse events [16].

31.6.3 Dexmedetomidine

Dexmedetomidine (Dex) is a highly selective alfa2 adrenoceptor agonist that provides anxiolysis, sedation, modest analgesia with minimal respiratory depression, opioid-sparing properties, and decreases anesthetic requirements. In ICU patients, Dex has been reported to reduce delirium, effect debated during surgical procedures [17].

31.6.4 Neuromuscular Blocking Agents

Profound muscle paralysis improves abdominal distension and is an important component for laparoscopy. Vecuronium and rocuronium, undergoing organ-dependent elimination, have prolonged duration, and appropriate changes must be made in dosing and intervals [18].

Atracurium and cisatracurium, eliminated by Hoffman degradation, have prolonged onset time but normal clinical duration in the elderly [18]. There is no alteration with succinylcholine, while mivacurium effect is prolonged, probably due to the decreased plasma acetylcholinesterase [18]. NMB monitoring is strongly advised, and pharmacological reversal must be a standard procedure in the elderly, to avoid pulmonary complications because of muscle weakness (airway obstruction, hypoxemia, atelectasis, pneumonia, acute respiratory failure) [19]. Old patients require more time to recover from NMB following reversal with anticholinesterase agents. Even with sugammadex, time to recovery is prolonged, and if immediate reversal is required, a greater dose of sugammadex may be considered [20].

31.7 Risk of Aspiration and Rapid Sequence Induction

Pulmonary aspiration risk (reduced protective airway reflexes from muscular/neural degenerative changes) is increased in intestinal obstruction, and gastric emptying is mandatory before anesthesia. To counterbalance this risk, rapid sequence induction is used, and tracheal intubation is performed with 1.0 mg/kg succinylcholine or 1.0–1.2 mg/kg rocuronium.

31.8 Intraoperative Fluid Management

Fluid strategy should aim to a near-zero balance in normovolemic patients at the beginning of surgery, and a slight positive fluid balance may be allowed to protect renal function [21].

31.9 Regional Anesthesia Techniques

RA includes neuraxial blockade (spinal, epidural) and peripheral nerve blocks. Neuraxial blockade has been used in elective laparoscopy mainly in fit patients [22] and occasionally in high-risk patients [23]; its use in emergency surgical old patients has a different risk–benefit profile. Combined RA techniques and GA in laparoscopy are beneficial for postoperative analgesia, reducing systemic analgesic side effects, and several peripheral nerve blocks (transversus abdominis plane (TAP), subcostal TAP, paravertebral, inguinal block, etc.) have become increasingly popular for postoperative analgesia [24].

31.10 Postoperative Care

Postoperative care should include adequate monitoring of vital organ functions: continuous monitoring of SpO_2 and respiratory rate, HR, and rhythm (ECG); intermittent BP measurements and urinary output are obligatory, and nausea and vomiting, pain, and POD need to be evaluated and treated as necessary. After emergency laparotomy, intermediary 24 hours care in the postoperative care unit (PACU) improves patients' outcome and has been included in several pathway care bundles. Enhanced recovery after surgery (ERAS) has become the standard of care for colorectal operations, even in emergencies [25].

Our PriME recommendations include the following [4]:

- Optimal postoperative pain control
- Early mobilization and walking
- Early resumption of feeding
- Conservation of the sleep–wake rhythm
- Reducing use of nasogastric tube and bladder catheters
- Antithrombotic prophylaxis

31.10.1 Pain Management

Pain increases POD, cardiorespiratory complications, and failure to mobilize, and needs to be assessed with specific scales, in case patients lose their ability to communicate (e.g., PAINAD, NOPPAIN) [4]. Older adults are at increased risk with systemic analgesics, and efficient pain relief includes combination of regional analgesic techniques and drugs [24]. Paracetamol is safe and is considered first-line drug (<3 g/day in frail

Table 31.6 Prevention, screening, and treatment of postoperative delirium

POD	To do and not to do
Prevention	Tailor anesthesia treatment (type, drug, dosage) Avoid medications that promote POD (e.g., anticholinergic drugs) Avoid deep anesthesia (monitoring depth of anesthesia, e.g., avoid BIS <55) Avoid hypothermia Pain assessment and adequate treatment Provision of visual and auditory aids soon after awakening from anesthesia Avoid constipation or urinary retention
Screening	CAM (Confusion Assessment Method) or 4AT (4 'A's test) tests (5 postoperative days starting in RR)
Management	Non-pharmacological (reorientation, cognitive exercises, sleep optimization, early mobilization, adequate nutrition, and hydration) Pharmacological: limited treatment options (low-dose haloperidol)

BIS Bispectral Index, *POD* postoperative delirium, *RR* recovery room

patients). NSAIDs should be used at the lowest possible dose and for the shortest possible duration, with concomitant proton pump inhibitors, and monitoring for gastric and renal damage. Morphine should be administered cautiously, particularly in patients with poor renal or respiratory function and/or cognitive impairment [4].

Instillation and/or laparoscopic access sites of local anesthetics infiltration provide limited pain relief. Abdominal wall blocks are the main components of multimodal pain strategy, and epidural analgesia has lost its status as the gold standard, especially in the presence of anticoagulation [24]. A relatively new technique is continuous TAP blocks via catheters which provides continuous analgesia, improves gastrointestinal motility, and shortens LOS [26]. Since the catheter can be inserted only after surgery, this can prove useful when emergency does not allow preoperative regional or neuraxial analgesia.

31.10.2 Postoperative Delirium

A common complication of surgery, POD, is often underdiagnosed in elderly. POD presents as agitation (hyperactive) or withdrawal (hypoactive) and tends to fluctuate significantly. Its pathogenesis is not completely understood, is associated with poor outcome, and can anticipate the development of permanent cognitive disturbances.

Recently, the European Society of Anaesthesiology, an Italian intersociety consensus, and PriME have highlighted recommendations for the prevention, diagnosis, and treatment of POD in old patients (Table 31.6) [4, 27, 28].

31.11 Conclusions

Emergency laparoscopic surgery appears to be safe for the geriatric population, although the frail patient is at higher risk of postoperative morbidity and mortality. The implementation of collaborative bundles, specifically designed to improve the reliable delivery of evidence-based perioperative care, can improve the outcome of frail elderly patients. Good communication and teamwork, involving anesthesiologist, surgeon, and geriatrician, when available, are of paramount importance to optimize the perioperative care of the elderly patient undergoing emergency surgery, and a key part in *doing the right things in a reliable and timely fashion.*

Five Things You Should Know About Anesthesia and Emergency Laparoscopy in the Elderly Patient

- **Pre-optimization**: Correct physiological derangements (anemia, water and electrolyte disturbances, prompt treatment of sepsis, glycemic control)

- **Anesthesia**: Individualize and tailor the best anesthesia management (type, drug, dosage). Avoid deep level of anesthesia (depth of anesthesia monitor, e.g., BIS 55–60)
- **Pneumoperitoneum**: Use the lowest possible IAP (<12 mm Hg)
- **Delirium**: Prevention, recognition (CAM, 4AT), and treatment of postoperative delirium must be an objective of the multidisciplinary team
- **Pain**: Personalized prevention and treatment of postoperative pain are mandatory. Multimodal strategy (combination of locoregional analgesic techniques and drugs (short-acting opioids, NSAIDs, paracetamol in appropriate dosage and timing))

References

1. Engelhardt KE, Reuter Q, Liu J, et al. Frailty screening and a frailty pathway decrease length of stay, loss of independence, and 30-day readmission rates in frail geriatric trauma and emergency general surgery patients. J Trauma Acute Care Surg. 2018;85(1):167–73.
2. Tommasino C, Corcione A. Anesthesia for the elderly patient. In: Crucitti A, editor. Surgical management of elderly patients. Springer International Publishing; 2018. pp 9–29.
3. Brunt LM, Quasebarth MA, Dunnegan DL, et al. Outcomes analysis of laparoscopic cholecystectomy in the extremely elderly. Surg Endosc. 2001;15:700–5.
4. Aceto P, Antonelli Incalzi R, Bettelli G, et al. Perioperative management of Elderly patients (PriME): recommendations from an Italian intersociety consensus. Aging Clin Exp Res. 2020;32(9):1647–73.
5. Rockwood K, Mitnitski A. Frailty in relation to the accumulation of deficits. J Gerontol A Biol Sci Med Sci. 2007;62:722–7.
6. Søreide K, Desserud KF. Emergency surgery in the elderly: the balance between function, frailty, fatality and futility. Scand J Trauma Resusc Emerg Med. 2015;23:10.
7. Poulton T, Murray D. Pre-optimisation of patients undergoing emergency laparotomy: a review of best practice. Anaesthesia. 2019;74(Suppl 1):100–7.
8. Tommasino C. Fluids and electrolyte management. In: Bettelli G, editor. Perioperative care of the elderly. Clinical and organizational aspects. Cambridge University Press; 2018. pp. 137–143.
9. Canty DJ, Royse CF, Kilpatrick D, et al. The impact on cardiac diagnosis and mortality of focused transthoracic echocardiography in hip fracture surgery patients with increased risk of cardiac disease: a retrospective cohort study. Anaesthesia. 2012;67:1202–9.
10. Whalley DG, Berrigan MJ. Anesthesia for radical prostatectomy, cystectomy, nephrectomy, pheochromocytoma, and laparoscopic procedures. Anesthesiol Clin North Am. 2000;18:899–917.
11. Sun GC, Hsu MC, Chia YY, et al. Effects of age and gender on intravenous midazolam premedication: a randomized double-blind study. Br J Anaesth. 2008;101:632–9.
12. Kowark A, Rossaint R, Keszei AF, et al. Impact of PReOperative Midazolam on OuTcome of Elderly patients (I-PROMOTE): study protocol for a multicentre randomised controlled trial. Trials. 2019;20(1):430.
13. Fritz BA, Kalarickal PL, Maybrier HR, et al. Intraoperative electroencephalogram suppression predicts postoperative delirium. Anesth Analg. 2016;122:234–42.
14. McCormick PJ, Levin MA, Lin HM, et al. Effectiveness of an electronic alert for hypotension and low Bispectral index on 90-day postoperative mortality: a prospective, randomized trial. Anesthesiology. 2016;125:1113–20.
15. Shafer SL. The pharmacology of anesthetic drugs in elderly patients. Anesthesiol Clin North Am. 2000;18:1–29.
16. Lugo RA, Kern SE. Clinical pharmacokinetics of morphine. J Pain Palliat Care Pharmacother. 2002;16:5–18.
17. Hu J, Zhu M, Gao Z, et al. Dexmedetomidine for prevention of postoperative delirium in older adults undergoing oesophagectomy with total intravenous anaesthesia: a double-blind, randomised clinical trial. Eur J Anaesthesiol. 2021;38(Suppl 1):S9–S17. https://doi.org/10.1097/EJA.0000000000001382.
18. Cope TM, Hunter JM. Selecting neuromuscular-blocking drugs for elderly patients. Drugs Aging. 2003;20:125–40.
19. Bablekos GD, Michaelides SA, Analitis A, et al. Effects of laparoscopic cholecystectomy on lung function: a systematic review. World J Gastroenterol. 2014;20:17603–17.
20. Carron M, Bertoncello F, Ieppariello G. Profile of sugammadex for reversal of neuromuscular blockade in the elderly: current perspectives. Clin Interv Aging. 2017;13:13–24.
21. Myles PS, Bellomo R, Corcoran T, et al. Restrictive versus liberal fluid therapy for major abdominal surgery. N Engl J Med. 2018;378(24):2263–74.

22. Yuksek YN, Akat AZ, Gozalan U, et al. Laparoscopic cholecystectomy under spinal anesthesia. Am J Surg. 2008;195:533–6.
23. Bayrak M, Altıntas Y. Comparing laparoscopic cholecystectomy in patients with chronic obstructive pulmonary disease under spinal anesthesia and general anesthesia. BMC Surg. 2018;18:65.
24. Hemmerling TM. Pain management in abdominal surgery. Langenbecks Arch Surg. 2018;403:791–803.
25. Lohsiriwat V. Enhanced recovery after surgery for emergency colorectal surgery: are there any differences between intra-abdominal infection and other indications? J Visc Surg. 2019;156:489–96.
26. Xu YJ, Sun X, Jiang H, et al. Randomized clinical trial of continuous transversus abdominis plane block, epidural or patient-controlled analgesia for patients undergoing laparoscopic colorectal cancer surgery. Br J Surg. 2020;107:e133–41.
27. Aldecoa C, Bettelli G, Bilotta F, et al. European Society of Anaesthesiology evidence-based and consensus-based guideline on postoperative delirium. Eur J Anaesthesiol. 2017;34:192–214.
28. Bellelli G, Morandi A, Trabucchi M, et al. Italian intersociety consensus on prevention, diagnosis, and treatment of delirium in hospitalized older persons. Intern Emerg Med. 2018;13:113–21.

PONV and Pain Management

32

Roberta Monzani

32.1 PONV

The incidence of nausea and vomiting in the postoperative period is estimated to be 30% in the general surgical population and can rise to 80% in high-risk cohorts [1]. Postoperative nausea and vomiting (PONV) is also associated with a significantly longer stay in the post-anaesthesia care unit, unanticipated hospital admission and increased health care costs [2, 3]. One of the goals of the current guidelines is to understand how effective the treatment is in the cases of PONV and postdischarge nausea and vomiting with or without prophylaxis, that is, emergency scenarios [4].

In an evidence-based analysis, the authors claim that there are patient-specific risk factors for PONV in adults: female sex, a history of PONV and/or motion sickness, non-smoking status and younger age. Moreover, in a randomized trial, Leslie et al. point out that laparoscopic surgery (in particular, bariatric surgery, gynaecological surgery and general surgery, such as cholecystectomy), duration of anaesthesia with volatile anaesthetics and postoperative opioids, may be associated with an increased risk of PONV [5, 6]. The effect of volatile anaesthetics on PONV was shown to be dose-dependent, particularly 2–6 h after surgery. The use of opioids in the postoperative period increases the risk for PONV in a dose-dependent fashion, and the effect lasts as long as the drugs are taken in the postoperative period. The incidence of PONV is lower for opioid-free anaesthesia and total intravenous anaesthesia. With the choice of multimodal pain management, with opioid-free regional anaesthesia, perioperative administration of alpha$_2$ agonist and beta-blockers helps to reduce the incidence of PONV [7–9]. The administration of nitrous oxide analgesia can increase the risk of PONV if the duration of exposure is more than 1 h [10]. In contrast to planned surgery, in emergency situations, there is less time to prepare patients preoperatively; however, it is helpful to apply a risk score to reduce the rate of PONV at an institutional level and can be important to draw up protocols and standardize behaviours.

The Apfel-simplified risk score is based on four predictors [11], and the Koivuranta score includes the four Apfel risk predictors as well as length of surgery >60′ [12]. Age is not an independent risk factor for PONV, and there is a 10% decreasing risk for every decade of age in adults, starting at age 30. This could be related to a decreasing dose of anaesthetic agents administered as a result of decreased lean body mass, reduction in cardiac output and metabolism and reduction of brain neurons, all lead to

R. Monzani (✉)
Department of Anaesthesia and Intensive Care Units, Humanitas Research Hospital and Humanitas University, Milan, Italy
e-mail: roberta.monzani@humanitas.it

F. Agresta et al. (eds.), *Emergency laparoscopic surgery in the elderly and frail patient*,
https://doi.org/10.1007/978-3-030-79990-8_32

an altered pharmacokinetic and pharmacodynamic response [13].

In an emergency setting, when there is not sufficient time to prepare the elderly and frail patient for surgery, another goal is to reduce baseline risk for PONV. Select multimodal systemic analgesia to minimize the use of perioperative opioids, use regional anaesthesia when possible, choose propofol infusions as the primary anaesthetic, avoid volatile anaesthetics and ensure proper preoperative and intraoperative hydration. In addition, during laparoscopic surgery, it is necessary to administer a neuromuscular blockade and a reversal at the end of surgery to avoid postoperative residual curarization, and different meta-analyses show that the choice of sugammadex instead of neostigmine is supported by evidence [14–18].

To apply multimodal prophylaxis, we have different classes of drugs: 5-HT_3 receptor antagonists (ondansetron, dolasetron, granisetron, tropisetron, ramosetron, palonosetron), NK1 receptor antagonists (aprepitant, casopitant, rolapitant, vestipitant), corticosteroids (dexamethasone, methylprednisolone), antidopaminergics (amisulpride, droperidol, haloperidol, metoclopramide, perphenazine), antihistamines (dimenhydrinate, promethazine) and anticholinergics (scopolamine transdermal patch) [19–38]. Some drugs have significant side effects and do not have an food and drug administration (FDA) indication for PONV, so it is difficult to define the best timing of administration or indication based only on the type of surgery (i.e. orthopaedic surgery).

Metoclopramide should not be used in elderly and Parkinson's patients due to significant central nervous system (CNS) side effects such as dyskinesia, drowsiness and agitation. Scopolamine is highly associated with delirium and should be avoided in elderly patients. Prophylactic antiemetics should be used based on a risk score; thus, they are not recommended in elderly patients [39]. Gabapentin, when given preoperatively in patients undergoing abdominal surgery, reduces PONV [40] but was associated with respiratory depression in patients undergoing laparoscopic surgery [41]. When they are part of a multimodal analgesic approach, intraoperative use should be reduced, especially in elderly patients [42].

PONV prophylaxis can be obtained even with a nonpharmacologic approach: many trials confirm that stimulation of the pericardium 6 acupuncture point (PC6) significantly reduces the risk of nausea and vomiting and the need for rescue therapies [43].

The evidence supports the use of two or more antiemetics, but there is insufficient evidence to allow the clinician to select the most effective individual antiemetic, with the exception of choosing agents from a different pharmacologic class [44]. Nausea and vomiting may be driven by a variety of central and peripheral mechanisms, so the right combination of choice of drug, dose and timing has not yet been identified [45, 46].

In emergency laparoscopic surgery, if the patient did not receive PONV prophylaxis, 5-HT_3 receptor antagonists are the first choice for treating PONV: ondansetron 4 mg per os or iv and ramosetron 0.3 mg iv [47]. A combination of multiple antiemetics may be more effective in treating established PONV [48].

Unfortunately, adherence to PONV prophylaxis guidelines is still poor, with less than half of medium- to high-risk patients receiving the appropriate prophylaxis [49].

32.2 Pain Management

Frequently, the problem of PONV is related to pain management; elderly patients may be receiving chronic treatment with opioids (e.g. for arthrosis), and the intra-postoperative administration of more opioids can worsen the situation. Perioperative pain management should be tailored to the needs of the individual patient, taking into account the patient's age, medical and physical condition, level of fear/anxiety, whether the surgery is elective or emergency, and the type of surgical procedure. Inadequate treatment of postoperative acute pain leads to increased sympathetic activity, which brings tachycardia and hypertension; in elderly patients with coronary artery disease, the risk of myocardial infarction is increased. Regional blood flow can be depressed and may increase the risk of postoperative infection; moreover, fear and anxiety due to inadequate pain control can impair sleep and rehabilitation in the immediate postoperative period. Generally, patients with pain have shallow breathing that in the postoperative period can lead to hypoxemia, atelectasis and pneumonia [50]. Moreover, postoperative pain increases the risk of postoperative delirium, and only high levels of rest pain are associated with postoperative delirium. About opioids, there is insufficient evidence to assert which do not cause this symptom, except meperidine, which has an influence on brain cholinergic activity [51]. However, inadequate postsurgical acute pain management could facilitate the development of a chronic pain syndrome that can, especially in the elderly population, affect the quality of life [52]. Regional anaesthesia, including neuraxial techniques (spinal and epidural anaesthesia) and peripheral nerve blocks, can prevent chronic pain and is the best choice for pain control during and/or after surgery, improving pain relief and functional outcomes, and reducing the hospital stay for selected patients. Epidural analgesia can be employed postoperatively to obtain better pain control from large abdominal and thoracic incisions; the advantages over systemic narcotics include less sedation and improved respiratory mechanics. Absolute contraindications to neuraxial anaesthesia/analgesia, even more so in emergency cases, are anticoagulation and antiplatelet medication; other situations include sepsis, bacteraemia and hypovolemia.

In the CNS of elderly patients, dementia, memory loss and degenerative diseases are present at higher frequencies. Alterations in neurotransmitter levels and neuronal circuits cause pharmacodynamic changes that can result in increased sensitivity to some classes of drugs, for example midazolam and some opioids [53]. Therefore, modifications in pain perception result from age-related changes in the peripheral nervous system (PNS). Generally, elderly patients have increased pain thresholds, which contribute to delayed presentation in the emergency room (ER) in cases of painful conditions (i.e. peritonitis).

With regard to laparoscopic surgery, the significant advantages in elderly patients are more rapid recovery, less pain in the postoperative period and reduced fluid requirements [54]. For opioids, age-related increased sensitivity seems more tied to changes in the pharmacodynamics and sensitivity of the receptors as opposed to an alteration in the distribution or clearance of the medications [55]. In general, all initial opioid doses should be reduced in older patients [56], but in the case of morphine, the initial postoperative requirement is the same as in a younger patient, changing the maintenance doses that should be reduced [57]. However, patients who requested parenteral morphine for pain had four times the risk of myocardial ischaemia and tachyarrhythmias than those whose pain was well controlled with epidural analgesia [58]. Thoracic epidural analgesia significantly reduced the incidence of myocardial injury and ameliorated pain compared with parenteral analgesia after major abdominal surgery [59].

When a multimodal opioid-sparing pain approach is chosen, acetaminophen is frequently overlooked intra- and postoperatively but should be used with caution in older patients with liver dysfunction and matched with low doses of non steroidal anti inflammatory drugs (NSAID) [60], as this drug category has ceiling dose effects above which no further analgesia is obtained. In general, elderly patients are most appropriately treated with agents with short half-lives (ibuprofen); for patients with a history of dyspepsia, ulcer disease or bleeding diatheses, acetyl salicylic acid (ASA) and choline magnesium trisalicylate should be used if a traditional NSAID is indicated [61]. Many physicians in the ER are reluctant to prescribe any analgesia when a patient arrives with acute abdominal pain, due to the risk of impairment of diagnostic accuracy, but it is possible to affirm that opioids can also be used safely [62].

The attention to certain measures in laparoscopic surgical techniques can reduce postoperative pain and improve its management. Low pressure, saline lavage followed by suction, aspiration of pneumoperitoneum gas, mini-port technique and port site local anaesthetic infiltration preferably with long-acting agents and prior to incision are recommended [63, 64].

Good practice for acute perioperative pain management is a multimodal therapy to minimize the need for opioids, and it is suitable to select regional anaesthesia and administer NSAIDs and to choose acetaminophen before the induction of general anaesthesia when possible. In the case of locoregional analgesia, transversus abdominis plane blocks or other interfascial plane blocks are indicated, and local anaesthetic wound infiltration and postoperative patient-controlled analgesia using iv opioids are suggested [65, 66]. It is known that patients receiving emergency surgery have significantly higher pain severity than those hospitalized in the scheduled mode. These patients have a high likelihood of developing postoperative wound complications, such as superficial or deep wound infections that affect pain severity and can require wound drains [39, 67]. For frail elderly patients and those with cognitive impairment undergoing major complex abdominal surgery, epidural anaesthesia/analgesia is probably the best choice for pain management for good reporting of efficacy/side effects [68]. Importantly, one of the causes of acute confusion in surgical patients is stress resulting from pain, and improved pain management can prevent postoperative delirium [39, 69].

Elderly patients should receive tailored pain therapy, and a multimodal analgesic plan should be developed. Potentially inappropriate medications such as barbiturates, benzodiazepines, non-benzodiazepine hypnotics, pentazocine and meperidine should be avoided. Opioid-sparing techniques should be used [70].

References

1. Eberhart LHJ, Mauch M, Morin AM, et al. Impact of a multimodal anti-emetic prophylaxis on patient satisfaction in high-risk patients for postoperative nausea and vomiting. Anaesthesia. 2002;57:1022–7.
2. Habib AS, Chen YT, Taguchi A, et al. Postoperative nausea and vomiting following inpatient surgeries in a teaching hospital: a retrospective database analysis. Curr Med Res Opin. 2006;22:1093–9.
3. Hill Robert P, Lubarsky David A, Phillips-Bute B, et al. Cost-effectiveness of prophylactic antiemetic therapy with ondansetron, droperidol, or placebo. Anesthesiology. 2000;92:958–67.
4. Gan TJ, Belani KG, Bergese S, et al. Fourth consensus guidelines for the management of postoperative nausea and vomiting. Anesth Analg. 2020;131:411–48.
5. Apfel CC, Heidrich FM, Jukar-Rao S, et al. Evidence-based analysis of risk factors for postoperative nausea and vomiting. Br J Anaesth. 2012;109:742–53.
6. Leslie K, Myles PS, Chan MTV, et al. Risk factors for severe postoperative nausea and vomiting in a randomized trial of nitrous oxide-based vs nitrous oxide-free anaesthesia. Br J Anaesth. 2008;101:498–505.
7. Bhakta P, Ghosh BR, Singh U, et al. Incidence of postoperative nausea and vomiting following gynecological laparoscopy: a comparison of standard anesthetic technique and propofol infusion. Acta Anaesthesiol Taiwanica. 2016;54:108–13.
8. Liu SS, Strodtbeck WM, Richman JM, et al. A comparison of regional versus general anesthesia for ambulatory anesthesia: a meta-analysis of randomized controlled trials. Anesth Analg. 2005;101:1634–42.
9. Collard V, Mistraletti G, Taqi A, et al. Intraoperative esmolol infusion in the absence of opioids spares postoperative fentanyl in patients undergoing ambulatory laparoscopic cholecystectomy. Anesth Analg. 2007;105:1255–62.
10. Peyton PJ, Wu CY. Nitrous oxide–related postoperative nausea and vomiting depends on duration of exposure. Anesthesiology. 2014;120:1137–45.
11. Apfel Christian C, Läärä E, Koivuranta M, et al. A simplified risk score for predicting postoperative nausea and vomiting. Anesthesiology. 1999;91:693–700.
12. Koivuranta M, Läärä E, Snåre L, et al. A survey of postoperative nausea and vomiting. Anaesthesia. 1997;52:443–9.
13. Martin G, Glass PSA, Breslin DS, et al. A study of anesthetic drug utilization in different age groups. J Clin Anesth. 2003;15:194–200.
14. Schraag S, Pradelli L, Alsaleh AJO, et al. Propofol vs. inhalational agents to maintain general anaesthesia in ambulatory and in-patient surgery: a systematic review and meta-analysis. BMC Anesthesiol. 2018;18:162.
15. Schaefer MS, Kranke P, Weibel S, et al. Total intravenous anaesthesia versus single-drug pharmacological antiemetic prophylaxis in adults. Eur J Anaesthesiol. 2016;33:750–60.
16. Jewer JK, Wong MJ, Bird SJ, et al. Supplemental perioperative intravenous crystalloids for postoperative nausea and vomiting. Cochrane Database Syst Rev. 2019;3:CD012212. https://doi.org/10.1002/14651858.pub2.
17. Kim HJ, Choi SH, Eum D, et al. Is perioperative colloid infusion more effective than crystalloid in preventing postoperative nausea and vomiting?: a systematic review and meta-analysis. Medicine. 2019;98:e14339.
18. Hristovska AM, Duch P, Allingstrup M, et al. Efficacy and safety of sugammadex versus neostigmine in reversing neuromuscular blockade in adults. Cochrane Database Syst Rev. 2017;8:CD012763. https://doi.org/10.1002/14651858.

19. Gan TJ, Kranke P, Minkowitz HS, et al. Intravenous amisulpride for the prevention of postoperative nausea and vomiting. Anesthesiology. 2017;126:268–75.
20. Singh PM, Borle A, Rewari V, et al. Aprepitant for postoperative nausea and vomiting: a systematic review and meta-analysis. Postgrad Med J. 2015;92:87–98.
21. Liu M, Zhang H, Du BX, et al. Neurokinin-1 receptor antagonists in preventing postoperative nausea and vomiting: a systematic review and meta-analysis. Medicine. 2015;94:e762.
22. De Oliveira GS, Castro-Alves LJS, Ahmad S, et al. Dexamethasone to prevent postoperative nausea and vomiting. Anesth Analg. 2013;116:58–74.
23. Kranke P, Morin AM, Roewer N, et al. Dimenhydrinate for prophylaxis of postoperative nausea and vomiting: a meta-analysis of randomized controlled trials. Acta Anaesthesiol Scand. 2002;46:238–44.
24. Le TP, Gan TJ. Update on the management of postoperative nausea and vomiting and postdischarge nausea and vomiting in ambulatory surgery. Anesthesiol Clin. 2010;28:225–49.
25. Henzi I, Sonderegger J, Tramèr MR. Efficacy, dose-response, and adverse effects of droperidol for prevention of postoperative nausea and vomiting. Can J Anesth. 2000;47:537–51.
26. Damevski V, Damevska G, Krivasija M, et al. Caesarean section in isobaric spinal anesthesia with and without direct preoperative hydration with crystalloids. Bratisl Lek Listy. 2011;112:459–62.
27. Dua N, Sethi N, Sood J, et al. Randomized double blind comparative study comparing efficacy of granisetron and ondansetron for the prophylactic control of postoperative nausea and vomiting in patients undergoing middle ear surgery. Indian J Otolaryngol Head Neck Surg. 2014;66:252–6.
28. Büttner M, Walder B, von Elm E, et al. Is low-dose haloperidol a useful antiemetic? Anesthesiology. 2004;101:1454–63.
29. Aghadavoudi O, Mirkheshti M. Evaluating the effect of intravenous haloperidol and midazolam on postoperative nausea and vomiting after strabismus surgery. J Isfahan Med School. 2019;32:281.
30. Liu G, Gong M, Wang Y, et al. Effect of methylprednisolone on pain management in total knee or hip arthroplasty. Clin J Pain. 2018;34:967–74.
31. De Oliveira GS, Castro-Alves LJ, Chang R, et al. Systemic metoclopramide to prevent postoperative nausea and vomiting: a meta-analysis without Fujii's studies. Br J Anaesth. 2012;109:688–97.
32. Singh PM, Borle A, Gouda D, et al. Efficacy of palonosetron in postoperative nausea and vomiting (PONV)—a meta-analysis. J Clin Anesth. 2016;34:459–82.
33. Schnabel A, Eberhart LH, Muellenbach R, et al. Efficacy of perphenazine to prevent postoperative nausea and vomiting: a quantitative systematic review. Eur J Anaesthesiol. 2010;27:1044–51.
34. Gan TJ, Candiotti KA, Klein S, et al. Double-blind comparison of granisetron, promethazine, or a combination of both for the prevention of postoperative nausea and vomiting in females undergoing outpatient laparoscopies. Can J Anesth. 2009;56:829–36.
35. Choi EK, Kim DG, Jeon Y. Comparison of the prophylactic antiemetic efficacy of aprepitant plus palonosetron versus aprepitant plus ramosetron in patients at high risk for postoperative nausea and vomiting after laparoscopic cholecystectomy. Surg Laparosc Endosc Percutan Tech. 2016;26:354–7.
36. Gan TJ, Gu J, Singla N, et al. Rolapitant for the prevention of postoperative nausea and vomiting. Anesth Analg. 2011;112:804–12.
37. Apfel CC, Zhang K, George E, et al. Transdermal scopolamine for the prevention of postoperative nausea and vomiting: a systematic review and meta-analysis. Clin Ther. 2010;32 1987–2002.
38. Papadima A, Gourgiotis S, Lagoudianakis E, et al. Granisetron versus tropisetron in the prevention of postoperative nausea and vomiting after total thyroidectomy. Saudi J Anaesth. 2013;7:68–74.
39. Rosenthal RA, Zenilman ME, Katlic MR. Principles and practice of geriatric surgery. New York: Springer; 2011. isbn:978144 96998 9.
40. Achuthan S, Singh I, Varthya SB, et al. Gabapentin prophylaxis for postoperative nausea and vomiting in abdominal surgeries: a quantitative analysis of evidence from randomized controlled clinical trials. Br J Anaesth. 2015:114:588–97.
41. Pandey CK, Priye S, Ambesh SP, et al. Prophylactic gabapentin for prevention of postoperative nausea and vomiting in patients undergoing laparoscopic cholecystectomy: a randomized, double blind, placebo-controlled study. J Postgrad Med. 2006;52:97–100.
42. FDA. In: FDA requires new warnings for gabapentinoids about risk of respiratory depression. 2019. https://www.fda.gov/drugs/drug-safety-and-availability/fda-warns-about-serious-breathing-problems-seizure-and-nerve-pain-medicines-gabapentin-neurontin.
43. Lee A, Chan SKC, Fan LTY. Stimulation of the wrist acupuncture point PC6 for preventing postoperative nausea and vomiting. Cochrane Database Syst Rev. 2015;2015(11):CD003281. https://doi.org/10.1002/14651858.CD003281.
44. Rüsch D, Eberhart LHJ, Wallenborn J, et al. Nausea and vomiting after surgery under general anesthesia: an evidence-based review concerning risk assessment, prevention, and treatment. Dtsch Arztebl Int. 2010;107:733–41.
45. Kranke P, Bergese SD, Minkowitz HS, et al. Amisulpride prevents postoperative nausea and vomiting in patients at high risk. Anesthesiology. 2018;128:1099–106.
46. Gupta R, Srivastava S, Dhiraaj S, et al. Minimum effective dose of dexamethasone in combination with midazolam as prophylaxis against postoperative nausea and vomiting after laparoscopic cholecystectomy. Anesth Essays Res. 2018;12:396–401.
47. Choi YS, Sohn HM, Do SH, et al. Comparison of ramosetron and ondansetron for the treatment of established postoperative nausea and vomiting after

laparoscopic surgery: a prospective, randomized, double-blinded multicenter trial. Ther Clin Risk Manag. 2018;14:601–6.
48. Ormel G, Romundstad L, Lambert-Jensen P, et al. Dexamethasone has additive effect when combined with ondansetron and droperidol for treatment of established PONV. Acta Anaesthesiol Scand. 2011;55:1196–205.
49. Gillmann HJ, Wasilenko S, Züger J, et al. Standardised electronic algorithms for monitoring prophylaxis of postoperative nausea and vomiting. Arch Med Sci. 2019;15:408–15.
50. Sinatra R. Role of COX-2 inhibitors in the evolution of acute pain management. J Pain Symptom Manag. 2002;24:S18–27.
51. Fong HK, Sands LP, Leung JM. The role of postoperative analgesia in delirium and cognitive decline in elderly patients: a systematic review. Anesth Analg. 2006;102:1255–66.
52. McCleane G. Pain and the elderly patient. In: McCleane G, Smiths H, editors. Clinical management of the elderly patient in pain. New York: Haworth Medical Press; 2006. isbn:0789026201.
53. Silverstein Jeffrey H, Timberger M, Reich David L, et al. Central nervous system dysfunction after noncardiac surgery and anesthesia in the elderly. Anesthesiology. 2007;106:622–8.
54. White PF, Kehlet H, Neal JM, et al. The role of the anesthesiologist in fast-track surgery: from multimodal analgesia to perioperative medical care. Anesth Analg. 2007;104:1380–96.
55. Lortat-Jacob B, Sevrin F. Pharmacology of intravenous drugs in the elderly. In: Seiber FE, editor. Geriatric anesthesia. New York: McGraw Hill; 2006.
56. Moore RA, Mc Quay HJ. Prevalence of opioid adverse events in chronic non-malignant pain: systematic review of randomized trials of oral opioids. Arthritis Res Ther. 2005;7:R1046–51.
57. Aubrun F. Management of postoperative analgesia in elderly patients. Reg Anesth Pain Med. 2005;30:363–79.
58. Guay J, Kopp S. Epidural pain relief versus systemic opioid-based pain relief for abdominal aortic surgery. Cochrane Database Syst Rev. 2016;2016(1):CD005059. https://doi.org/10.1002/14651858.CD005059.
59. Mohamad MF, Mohammad MA, Hetta DF, et al. Thoracic epidural analgesia reduces myocardial injury in ischemic patients undergoing major abdominal cancer surgery. J Pain Res. 2017;10:887–95.
60. Remy C, Marret E, Bonnet F. Effects of acetaminophen on morphine side effects and consumption after major surgery: meta-analysis of randomized controlled trials. Br J Anaesth. 2005;94:505–13.
61. Morrison R, Carney M, Manfredi P. Pain management. In: Rosenthal RA, Zenilman ME, Katlic MR, editors. Principles and practice of geriatric surgery. New York: Springer; 2001. https://doi.org/10.1007/978-1-4757-3432-4_12.
62. Gavriilidis P, de'Angelis N, Tobias A. To use or not to use opioid analgesia for acute abdominal pain before definitive surgical diagnosis? A systematic review and network meta-analysis. J Clin Med Res. 2019;11:121–6.
63. Barazanchi AWH, MacFater WS, Rahiri JL, et al. Evidence-based management of pain after laparoscopic cholecystectomy: a PROSPECT review update. Br J Anaesth. 2018;121:787–803.
64. Lirk P, Thiry J, Bonnet MP, et al. Pain management after laparoscopic hysterectomy: systematic review of literature and PROSPECT recommendations. Reg Anesth Pain Med. 2019;44:425–36.
65. Mariano E. Management of acute perioperative pain. Fishman S, Crowley M, editors. Wolters Kluwer. 2020. https://www.uptodate.com/.
66. Gagliese L, Jackson M, Ritvo P, et al. Age is not an impediment to effective use of patient-controlled analgesia by surgical patients. Anesthesiology. 2000;93:601–10.
67. Sierżantowicz R, Lewko J, Bitiucka D, et al. Evaluation of pain management after surgery: an observational study. Medicine. 2020;56:65.
68. Mann C, Pouzeratte Y, Boccara G, et al. Comparison of intravenous or epidural patient-controlled analgesia in the elderly after major abdominal surgery. Anesthesiology. 2000;92:433.
69. Marcantonio ER, Flacker JM, Wright RJ, et al. Reducing delirium after hip fracture: a randomized trial. J Am Geriatr Soc. 2001;49:516–22.
70. Chow WB, Rosenthal RA, Merkow RP, et al. Optimal preoperative assessment of the geriatric surgical patient: a best practices guideline from the American College of Surgeons National Surgical Quality Improvement Program and the American Geriatrics Society. J Am Coll Surg. 2012;215:453–66.

The Geriatrician Point of View

33

Stefano Volpato

33.1 Introduction

A growing number of older patients are undergoing emergency surgery worldwide. This is the consequence of three main factors: first, the demographic transition, with people older than 75 years now representing the largest cohort in the so-called developed countries; second, the increasing prevalence in the oldest population of degenerative, infective, and neoplastic conditions for which surgery might represent the first-choice treatment; third, continuous advance in anesthesiological and surgical approach, including minimally invasive techniques, that are associated with less perioperative burden and stress In addition, because of patients' and relatives' change in attitude and expectations, older patients increasingly seek surgical interventions [1].

Current literature suggests that, although more prone to peri- and postoperative complications or long-term adverse outcomes, older patients may equally benefit from surgical intervention for both symptom relief (palliative surgery) and increasing survival compared to younger people. Furthermore, it has been demonstrated that it is not chronological age *per sè* which confers a poor prognostic profile but the impact of age-related pathophysiological changes which combined with the burden of multimorbidity on overall health status and patient's functional status [2, 3]. From this point of view, including comprehensive geriatric assessment into the perioperative process might facilitate the overall decision-making process improving prognostic stratification, perioperative care, and patient's outcomes [4].

33.2 Geriatric Patients: Clinical Characteristics

At the beginning of the twenty-first century, the surgical risk was mostly determined by age and medical comorbidities [5]. This approach, however, was limited by either the insensitivity of chronological age alone or the inability to evaluate sub-clinical physiologic impairments and vulnerability to stress, which renders distinction between high- and higher-risk patients very challenging in older people [6]. The aging process is indeed characterized by a multisystem physiologic decline with reduction of functional reserve and increased vulnerability to stress From this point of view, the geriatric patient candidate to surgery is characterized by three main features (Figs. 33.1 and 33.2):

1. The acute conditions requiring surgery
2. Reduction in functional reserve and increased vulnerability
3. Multimorbidity and polypharmacotherapy.

S. Volpato (✉)
Department of Medical Sciences, University of Ferrara, Ferrara, Italy
e-mail: vlt@unife.it; stefano.volpato@unife.it

F. Agresta et al. (eds.), *Emergency laparoscopic surgery in the elderly and frail patient*,
https://doi.org/10.1007/978-3-030-79990-8_33

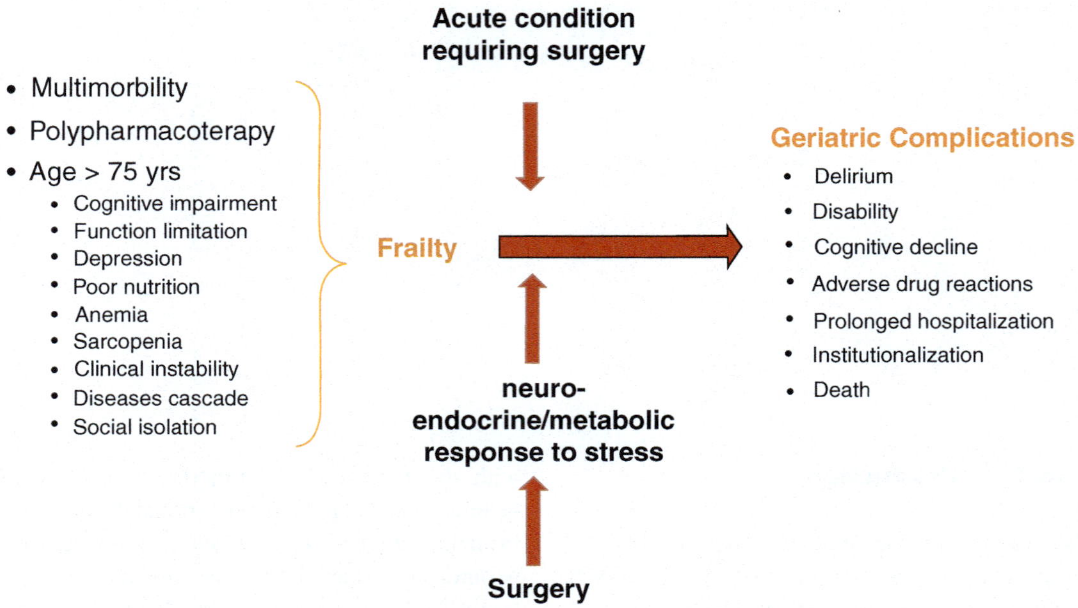

Fig. 33.1 Main clinical characteristics of the geriatric patient with surgical indication

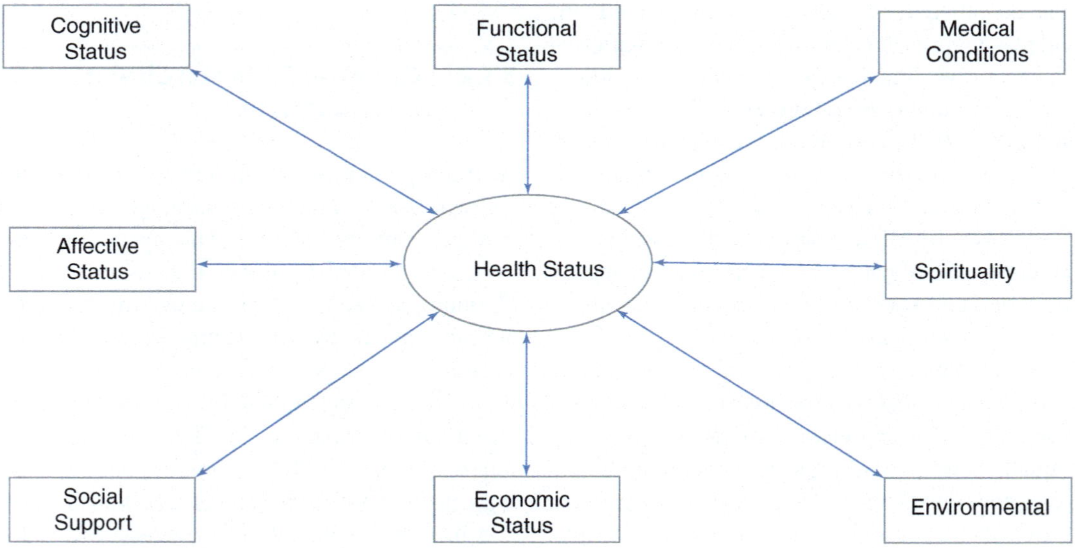

Fig. 33.2 Main determinants of health status of older people

Older patients with these characteristics, often defined as *frail*, are at high risk of worsening mobility or disability, accidental falls, morbidity, hospitalization, and mortality [7]; furthermore, surgical procedures have been consistently associated with unfavorable postoperative outcomes in different surgical specialties and settings [5]. These postoperative complications, however, are predominantly medical or "geriatrics" as opposed to surgical: for example, in colorectal surgery it has been reported no increase in risk of anastomotic leak with advancing age but higher rates of respiratory failure, congestive heart failure, acute kidney injury, and postoperative delirium.

Furthermore, observational studies demonstrated that common chronic conditions of older people, including congestive heart failure, renal failure, depression, and Parkinson's disease, are associated with perioperative adverse events, independent of age. These adverse events are more likely when predisposing factors, including but not limited to functional impairment, multimorbidity, and geriatric syndromes, are not recognized and treated before surgery and in the perioperative period [8].

33.3 Establishing Goals of Care and Surgery

Usual assessment of adults and resilient patients undergoing surgery is centered on identification of the key surgical problem and the most appropriate technical approach. Patient's involvement is usually limited to discussing procedure-related technical issues and evaluating morbidity and mortality statistics associated with the underlying disease and surgical approach. The ultimate goal of surgery is to make complete recovery and extension of the lifespan for these patients.

Establishing patient-centered treatment goals in older patients' candidate to surgery is much more challenging as should extend to the concept of quality of life and healthspan, defined as the time during which an individual retains health and well-being [9]. In older people, health and well-being are not synonyms of the absence of disease but are conceptualized as the capability of living independently regardless of the coexistence of one or more chronic conditions [10]. Healthspan and lifespan are therefore contrasting concepts, as increase in lifespan is often associated with relative reduction in healthspan time; indeed, major operations can easily prolong lifespan but at the same time can dramatically decrease the quality of life and healthspan [11]. From this point of view, patients, relatives, and surgeons must make a tradeoff between these two clinical endpoints. Therefore, besides a careful evaluation of patient health and functional status through an accurate geriatric risk assessment, a key domain of the initial preoperative assessment is a net identification of patient's overall healthcare goals. This task is often challenging in very old patients and even more difficult in emergency situations and among patients with cognitive impairment. The surgeon and the anesthesiologist must advise patients and caregivers of the potential impact of the available procedures (i.e. laparoscopic or laparotomic) on symptoms, functional status, burden of care, and eventually survival. This approach should allow the healthcare professionals aligning surgical and patients' goals. The first step of this process is a careful assessment of patient's risk profile to better foresee potential risk and benefit of different surgical approaches.

Before surgery, patients and surgeons should discuss clearly what they hope to achieve with the intervention, and what secondary strategy should be adopted if these objectives are not achieved or complications occur. All members of the multidisciplinary team should take into consideration advance directives, such as "do not resuscitate" orders. The patient's autonomy must always be respected, to avoid a paternalistic approach, and it should not be assumed that the patient will accept all postoperative treatments should complications occur [12].

33.4 Preoperative Assessment: Risk Stratification

Usually, preoperative assessment evaluates global patient's health status to assess surgical and anesthesiological risk, increase functional reserves, manage vulnerability, and anticipate, minimize, or even prevent possible complications [3]. Although in an emergency situation increasing functional reserves is obviously unfeasible, identification of older individuals who are frail or at risk of poor health outcomes, followed by appropriate subsequent evaluation and intervention, must be considered a fundamental step of perioperative geriatric medicine and quality of care for older patients' candidate to surgery. In the geriatric population, clinical decision-making, including diagnosis, treatment, and outcomes selection, may be particularly challenging. Indeed, older patients are often frail and complex because of the interplay of the multisystemic effects of the aging process with multimorbidity and polytherapy and because of the important contribution of psychological, social, economic, and environmental factors as key determinants of older people's health status [7].

Comprehensive geriatric assessment (CGA) is a multimodal, multidisciplinary process aimed at identifying care needs, planning care, and improving clinical and functional outcomes for older people. This process includes both clinical data and functional measures of physical, cognitive, psychological, nutritional, and behavioral status, and evaluation of family and social network availability. The overall aims of CGA are to improve diagnostic accuracy, optimize medical treatment, improve medical outcomes, minimize unnecessary service use, and arrange long-term management [13].

Frailty and CGA evaluation are extremely useful in surgical risk evaluation of older patients and in making decisions about elective surgery [4]. Although this multidisciplinary assessment is time-consuming and might be more troublesome in urgent situation, including emergency department and acute complications of already hospitalized patients, there are several popular frailty and risk stratification tools (i.e., Clinical Frailty Scale, Identification of Senior At Risk, Silver Code) that are simple and quick and are suitable for use in the emergency setting. Regarding CGA, many different models of care and multiple instruments have been developed and validated over the last 40 years, but the majority of CGA tools include similar measurable dimensions, usually grouped into four main domains:

- Physical health
- Functional status
- Psychological health
- Socioenvironmental status [14].

Many simple and quick scales have been developed and validated to assess these key domains (Table 33.1). These instruments can be used also in emergency setting to achieve a complete and more relevant picture of patients' needs and refining the diagnosis of medical conditions, development of personalized treatment and follow-up [15] (Table 33.2).

Table 33.1 Brief geriatric assessment in the emergency preoperative setting

Domain	Aim	Tools
Physical health	Identify and optimize recognized and unrecognized diseases	Medical history; medication review
Functional status	Establish functional capability	Functional status (BADL IADL)
Psychological health	Establish cognitive function	SPMSQ; 4AT
Socioenvironmental status	Assess social network	Relatives and/or caregiver interview

BADL Basic Activities of Daily Living, *IADL* Instrumental Activities of Daily Living, *SPMSQ* Short Portable Mental Stated Questionnaire, *4AT* Rapid clinical test for delirium

Table 33.2 Main strategies of postoperative care in older surgical patients

Interventions	Objectives
• Optimal postoperative pain control	• Reduce delirium risk; favor mobilization
• Early mobilization and walking	• Reduce disability, reduce risk of cardiovascular and respiratory complications, reduce pressure ulcer risk
• Early resumption of feeding	• Reduce malnutrition risk
• Conservation of the sleep–wake rhythm	• Reduce delirium risk
• Planning personalized discharge plan	• Reduce the length of hospital care and favor continuity of care

33.5 Postoperative Care and Prevention of Geriatric Complications

The benefits of multidisciplinary team management for geriatric patients have been shown in multiple specialties, including surgery, where it has been associated with lower morbidity, short-term mortality, and hospital readmission rates [7]. The main

Table 33.3 Common perioperative and postoperative complication in geriatric patients

- Postoperative delirium (POD)
  - Cognitive decline
- Malnutrition
  - Anorexia
  - Acute sarcopenia
- Mobility disability
- Pressure ulcers
- Respiratory failure
- Congestive heart failure
- Urinary tract infection

goals of postoperative care in older surgical patients are the prevention of geriatric complications, including but not limited to functional decline, delirium, malnutrition, and the definition of a personalized hospital discharge plan (Table 33.3).

Enhanced Recovery After Surgery (ERAS) protocols have been associated with lower length of hospital stay and faster recovery. These protocols, which aim at reducing postoperative morbidity, cover the whole perioperative period [16] and decrease post-surgery complications, length of hospital stay, and healthcare costs. In a systematic review of 24 studies, the ERAS items that most strongly predicted shorter hospitalization and lower morbidity were the absence of a nasogastric tube; early mobilization, oral nutrition, and removal of the urinary catheter; and use of nonopioid analgesia [17]. More importantly, reduction in surgical stress through ERAS appears to be particularly effective in reducing complications and supporting recovery in older and frail patients.

33.5.1 Function and Mobility Preservation

In older people, hospitalization is associated with functional decline and new disability [18] and among surgical patients, up to 50% of them do not regain baseline functional status [19]. Prolonged bed rest with limited ambulation has been associated with increased risk of incident mobility disability. Early mobilization and walking, as recommended by ERAS protocols, are essential interventions to prevent several complications including loss of muscle mass and strength (acute sarcopenia), disability, bed rest syndrome, and pressure ulcers. Selected patients with more severe physical impairment might benefit from early physiotherapy interventions to reinforce muscle function and regain mobility.

33.5.2 Delirium

Delirium is an acute fluctuating alteration of mental state, reduced awareness, and disturbance of attention, which may be triggered by acute medical illness, surgery, trauma, or drugs [20]; multiple factors often coexist in an individual older patient. Postoperative delirium affects 20–80% of geriatric surgical patients; preexisting cognitive impairment is the major risk factor, but delirium can develop also in patients with normal cognitive function [21]. Delirium is independently linked with poor postoperative outcomes, including medical complications, falls, prolonged hospitalization, permanent cognitive dysfunction, need for institutionalization, and death, and can cause significant patient and caregiver distress.

Perioperative delirium assessment should be performed, and after surgery should be repeated over 3–5 days. Validated screening tools, such as the 4AT and the confusion assessment method (CAM), facilitate recognition of delirium and should be used in both the pre- and postoperative periods [22]. The 4AT that can be used in various care settings without specific training allows the assessment of patients who are unable to complete more demanding cognitive tests because of drowsiness or agitation [23].

All patients with delirium should receive an individualized treatment plan, including identification of underlying acute diseases and other clinical conditions that may trigger delirium. Medication reconciliation, early mobilization, promotion of physiologic sleep–wake rhythm, maintenance of adequate nutrition and hydration, and the provision of visual and auditory aids are effective interventions to prevent delirium and to facilitate its resolution when present. It is also important to recognize the potential role of family and caregivers in supporting the patient. Flexibility of hospital visiting schedules should be encouraged. These complex interventions require a multidisciplinary, coordinated approach, coordinated where possible by the geriatrician. Avoiding episodes of deep anesthesia during surgery lasting more than 1 h can significantly reduce the risk of postoperative delirium [24].

33.5.3 Malnutrition

Several studies have highlighted the association between malnutrition and adverse outcomes in older patients, and systematic reviews have reported that early feeding in selected patients is not harmful [25]. Thus, also in emergency situations, nutritional support should be instituted early after surgery, to improve wound healing and recovery. Enteral nutrition is associated with better outcomes as compared to parental nutrition. Postoperative nausea and vomiting reduce oral caloric intake and increase the risk of malnutrition; risk factors for postoperative nausea and vomiting should be assessed in all older surgical patients. Patients at moderate or high risks should receive appropriate prophylactic interventions.

Oral feeding ability and aspiration risk should be assessed daily in older patients along with a formal swallowing assessment; this intervention is of pivotal importance in patients with dysphagia, cognitive impairment, Parkinson's disease, and abnormal conscious level. During oral feeding, the head of the bed should always be elevated, and the patient should be sitting upright while eating and for 1 h after each meal, to prevent aspiration and *ab-ingestis* or aspiration pneumonia [26]. Voluntary oral intake in the postoperative phase is often inadequate in older frail patients, and hence, rapid deterioration of nutritional status and impaired recovery are common; therefore, oral nutritional supplements postoperatively should be offered. Nutritional support should be part of an individually tailored, multimodal, and multidisciplinary intervention to ensure adequate dietary intake, improve clinical outcomes, and maintain quality of life [27].

33.5.4 Postoperative Pain

Persistent postoperative pain is a powerful risk factor for postoperative morbidity, including delirium, cardiorespiratory complications, and failure to mobilize. Pain, however, is often poorly assessed and treated in older patients, particularly in those with cognitive impairment and multimorbidity. Pain should be assessed daily and should be evaluated using the numerical rating scale, visual analogic scale, or verbal rating scale in patients with mild-to-moderate cognitive impairment. Analgesic plans for older adults should be multimodal to avoid adverse effects of opioid analgesics and anxiolytics. Non-pharmacological methods (e.g., positioning, acupuncture, music therapy, massage) are important adjunctive analgesic modalities. Paracetamol is safe and should be considered first-line pain therapy, with only minor concerns about dosage (up to 3 g/day in older patients). If paracetamol is ineffective, nonsteroidal anti-inflammatory drugs should be used at the lowest possible dose and for the shortest possible duration, with concomitant proton pump inhibitor therapy and monitoring for gastric and renal damage. Older patients are more sensitive to adverse effects of opioids and nonsteroidal anti-inflammatory drugs, and more prone to postoperative morbidity. The combination of opioid-free general anesthesia with neuraxial or regional local anesthesia, according to ERAS principles, is indicated in this situation. Morphine is an effective analgesic for moderate or severe pain but should be administered cautiously, particularly in patients with poor renal or respiratory function, cognitive impairment, or both [28].

33.5.5 Postoperative Pulmonary Complications

Postoperative pulmonary complications, including atelectasis and pneumonia, are common and increase postoperative length of hospital stay, disability, mortality, and healthcare costs. Periodic evaluation of oxygen saturation, respiratory rate, and arterial blood gases should be performed regularly in older patients, regardless of the type of intervention undergone. Onset of fever, dyspnea, or peripheral oxygen desaturation should be always triggering a careful pulmonary evaluation including chest X-rays. Several postoperative strategies can be used to prevent postoperative pulmonary complications including early mobilization, adequate bed posture, screening for signs and symptoms of dysphagia incentive spirometry, chest physical therapy, and deep breathing exercises [29].

33.5.6 Postoperative Cardiovascular Complications

Congestive heart failure, parossistic atrial fibrillation, and deep venous thrombosis are the most common cardiovascular complications. Acute myocardial infarction is not common after surgery; nevertheless, it is a strong risk factor for perioperative mortality in older patients [30]. Periodic evaluation of oxygen saturation, respiratory rate, and cardiac rate should be performed regularly in older patients; electroencephalography should be performed in case of any new arrhythmia. In patients at risk of congestive heart failure, liquid balance must be carefully evaluated daily. Thromboprophylaxis to prevent deep venous thrombosis is usually based on low-molecular-weight heparins. Graduated compression stockings or intermittent pneumatic compression is a valuable alternative in selected situations for patients in which antithrombotic therapy is contraindicated.

33.5.7 Urinary Tract Infection

Geriatric patients are at high risk for urinary tract infection, particularly if immobilized and with urinary catheter. Guidelines for the prevention and management of urinary tract infection recommend limited use of urinary catheters, aseptic insertion of catheters, and maintenance of a closed drainage system. Clinical evidence suggests that early removal of urinary catheters, whenever possible, is related to a lower risk of urinary infection, lower incidence of delirium, and faster hospital discharge [31].

33.5.8 Pressure Ulcers

Hospitalized older patients, particularly frail patients with limited mobility and/or cognitive impairment [32], are at high risk of pressure ulcers. Healthcare teams should, therefore, assess the risk of pressure ulcers in all older postoperative patients and should implement multimodal interventions to prevent and treat pressure ulcers, according to local guidelines.

33.6 Hospital Discharge and Continuity of Care

Older frail patients often need prolonged hospitalization, sometimes in non-surgical wards, or a period of care in intermediate care facilities, before returning home. For some patients, worsening health and functional status resulting from negative effects of the disease and surgery makes it impossible to return home. Discharge to a residential care facility, and inability to maintain independence after surgery, may be significant and unacceptable outcomes for many older patients. Anticipating which adults will require discharge to an additional care facility, rather than to their home, following a major operation is important for preoperative counseling of expected outcomes, and preoperative care planning for both the patient and their family. Therefore, throughout the perioperative period, attention should be paid as to how the patient can be discharged into the better healthcare setting to guarantee continuity of care and adequate support. Indeed, the lack of an appropriate and tailored discharge plan and transition program increases the risk of early readmission and may negatively affect functional status and quality of life of both patients and caregivers [33]. To reduce the risk of negative outcomes, it is essential to establish an organizational framework that incorporates appropriate assessment of the patient's clinical, social, and care status; recognition of the expectations of the patient and their relatives; formalization of institutional roles or teams dedicated to the planning and coordination of discharge; good knowledge of transitional management programs; and strong communication between the hospital, home care, and community setting.

The available evidence shows that CGA of frail elderly patients in community settings can reduce the risk of readmission in those recently discharged. Key elements of post-hospital discharge CGA include targeting criteria to identify vulnerable patients, a program of multidimensional assessment, and home follow-up.

There is evidence that some fragile patients may develop a transient period of health vulnerability following hospitalization for acute illness, known as the post-hospital syndrome. This syndrome is characterized by the risk of early rehospitalization due to physiologic stressors resulting from the initial admission, including disruption in sleep–wake cycles, inadequate pain control, deconditioning, and changes in nutritional status. Patients hospitalized within 90 days of elective surgery are at increased risk of postoperative adverse event characteristics of post-hospital syndrome [28].

33.7 Conclusions

Emergency surgery, regardless of technical approach, is always a stressful event for older patients; frail patients are therefore at the highest risk of several perioperative complications, including delirium, functional decline, loss of independence, and mortality. Where feasible, laparoscopic surgery should be considered the standard treatment for many conditions that commonly affect older patients. Benefits of laparoscopy include less severe neuroendocrine/metabolic response to stress, avoiding general anesthesia, less blood loss, decreased postoperative pain, shorter hospitalizations, and therefore a quicker return to full mobility and normal activity. However, laparoscopy may be technically challenging and might also impose specific physiologic demands on older patients; therefore, any choice regarding decision to operate and regarding the most appropriate technical approach should be based on a preliminary multidimensional and multidisciplinary geriatric assessment, including, when feasible, evaluation of patients' preferences and goals.

The Five Things You Should Know About the Geriatrician Point of View About Emergency Abdominal Surgery in the Elderly and Frail Patient

- Ensure multidisciplinary team approach
- Identify patients at high risk by comprehensive geriatric assessment
- Assess patient's and caregiver's preference
- Preserve mobility and walking ability
- Establish a discharge planning early in the perioperative phase

References

1. Aucoin S, McIsaac DI. Emergency general surgery in older adults: a review. Anesthesiol Clin. 2019;37:493–505. https://doi.org/10.1016/j.anclin.2019.04.008.
2. Fowler AJ, Abbott TEF, Prowle J, et al. Age of patients undergoing surgery. Br J Surg. 2019;106:1012–8.
3. Makary MA, Segev DL, Pronovost PJ, et al. Frailty as a predictor of surgical outcomes in older patients. J Am Coll Surg. 2010;210:901–8. https://doi.org/10.1016/j.jamcollsurg.2010.01.028.
4. Aceto P, Antonelli Incalzi R, Bettelli G, et al. Perioperative Management of Elderly patients (PriME): recommendations from an Italian intersociety consensus. Aging Clin Exp Res. 2020;32:1647–73. https://doi.org/10.1007/s40520-020-01624-x.
5. Joseph B, Zangbar B, Pandit V, et al. Emergency general surgery in the elderly: too old or too frail? J Am Coll Surg. 2016;222(5):805–13. https://doi.org/10.1016/j.jamcollsurg.2016.01.063.
6. McIsaac DI, MacDonald DB, Aucoin SD. Frailty for perioperative clinicians: a narrative review. Anesth Analg. 2020;130:1450–60. https://doi.org/10.1213/ANE.0000000000004602.
7. Clegg A, Young J, Iliffe S, et al. Frailty in elderly people. Lancet. 2013;381:752–62. https://doi.org/10.1016/S0140-6736(12)62167-9.
8. Chang C-M, Yin W-Y, Wei C-K, et al. Adjusted age-adjusted Charlson comorbidity index score as a risk measure of perioperative mortality before cancer surgery. PLoS One. 2016;11:e0148076. https://doi.org/10.1371/journal.pone.0148076.
9. Jones TS, Moore JT, Robinson TN. Perioperative care strategy for older adults. Med Clin North Am. 2020;104:895–908. https://doi.org/10.1016/j.mcna.2020.06.010.
10. Tinetti ME, Fried T. The end of the disease era. Am J Med. 2004;116:179–85. https://doi.org/10.1016/j.amjmed.2003.09.031.

11. Crimmins EM. Lifespan and Healthspan: past, present, and Promis. Gerontologist. 2015;55:901–11. https://doi.org/10.1093/geront/gnv130.
12. Krumholz HM. Post-hospital syndrome–an acquired, transient condition of generalized risk. N Engl J Med. 2013;368:100–2. https://doi.org/10.1056/NEJMp1212324.
13. Pilotto A, Cella A, Pilotto A, et al. Three decades of comprehensive geriatric assessment: evidence coming from different healthcare settings and specific clinical conditions. J Am Med Dir Assoc. 2017;18:192.e1–192.e11. https://doi.org/10.1016/j.jamda.2016.11.004.
14. Ellis G, Whitehead MA, Robinson D, et al. Comprehensive geriatric assessment for older adults admitted to hospital: meta-analysis of randomised controlled trials. BMJ. 2011;343:d6553. https://doi.org/10.1136/bmj.d6553.
15. Carpenter CR, Shelton E, Fowler S, et al. Risk factors and screening instruments to predict adverse outcomes for undifferentiated older emergency department patients: a systematic review and meta-analysis. Acad Emerg Med. 2015;22:1–21. https://doi.org/10.1111/acem.12569.
16. Ljungqvist O, Scott M, Fearon KC. Enhanced recovery after surgery: a review. JAMA Surg. 2017;152:292–8. https://doi.org/10.1001/jamasurg.2016.4952.
17. Parks L, Routt M, De Villiers A. Enhanced recovery after surgery. J Adv Pract Oncol. 2018;9:511–9.
18. Volpato S, Onder G, Cavalieri M, et al. Characteristics of nondisabled older patients developing new disability associated with medical illnesses and hospitalization. J Gen Intern Med. 2007;22:668–74. https://doi.org/10.1007/s11606-007-0152-1.
19. Lawrence VA, Hazuda HP, Cornell JE, et al. Functional independence after major abdominal surgery in the elderly. J Am Coll Surg. 2004;199:762–72. https://doi.org/10.1016/j.jamcollsurg.2004.05.280.
20. American Psychiatric Association. Diagnostic and statistical manual of mental disorders: DSM-5™. 5th ed. Arlington: American Psychiatric Publishing; 2013.
21. Robinson TN, Wu DS, Pointer LF, et al. Preoperative cognitive dysfunction is related to adverse postoperative outcomes in the elderly. J Am Coll Surg. 2012;215:12–8. https://doi.org/10.1016/j.jamcollsurg.2012.02.007.
22. Inouye SK, van Dyck CH, Alessi CA, et al. Clarifying confusion: the confusion assessment method. A new method for detection of delirium. Ann Intern Med. 1990;113:941–8. https://doi.org/10.7326/0003-4819-113-12-941.
23. Bellelli G, Morandi A, Davis DH, et al. Validation of the 4AT, a new instrument for rapid delirium screening: a study in 234 hospitalised older people. Age Ageing. 2014;43:496–502. https://doi.org/10.1093/ageing/afu021.
24. National Institute for Health and Care Excellence (NICE). Delirium: prevention, diagnosis and management. Clinical guideline [CG103]. 2019. https://www.nice.org.uk/guidance/cg103. Accessed 7 Nov 2020.
25. Lim SC, Koh IAJH. Nutrition and the elderly surgical patients. MOJ Surg. 2017;4:114–20.
26. Mohanty S, Rosenthal RA, Russell MM, et al. Optimal perioperative management of the geriatric patient: a best practices guideline from the American College of Surgeons NSQIP and the American Geriatrics Society. J Am Coll Surg. 2016;222:930–47. https://doi.org/10.1016/j.jamcollsurg.2015.12.026.
27. Volkert D, Beck AM, Cederholm T, et al. ESPEN guideline on clinical nutrition and hydration in geriatrics. Clin Nutr. 2019;38:10–47. https://doi.org/10.1016/j.clnu.2018.05.024.
28. Zurlo A, Zuliani G. Management of care transition and hospital discharge. Aging Clin Exp Res. 2018;30:263–70. https://doi.org/10.1007/s40520-017-0885-6.
29. Las Vegas Investigators. Epidemiology, practice of ventilation and outcome for patients at increased risk of postoperative pulmonary complications: LAS VEGAS—an observational study in 29 countries. Eur J Anaesth. 2017;34:492–507. https://doi.org/10.1097/EJA.0000000000000646.
30. Sieber FE, Barnett SR. Preventing postoperative complications in the elderly. Anesthesiol Clin. 2011;29:83–97.
31. Conway LJ, Larson EL. Guidelines to prevent catheter associated urinary tract infection: 1980 to 2010. Heart Lung. 2012;41:271–83. https://doi.org/10.1016/j.hrtlng.2011.08.001.
32. Chiari P, Forni C, Guberti M, et al. Predictive factors for pressure ulcers in an older adult population hospitalized for hip fractures: a prognostic cohort study. PLoS One. 2017;12:e0169909. https://doi.org/10.1371/journal.pone.0169909.
33. Goncalves-Bradley DC, Lannin NA, Clemson LM, et al. Discharge planning from hospital. Cochrane Database Syst Rev. 2016;2016(1):CD000313. https://doi.org/10.1002/14651858.CD000313.pub5.

34 Perioperative Nutritional Management of Elderly Patients

Nicolò Pecorelli, Maria Teresa Salvioni, Alessia Vallorani, and Giovanni Guarneri

34.1 Introduction

The importance of patient perioperative nutritional status could be summed up in a single statement; malnutrition is a strong predictor of postoperative outcomes including morbidity, mortality, and length of hospital stay (LOS), but it represents one of the only modifiable risk factors before surgery.

It is estimated that up to two-thirds of patients undergoing surgery are at nutritional risk [1]. A study including 26 hospitals across the European Union using the nutritional risk screening tool 2002 (NRS-2002) found that one-third of patients were at "high risk" of malnutrition. Compared to patients "not-at-risk", these patients developed greater morbidity (31% vs. 11%) and increased mortality rates (12% vs. 1%), with a 3-day longer LOS (median 9 vs. 6 days) [2]. However, despite the large body of evidence accumulated in the last two decades regarding the positive impact of nutritional interventions on postoperative results, healthcare systems still disregard this important issue. A recent study revealed significant deficiencies in nutritional screening and intervention in US colorectal and oncologic surgical patients with only about one in five hospitals currently utilizing a formal nutrition screening process, and only 20% of these patients receive any nutritional supplements in the preoperative or postoperative setting [3].

Recent literature showed that the surgical population in the UK tends to be older than the general population, and that the age gap is increasing with time. Between 1999 and 2015, the percentage of people aged 75 years or more undergoing surgery increased from 15 to 23%, and this figure is expected to increase further [4]. Advanced age is associated with underlying chronic diseases (e.g., hypertension, diabetes, heart disease, chronic kidney dysfunction) but also a diminished functional (physiologic) reserve capacity that accompanies aging and declines rather steadily as age advances. The increased vulnerability to stressors as a result of decreased physiologic reserves, which leads to the dysregulation of multiple physiologic systems and a higher risk of adverse outcomes, is commonly known as frailty [5]. Although there is a lack of consensus on the definition of frailty, according to Fried et al., a frailty phenotype can be identified if three of the following five indicators are present: weight loss, self-reported exhaustion, low energy expenditure, slow gait speed, weak grip strength [6]. Another syndrome frequently affecting elderly patients is sarcopenia, described as "the

N. Pecorelli (✉) · G. Guarneri
Division of Pancreatic Surgery, Pancreas Translational and Clinical Research Center, IRCCS San Raffaele Scientific Institute, Milan, Italy

Vita-Salute San Raffaele University, Milan, Italy
e-mail: pecorelli.nicolo@hsr.it

M. T. Salvioni · A. Vallorani
Vita-Salute San Raffaele University, Milan, Italy

F. Agresta et al. (eds.), *Emergency laparoscopic surgery in the elderly and frail patient*,
https://doi.org/10.1007/978-3-030-79990-8_34

loss of skeletal muscle mass and strength as a result of ageing." There are many definitions available for sarcopenia, relying on the measurement of both muscle function and muscle mass [7]. In recent years, preoperative cross-sectional images at the third lumber vertebral level (L3) have been increasingly used to analyze body composition, and the term "sarcopenia" has been used to describe reduced skeletal muscle area, without assessment of patient's functional status. In these terms, sarcopenia has been linked to adverse outcomes such as increased postoperative morbidity and reduced survival in most oncologic surgery contexts [8, 9].

Frailty, comorbidity, sarcopenia, and malnutrition often overlap, as they involve correlated domains of patient's health and identify patients with increased vulnerability and reduced reserves. These premises are fundamental to understand why elderly patients are at increased risk of postoperative poor outcomes, especially after emergency surgery. In fact, evidence demonstrates nearly tenfold higher mortality rates in the elderly undergoing major emergency surgery when compared to younger patients [10], mostly due to a significantly higher failure-to-rescue rates in the elderly [11]. Failure to rescue measures the ability of a hospital to respond to a major complication, but also the patient's physiological reserves to tolerate and survive a life-threatening complication. In a large Michigan statewide database analysis, a twofold higher failure-to-rescue rate in elderly was found compared to younger patients, highlighting a diminished physiological reserve for surviving critical illness in these patients [12].

In this chapter, we will discuss preoperative nutritional screening and interventions, potentially useful intraoperative strategies and postoperative nutritional management with a focus on elderly patients undergoing emergency surgery.

34.2 Preoperative Nutritional Screening and Assessment

Nutritional screening before major surgery is essential to identify undernourished patients or those at risk of malnutrition who may benefit from a nutritional intervention preoperatively.

Four central criteria have been proposed to identify those at high nutritional risk: body mass index (BMI) and a detailed nutritional history, the presence of pathological weight loss, appetite and food intake, and the severity of the underlying disease. Several validated nutritional screening questionnaires are available, such as the Malnutrition Universal Screening Tool (MUST) [13], the NRS-2002 [14], the Subjective Global Assessment (SGA) [15], and the Mini-Nutritional Assessment (MNA) [16]. Expert consensus considers MUST superior in the community, NRS-2002 for inpatients and MNA for those in older adult care homes [17].

The most recent European Society for Clinical Nutrition and Metabolism (ESPEN) guidelines [18] suggest that criteria for the diagnosis of severe nutritional risk should include the following:

- Weight loss exceeding 10–15% within the preceding 6 months;
- BMI less than 18.5 kg/m^2, over 75 years, BMI less than 20 kg/m^2;
- NRS-2002 > 5;
- SGA grade C;
- Preoperative serum albumin concentration less than 30 g/L (in the absence of hepatic or renal dysfunction).

If one of these criteria is present, nutritional therapy should be immediately initiated to prevent adverse surgical outcomes.

Very recently, the American Society for Enhanced Recovery (ASER) and Perioperative Quality Initiative (PQI) developed and proposed a simple and easily applicable tool named perioperative nutrition screen (PONS), which is a modified version of the MUST [19]. PONS evaluates the presence of nutrition risk based on four different parameters: patient's body max index (BMI), recent body weight changes, decrease in dietary intake, and preoperative albumin level. The PONS tool suggests a formal nutritional evaluation if the patient has any of the following risk factors:

- BMI lower than 18.5 (or lower than 20 if the patient is 65 or older).
- Unplanned weight loss exceeding 10% over the previous 6 months.

- Dietary intake was less than 50% in the previous week.
- Albumin levels are below 3.0 g/dL.

Serum albumin has been consistently reported in the literature as a valid predictor of postoperative complications. However, recent studies showed controversial results. In fact, albumin levels are influenced by a series of factors outside of its plain synthesis and degradation. Most of all, inflammation induces a shift in protein synthesis toward acute-phase proteins that increase vascular permeability and extravascular leakage.

In the setting of emergency surgery, a thorough nutritional and functional assessment is usually not possible, but the screening is essential to guide intraoperative strategies and postoperative nutritional interventions. In the elective setting, a formal and extensive nutritional assessment by a trained professional is recommended to tailor the dietary approach and nutritional therapy upon patients' characteristics. This includes the use of a plate chart or 24-h dietary recall; estimation of body composition (subcutaneous fat, visceral adiposity and skeletal muscle mass via CT scan or dual X-ray absorptiometry, or bioelectrical impedance analysis); measurement of hand-grip strength as a test of muscle function or performance of the 6-min walking test for functional status. For elderly patients, the use of the comprehensive geriatric assessment (CGA) would be the recommended multidisciplinary approach to evaluate their general health status. The CGA evaluates comorbidities, cognition, mental health status, functional status, nutrition, social status, and support. Especially the functional status and nutrition allow focusing on frailty, sarcopenia, cachexia, and malnutrition variables that may affect patient outcome. As mentioned before, the MNA should be the nutritional assessment tool, as it appears to have a significantly higher sensitivity compared to other metrics in the elderly [20].

34.3 Preoperative Nutritional Interventions

After assessing the nutritional and functional status, as discussed in the previous paragraph, attention needs to be focused on implementing strategies and interventions to prepare patients to face the surgical stress and favor their recovery process. Preoperative conditioning, also known as prehabilitation, is defined as the process of enhancing physical fitness and well-being via a multimodal intervention including exercise training, diet, and psychological support. Although it is clear that, in emergency situations, there is no time for prehabilitation as described in elective settings, there is plenty of evidence supporting preoperative nutritional interventions that will be discussed in this section [21].

First, preoperatively it is not only about reaching the adequate caloric intake, but it is necessary to meet an adequate protein target, since proteins are the most used substrate in surgical stress situations. For this purpose, the best solution is enriching daily diet with high-quality proteins (e.g., whey proteins and casein) that demonstrated to increase anabolism and muscle synthesis. The aim is to reach an intake of at least 1.2–2.0 g of protein/kg/day that is approximately 25–35 g of proteins for each meal. However, if the goal is not met with the oral diet alone, it should be integrated with high-protein oral nutritional supplements (ONS).

Additionally, it is still debated if there is a role for preoperative immunonutrition (IMN). IMN is an oral supplementation of specific nutrients such as arginine, glutamine, nucleotides, and omega-3 fatty acids. Arginine and glutamine are conditional amino acids, as they represent more than 70% of the amino acids mobilized during the stress response. Their biological functions include stimulation of the immune system and promotion of wound healing. They also serve as nitric oxide precursors whose action is to improve microvascular perfusion through vasodilation.

Omega-3 fatty acids comprising docosahexaenoic acid (DHA) and eicosapentaenoic acid (EPA) are known to be positive modulators of the inflammatory response. Combined IMN formulas have a positive influence on the immune and inflammatory response as well as encouraging protein synthesis, suggesting a synergic effect. A recent meta-analysis on preoperative IMN in gastrointestinal cancer only has demonstrated a significant reduction in postoperative infectious complications [22]. However, there is conflicting evidence regarding the actual benefit of IMN in a modern perioperative care setting such as enhanced recovery after surgery (ERAS) programs. For this reason, ESPEN guidelines suggest that peri- or at least postoperative administration of IMN should be given in malnourished patients undergoing major cancer surgery [17]. Although further research is needed to determine the benefit and optimal duration of IMN, current data suggest that administration should be initiated at least 5–7 days before surgery, and a minimum treatment of 14 days in patients with severe malnutrition.

When supplementation is not possible via the oral route, a preoperative nutritional intervention can be administered via enteral route following the positioning of a feeding tube for a period of at least 7 days. The enteral route is always preferable, when feasible, due to the many benefits in terms of intestinal barrier permeability and preservation of the gut immune system and microbiota. If neither oral nutrition supplementation via ONS nor enteral nutrition is possible, or when protein or calories requirement cannot be adequately reached by the discussed strategies, meaning at least 50% of the recommended intake, parenteral nutrition should be administrated for a period of 7–14 days.

In the emergency setting, if a patient is deemed malnourished, it is crucial to evaluate the possibility of delaying surgery to allow a preoperative nutritional intervention until the patient has reached an adequate target. The decision-making process should also take into account overall patient conditions, the expected extent of the anticipated surgical procedure, and the underlying disease, as these represent key risk factors for postoperative outcomes. For example, an elderly undernourished patient presenting with acute cholecystitis planned for emergency cholecystectomy has far less chances of postoperative morbidity compared to the same patient presenting with a left colonic obstructive cancer candidate for emergency left colectomy. In the latter situation, an endoscopic palliation with a colonic stent should be considered as a bridge to surgery, as it may allow patient preoperative optimization and potential improvement of surgical outcome. Anyhow, each case should be evaluated individually, and a tailored approach should continue intraoperatively and after surgery.

34.4 Intraoperative Strategies

The ability to mobilize nutrients is particularly important in response to surgical stress, which like injuries or traumas induce a hypercatabolic metabolism, depletion of muscle mass, and increase in hepatic acute-phase protein synthesis [23]. In this context, intraoperative nutritional management should pursue two objectives: minimize surgical stress and allow an adequate and timely postoperative nutrition. In an emergency setting, factors related to the disease, trauma, or other causes, which lead the patient to surgery, are difficult to modify; therefore, intraoperative and postoperative strategies acquire even more importance than in elective surgery.

The laparoscopic approach has become the treatment of choice for most diseases due to its many advantages, such as reduction of surgical stress, better postoperative pain control, and faster time to functional recovery. Laparoscopic surgery was initially withheld from elderly patients due to concerns over the unique physiological demands of pneumoperitoneum. However, there are more and more clinical evidences showing that also this group benefits from a laparoscopic approach [24].

Intraoperative management should anticipate the nutritional support needed postoperatively. For example, in case of major abdominal surgery involving digestive tract, positioning a feeding naso-enteric tube or needle catheter jejunostomy (NCJ) should always be considered. In procedures involving upper GI tract, such as esophageal, gastric, or a part of pancreato-biliary surgery, enteral nutrition via jejunostomy or nasojejunal tube could represent a valid alternative to parenteral support, which could be particularly useful if complications are encountered.

The ESPEN guidelines recommend the placement of a nasojejunal tube (NJ) or NCJ in all malnourished patients, candidates to major upper gastrointestinal and pancreatic surgery [18]. The benefits and feasibility of a feeding tube either inserted directly in the jejunum or inserted through the nose and placed intraoperatively with the tip in the stomach, small bowel, or distally to an eventual anastomosis are well demonstrated [25–31]. However, the question is which route of enteral nutrition should be preferred as both feeding routes carry additional costs and complications.

In terms of postoperative complications, an observational study in esophageal surgery showed a reduced incidence of anastomotic leakage in the NCJ group compared to nasojejunal tube [32]. For this type of surgery, the catheter-associated complications were absolutely similar among the two techniques [33]. Conversely, in pancreaticoduodenectomy, the rate of catheter-related complications and time to tube removal have been reported as higher in NCJ patients [34]. A randomized trial showed no difference in terms of overall postoperative complications between the two techniques but also reported a lower incidence of mechanical bowel obstruction and delayed gastric emptying in nasojejunal patients [34].

Some authors consider the routine use of NCJ an overtreatment and propose to consider NCJ only in high-risk patients [35–37] for postoperative complications, which should be stratified using available predictive risk scores. On the other hand, nasojejunal and nasoduodenal tubes are associated with a significant rate of displacement or early accidental dislodgement [36, 38]. Keeping all of these observations in mind, in all frail patients with an impaired nutritional status who undergo emergency major surgery, an enteral feeding route is mandatory.

34.5 Postoperative Nutritional Management

The consequence of protein catabolism triggered by the surgical stress response is muscle wasting which represents an obstacle for functional recovery, the most valued clinical objective [39]. This catabolic response is proportional to the magnitude of the procedure, but traditional perioperative care has been characterized by measures that also tended to amplify catabolism such as prolonged fasting, fluid and salt overload, and bed rest. Nutritional therapy may provide the energy for optimal healing and recovery but in the immediate postoperative phase may only minimally counteract muscle catabolism, or not at all. To restore peripheral protein mass, the body needs to deal with the surgical trauma and possible infection adequately. Nutritional support/intake and physical exercise are prerequisites to rebuild peripheral protein mass.

The mode of nutritional delivery in the early postoperative period has been a subject of much debate, especially in procedures involving the formation of bowel anastomosis. However, several systematic reviews with meta-analysis have concluded that the oral and/or enteral route is the preferred mode of nutrition for surgical patients. From a clinical point of view, return to oral feeding and recovery of gastrointestinal function after surgery represent key outcomes for patient recovery and are also considered as common criteria for patient discharge after bowel surgery along with resumption of mobilization out of bed and adequate pain control [40]. Randomized controlled trials (RCTs) demonstrated that early oral feeding after elective surgery is safe and associated with multiple benefits on postoperative outcomes such as earlier return of bowel movements and shorter length of hospital stay [41]. A Cochrane review on early enteral nutrition also showed no difference in risk of postoperative complications in patients fed within 24 h after surgery and those fed later. Importantly, the authors found that patients who were fed early had a reduction in mortality (relative risk (RR) 0.41, 95% CI 0.18–0.93) [41]. A recently updated review from the Cochrane database confirmed a consistent reduction in LOS but was inconclusive on other postoperative outcomes and patient quality of life [42].

Avoidance of postoperative nasogastric tube (NGT) decompression is a pre-requisite for early return to oral nutrition. A 2007 Cochrane review of RCTs in elective abdominal surgery showed that prophylactic NGT led to delayed return of bowel function, and increased pulmonary complications compared to no NGT, suggesting that routine decompression should be abandoned in favor of a selective use policy [43]. Avoidance of postoperative nasogastric tube and oral nutrition as soon as tolerated are cornerstones of ERAS programs. In the context of elective abdominal surgery, ERAS pathways represent the best available care bundle and are associated with a faster return of bowel function and reduced medical morbidity [44, 45].

Not all patients can rely solely on oral nutrition. According to 2020 ESPEN perioperative nutrition guidelines [18], nutritional support therapy (i.e., enteral or parenteral) is indicated upfront in patients with preoperative malnutrition and those at nutritional risk. Artificial nutrition should also be initiated, if it is anticipated that the patient will be unable to eat for more than 5 days perioperatively, and in patients expected to have low oral intake and who cannot maintain above 50% of recommended intake for more than 7 days. In these situations, it is recommended to initiate nutritional support therapy without delay. This approach is supported by data from systematic reviews and meta-analyses on several gastrointestinal surgical procedures including emergency surgery, reporting no benefit of food avoidance, and sustained improved outcomes in patients who received oral nutrition and those fed via enteral route [36, 41, 46].

In the postoperative setting, the patient's objective is to reach daily calorie (25–30 kcal/kg/day) and protein (1.5–2 g/kg/day) targets by tolerating oral intake [17]. A practical approach from a recent publication by the ASER suggests that patients tolerating 50–100% of nutrition goals should receive high-protein ONS to meet protein needs at least twice a day. In patients consuming <50% via the oral route, enteral nutrition via tube feeds (i.e., NGT or naso-enteric tube, or feeding jejunostomy) should be given. Parenteral nutrition should be utilized if more than 50% of protein/calories needs are not met via oral or enteral nutrition for more than 7 days, even in well-nourished patients [19].

Using the gut to feed the patients is extremely important in order to preserve the immune response. The bowel provides a physical barrier to infection and is home to the largest source of immune tissue in the body, producing antibodies that prevent bacterial translocation. Importantly, gut starvation and critical illness induce changes to the immune function of the gastrointestinal tract leading to increased mucosal permeability, potentially allowing bacterial translocation and bacteremia [47]. However, while parenteral nutrition is undoubtedly capable of providing excellent nutrition, there are additional risks to take into account with this form of supplementation. First, patients require a central venous access creating the potential for line complications. Next, hyperglycemia is frequently encountered and close attention to glycemic control is necessary [48]. In undernourished patients or those at risk for malnutrition, if nutrition goals are not met via the enteral route, it is now recommended to start parenteral nutrition early, in combination with enteral nutrition if possible. Despite concerns for infection risks that have limited the use of parenteral nutrition in the past, recent RCTs in ICU patients clearly demonstrated that parenteral administration is no longer associated with an increased risk of infection, and suggest that late infections are reduced in patients supplemented early by parenteral nutrition in addition to enteral feeding [49–51].

Elderly patients undergoing emergency surgery represent a peculiar category where ERAS interventions and especially postoperative oral nutrition can be hampered by several factors. First, emergency surgery may involve patients with gastrointestinal mechanical obstruction or perforation which require longer perioperative

NGT decompression and bowel rest. Second, the emergency setting is a recognized risk factor for prolonged postoperative ileus after bowel resection [52]. Finally, it should be mentioned that both advanced age and emergency surgery are associated with increased postoperative morbidity and infections, which significantly delay postoperative recovery and influence the ability to resume oral feeding.

In the only RCT focused on early oral nutrition following emergency surgery, by Klappenbach et al. [53], 295 patients were allocated after emergency surgery to early versus delayed feeding. Patients were stratified as high or low risk depending on whether they presented with generalized peritonitis, intestinal obstruction, gastrointestinal perforation, required bowel resection with anastomosis (high risk) or not (low risk). All patients assigned to the early oral-feeding group commenced a soft diet within 24 h after surgery. In the low-risk routine care group, a liquid diet was started upon passage of flatus and diet progressively advanced thereafter. High-risk patients were fasted for at least 3 days, and a liquid diet was then commenced only if patients had already passed flatus. The overall morbidity rate was 41% without any significant difference among groups. Nevertheless, the authors observed a significant difference in postprandial vomiting with an increased risk in the early-feeding group [13.5% versus 6.1%; odds ratio (OR) 2.4; 95% CI 1.05–5.40; $P = 0.03$]. Conversely, a retrospective propensity score-matched study performed in Korea, including 484 patients who had undergone bowel resection and/or anastomosis or primary intestinal repair, demonstrated that early enteral nutrition (i.e., oral or tube feeding within 3 days postoperatively) was associated with the reduction of in-hospital mortality rate, pulmonary complication, length of hospital stay, and longer 28-day ICU-free days when compared with late enteral nutrition [46]. Results from studies in the emergency surgery context suggest that early enteral feeding is safe and feasible but it is difficult to draw conclusion on the actual clinical benefit that these patients derive.

34.6 Post-discharge Follow-Up

In a considerable number of patients after major gastrointestinal surgery, oral calorie intake will be inadequate for a longer period with a risk for postoperative malnutrition. In patients who have lost significant weight after surgery, a considerable period of significant increases in calorie and protein delivery is required for recovery. Furthermore, patients who developed postoperative complications will continue to lose weight and are at risk for serious further deterioration of nutritional status. Thus, regular reassessment of nutritional status during hospital stay and, if necessary, continuation of nutrition therapy after discharge, is advised for patients who have received nutrition therapy perioperatively and still do not cover appropriately their energy requirements via the oral route [18].

Recovering postoperative patients, especially elderly individuals, are challenged by decreased appetite, persistent nausea, constipation from opioid medications, and lack of education about how to optimize their diet [54].

To address this, a large body of data demonstrates that high-protein ONS should be a fundamental part of our postoperative discharge care plan [55, 56]. In all patients who underwent major surgery, it is suggested to continue postoperative high-protein ONS for 4–8 weeks minimum and as long as 3–6 months postoperatively in more severely malnourished patients or those with prolonged hospital stays. Follow-up of the nutritional status can be easily performed by observation of the weight and BMI. However, the BMI is not sensitive for differences in body composition without change of BMI. Bioimpedance analysis (BIA) is a feasible non-invasive tool which is also convenient for outpatients and may give reliable information on body composition parameters.

Five Things You Should Know About Perioperative Nutritional Management of Elderly Patients

- Malnutrition often overlaps with frailty in the elderly patient and represents one of the few modifiable preoperative risk factors for poor postoperative outcomes.

- Screening for nutritional status is simple and should be performed in all patients undergoing surgery, utilizing validated questionnaires such as the Mini-Nutritional Assessment (MNA) or the Nutritional Risk Screening-2002 (NRS-2002).
- In the emergency setting, it is crucial to evaluate the chance of delaying surgery in a malnourished patient to allow a preoperative nutritional intervention to optimize patient status. The decision-making process should also take into account overall patient conditions, the expected extent of the anticipated surgical procedure, and the underlying disease.
- Intraoperatively, the nutritional support needed during recovery should be anticipated, and tailored strategies including positioning of a naso-enteric feeding tube or a needle catheter jejunostomy should be carried out.
- Postoperatively, oral or enteral feeding should be commenced as early as possible to reach calorie and protein targets, which are essential to promote anabolism and functional recovery.

References

1. Correia MI, Waitzberg DL. The impact of malnutrition on morbidity, mortality, length of hospital stay and costs evaluated through a multivariate model analysis. Clin Nutr. 2003;22:235–9.
2. Sorensen J, Kondrup J, Prokopowicz J, et al. EuroOOPS: an international, multicentre study to implement nutritional risk screening and evaluate clinical outcome. Clin Nutr. 2008;27:340–9.
3. Williams JD, Wischmeyer PE. Assessment of perioperative nutrition practices and attitudes—a national survey of colorectal and GI surgical oncology programs. Am J Surg. 2017;213:1010–8.
4. Fowler AJ, Abbott TEF, Prowle J, et al. Age of patients undergoing surgery. Br J Surg. 2019;106:1012–8.
5. Clegg A, Young J, Iliffe S, et al. Frailty in elderly people. Lancet. 2013;381:752–62.
6. Fried LP, Tangen CM, Walston J, et al. Frailty in older adults: evidence for a phenotype. J Gerontol A Biol Sci Med Sci. 2001;56:M146–56.
7. Cruz-Jentoft AJ, Baeyens JP, Bauer JM, et al. Sarcopenia: European consensus on definition and diagnosis: report of the European Working Group on Sarcopenia in Older People. Age Ageing. 2010;39:412–23.
8. Pecorelli N, Carrara G, De Cobelli F, et al. Effect of sarcopenia and visceral obesity on mortality and pancreatic fistula following pancreatic cancer surgery. Br J Surg. 2016;103:434–42.
9. Kamarajah SK, Bundred J, Tan BHL. Body composition assessment and sarcopenia in patients with gastric cancer: a systematic review and meta-analysis. Gastric Cancer. 2019;22:10–22.
10. Lidsky ME, Thacker JKM, Lagoo-Deenadayalan SA, et al. Advanced age is an independent predictor for increased morbidity and mortality after emergent surgery for diverticulitis. Surgery. 2012;152:465–72.
11. Sheetz KH, Krell RW, Englesbe MJ, et al. The importance of the first complication: understanding failure to rescue after emergent surgery in the elderly. J Am Coll Surg. 2014;219(3):365–70.
12. Sheetz KH, Waits SA, Krell RW, et al. Improving mortality following emergent surgery in older patients requires focus on complication rescue. Ann Surg. 2013;258(4):614–8.
13. Stratton RJ, Hackston A, Longmore D, et al. Malnutrition in hospital outpatients and inpatients: prevalence, concurrent validity and ease of use of the 'malnutrition universal screening tool' ('MUST') for adults. Br J Nutr. 2004;92:799–808.
14. The Veterans Affairs Total Parenteral Nutrition Cooperative Study Group. Perioperative total parenteral nutrition in surgical patients. The Veterans Affairs Total Parenteral Nutrition Cooperative Study Group. N Engl J Med. 1991;325:525–32.
15. Detsky AS, McLaughlin JR, Baker JP, et al. What is subjective global assessment of nutritional status? Nutr Hosp. 2008;11:8–13.
16. Cohendy R, Rubenstein LZ, Eledjam JJ. The mini nutritional assessment-short form for preoperative nutritional evaluation of elderly patients. Aging Clin Exp Res. 2001;13:293–7.
17. Weimann A, Braga M, Carli F, et al. ESPEN guideline: clinical nutrition in surgery. Clin Nutr. 2017;36(3):623–50.
18. Lobo DN, Gianotti L, Adiamah A, et al. Perioperative nutrition: recommendations from the ESPEN Expert Group. Clin Nutr. 2020;39(11):3211–27.
19. Wischmeyer PE, Carli F, Evans DC, et al. American Society for Enhanced Recovery and Perioperative Quality initiative joint consensus statement on nutrition screening and therapy within a surgical enhanced recovery pathway. Anesth Analg. 2018;126(6):1883–95.
20. Vigano A, Kasvis P, Di Tomasso J, et al. Pearls of optimizing nutrition and physical performance of older adults undergoing cancer therapy. J Geriatr Oncol. 2017;8(6):428–36.
21. Gillis C, Buhler K, Bresee L, et al. Effects of nutritional prehabilitation, with and without exercise, on outcomes of patients who undergo colorectal

surgery: a systematic review and meta-analysis. Gastroenterology. 2018;155(2):391–410.
22. Adiamah A, Skořepa P, Weimann A, et al. The impact of preoperative immune modulating nutrition on outcomes in patients undergoing surgery for gastrointestinal cancer: a systematic review and meta-analysis. Ann Surg. 2019;270:247–56.
23. Folwarski M, Bartoszewska L, Figuła K, et al. Home enteral nutrition in adults—nationwide multicenter survey. Nutrients. 2020;12(7):2087.
24. Weber DM. Laparoscopic surgery: an excellent approach in elderly patients. Arch Surg. 2003;138(10):1083–8.
25. Gianotti L, Braga M, Vignali A, et al. Effect of route of delivery and formulation of postoperative nutritional support in patients undergoing major operations for malignant neoplasms. Arch Surg. 1997;132:1222–9.
26. Braga M, Gianotti L, Gentilini O, et al. Feeding the gut early after digestive surgery: results of a nine-year experience. Clin Nutr. 2002;21:59–65.
27. Daly JM, Bonau R, Stofberg P, et al. Immediate postoperative jejunostomy feeding. Clinical and metabolic results in a prospective trial. Am J Surg. 1987;153:198–206.
28. Delany HM, Carnevale N, Garvey JW, et al. Postoperative nutritional support using needle catheter feeding jejunostomy. Ann Surg. 1977;186:165–70.
29. Gabor S, Renner H, Matzi V, et al. Early enteral feeding compared with parenteral nutrition after oesophageal or oesophagogastric resection and reconstruction. Br J Nutr, 13. 2005;93:509.
30. Gupta V. Benefits versus risks: a prospective audit: Feeding jejunostomy during esophagectomy. World J Surg. 2009;33:1432–8.
31. Kemen M, Senkal M, Homann HH, et al. Early postoperative enteral nutrition with arginine-ω-3 fatty acids and ribonucleic acid-supplemented diet versus placebo in cancer patients: an immunologic evaluation of impact®. Crit Care Med. 1995;23:652–9.
32. Sica GS, Sujendran V, Wheeler J, et al. Needle catheter jejunostomy at esophagectomy for cancer. J Surg Oncol. 2005;33:1432–8.
33. Han-Geurts IJM, Hop WC, Verhoef C, et al. Randomized clinical trial comparing feeding jejunostomy with nasoduodenal tube placement in patients undergoing oesophagectomy. Br J Surg. 2007;94:31–5.
34. Zhu X, Wu Y, Qiu Y, et al. Comparative analysis of the efficacy and complications of nasojejunal and jejunostomy on patients undergoing pancreaticoduodenectomy. J Parenter Enter Nutr. 2014;38:996–1002.
35. Yermilov I, Jain S, Sekeris E, et al. Utilization of parenteral nutrition following pancreaticoduodenectomy: is routine Jejunostomy tube placement warranted? Dig Dis Sci. 2009;54:1582–8.
36. Gerritsen A, Besselink MG, Cieslak KP, et al. Efficacy and complications of nasojejunal, jejunostomy and parenteral feeding after pancreaticoduodenectomy. J Gastrointest Surg. 2012;16:1144–51.
37. Dann GC, Squires MH, Postlewait LM, et al. An assessment of feeding jejunostomy tube placement at the time of resection for gastric adenocarcinoma: a seven-institution analysis of 837 patients from the U.S. gastric Cancer collaborative. J Clin Oncol. 2015;112:195–202.
38. Markides GA, Al-Khaffaf B, Vickers J. Nutritional access routes following oesophagectomy—a systematic review. Eur J Clin Nutr. 2011;65:565–73.
39. Alazawi W, Pirmadjid N, Lahiri R, et al. Inflammatory and immune responses to surgery and their clinical impact. Ann Surg. 2016;64:73–80.
40. Fiore JF, Bialocerkowski A, Browning L, et al. Criteria to determine readiness for hospital discharge following colorectal surgery: an international consensus using the Delphi technique. Dis Colon Rectum. 2012;55(4):416–23.
41. Lewis SJ, Andersen HK, Thomas S. Early enteral nutrition within 24 h of intestinal surgery versus later commencement of feeding: a systematic review and meta-analysis. J Gastrointest Surg. 2009;13(3):569–75.
42. Herbert G, Perry R, Andersen HK, et al. Early enteral nutrition within 24 hours of lower gastrointestinal surgery versus later commencement for length of hospital stay and postoperative complications. Cochrane Database Syst Rev. 2019;10:CD004080.
43. Nelson R, Edwards S, Tse B. Prophylactic nasogastric decompression after abdominal surgery. Cochrane Database Syst Rev. 2007;2007(3):CD004929.
44. Lau CSM, Chamberlain RS. Enhanced recovery after surgery programs improve patient outcomes and recovery: a meta-analysis. World J Surg. 2017;41(4):899–913.
45. Greco M, Capretti G, Beretta L, et al. Enhanced recovery program in colorectal surgery: a meta-analysis of randomized controlled trials. World J Surg. 2014;38(6):1531–41.
46. Lee SH, Jang JY, Kim HW, et al. Effects of early enteral nutrition on patients after emergency gastrointestinal surgery: a propensity score matching analysis. Medicine. 2014;93:e323.
47. Fukatsu K, Kudsk KA. Nutrition and gut immunity. Surg Clin N Am. 2011;91(4):755–70.
48. Abunnaja S, Cuviello A, Sanchez JA. Enteral and parenteral nutrition in the perioperative period: state of the art. Nutrients. 2013;5(2):608–23.
49. Doig GS, Simpson F, Sweetman EA, et al. Early parenteral nutrition in critically ill patients with short-term relative contraindications to early enteral nutrition: a randomized controlled trial. JAMA. 2013;309:2130–8.
50. Harvey SE, Parrott F, Harrison DA, et al. Trial of the route of early nutritional support in critically ill adults. N Engl J Med. 2014;371:1673–84.
51. Heidegger CP, Berger MM, Graf S, et al. Optimisation of energy provision with supplemental parenteral nutrition in critically ill patients: a randomised controlled clinical trial. Lancet. 2013;381:385–93.

52. Chapuis PH, Bokey L, Keshava A, et al. Risk factors for prolonged ileus after resection of colorectal cancer: an observational study of 2400 consecutive patients. Ann Surg. 2013;257(5):909–15.
53. Klappenbach RF, Yazyi FJ, Alonso Quintas F, et al. Early oral feeding versus traditional postoperative care after abdominal emergency surgery: a randomized controlled trial. World J Surg. 2013;37:2293–9.
54. Wischmeyer PE. Are we creating survivors … or victims in critical care? Delivering targeted nutrition to improve outcomes. Curr Opin Crit Care. 2016;22:279–84.
55. Cawood AL, Elia M, Stratton RJ. Systematic review and meta-analysis of the effects of high protein oral nutritional supplements. Ageing Res Rev. 2012;11:278–96.
56. Stratton RJ, Hébuterne X, Elia M. A systematic review and meta-analysis of the impact of oral nutritional supplements on hospital readmissions. Ageing Res Rev. 2013;12:884–97.

35 Emergency Laparoscopy in the Elderly and Frail Patient: Perioperative Nursing Considerations

Salvatore Casarano, Pierpaolo Pizzolante, and Dario Galati

35.1 Introduction

Emergency surgery in the elderly patient, despite being increasingly recurrent due to the demographic curve of the world population [1], is actively among the most delicate intraoperative approaches due to the particular logistical needs that frailty imposes throughout the surgical process [2]. The advantages of laparoscopic technique are well established, with better postoperative outcomes and pain management and significant reduction in the duration of hospitalization. Also, the application of laparoscopy technique in emergency surgery involves several organizational problems. First, surgeons should have large experience in laparoscopic techniques. While good preparation by the surgeon is required, the same basket of experience is also required from the operating room nursing team. Nurses at the end of university courses are trained in the management of surgical patients; however, further in-depth studies would be required with regard to assistance to patients in an emergency regime, having to manage complex technology operating situations (Laparoscopy).

Geriatric culture has traditionally been oriented toward the prevention of frailty, minimizing the clinical consequences of chronic diseases and optimizing residual functions in compromised patients. From a clinical point of view, the very classification of the fragile patient presents the overlap between comorbidities and chronicity not so much as a nomenclature but rather as the need to make clinical or prognostic decisions in a limited period of time. The operating room, also thanks to the ageing of the population and the increase in the incidence of laparoscopic cases in the elderly, represents the full summary of the evolution of an increasingly "old" society and the need to implement logistical and organizational standards that allow the team to deal with this type of urgency on a daily basis and with the aim of a prognostic favour as positive as possible. All this would seem almost in contrast with some numbers, if we consider that on one hand 50% of routine surgeries are represented by patients over 65 years old, with a more organized operating room and increasingly able to actively deal with the laparoscopic emergency: it is the unpredictability of the postoperative phase that puts the outcomes back to variables that go beyond the problems of persistence caused by multifactoriality and chronicity

S. Casarano (✉) · P. Pizzolante · D. Galati
Associazione Italiana Infermieri di Camera Operatoria ed Area Chirurgica, Verona, Italy

Surgical Theatre Pia Fondazione C. Panico Azienda Ospedaliera, Tricase, Italy
e-mail: presidente@aicoitalia.it; info@aicoitalia.it

F. Agresta et al. (eds.), *Emergency laparoscopic surgery in the elderly and frail patient*,
https://doi.org/10.1007/978-3-030-79990-8_35

35.2 Operative Nursing

Preoperative education is an integral part of the assistance provided by nurses, capable through therapeutic communication of preparing and instructing the person with the aim of obtaining their collaboration in the self-care process. Considering that the postoperative course is not only influenced by the physiological outcomes of the disease, biopsychosocial responses given by the health-disease continuum are expected as an outcome for the improvement of the quality of life even in critical clinical conditions given by the emergency surgical situation.

The evolution of nursing is related to certain levels of education and practice to fill the important roles within the multi-professional team in the surgical area.

The preoperative evaluation of the fragile patient requires multidisciplinary vision skills: the preoperative execution of diagnostic investigations, which do not have a predictive role in the context of emergency surgery, can negatively affect the intervention times. In this case, the figure of the anaesthetist plays a key role in the predictive clinical assessment of risk [3], in the preparation time of the operating room for any surgery and coordinates both pre- and postoperative logistical and support activities. It is always at this stage that the operating team becomes aware of the surgical needs of the intervention itself. Given the indication of the minimally invasive surgical urgency—both diagnostic and therapeutic—the patient's care in the perioperative phase involves the methodological application of assistance models with a holistic approach, as clearly highlighted by the functional model of Marjory Gordon. This methodology lends itself perfectly to complex healthcare situations that arise daily in emergency medicine.

Emergency medicine for the elderly with frailty provides for a careful approach with the highest degree of customization, in consideration of the complex nursing problems given both by the combination of ordinary logistics problems and by the extraordinary nature of multifactorial variables of the fragile that make urgency laparoscopic a "care situation" which, by methodology applied, recognizes the personalization of the clinical case, the person, different from each other, and therefore a specific approach. In the emergency–urgency regime, the sign-in phase is sometimes compressed due to lack of time. This situation can translate into a gap of useful data/information in the first approach; therefore, a strong attention must be paid to the emergency situation as part of the criticality. In emergency situations, the risk assessment scales are effective. With a multidisciplinary approach, the measurements taken provide responses to the management of perioperative risks in an appropriate way.

The aim is to prevent all potential risk conditions such as infections, damage from posture and damage from hypothermia useful for reducing perioperative complications. For this purpose, the "care bundles" provide a few clear rules to follow and are to be considered "golden" rules which on the basis of the evidence obtain significant improvements in health outcomes.

The nursing care of anaesthesia constitutes the trait d'union between the initial medical-nursing diagnosis and the identification of the conditions of risk and vulnerability, an approach aware of the situation of unstable equilibrium and of the possible outcome, even intraoperative, which is why aims to apply or integrate care models entirely aimed at the prevention of clinical risk and complications, starting with the highest level of the operative stress score (OSS).

The fragile patient has a very high sensitivity toward normal surgical procedures, even those that are normally labelled as "low risk", so the time and space in which the team moves, the choices of each individual operator affect substantially in the postoperative period even in the medium-long term. Some practical findings are represented by postural injuries that can occur as a result of incorrect positioning on the operating table. For example, we should know the "anatomical-functional limits" of walking, which would be evident only through an appropriate acquisition of preoperative information provided by the caregiver or by the person.

The anaesthetist and the nurse dedicated to anaesthesia mark the approach times, prepare, implement and evaluate the care interventions of all the perioperative phases. From the knowledge and preparation of all the clinical examinations to be carried out during the surgery, to the recognition of Mallampati, the management of the airways and the assessment of the pain scale (just to name few of them), the anaesthetist nurse becomes the fulcrum of all activities and the trait d'union of the other figures that revolve around the patient's life in the peri- and intraoperative phase: the time lapse between the call and the urgent request for surgery until the patient arrives in the room is time gold that the nursing has to activate for all the procedures and anaesthetic settings necessary for the best possible assistance. From a logistical point of view, the anaesthetist nurse must verify that all the equipment has been checked and correctly operated before its use on the patient, as well as the availability of drugs and all technological and instrumental devices for the emergency, including status of the pulmonary ventilator. The theatre nurse and the scrub nurse maintain and implement the emergency/urgency standards that are expressed in the preparation of the electromedical devices necessary for the execution of the surgery, the availability of both laparoscopic and open surgical instruments for any conversion, the preparation of the operating table, as well as the activation of other health professionals, the radiology technician (TRSM) or the interventional radiologist.

If the patient is conscious, the anaesthetist nurse represents the first contact of the elderly with the operating reality and is able to quantify stress, psycho-motor conditions and difficulties in managing the airways, comparing them with the real capacity of the patient to recover after waking up. The condition of fragility is an indisputable priority element for a careful assessment and taking charge of the person. The need to carefully evaluate the patient's physical and motor conditions, proceeding in order from dyspnoea to confusion, from chronic pain and difficulty in walking up to infectious risk become the priority and characterizing care interventions. Upon arrival in the operating room, the theatre nurse coordinates the patient's transfer activities from the hospital bed to the operating table, which correctly identifies the patient, the surgical site, the possible presence of allergies and factors that could counteract anaesthesia.

The signs and symptoms detected during the approach phase are fundamental for the management of processes given by the perioperative times and risks.

It has been demonstrated that a surgical safety checklist may reduce morbidity and mortality. Haynes BN and colleagues collected data from a large prospective database on clinical processes and outcomes after non-cardiac surgery. The rate of death was 1.5% before the checklist was introduced and decreased to 0.8% afterward (PD0.003). Similarly, inpatient complications occurred in 11.0% of patients at baseline and in 7.0% after introduction of the checklist ($P < 0.001$) [4, 5]. The WHO recommendations suggest that "Sign in timeout and sign out" are the predictive phases of potential risk conditions that the patient runs in the intraoperative period. Therefore, the preparation of the patient for surgery considers numerous risk factors: clinical, communication, technological, organizational and managerial [1].

35.3 Intraoperative Phase

In this context, patient monitoring represents, together with the correct risk assessment, the extra point that also allows to evaluate the (possible) progressive accumulation of deficits, thanks to the multidimensional assessment (the comprehensive geriatric assessment (CGA) with its Italian acronym VMD—Valutazione Multidimenzionale) as a first-choice tool for the qualitative and quantitative evaluations of the various biological, functional, cognitive and clinical aspects of the elderly subject throughout the emergency care path. The control of the state of consciousness, the management of cardiovascular risk [6, 7], the reduction of pain or the prevention of venous thromboembolism are all elements of an unstable balance in which the technological aid of an increasingly specific monitoring allows to combine the need for a laparoscopic access, specific to the high surgical risk that falls within the anaesthetic field.

The multifactorial evaluation described in the literature by numerous scientific papers provides the basis on which to start a clinical reasoning to direct to a diagnosis and prognosis of the clinical case of surgical interest [5].

Due to the considerable variables involved, it is difficult to estimate the effects of the frailty condition during the operative phase, and despite this, frailty looms large in most of the postoperative courses of subjects at risk. It is, however, correct to believe that the initial choices made during the induction of anaesthesia play a fundamental role in limiting the damage common to multi-organ dysfunction and pre-existing or decompensated multifactorial pathologies, conditions that are considered and measured because they predict criticalities expected in the postoperative period. From this point of view, it is the very important concept of emergency–urgency that imposes specific models and levels of interventions, aiming at the preset setting of the operating room intended for laparoscopic emergencies. The condition in which the training and experience gained work together, placing the various health professionals in the field of laparoscopic emergency on an equal level, with the awareness that the indicators of fragility and their correlation with the incidence of some complications, especially non-surgical, determine a fundamental contribution to the situation [8–13].

Anaesthesiology nursing acts as an assistant specialist and uses multi-parametric detection technology of vital signs useful for the early detection of conditions of critical instability to determine the risk of adverse events related to the deterioration of vital signs, such as the early warning score [11, 12].

For this reason, the alterations detected promptly provide timely corrective interventions useful for the result.

In this perspective, speaking of holistic assessment of frailty indices, the functional state of the patient and the nursing diagnosis are well combined: social isolation, lack of family relationships and total dependence in daily activities are all elements related to nutritional status of the patient; without forgetting weight loss or hypoalbuminemia, for example, or the american society of anesthesiologists scale (ASA), age, body mass index (BMI), comorbidities such as diabetes mellitus, chronic obstructive pulmonary disease (COPD), arterial hypertension and kidney failure [12]. Still in this perspective, the theatre nurse interprets the indicators in the logic of continuity of care, for example, a single model for managing the fragile patient within a multidisciplinary and multi-step protocol, in which the different care contexts determine a shared evaluation track in which multidimensionality takes on concrete and truly quantifiable characteristics [9].

The clinical risk management systems, in the clinical-assistance pathways, provide for the application of single nursing documentation, for the frail and elderly person, which documents the nursing diagnoses for continuity of care/taking charge between the operating room and the hospitalization. As part of the perioperative nursing assessments in the anaesthetic induction phase, due attention must be paid to the detection, measurement and treatment of pain and the patient's motor ability; all elements must be evaluated for the correct positioning of the frail elderly on the operating table [8–12].

The need to make our patient assume specific positions on the operating table during surgery, for example, the extreme Trendelenburg and reverse Trendelenburg positions, or a lateral position, can compromise the patient's hemodynamic status by influencing the conditions of respiratory and cardiovascular homeostasis. It is necessary to manage the patient's head during positioning, to ensure the protection of the joint compression points (occiput, elbows, wrists, sacrum and heels) to avoid and prevent any transient or permanent damage. In the elderly, this prevention becomes a nursing diagnosis in the preoperative education phase through physical examination, inspection of every single part of the body to avoid stretching or nerve compression to which it must be added the awareness of high bone fragility and a limited range of motion of joint movements. A Trendelenburg position involves a strong increase in venous return, intracranial and intraocular pressure with possible complications such as headache, cerebral oedema and retinal detachment, without forgetting an alteration of the relationship between mechanical ventilation and perfusion, with a decrease in functional residual capacity (FRC) and increased gastric pressure. Conversely, an anti-Trendelenburg position involves a decrease in venous return, range and blood pressure, while improving lung capacity and the quality of respiratory exchanges. Urgently implementing all the manoeuvres to ensure the spine or the extension of the upper limbs, the lower ones and the trunk reach the maximum degree of difficulty because the time factor often comes into play [2, 4, 9].

35.4 Continuity of Care

The role of the nurse is fundamental both in the early recognition of signs and symptoms of any complications and in assisting the anaesthesiologist in the difficult maintenance, in an emergency regime, of all the standards necessary to ensure patient comfort. It is essential to keep the monitoring of the patient's vital parameters under control throughout the surgery; in this regard, the technology available today is extremely punctual and varied. Nursing surveillance includes the management of venous access, the assessment of the correct functioning of the drainage of the surgical site, infusion therapy, the management of abdominal stoma, the assessment of diuresis and continuous monitoring. All surveillance and care management activities must find the right communication channel in the transfer of the patient from the operating room to the ward of origin, or to the post-anaesthesia care unit (PACU) or intensive care through adequate communication and handover. Specifically, postoperative monitoring should include a set of assessments that are also the result of a continuum between nursing services in the operating room and subsequent clinical steps. In the emergency laparoscopy of the elderly and frail patient, all the independent variables of multi-chronic disease could be taken into consideration; therefore, the information relating to the surgical postures must be taken into account, for a subsequent evaluation of pain and any syndrome related to incorrect positioning on the operating table

The postoperative evaluation of the patient must be constant and punctual to avoid risky situations. It is necessary to a constant and repeated control of vital signs, the patency of the drainages, inspection of the surgical site to detect the presence of any blood loss. The postoperative assistance activities include infusion therapy checks, painkillers, pain measurement and treatment, evaluation of the hydroelectrolytic balance, blood chemistry checks, and evaluation of the state of consciousness [6–12].

Acute postoperative pain is assessed on the basis of pre-existing pain, plus pain caused by the surgical procedure and the presence of drains, nasal tubes or complications. Severe pain, especially if associated with the patient's agitation, leads to lower respiratory compliance and bronchial spasm, with atelectasis and hypoxia. Even in laparoscopy, which largely involves the abdomen, especially in the upper portion, the pain makes breathing difficult, and a lower cough reflex favours the accumulation of secretions, an excellent ground for lung infections.

Untreated postoperative pain increases the risk of cardio-circulatory, pulmonary, metabolic, gastrointestinal and urinary complications, often leading the patient to a state of stress and excessive agitation [8–13].

The need for a multidisciplinary and multiprofessional approach, with a precise location within the in-hospital path, provides the specific resources and paths The fragile patient requires a more accurate preoperative evaluation and a constant and more intense postoperative control. Perhaps, the most profound problem in the control phase of healing refers to an associated and increased morbidity and mortality during major surgery, especially in an emergency, regardless of age. The fact that many complications can arise even 30 days after surgery clarifies how complex it is to draw up a specific care plan for the fragile patient, given the wide list of comorbidities with which the patient has to live. However, it is increasingly unanimous to consider the moments following surgery, the awakening and postoperative stationing phase before discharge, as the most important moment for a successful perioperative strategy. Good monitoring in the patient's awakening phase helps, in most cases, to achieve a good and early recognition of the most common postoperative symptoms, as well as the most serious vital alterations [8].

35.5 Teamwork and Multidisciplinary

Laparoscopic surgery in the elderly/frail patient revolves around maintaining the state of equilibrium of the clinical conditions, made precarious by the multifactorial itself at the origin of the fragility. The patient's ability to tolerate, during the surgical phase, between incision and suture, the type of urgency that is being faced, the mix of analgesic therapy applied: time plays the most important role. From this point of view, the presence of a stable and constantly trained nursing team, available to the surgical team, is certainly a winning team, because surgery plays many of its chances also on the time factor. However, the reduction of downtime between one step and another, the ability to know how to anticipate and correctly read the surgical needs in the operating field, are only the first step in managing emergencies. It is implausible to talk about the management of non-postponable cases simply by drawing on the rigid application of one or more checklists: it is the unpredictability of the fragile that identifies skills, to which must be added the difficulties of an intervention that, although minimally invasive, is almost never free from intrinsic complications. The ability of a nursing team to be flexible, dynamic and prepared for the unexpected places the surgeon in the best conditions to be able to release his or her potential, a security that is also reflected in a better ability to perform. For these reasons, a team dedicated to surgical emergencies in laparoscopy must have the typical skills of urgencies/emergencies, stratified in the multifactorial of the fragile. A good nursing team will hardly waste time due to the redundancy of care practices, which in everyday life are often the result of poor communication, precisely because it is clearly divided into roles and responsibilities, skills and specializations [5, 8, 9, 12].

Five Things You Should Know About Perioperative Nursing in Elderly and Frail Patient

The objectives of the protocol for the management of frail patients in emergency laparoscopic surgery must guarantee the following:

- Knowledge/preparation/preoperative education. Adequate clinical and technical preparation for surgery, with the aim of optimizing time by minimizing postoperative stress and complications from both surgical and anaesthetic stresses. Application of functional models of assistance through the case manager is useful for promoting the effectiveness and control of costs through the maximum individualization of responses to care needs.
- Experienced multidisciplinary nursing team (primary nurse) in consideration of the surgical and anaesthetic needs, which has as a prerequisite the ability to face the unpredictability of the fragile patient.
- Attention to care for a better functional recovery, even residual, in the patient.
- Detection and management of communication obstacles useful for the control of clinical risk in the perioperative period.
- Improvement of outcomes, thanks to unique clinical management protocols of different professional figures in the perioperative, with the use of assessment scales that allow operators to integrate data.

References

1. World Health Organization. The world health report 2008: primary health care now more than ever. Geneva: WHO Press; 2008.
2. Ergina P, Gold S, Meakins J. Perioperative care of the elderly patient. World J Surg. 1993;17:192–8.
3. AAGBI safety guideline. Pre-operative assessment and patient preparation: the role of the anaesthetist.

London: Association of Anaesthetists of Great Britain and Ireland (AAGBI); 2010.

4. Haynes AB, Weiser TG, Berry WR, et al. A surgical safety checklist to reduce morbidity and mortality in a global population. N Engl J Med. 2009;360(5):491–9.
5. Agresta F, Campanile FC, Anania G, Bergamini C. Emergency laparoscopy; 2016. isbn:978-3-319-29618-0 234-236.
6. Leung JM, Dzankic S. Relative importance of preoperative health status versus intraoperative factors in predicting postoperative adverse outcomes in geriatric surgical patients. J Am Geriatr Soc. 2001;49:1080.
7. Polanczyk CA, Marcantonio E, Goldman L, et al. Impact of age on perioperative complications and length of stay in patients undergoing noncardiac surgery. Ann Intern Med. 2001;134:637–43.
8. Ossevatorio Regionale Ospedale Per Intensita' Di Cure (Mario Cecchi, Andrea Valeri) Percorso Perioperatoriodel Paziente Adulto Critico E/O Fragile. https://www.regione.toscana.it/documents/10180/12158927/Allegato+Parere+n.+52-2013.pdf/9c4b8160-6033-4091-b6be-ce5ce582413f;jsessionid=73BAEAB6F3821A773355BA969B73F3DD.web-rt-as01-p2?version=1.0.
9. Bergman H, et al. Frailty: an emerging research and clinical paradigm–issues and controversies. J Gerontol A Biol Med Sci. 2007;62(7):731–7.
10. Fiore V, Boemi M. Riconoscere la fragilità: gli strumenti della valutazione multidimensionale. Il Giornale di AMD. 2013;16(S1):11–4.
11. Ferrucci L, et al. Linee-Guida per la Valutazione Multidimensionale per l'Anziano Fragile nella Rete dei Servizi. Giornale di Gerontologia. 2001;49(Suppl. 11).
12. Evans SJ, Sayers M, Mitnitski A, Rockwood K. The risk of adverse outcomes in hospitalized older patients in relation to a frailty index based on a comprehensive geriatric assessment. Age Ageing. 2014;43:127–32.
13. Abete P, Testa G, Della Morte D, Mazzella M, Galizia G, D'ambrosio D, Visconti C, Gargiulo G, Cacciatore F, Rengo F. La comorbilità nell'anziano: epidemiologia e caratteristiche cliniche. G Gerontol. 2004;52:267–72.

Shared Decision-Making at the End of Life

36

Antonio G. Spagnolo, Barbara Corsano, and Dario Sacchini

36.1 Introduction: The Age as a Decisional Criterion

A critical transformation of the current era seems to be medicine's conquest of old age, beginning with its acquired ability to prolong human life. Providing increasingly effective health care for the elderly has become the most extensive of medicine's frontiers. This is also an ideal of a moral nature: it is a discrimination unworthy of medicine the idea that the age of the patient can be a variable to be taken into account, if there are the technical means to be able to bring him the benefits (the standards of treatment should not take into account the age). However, not everyone considers this orientation justified. There are those who [1] have been questioning the fundamental assumptions of this concept for some time, proposing to withdraw medical care from the elderly after a certain age: first, because it is doubtful that this care would give a tolerable quality to the last years snatched from death, and then because, even if we wanted it, very soon we could no longer afford it, due to the increase in healthcare costs and the change in the demographic curve.

More recently, following the current pandemic of COVID-19, even the SIAARTI [2] has indicated the age as a limit to entry into intensive care, stating that "health care resources should be reserved for those who have first of all a higher probability of survival and secondarily for those who can have more years of life saved, with a view to maximizing the benefits for the greatest number of people."

The question of whether laparoscopic surgery should also be applied to the elderly patient also arose at first, and the conclusion was reached [3] that despite underlying comorbidities, individuals older than 65 years tolerate laparoscopic procedures extremely well. Therefore, denial of laparoscopic surgery should never be based solely on age.

From these preliminary considerations, we want to conclude with the consideration that sickness speaks to us of our limitations and human frailty. It can take the form of infirmity resulting from the simple passing of years or injury from the exuberance of youthful energy. It can be temporary or chronic, debilitating, and even terminal, but ethical principles that govern medical decisions in elderly and frail patients should be no different from those that guide all medical choices in all patients, although any decision cannot fail to take into account the condition of the elderly and frail patient as a contextual aspect and not as a decisional criterion.

A. G. Spagnolo (✉) · B. Corsano · D. Sacchini
Department of Healthcare Surveillance and Bioethics, "A. Gemelli" School of Medicine, Università Cattolica del Sacro Cuore, Rome, Italy
e-mail: antoniogioacchino.spagnolo@unicatt.it

F. Agresta et al. (eds.), *Emergency laparoscopic surgery in the elderly and frail patient*,
https://doi.org/10.1007/978-3-030-79990-8_36

The same considerations also apply when faced with the final phase of a patient's life, when they can no longer be cured but much can still be done to accompany them and provide palliative care. It is precisely at this time that it is necessary to understand when it is ethically justified to move from healing to curing. In surgery, it has been more difficult than in medicine to understand that when surgery is no longer possible, the surgeon's task is not yet finished and he can offer palliative treatment to accompany patient. At this point, the ethical question arises as to whether what is technically possible is also ethically right.

36.2 The Ethical Value of Palliative Surgery at the End of Life (EOL)

In 1975, Canadian surgeon Balfour Mount introduced the term "palliative care," after a meeting with Dame Cicely Saunders of St Christopher's Hospital in London, the English Doctor who first conceived Hospices as a place and method of treatment for the sick and terminal illnesses. Attention to palliative care has grown over time, gradually acquiring the need for a more incisive reflection on the matter, embedding not only scientific aspects but also ethical–social and medical–legal ones relating to the use of palliation as a global personal care. Nevertheless, the literature on palliative surgery is scarce, particularly on ethical issues [4, 5]] and mostly consists of retrospective studies [6–8]], even if in the last year the literature is slightly rising. Moreover, studies around ethical issues about palliative surgery, including emergency laparoscopic surgery in the elderly and frail patient, are even rarer.

In a document of 1990, the World Health Organization made this concept explicit, giving the following definition: "the active and global care of patients whose illness is no longer responsive to curative treatment. The control of pain, other symptoms and psychological, social and spiritual aspects is of primary importance. The aim of palliative care is to achieve the best possible quality of life for patients and their families."

In 2002, the World Health Organization updated and expanded its previous definition of palliative care to emphasize the unique and novel aspects of contemporary medicine introduced by palliative care, thereby clarifying and reaffirming the concept of "global care" [9]. As is clear from these definitions, palliative care also includes palliative surgery when it represents a means, if not the means, of reducing suffering and when the benefits that can be derived from it are greater or at least equal to the risks of the intervention itself. Surgery therefore represents a valid aid in the management of symptoms or complications resulting from the progression of the disease and its worsening.

When we talk about palliative surgery, a distinction should be made between "surgical palliative care" and "palliative surgery." Surgical palliative care is defined as treatments that promote quality of life and reduction of suffering in patients with a severe or terminal clinical condition through the use of surgical techniques [10] (e.g., Percutaneous Endoscopic Gastrostomy (PEG) in patients who are not necessarily terminal but in severe clinical conditions unable to feed themselves).

Palliative surgery, on the other hand, aims to relieve symptoms and improve quality of life (QoL) with minimal impact on survival [11] (e.g., the removal of a mass obstructing the intestine, or an appendectomy in a patient with metastasis, or the removal of a metastasis—a tumor located in a different location—that compresses the spinal cord and prevents natural movement). Palliative surgery, therefore, indicates a surgical procedure of a non-curative nature, used with the primary intention of preserving or improving the QoL and alleviating the symptoms caused by an advanced disease [12].

The effectiveness of palliative surgery is judged by the resolution of the symptoms as an expression of multifactorial discomfort (and the duration of such resolution) as recognized by the patient. However, there is no unanimous consensus in the literature on the definition of "palliative surgery." A study conducted in 2002 by MC Cahill et al. [13] (albeit in some respects dated) has highlighted this criticality, demonstrating that the palliative surgery is still little beaten in the literature. Particularly, the following points rise: the lack of clarity regarding the definition of "palliative care" and therefore its classification within patient's therapies. In fact, 41% of those interviewed consider that palliative surgery should be based on pre-operative intentions of the procedure, that is, the intention is to perform surgery to remove (for example) a part of a large tumor mass in order to be able to apply, afterward, other treatments necessary for the pathology. Twenty-seven percent of those interviewed base palliative surgery on factors, on the contrary, post-operative, that is, surgery can be considered palliative if a tumor mass or metastases remain after the operation. The remaining 32% rely on the prognosis, and therefore on the possibilities of healing or treatment that can improve the clinical situation.

This study is also interesting with regard to knowledge of palliative surgery. In fact, 20.7% of the respondents state that the oncological surgery they have performed is for palliative purposes, 76.8% for curative purposes, and the remaining 2.5% have other purposes.

Second, the study reveals the parameters most considered and the objectives considered important in the application of palliation (specifically, the study refers to oncological surgery, but the considerations remain valid at all): in fact, greater attention is paid to symptom relief, pain relief, and the maintenance of a certain patient's autonomy. Survival is not the decisive parameter.

The recommendation that surgeons should be more involved in this specific field of palliative medicine is significant, precisely because of the fundamental role that palliative surgery often plays in improving the patient's symptoms.

Returning to the more general discourse of palliative surgery and with regard to its indications, the nebulosity surrounding the palliation begins to dissolve. The advent of minimally invasive surgery techniques has, in fact, allowed more patients to undergo surgery. This is mainly due to the lower degree of risk that these techniques present. This degree of risk makes eligible even patients who do not have a chance of recovery, but whose QoL would be improved if they were able to undergo surgery. The reduction of tumor masses is the most frequent aspect of palliative surgery. The indications are all causes of obstruction of vital structures caused by neoplasia, such as masses occluding the urethra, ureters, or rectum (through the application of stents). Another example is the stabilization of pathological fractures, which can relieve the pain related to them. The indication therefore is the reduction of pain caused by the underlying pathology (e.g., the pain caused by a tumor mass); or the reduction or elimination of problems caused by the pathology (e.g., an intestinal blockage caused by the presence of a tumor mass compressing the intestine).

Any surgical intervention has in itself ethical issues generally due to the risk of the procedure and to a correct balance of this risk with the actual/potential benefit of the intervention. In surgical palliation, the ethical reflection on "doing" or "not doing," and therefore on whether or not the patient should undergo surgery, is charged with deep significance, as healing is no longer a goal. In this regard, we consider three issues: (1) The risk of the intervention itself and therefore the appropriateness or, on the contrary, its futility; (2) The quality/completeness of patient information; and (3) The "sham/placebo surgery" issue.

Appropriateness and futility as an ethical issue. Compared to pain therapy, which can generate the acceleration of the death process or the decrease in the patient's consciousness due to the need to increase the dosage of analgesics, palliative surgery poses a further ethical concern represented by the risk for the patient's life by surgery itself.

As Grant et al. [14] reminded us, when we talk about surgery, and obviously also regarding a less complex medical act, we are referring to a balance between beneficence and non-maleficence. In particular, surgery in itself represents a high source of risk due to the intervention on the human body (for curative purposes). Therefore, the medical act, in general, and the surgical intervention, in particular, are called to confront with the concept of futility, both quantitative (as a likelihood that the intervention will bring a very low benefit to the patient) and qualitative (and, as a consequence, the intervention will bring a low benefit to the patient's QoL).

Palliative surgery is called in an even more urgent way to confront with the appropriateness of such an act, precisely because it is not aimed at curing or restoring but rather at soothing and treating the symptoms. In fact, this concept refers to an assessment of the actual achievement of the medical goal and of the patient, calling into question the concepts of burdensomeness and risk for the sick.

About futility, Edmund D. Pellegrino makes it clear that it should be a guide to balance three criteria:

(a) The criterion of effectiveness: the ability to positively modify the natural history of the disease or the symptoms (the key question is whether or not the intervention in object produces a difference in terms of morbidity, mortality, and function, and the answer is in charge of the medical experience that seeks the biomedical good);
(b) The criterion of global benefit: what the patient/proxy perceives as patient's good (the key question is whether the intervention is worthwhile for that specific patient, and therefore the domain of the response is predominantly in charge of the patient/proxy);
(c) The criterion of burdensomeness: physical, emotional, financial, or social costs that arise for the patient (and in some circumstances also for the physician and society) from the treatment (the key question is how much cost—not only economically but in a global sense for the patient—the effectiveness and benefits brought by the medical intervention. The answer to this question should look to the patient's good as such and in a sense to also his/her spiritual good) [15].

The quality/completeness of patient information. The process of communication–information with the patient is known for its complexity and necessity for the correct application of a medical art. The condition of terminality or in any case of chronicity that characterizes certain pathologies makes this process even more delicate. In fact, it is a matter of keeping the patient aware that the consequence of surgery will not be healing but relieving pain and other symptoms. So, the major problem is to give the patient correct information while keeping hope alive. As recalled by McCahill et al., this is a delicate issue in which the training itself of the surgeon takes on considerable weight, which should inform the patient about the benefits of the proposed intervention, making the patient aware that through that act he is seeking an improvement in the QoL. On the other hand, the surgeon himself should be able to recognize the limitations of the treatment in order to prevent that his/her professional authority and skill can influence the patient's decision in any way.

The "sham/placebo surgery" issue. The last, but not the least, ethical question concerning the use of surgery for palliative purposes is "sham/placebo surgery": the patient is anesthetized; the surgeon makes incisions, which are then sutured: the patient is convinced that he has undergone surgery [16]. Although some consider sham/placebo surgery to be justified because it would have a positive effect, others are strongly opposed to it. One of the reasons for opposing such procedure is the problem of an adequate informed consent because, as in clinical trials, the use of placebo is ethically acceptable where it is necessary to determine the efficacy of the drug in the study, provided that the patient is not exposed to excessive risk. This problem is even more acute in the case of sham/placebo surgery since the subject undergoes surgery (which in itself is always invasive and always poses risks) from which he/she will have no real benefit.

Like any surgical intervention, palliative surgery also raises important medical–legal issues that can be traced back to two categories, both of which can lead to the established practice of "defensive medicine," that is, the fear of incurring medical–legal litigation.

On the one hand, there are the risks associated with soothing the patient's suffering "too much," in which the danger of incorrect application of opiates (in the case of severe palliation) administered in overdose may actually cause an acceleration of the patient's death or lead to useless overtreatment and thus cause the onset of medical–legal responsibilities.

On the other hand, not wanting that patient to undergo palliative surgery or not wanting to apply severe palliation—for example, palliative sedation (for fear of the consequences linked to the administration of opiates)—is an expression of the now considerably widespread risk of unjustified therapeutic abandonment for fear of a not real anticipation of patient's death.

36.3 Ethical Principles Governing Clinical Decisions at the EOL

In medicine, also in palliative care aimed at the relief of symptoms linked to critical clinical situations, "doing the good," understood as starting treatments to restore the functions of the body (but not only), has already been put in place. In the palliation phase, "not maleficence" through risky or harsh or even futile treatments represents the "guiding principle" of the medical act, since the disease is no longer responsive to active treatments for healing and its aggressiveness or in any case its inevitable progression requires the activation of continuous therapies in which the objective has changed.

What must guide the implementation of medical treatments is, on the one hand, the therapeutic principle that justifies their use. On the other hand, there is the corollary, from that derived principle, of the therapeutic proportionality which justifies the application or continuation of the treatment even if it is risky and/or burdensome in view of a greater good for the patient himself and, vice versa, justifies desisting when the "burdensomeness" is too high compared to the benefits for that patient. The decision in these cases is a decision of value rather than a simple medical decision, and therefore the involvement of the patient or his substitutes is an essential duty.

More complicated, however, is the decision-making process in palliative surgery when trying to apply to it the well-known criteria of clinical ethics, such as (1) indications for medical intervention, (2) patient preferences, (3) quality of life, and (4) contextual aspects [17].

Diagnostic and therapeutic interventions and, therefore, the clinical, objective evaluation of the medical act certainly represent the starting point in the decision-making process, but they are not sufficient for determining the therapeutic decision. In order to reach the latter, the patient's expressed preferences (where possible) cannot be overlooked, since they constitute the patient's own values. In the case of palliation at EOL, these values and preferences play an important, if not decisive, role precisely because there is no cure on the horizon, but an improvement in the QoL in the illness. This QoL (as a balance between physical, psychological, and moral factors) leads one to wonder strongly about the current prospects in the absence of further treatment for the patient or what would be determined in the presence of treatments such as palliative surgery.

Finally, a fundamental role in the decision-making process is not only played by the contextual and, therefore, social, economic, and psychological aspects that concern the patient but also his/her family, aspects that in certain situations can be pressing and therefore become crucial.

36.4 "Shared Care Planning" as a Tool for Decision in EOL Setting

Which is the best way to manage clinical and ethical issues in EOL issues between physician and patient? Literature agrees that paternalistic approach is inappropriate as well as a mere informative approach [18].

The "shared care planning" (SCP) [19] can be a way to solve this ethical and relational dilemma. SCP is rooted in both shared decision-making (SDM) and advance care planning (ACP). The first one is defined as "a process where healthcare professionals and patients make decisions together, using the best available evidence [aimed at]… a framework for care planning" [20]. So, SDM is an intermediate among a "right" paternalism (strongly

"Doctor knows best,", not necessarily contemplating patient's will and wishes) and patient informed choice (where the patient makes his/her decision based on information received from the physician with no possible interference of professional's own preferences) [21]. SDM is carried out in different clinical settings: EOL, emergency department (ED), intensive care unit (ICU), advanced dementia patients, critically ill patients with cardiac disease, frail elderly with end-stage renal disease, oncology, policymakers, and evidence based medicine (EBM). Particularly in EOL setting, the literature shows that a long-lasting relationship appeared to facilitate the end-of-life decision-making (EoLDM) process; eventual disagreements during the EoLDM process could also improve DM process; previous negative health-care encounters could also lead to distrust. The stakeholders preferred an SDM approach, although they differed in what they actually meant by this concept; for advanced dementia patients, integrating concepts of patient-centered care, shared decision- making, health literacy, and teach-back method of education enhance the desired outcome of ethical dilemma prevention [22].

On the other hand, advance care planning is "a way to inform care choices when the patient cannot express a preference but it is also a planning tool" [23]. Literature highlights: large variations in definitions and content of ACP; variation in ACP definitions may be related to cultural and legal differences; seriously ill patients' preferences regarding life-sustaining interventions depend on their goals for care; religious and spiritual values and beliefs may also affect goals of care [24, 25]. Particularly in EOL setting, the points of discussion are as follows: patients with advanced cancer may benefit from EOL planning, but there is evidence that their willingness and desire to engage in ACP varies; the complex social and emotional environments within which EOL planning is initiated and actioned are not sufficiently embedded within standardized ACP; the notion that ACP is concerned principally with the "right" to self-determination through control over treatment choices at the EOL may misrepresent the way that ACP actually occurs in cancer care.

36.5 The Role of Clinical Ethics Consultation in Decision-Making

Clinical ethics consultation (CEC) can help identify areas of conflict and ethical doubts that individual healthcare workers, patients, and family members may experience in clinical practice, thus facilitating their resolution by diagnostic and therapeutic decisions shared at the patient's bedside, within the framework of values proper to medicine and ethics. CEC can promote an effective "shared" advanced care planning in EOL care setting and can be an effective support to get it. Clinical bioethics, as ethics "at the patient's bedside," deals not only with general issues arising from questions of logical coherence but also with problems arising in clinical practice from the care of a particular patient, with his/her concrete suffering, problems, feelings, as is the case with end-of-life setting [26–28].

CEC is "a service provided by an individual consultant, team, or committee to address the ethical issues involved in a specific clinical case. Its central purpose is to improve the process and outcomes of patient care by helping to identify, analyze, and resolve ethical problems" [29]. It is a special skill which, as also the *New Charter for Health Care Workers* [30] emphasizes, helps to identify conflicts and ethical doubts which individual healthcare workers, patients, and relatives may experience in clinical practice, thereby facilitating their resolution by means of shared diagnostic and therapeutic choices at the patient's bedside, within the value framework of medicine and ethics. The ultimate aim is to improve the performance and results of health care, limiting the inappropriate use of medical technologies, promoting palliative care, focusing on what the doctor can do for the patient, to mitigate his/her physical, psychosocial, and spiritual suffering. Indeed, this is true in the context of the accompaniment of pain and suffering, in situations which are often at the EOL or in any case of chronic evolution of the disease, and in order to facilitate the practice of care [31].

Most ethical and professional assessments are simple and straightforward and, like many of our actions, are the result of good habits other than deeply considered choices. However, in view also of the ever-increasing complexity in everyday clinical practice, it is necessary to carefully rethink one's professional and moral habits and to consider the need to weigh up, analyze, and justify decisions. Not to mention that today clinical ethics has also become a public issue: every decision cannot fail to be justified to the patient, his family, his colleagues, and sometimes, unfortunately also to the courts!

This is why it may be useful for ethics consultants to facilitate decision-making processes so that decisions can be weighed up, analyzed in all their various aspects, and clarified with regard to the values involved and the consequences they may entail. There is, however, a need for greater systematic and formal knowledge of the ethical analysis of individual cases on the part of the medical doctor, starting by learning how to use the tools and methodologies of clinical bioethics.

36.6 Concluding Remarks

Palliative care is the medical field where there is the greatest lack of specific training for surgeons. A better and more appropriate implementation of palliative surgery cannot fail to take into account the role of proper professional training. This goal can be achieved by creating a real palliation culture, leading to a result that will benefit the patient above all, but also the family and health professionals, thus humanizing suffering and illness.

Finally, as recalled in a document of the Italian National Committee for Bioethics (CNB) "adequate support for ars moriendi requires that the rigorous technical-scientific preparation of personnel be supplemented by a corresponding bioethical preparation, which enriches the scientific tradition (often reductionist) of modern medicine with a dutiful anthropological-relational sensitivity" [32].

This dutiful sensibility is strongly advocated by the CNB which expresses itself as follows: "The incurable patient, precisely because of his suffering condition, needs continuous care aimed not at prolonging life at any cost and by any means, but at improving its quality: attention to psychological assistance to the patient and family, spiritual support, treatment of symptoms, pain therapy." This sensitivity is required to a greater extent by those who deal with pain and suffering, doctors and, because of their specific skills, surgeons, so that palliative care fully exploits its meaning of humanization of suffering, giving "support and meaning to the accompaniment of the dying person" and as such therapies "expression of a medicine that is repositioned at the service of the sick person."

On the other hand, there is a need to improve awareness of what palliative surgery represents, since in general, palliative care is presented as one of the fields in which modern medicine shows its deep vocation to care, in a global sense, therefore not only physical but also psychological and existential, for the suffering person.

In this way, surgery will play a greater role in the management of patients in critical conditions and at EOL, contributing to the improvement of their QoL and giving them (where possible) a certain degree of autonomy.

References

1. Callahan D. False hopes. New York: Simon & Schuster; 1998.
2. The Italian Society of Anesthesiology, Analgesia, Resuscitation and Intensive Care (SIAARTI). Clinical ethics recommendations for the allocation of intensive care treatments, in exceptional, resource-limited circumstances. Recenti Prog Med. 2020;111:207–11.
3. Weber DM. Laparoscopic surgery. An excellent approach in elderly patients. Arch Surg. 2003;138(10):1083–8.
4. Krouse RS, Easson AM, Angelos P. Ethical considerations and barriers to research in surgical palliative care. J Am Coll Surg. 2003;196(3):469–74.
5. Pawlik TM, Curley SA. Ethical issues in surgical palliative care: am I killing the patient by "letting him go"? Surg Clin N Am. 2005;85(2):273–86, vii.
6. McCahill L, Krouse RS, Chu DZJ, et al. Indications and use of palliative surgery—results of Society of Surgical Oncology survey. Ann Surg Oncol. 2002;9(1):104–12.
7. Foster D, Shaikh MF, Gleeson E, Babcock BD, Ringold D, Bowne WB. Palliative surgery for advanced cancer: identifying evidence-based criteria

for patient selection: case report and review of literature. J Palliat Med. 2016;19(1):22–9.
8. Lilley EJ, Khan KT, Johnston FM, et al. Palliative care interventions for surgical patients: a systematic review. JAMA Surg. 2016;151:172–83.
9. World Health Organization. National cancer control programs: policies and managerial guidelines. Ginevra: WHO; 2002.
10. Cameron JL, editor. Current surgical therapy. 9th ed. Philadelphia: Mosby; 2007. p. 1179.
11. Osaba D. Rationale for the timing of health-related quality of life (HQL) assessments in oncologic palliative therapy. Cancer Treat Rev. 1996;22(suppl A):69–73.
12. American College of Surgeons. Surgical palliative care: a resident's guide. Cunniff Dixon Foundation; 2009.
13. McCahill L, Krouse RS, Chu D ZJ, et al. Ref. [6]
14. Grant SB, Modi PK, Singer EA. Futility and the care of surgical patients: ethical dilemmas. World J Surg. 2014;38(7):1631–7. [Epub ahead of print].
15. Pellegrino ED. Decisions at the end of life: the use and abuse of the concept of futility. In: Vial Correa J, Sgreccia E, editors. The dignity of dying, Pontificia Academia Pro Vita-Libreria Editrice Vaticana: Città del Vaticano; 2000. pp. 219–241.
16. Tambone V, Sacchini D, Spagnolo AG, et al. A proposed road map for the ethical evaluation of sham (placebo) surgery. Ann Surg. 2017;265(4):658–61.
17. Jonsen AR, Siegler M, Winslade WJ. Clinical ethics: a practical approach to ethical decisions in clinical medicine. 8th ed. New York: McGraw-Hill; 2015.
18. Emanuel E, Emanuel L. Four models of the physician-patient relationship. JAMA. 1992;267(16): 2221–6.
19. Spagnolo AG, Corsano B, Sacchini D. La consulenza bioetica al letto del malato: l'esperienza del Servizio di Etica clinica presso la Fondazione Policlinico Universitario "Agostino Gemelli" IRCCS—Roma. Medicina e Morale. 2019;4:375–95.
20. Mariani E, Engels Y, Koopmans R, et al. Shared decision-making on a 'life-and-care plan' in long-term care facilities: research protocol. Nurs Open. 2016;3(3):179–87.
21. D'Aloja E, et al. Shared decision-making in neonatology: an utopia or an attainable goal? J Matern Fetal Neonatal Med. 2010;23(Suppl 3):56–8.
22. Schwartz DB, et al. Gastrostomy tube placement in patients with advanced dementia or near end of life. Nutr Clin Pract. 2014;29(6):829–40.
23. Butler M, Ratner E, McCreedy E, et al. Decision Aids for Advance Care Planning, Agency for Healthcare Research and Quality. Technical Brief, No. 16. U.S. Department of Health and Human Services, Agency for Healthcare Research and Quality; 2014.
24. Flo E, et al. A review of the implementation and research strategies of advance care planning in nursing homes. BMC Geriatr. 2016;16:24.
25. Johnson S, et al. Advance care planning for cancer patients: a systematic review of perceptions and experiences of patients, families, and healthcare providers. Psychooncology. 2016;25(4):362–86.
26. Kanoti GA, Youngner SY. Clinical ethics: clinical ethics consultation. In: Reich WT, editor. Encyclopedia of bioethics, vol. 1. New York: McMillan-Schuster; 1995. p. 404–8.
27. Rasoal D, Skovdahl K, Gifford M, Kihlgren A. Clinical ethics support for healthcare personnel: an integrative literature review. HEC Forum. 2017;29(4):313–46.
28. Orr RD, de Leon DM. The role of the clinical ethicist in conflict resolution. J Clin Ethics. 2000;11(1):21–30.
29. Society for Health And Human Values—Society for Bioethics Consultation, Task Force on Standards for Bioethics Consultation. Core competencies for health care ethics consultation. The report of the American Society for Bioethics and Humanities. Glenview: American Society for Bioethics and Humanities; 2011.
30. Pontifical Council for Pastoral Assistance to Health Care Workers, New Charter for Health Care Workers. Philadelphia: The National Catholic Bioethics Center; 2017. n. 140.
31. Schneiderman LJ, Gilmer T, Teetzel HD, et al. Effect of ethics consultations on nonbeneficial life-sustaining treatments in the intensive care setting. A randomized controlled trial. JAMA. 2003;290:1166–72.
32. Italian National Committee for Bioethics. End-of-life issues in bioethics; 1995.

37 Minimally Invasive Surgery in the Elderly and Frail Patient in the COVID-19 Era

Emanuele Botteri, Alberto Sartori, Marco Giovenzana, Beatrice Giuliani, Giacomo Piatto, Andrea Balla, Fabio Cesare Campanile, Gabriele Anania, Mauro Podda, Alberto Arezzo, and Ferdinando Agresta

Surgery, especially in elderly and frail patients, can potentially cause the development of many types of post-operative complications. The SARS-Cov2 infection has shown to be related with increased post-operative morbidity and mortality in patients undergoing surgery, with direct implications for clinical practice worldwide [1].

It is common knowledge that surgical stress is associated with changes in the immunological profile. Specifically, patients undergoing major surgery present increased pro-inflammatory cytokines levels, particularly IL-6, which expose patients to the risk of post-operative complications. Moreover, surgical patients often present with a deranged leukocyte profile, with the shift of lymphocytes from the vascular district to lymphatic tissues, causing the development of lymphopenia.

COVID-19 patients present an immunological profile with lymphopenia, an increase in the neutrophil/lymphocyte ratio, and an unbalanced cytokine profile with a predominantly pro-inflammatory response, driven by IL-6 [2].

All these elements suggest that adding surgical stress to COVID-19 patients may be harmful

E. Botteri (✉)
Montichiari Surgery, ASST Spedali Civili Brescia, Brescia, Italy

A. Sartori · G. Piatto
Department of General Surgery, San Valentino Hospital, Montebelluna, Italy

M. Giovenzana · B. Giuliani
UOC Chirurgia Epato-bilio-pancreatica e Digestiva, ASST Santi Paolo e Carlo, Ospedale San Paolo, University of Milan, Milan, Italy

A. Balla
General Surgery Unit, San Paolo Hospital, Rome, Italy

F. C. Campanile
Division of General Surgery, Ospedale San Giovanni Decollato, Civita Castellana, Italy

G. Anania
Division of General Surgery, S. Anna University Hospital of Ferrara, Ferrara, Italy

M. Podda
Policlinico Universitario Duilio Casula, AOU Cagliari, Department of Emergency Surgery, Monserrato, Italy

A. Arezzo
Department of Surgical Sciences, University of Torino, Torino, Italy

F. Agresta
Department of General Surgery, ULSS2 Trevigiana del veneto, Vittorio Veneto (TV), Italy

F. Agresta et al. (eds.), *Emergency laparoscopic surgery in the elderly and frail patient*,
https://doi.org/10.1007/978-3-030-79990-8_37

to those undergoing major surgery, especially in terms of increased rate of pulmonary complications.

Moreover, SARS-Cov2-infected patients with post-operative pulmonary complications have the same mortality rate as the most compromised patients with community-acquired COVID-19 who needed intensive care support.

As a consequence, when to decide whether to operate a COVID-19 positive patient, all those variables should be considered, as men over 70 years are at high risk of mortality not only when undergoing emergency or major elective surgery, but also when minor elective surgery is scheduled.

In particular, according to a recent study published in the Lancet journal about 1128 patients [3], the overall 30-day mortality reaches 23.8% in COVID-19 patients undergoing surgery. Mortality rate is high across all patient subgroups. In fact, while all-cause mortality rates are 18.9% in elective surgery compared to 25.6% in emergency surgery, or 16.3% in minor surgery compared to 26.9% in major surgery, it is never negligible.

A study published by a Chinese team [4] also suggested that neoplastic patients are more susceptible to develop a severe SARS-Cov2 infection, probably because of their immunology status due to both the presence of a malignancy and possibly also a recent chemotherapy. Therefore, patients undergoing either surgery or chemotherapy during the month before a COVID-19 infection experienced a severe grade of pulmonary infection in 75% of cases.

Given the high risk of perioperative complications and the reduction of available operating rooms and medical staff during the COVID-19 era, the trend has been to postpone non-critical procedures and promote conservative treatment to delay or avoid a surgical operation.

Yet, the direct consequence of this approach is that almost 28 million or 72.3% of elective operations have been delayed or canceled during the first 3 months of the COVID-19 pandemic. More precisely, the overall 12-week cancellation rate or delay due to the pandemic has reached globally 81.7% of all surgery scheduled for benign disease, 37.7% for cancer, and 25.4% for elective cesarean sections [5].

Unfortunately, canceled surgeries will be added to already existing waiting lists. Postponing elective surgery at this scale will have a significant impact on patients and cumulative, potentially devastating consequences for health systems worldwide; delaying time-sensitive elective operations, such as cancer surgery, while waiting for the resolution of the pandemic, may lead to the progression of the disease and consequently to the worsening of patient's health status, productivity, and socio-economic costs [6].

For example, if countries increased their regular activity by 20% post-pandemic, it would take almost 45 weeks to overcome the backlog of surgical procedures resulting from COVID-19 interference.

It is necessary to promote patient's disease stratification to balance the perioperative risk of COVID-19 infection against the dangers of postponing surgery case-by-case. In this era, as the surgical indications are restricted, the surgeon should explore new strategies to safely maintain the regular or near-to-normal surgical activity during and immediately following the SARS-Cov2 pandemic. For example, time-sensitive surgery might be performed in designated non-COVID-19 units: patients should be selected according to their comorbidity and their potential need for post-operative intensive therapy, so that they can be safely operated in a COVID-free hub. Both patients and medical staff will require rigorous screening with pharyngeal swabs to reduce cross-infection risks.

The Italian Society of Endoscopic surgery and novel techniques (SICE—Società Italiana di Chirurgia Endoscopica e nuove tecnologie) developed a group of surgical response recommendations to COVID-19, based on those published by SAGES and EAES in April 2020 [7].

Five main aspects were identified: care services reorganization (a), general technical elements (b), measures to be implemented for surgical patients (c), efforts to be implemented for laparoscopic surgery (d), and steps to be implemented for endoscopic procedures (e).

These aspects are summarized below:

(a) ***Care services reorganization***:
   - Elective benign surgery and elective endoscopic procedures should be postponed at the end of the COVID emergency, while oncological surgery and emergency surgery must be granted within COVID-free pathways.
   - Surgeons should be ready to operate on COVID-19 patients when affected by undelayable oncological disease or by clinical conditions requiring emergency surgery.
   - All the other surgical and endoscopic procedure should be performed after the pandemic peak, to minimize the infectious risk and to save material resources as beds, ventilators, and personal protective equipment (PPE).

(b) ***General technical aspects***:
   - There is very little evidence regarding the risk of spreading the virus related to the use of laparoscopic surgery versus the open approach.
   - All the operating room staff members are at risk of viral contamination during endoscopic and surgical interventions; therefore, the rigorous use of appropriate PPE must be adopted by the whole team.
   - Coronavirus should be considered capable of aerosolizing; for this reason, the use of CO_2 filtering devices should be strongly considered.
   - The proven benefits of minimally invasive techniques in terms of reduced hospital stay and reduction of complications must be strongly considered, in addition to the potential advantages in ultrafiltration of aerosol particles.

(c) ***Measures to be implemented for surgical patients***:
   - Each patient undergoing surgery should be informed of the risk of COVID-19 exposure during hospitalization and should be tested for COVID-19 before surgery, even in emergency surgery.
   - If in the emergency settings COVID test is not feasible and the patient requires emergency surgery, the patient must be considered COVID-19 positive and must be treated with full PPE.
   - COVID-19 patients or COVID-19 suspected patients should be operated on in dedicated operating rooms that should be reserved for these types of patients.
   - Monopolar, bipolar, and ultrasonic electrical devices should be used as little as possible for their capacity to generate aerosol particles.

(d) ***Measures to be implemented for laparoscopic surgery***:
   - Skin incision should be as smallest as possible to prevent CO_2 leak.
   - CO_2 pressure should be reduced as much as possible and a smoke evacuation system should be used during all the interventions and during each procedure requiring CO_2 evacuation (specimen extraction, end of the intervention, conversion to open approach).

(e) ***Measures to be implemented for endoscopic procedures***:
   - All members of the endoscopic room must wear full PPE for both elective and emergency courses because of the possible presence of the virus in the gastrointestinal tract and biological fluids.

In September 2020, the European Association for Endoscopic Surgery published the recommendations for a recovery plan in minimally invasive surgery (MIS) during the COrona Virus Disease 2019 (COVID-19) pandemic after a Delphi among experts [8]. Eight domains were identified: (1) general, (2) hepatobiliary and pancreatic, (3) abdominal wall hernia, (4) upper gastrointestinal (GI), (5) lower GI, (6) bariatrics, (7) endocrine, and (8) new technologies and research, as briefly reported below:

1. ***General:*** For general anesthesia, a real-time polymerase chain reaction (RT-PCR) test is always required, or if it is not available, computed tomography scan or ultrasound is indicated. Local resources, pandemic control, and patients' conditions should be considered for the priority of surgery. Emergency surgery

should always be performed, while elective surgery, also in case of cancer, only after a negative COVID-19 test. In case of overutilization of hospital resources, alternative oncologic therapies can be employed in patients harmful for COVID-19. Regional anesthesia should be of choice in case of positive or suspected COVID-19 patients. MIS is not contraindicated in both positive and negative COVID-19 patients, apart from other contraindications or team inexperience [9]. Personal protection equipment (PPE) should be employed in case of patients negative for COVID-19. In the case of a SARS-Cov2 positive patient, it is necessary to use a high PPE level to reduce the gas leaks (evacuating system, low CO_2 pressure, minimize the use of energy devices, to have a dedicated operative room).

2. ***Hepatobiliary:*** Cholecystitis in patients positive for SARS-Cov2 should be treated by antibiotics or by transhepatic drainage in case of severe cholecystitis. In case of common bile duct stone with or without jaundice or cholangitis, the surgical treatment should be considered only if patients are not responsive to medical therapy, endoscopic retrograde cholangiopancreatography (ERCP), and percutaneous transhepatic biliary drainage (PTDB).

   Elective cholecystectomy in patients negative for COVID-19 should be performed in hospitals with sufficient local resources and safe pathways. In contrast, in patients positive for SARS-Cov2, cholecystectomy should be delayed after the pandemic period.

   Surgery in the case of liver or pancreatic cancer in patients negative for COVID-19 should not be delayed, while in positive patients it should be delayed until patients fully recover from SARS-Cov2.

3. ***Abdominal wall hernia:*** Laparoscopy, with mesh and bowel resection if necessary, can be performed in patients positive for COVID-19 with the incarcerated hernia.

   Elective surgery in asymptomatic patients should be postponed. In COVID-19 patients, both spinal and general anesthesia are safe.

4. ***Upper GI:*** In patients positive for COVID-19, endoscopy should be the first attempt in case of bleeding, obstructing esophageal or gastric cancer, benign esophageal perforation (surgery only after 24 h), and anastomotic leak. Laparoscopy should be performed only after endoscopic failure or perforated gastroduodenal ulcer.

   In patients positive for COVID-19 with early esophageal or gastric cancer, surgery should be delayed in favor of neoadjuvant treatment, if indicated. Patients with achalasia or gastroesophageal reflux disease should be a candidate for endoscopic treatment after the pandemic. Surgery, if indicated, should be delayed. Patients with the neoplastic disease are a candidate to MIS surgery after the pandemic.

5. ***Lower GI:*** Endoscopy should be the first attempt to obstruct colorectal carcinoma, uncomplicated volvulus, and low rectal anastomosis leak, while emergency surgery is indicated only after endoscopic failure. In the case of patients positive for COVID-19 and diverticular disease, laparoscopic lavage or resection with or without anastomosis is shown if PPE is available and performed by an experienced surgeon. Percutaneous drainage or stoma is indicated in unstable patients. Laparoscopy should be considered in patients positive for COVID-19 in the virgin abdomen and acute small bowel obstruction due to a single adhesion band. In patients with acute appendicitis, medical treatment should be the first choice, and laparoscopic surgery is indicated after failed conservative treatment.

   Neoadjuvant chemotherapy could be in early rectal cancer to postpone surgery after the pandemic. Chemoradiotherapy should not be offered as only therapy in rectal cancer except within a clinical trial testing the watch-and-wait policy. A liver first approach, in case of synchronous liver metastases from rectal cancer, is not recommended. After colorectal resection, anastomosis should be performed in patients positive for SARS-Cov2 if it is not otherwise contraindicated. Stoma creation should be preferred only in case of patients positive for SARS-Cov2 or medically unfit. Endoscopy, transanal endoscopic microsurgery, and transanal minimally invasive surgery should be considered in patients positive for COVID-19. High-risk procedures for post-operative complications should be performed in expert centers. MIS should always be considered.

6. ***Bariatrics:*** Endoscopic techniques should be employed as a bridge to surgery. In patients who experience complications after surgery, endoscopic treatment should be preferred. After pandemics, surgery should not be delayed further. In case of local restriction, more complex metabolic patients should be prioritized.
7. ***Endocrine:*** Elective adrenal surgery for cancer and functional tumors in patients negative for COVID-19 should not be delayed. In the case of patients positive for COVID-19, surgery should be postponed until patients recover from SARS-Cov2. Elective thyroid surgery in patients negative for COVID-19 should be delayed; instead of positive patients, surgery should be delayed until patients recover from SARS-Cov2.
8. ***New technologies and research:*** Research activity should focus on how to reduce unnecessary personnel, how to minimize production of waste dramatically increased by the need of PPE, how to develop new solutions for training, how to reduce the aerosol contamination in the operative room, and how to implement the safety of MIS. Research not related to COVID-19 should also restart as soon as possible.

In conclusion, the well-known benefits for patients offered by the extensive use of MIS should not be abandoned unless an increased risk for both patients and operators has been proven.

Five Things You Should Know About Minimally Invasive Surgery in the COVID-19 Era

- Minimally invasive surgery is not contraindicated in the COVID-19 era.
- Elective surgery for benign pathology in the elderly and frail patient should be postponed during the COVID-19 pandemic.
- Surgical interventions for oncological diseases should be centralized in COVID-free hospitals.
- Erring on the side of safety, SARS-CoV2 virus should be considered present in surgical plumes and CO_2 filtration systems should be used.
- Healthcare workers should implement all possible precautions in surgery, even with a negative rapid or molecular test, to decrease the risk of infection.

References

1. Huang C, et al. Clinical features of patients infected with 2019 novel coronavirus in Wuhan, China. Lancet. 2020;395:497. https://doi.org/10.1016/S0140-6736(20)30183-5.
2. Besnier E, Tuech JJ, Schwarz L. We asked the experts: Covid-19 outbreak: is there still a place for scheduled surgery? "Reflection from pathophysiological data". World J Surg. 2020;44(6):1695–8. https://doi.org/10.1007/s00268-020-05501-6.
3. COVIDSurg Collaborative. Mortality and pulmonary complications in patients undergoing surgery with perioperative SARS-CoV-2 infection: an international cohort study. Lancet. 2020;396. https://doi.org/10.1016/S0140-6736(20)31182-X.
4. Landman A, Feetham L, Stuckey D. Cancer patients in SARS-CoV-2 infection: a nationwide analysis in China. Lancet Oncol. 2020;21:335–7.
5. COVIDSurg Collaborative. Elective surgery cancellations due to the COVID-19 pandemic: global predictive modeling to inform surgical recovery plans. Br J Surg. 2020;107(11):1440–9. https://doi.org/10.1002/bjs.11746.
6. Glasbey JC, et al. Delaying surgery for patients with a previous SARS-CoV-2 infection. Br J Surg. 2020;107(12):e601–2. https://doi.org/10.1002/bjs.12050.
7. Francis N, Dort J, Cho E, Feldman L, Keller D, Lim R, Mikami D, Phillips E, Spaniolas K, Tsuda S, Wasco K, Arulampalam T, Sheraz M, Morales S, Pietrabissa A, Asbun H, Pryor A. SAGES and EAES recommendations for minimally invasive surgery during COVID-19 pandemic. Surg Endosc. 2020;34(6):2327–31. https://doi.org/10.1007/s00464-020-07565-w. Epub 2020 Apr 22.
8. Arezzo A, Francis N, Mintz Y, Adamina M, Antoniou SA, Bouvy N, Copaescu C, de Manzini N, Di Lorenzo

N, Morales-Conde S, Müller-Stich BP, Nickel F, Popa D, Tait D, Thomas C, Nimmo S, Paraskevis D, Pietrabissa A, EAES Group of Experts for Recovery Amid COVID-19 Pandemic. EAES recommendations for recovery plan in minimally invasive surgery amid COVID-19 pandemic. Surg Endosc. 2021;35(1):1–17. https://doi.org/10.1007/s00464-020-08131-0. Epub 2020 Nov 10. PMID: 33170335; PMCID: PMC7653984.

9. Mintz Y, Arezzo A, Boni L, Baldari L, Cassinotti E, Brodie R, Uranues S, Zheng M, Fingerhut A. Minimally invasive surgery is the key to patient and operating room team safety during the COVID19 pandemic as well as in the "new normal" or chronic pandemic state to come. Br J Surg. 2020;107(11):e461–2. https://doi.org/10.1002/bjs.11916. Epub 2020 Aug 18. PMID: 32809212; PMCID: PMC7461225.

The manufacturer's authorised representative in the EU is Springer Nature Customer Service Centre GmbH, Europaplatz 3, 69115 Heidelberg, Germany. If you have any concerns regarding our products, please contact ProductSafety@springernature.com

Printed and bound by CPI Group (UK) Ltd, Croydon, CR0 4YY
30/09/2026
02225594-0008